Current Therapy in Allergy, Immunology, and Rheumatology

CURRENT THERAPY SERIES

Bardin:
Current Therapy in Endocrinology and Metabolism
Bayless:
Current Therapy in Gastroenterology and Liver Disease
Brain, Carbone:
Current Therapy in Hematology–Oncology
Callaham:
Current Practice of Emergency Medicine
Cameron:
Current Surgical Therapy
Ernst, Stanley:
Current Therapy in Vascular Surgery
Fazio:
Current Therapy in Colon and Rectal Surgery
Garcia, Mastroianni, Amelar, Dubin:
Current Therapy of Infertility
Gates:
Current Therapy in Otolaryngology–Head and Neck Surgery
Glassock:
Current Therapy in Nephrology and Hypertension
Grillo, Austen, Wilkins, Mathisen, Vlahakes:
Current Therapy in Cardiothoracic Surgery
Hurst:
Current Therapy in Cardiovascular Disease
Johnson, Griffin:
Current Therapy in Neurologic Disease
Kadir:
Current Practice of Interventional Radiology
Kaplan:
Current Therapy in Pediatric Infectious Disease
Kassirer:
Current Therapy in Internal Medicine
Lichtenstein, Fauci:
Current Therapy in Allergy, Immunology, and Rheumatology
Myerson:
Current Therapy in Foot and Ankle Surgery
Nelson:
Current Therapy in Neonatal–Perinatal Medicine
Niederhuber:
Current Therapy in Oncology
Parrillo:
Current Therapy in Critical Care Medicine
Resnick, Kursh:
Current Therapy in Genitourinary Surgery
Rogers:
Current Practice in Anesthesiology
Schlossberg:
Current Therapy of Infectious Disease
Thrall:
Current Practice of Radiology
Torg, Shephard:
Current Therapy in Sports Medicine
Trunkey, Lewis:
Current Therapy of Trauma

CURRENT THERAPY IN ALLERGY, IMMUNOLOGY, AND RHEUMATOLOGY

FIFTH EDITION

LAWRENCE M. LICHTENSTEIN, M.D., Ph.D.
Professor of Medicine
The Johns Hopkins University School of Medicine
Director
Johns Hopkins Asthma and Allergy Center
Baltimore, Maryland

ANTHONY S. FAUCI, M.D.*
Director
National Institute of Allergy and Infectious Diseases
National Institutes of Health
Bethesda, Maryland

*Dr. Fauci's editing of this book was not done as part of his official government duties.

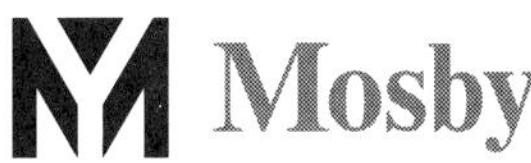

St. Louis Baltimore Boston Carlsbad Chicago Naples New York Philadelphia Portland
London Madrid Mexico City Singapore Sydney Tokyo Toronto Wiesbaden

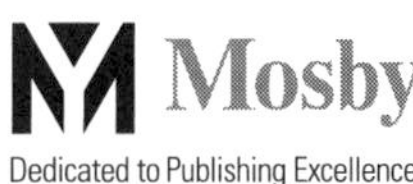

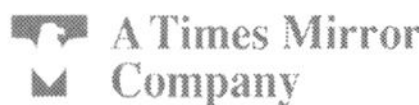

Vice President and Publisher: Anne S. Patterson
Senior Managing Editor: Lynne Gery
Production Editor: Jennifer Harper
Production: Graphic World Publishing Services
Assistant Editor: Carey Conover
Project Manager: Linda Clarke
Manufacturing Supervisor: Andrew Christensen

FIFTH EDITION

Printed in the United States of America
Composition by Graphic World, Inc.
Printing/binding by Maple–Vail Book Manufacturing Group

Mosby–Year Book, Inc.
11830 Westline Industrial Drive
St. Louis, Missouri 63146

96 97 98 99 00 / 9 8 7 6 5 4 3 2 1

CONTRIBUTORS

ELIZABETH M. ADAMS, M.D.

Arthritis and Rheumatism Branch, National Institute of Arthritis and Musculoskeletal and Skin Diseases, National Institutes of Health, Bethesda, Maryland

Dermatomyositis and Polymyositis

JUAN-MANUEL ANAYA, M.D.

Postdoctoral Research Fellow, Division of Clinical Immunology, University of Texas Health Science Center at San Antonio, San Antonio, Texas

Sjögren's Syndrome

GERALD B. APPEL, M.D.

Professor of Clinical Medicine, Columbia University College of Physicians and Surgeons; Director of Clinical Nephrology, Columbia-Presbyterian Medical Center, New York, New York

Immunologically Mediated Nephritic Renal Disease

JOHN G. BARTLETT, M.D.

Professor of Medicine, and Chief, Division of Infectious Diseases, Department of Medicine, The Johns Hopkins University School of Medicine, Baltimore, Maryland

Human Immunodeficiency Virus Infection

THEODORE M. BAYLESS, M.D.

Professor of Medicine, The Johns Hopkins University School of Medicine; Clinical Director, Meyerhoff Digestive Disease-Inflammatory Bowel Disease Center, Johns Hopkins Hospital, Baltimore, Maryland

Crohn's Disease

ZEINA E. BAZ, M.D.

Fellow in Allergy/Immunology, Children's Hospital, Boston, Massachusetts

Severe Combined Immunodeficiency Disease

JEAN BOUSQUET, M.D., Ph.D.

Professor of Pulmonary Medicine, Montpellier University, Montpellier, France

Asthma Provoked by Exposure to Allergens

REBECCA H. BUCKLEY, M.D.

J. Buren Sidbury Professor of Pediatrics, and Professor and Chief of Immunology, Duke University Medical Center, Durham, North Carolina

Congenital Immunodeficiency Diseases

JAMES F. BURDICK, M.D.

Professor of Surgery, The Johns Hopkins University School of Medicine, Baltimore, Maryland

Therapeutic Approaches to Renal Transplantation

LEONARD H. CALABRESE, D.O.

Vice Chairman, Department of Rheumatic and Immunologic Disease, and Head, Section of Clinical Immunology, The Cleveland Clinic Foundation, Cleveland, Ohio

Temporal Arteritis

JEFFREY P. CALLEN, M.D.

Professor of Medicine (Dermatology), and Chief, Division of Dermatology, University of Louisville School of Medicine, Louisville, Kentucky

Behçet's Disease

JOSEPH M. CASH, M.D.

Senior Staff Rheumatologist, Department of Rheumatic and Immunologic Diseases, The Cleveland Clinic Foundation, Cleveland, Ohio

Rheumatoid Arthritis

LAWRENCE S. CHAN, M.D.

Assistant Professor of Dermatology and Director of Immunodermatology, Northwestern University Medical School; Associate Staff Physician, Northwestern Memorial Hospital, and Attending Physician, Veterans Administration Lakeside Medical Center, Chicago, Illinois

Pemphigoid: Bullous and Cicatricial

H. PETER CHASE, M.D.

Professor of Pediatrics, and Clinical Director, Barbara Davis Center for Childhood Diabetes, University of Colorado Health Sciences Center, Denver, Colorado

Immunotherapy for Type I Diabetes

DANIEL J. CLAUW, M.D.

Assistant Professor of Medicine, Division of Rheumatology, Immunology, and Allergy, Georgetown University Medical Center, Washington, DC

Ankylosing Spondylitis

JOHN CONDEMI, M.D.

Clinical Professor of Medicine, University of Rochester School of Medicine and Dentistry, Rochester, New York

Food Allergy in Adults

JONATHAN L. COOK, M.D.

Resident, Department of Dermatology, Emory University School of Medicine, Atlanta, Georgia

Cutaneous Vasculitis

ANDREA M. CORSE, M.D.

Assistant Professor of Neurology, Johns Hopkins University School of Medicine, Baltimore, Maryland

Myasthenia Gravis

PETER S. CRETICOS, M.D.

Associate Professor, Division of Allergy and Clinical Immunology, Department of Medicine, The Johns Hopkins University School of Medicine; Medical Director, Asthma and Allergic Diseases, Johns Hopkins Asthma and Allergy Center, Baltimore, Maryland

Allergic Rhinitis
Asthma in Adults

DAVID C. DALE, M.D.

Professor of Medicine, University of Washington School of Medicine; Attending Physician, University of Washington Medical Center, Seattle, Washington

Autoimmune Leukopenia

GERALD S. DAVIS, M.D.

Professor of Medicine, University of Vermont College of Medicine; Director, Pulmonary Disease and Critical Care Medicine, Fletcher Allen Health Care, Burlington, Vermont

Idiopathic Pulmonary Fibrosis

VINCENT DeLEO, M.D.

Associate Professor and Vice-Chairman, Department of Dermatology, Columbia University College of Physicians and Surgeons; Director of Service, Dermatology, St. Luke's-Roosevelt Hospital Center, New York, New York

Contact Dermatitis

RICHARD D. DeSHAZO, M.D.

Professor of Medicine and Pediatrics, Director, Division of Allergy and Immunology, and Chairman, Department of Internal Medicine, University of South Alabama College of Medicine, Mobile, Alabama

Drug Reactions

EMMANUEL N. DESSYPRIS, M.D.

Professor of Medicine, Division of Hematology/Oncology, Virginia Commonwealth University Medical College of Virginia School of Medicine; Chief, Hematology/Oncology Section, Hunter Holmes McGuire Veterans Affairs Medical Center, Richmond, Virginia

Aplastic Anemia

LUIS A. DIAZ, M.D.

Professor and Chairman, Department of Dermatology, Medical College of Wisconsin, Milwaukee, Wisconsin

Pemphigus

HOWARD B. DICKLER, M.D.

Chief, Clinical Immunology Branch, Division of Allergy, Immunology and Transplantation, National Institute of Allergy and Infectious Diseases; Senior Attending, Clinical Center, National Institutes of Health, Bethesda, Maryland

New Vaccines for Immunologic Diseases

VIRGINIA H. DONALDSON, M.D.

Professor of Pediatrics and Medicine, University of Cincinnati College of Medicine; Attending Physician, Children's Hospital Medical Center, and Active Medical Staff, Internal Medicine and Pediatrics, University of Cincinnati Hospital, Cincinnati, Ohio

Hereditary Angioneurotic Edema

JEFFREY M. DRAZEN, M.D.

Parker B. Francis Professor of Medicine, Harvard Medical School; Chief, Respiratory Division, Brigham and Women's Hospital, Boston, Massachusetts

Treatment of Asthma and Rhinitis with Agents Active on the 5-Lipoxygenase Pathway

GEORGE F. DUNA, M.D.

Clinical Associate Staff, The Cleveland Clinic Foundation, Cleveland, Ohio

Temporal Arteritis

MARTHA M. EIBL, M.D.

Professor of Immunology, Institute of Immunology, University of Vienna Medical School; Consultant Immunologist of the Pediatric Hospitals of the City of Vienna, Vienna, Austria

Common Variable Immunodeficiency

MARK P. EPSTEIN, M.B., B.Ch.

Research Associate, Division of Geographic Medicine and Infectious Diseases, New England Medical Center, Boston, Massachusetts

Phagocyte Function Disorders

J. MARK FITZGERALD, M.B., F.R.C.P.C.

Assistant Professor, Department of Medicine, University of British Columbia Faculty of Medicine; Staff Physician, Respiratory Division, Vancouver General Hospital and Health Sciences Centre, Vancouver, British Columbia, Canada

Acute Life-Threatening Asthma

C. STEPHEN FOSTER, M.D., F.A.C.S.

Professor, Harvard Medical School; Director, Hilles Immunology Laboratory, and Director, Immunology Service, Massachusetts Eye and Ear Infirmary, Boston, Massachusetts

Autoimmune Uveitis

MICHAEL M. FRANK, M.D.

Samuel L. Katz Professor and Chairman, Department of Pediatrics, and Professor of Immunology and Medicine, Duke University Medical Center, Durham, North Carolina

Autoimmune Hemolytic Anemia

MALCOLM L. GEFTER, Ph.D.

Professor of Biology, Massachusetts Institute of Technology, Cambridge, Massachusetts

A New Generation of Antigens for Immunotherapy

RAIF S. GEHA, M.D.

Prince Turki bin Abdul Aziz Al-Saud Professor of Pediatrics, Harvard Medical School; Chief, Division of Immunology, Children's Hospital, Boston, Massachusetts

Severe Combined Immunodeficiency Disease

ALLAN C. GELBER, M.D., M.P.H.

Instructor of Medicine, The Johns Hopkins University School of Medicine, Baltimore, Maryland

Scleroderma

ERWIN W. GELFAND, M.D.

Professor of Pediatrics, and Professor of Microbiology and Immunology, University of Colorado Health Sciences Center; Chairman, Department of Pediatrics, National Jewish Center for Immunology and Respiratory Medicine, Denver, Colorado

Benefit of Intravenous Immunoglobulin in the Treatment of Steroid-Dependent Asthma

JAMES E. GERN, M.D.

Assistant Professor of Pediatrics, University of Wisconsin Medical School, Madison, Wisconsin

Childhood Asthma

JENS GILLE, M.D.

Post-Doctoral Research Fellow, Emory University School of Medicine, Atlanta, Georgia

Dermatitis Herpetiformis

RICHARD J. GLASSOCK, M.D.

Professor and Chairman, Department of Internal Medicine, University of Kentucky College of Medicine; Chairman, Department of Internal Medicine, Chandler Medical Center, University of Kentucky, Lexington, Kentucky

Immunologically Mediated Nephrotic Renal Disease

PHILIPPE GODARD, M.D.

Clinique des Maladies Respiratoires, Hospital Arnaud de Villeneuve, Centre Hospitalier Universitaire, Montpellier-Cedex, France

Asthma Provoked by Exposure to Allergens

DAVID F. GRAFT, M.D.

Clinical Associate Professor, University of Minnesota School of Medicine; Chairman, Allergy Department, Park Nicollet Medical Center, Minneapolis, Minnesota

Insect Sting Allergy in Adults

MALCOLM GREAVES, M.D., Ph.D., F.R.C.P.

Professor of Dermatology and Dean, St. John's Institute of Dermatology, University of London; Consultant Dermatologist, Guys and Thomas's NHS Trust, Saint Thomas's Hospital, London, United Kingdom

Chronic Urticaria

PAUL A. GREENBERGER, M.D.

Professor of Medicine, Division of Allergy-Immunology, Northwestern University Medical School; Attending Physician, Northwestern Memorial Hospital, Chicago, Illinois

Allergic Bronchopulmonary Aspergillosis

ANTON GRUNFELD, M.D., F.R.C.P.C.

Assistant Professor, Division of Emergency Medicine, Department of Surgery, University of British Columbia Faculty of Medicine, Vancouver, British Columbia, Canada

Acute Life-Threatening Asthma

RUSSELL P. HALL III, M.D.

Associate Professor and Vice-Chief, Division of Dermatology, and Assistant Professor, Department of Immunology, Department of Medicine, Duke University Medical Center; Chief, Dermatology Section, Department of Medicine, Durham Veterans Administration Medical Center, Durham, North Carolina

Herpes Gestationis

STEPHEN B. HANAUER, M.D.

Professor of Medicine and Clinical Pharmacology, and Co-Director, University of Chicago Inflammatory Bowel Disease Research Center, University of Chicago Pritzker School of Medicine, Chicago, Illinois

Ulcerative Colitis

PIA HAUK, M.D.

Pediatrician, University Childen's Hospital, Freiburg, Germany

Insect Sting Allergy in Children

STEPHEN L. HAUSER, M.D.

Professor and Chairman, Department of Neurology, University of California, San Francisco, School of Medicine, San Francisco, California

Multiple Sclerosis and Related Demyelinating Diseases

BARTON F. HAYNES, M.D.

Frederic M. Hanes Professor of Medicine, Director, Duke University Arthritis Center, and Chief, Division of Rheumatology, Allergy, and Clinical Immunology, Duke University School of Medicine, Durham, North Carolina

Systemic Necrotizing Vasculitis

PETER S. HEEGER, M.D.

Assistant Professor of Medicine, Case Western Reserve University School of Medicine, Cleveland Veterans Administration Medical Center, Cleveland, Ohio

Acute Hypersensitivity Interstitial Nephritis

GARY S. HOFFMAN, M.D.

Professor of Medicine, Ohio State University College of Medicine, Columbus; Chairman, Department of Rheumatic and Immunologic Diseases, The Cleveland Clinic Foundation, Cleveland, Ohio

Rheumatoid Arthritis

PAUL S. IMPERIA, M.D.

Rogue Valley Medical Center, Medford, Oregon

Immunologic Diseases of the External Eye

MARK D. INMAN, M.D., Ph.D.

Post-Doctoral Research Fellow, Department of Medicine, McMaster University School of Medicine, Hamilton, Ontario, Canada

Exercise-Induced Bronchoconstriction, Anaphylaxis, and Urticaria

MARCEL-FRANCIS KAHN, M.D.

Professor of Rheumatology, Bichat School of Medicine, University of Paris; Chief, Rheumatology Unit, Bichat Hospital, Paris, France

Mixed Connective Tissue Disease (Undifferentiated Tissue Disease)

MICHAEL S. KAPLAN, M.D.

Associate Clinical Professor of Pediatrics, University of California, Los Angeles, School of Medicine; Chief and Training Program Director, Kaiser Permanente, Los Angeles, California

Penicillin Allergy

MARSHALL M. KAPLAN, M.D.

Professor of Medicine, Tufts University School of Medicine; Chief, Division of Gastroenterology, New England Medical Center, Boston, Massachusetts

Primary Biliary Cirrhosis

LEE D. KAUFMAN, M.D., F.A.C.P.

Associate Professor of Medicine, and Director of Clinical Rheumatology, State University of New York at Stony Brook Health Sciences Center School of Medicine, Stony Brook, New York

The Eosinophilia-Myalgia Syndrome Associated with L-Tryptophan Ingestion

CLIFFORD J. KAVINSKY, M.D., Ph.D.

Assistant Professor of Medicine, Rush Medical College of Rush University; Assistant Director, Section of Cardiology, Rush-Presbyterian-St. Luke's Medical Center, Chicago, Illinois

Postcardiac Injury Syndrome

A. BARRY KAY, Ph.D., F.R.C.P.

Professor and Director, Department of Allergy and Clinical Immunology, National Heart and Lung Institute; Honorary Consultant Physician, Royal Brompton Hospital, London, United Kingdom

Immunosuppressive Treatment of Chronic Asthma

DILIP S. KITTUR, M.D., Sc.D.

Associate Professor of Surgery, The Johns Hopkins University School of Medicine; Attending Physician, and Director, Pancreas Transplant Program, Johns Hopkins Hospital, Baltimore, Maryland

Therapeutic Approaches to Renal Transplantation

MARK S. KLEMPNER, M.D.

Professor of Medicine, Microbiology and Molecular Biology, and Vice Chairman for Research Affairs, Department of Medicine, Tufts University School of Medicine; Physician, New England Medical Center, Boston, Massachusetts

Phagocyte Function Disorders

JOHN H. KLIPPEL, M.D.

Clinical Director, National Institute of Arthritis and Musculoskeletal and Skin Diseases, National Institutes of Health, Bethesda, Maryland

Reactive Arthritis

LAUREN B. KRUPP, M.D.

Associate Professor of Neurology, State University of New York at Stony Brook Health Sciences Center School of Medicine; Attending Physician, University Hospital, Stony Brook, and Northport Veterans Hospital, Northport, New York

The Eosinophilia-Myalgia Syndrome Associated with L-Tryptophan Ingestion

RALPH W. KUNCL, M.D., Ph.D.

Associate Professor of Neurology, The Johns Hopkins University School of Medicine; Attending Neurologist, Johns Hopkins Hospital, Baltimore, Maryland

Myasthenia Gravis

SMRITI K. KUNDU, M.D.

Senior Scientist, Division of Infectious Diseases and Geographic Medicine, Stanford University Medical Center, Stanford, California

Human Immunodeficiency Virus Infection: Potential Therapies for Immunologic Reconstruction

CAROL A. LANGFORD, M.D., M.H.S.

Immunologic Diseases Section, Laboratory of Immunoregulation, National Institute of Allergy and Infectious Diseases, National Institutes of Health, Bethesda, Maryland

Takayasu's Arteritis

THOMAS J. LAWLEY, M.D.

Professor and Chairman, Department of Dermatology, Emory University School of Medicine; Chief of Dermatology Service, Emory University Hospital, and Chief of Dermatology Section, The Emory Clinic, Atlanta, Georgia

Cutaneous Vasculitis

FRANCES LAWLOR, M.D., F.R.C.P.I., D.C.H.

Honorary Senior Lecturer in Dermatology, United Medical School of Guys and St. Thomas; Consultant Dermatologist, Health Authority, and Honorary Consultant Dermatologist, St. John's Institute of Dermatology, London, United Kingdom

Chronic Urticaria

ROBERT F. LEMANSKE Jr., M.D.

Professor of Medicine and Pediatrics, University of Wisconsin Medical School; Head, Division of Pediatric Allergy, University of Wisconsin Hospital, Madison, Wisconsin

Childhood Asthma

ALEXANDRA LEVINE, M.D.

Professor of Medicine, and Chief, Division of Hematology, University of Southern California School of Medicine, Los Angeles, California

Acquired Immunodeficiency Syndrome: Therapy for Neoplastic Complications

SARA H. LOCK, M.B., B.S., M.R.C.P.

Clinical Research Fellow, Department of Allergy and Clinical Immunology; Senior Registrar, General and Respiratory Medicine, Chelsea and Westminster Hospital, London, United Kingdom

Immunosuppressive Treatment of Chronic Asthma

VALERIE J. LUND, M.S., F.R.C.S., F.R.C.S.Ed.

Reader in Rhinology, Institute of Laryngology and Otology, University College London; Honorary Consultant Surgeon, Royal National Throat, Nose and Ear Hospital, London, United Kingdom

Perennial Non-Allergic Rhinitis

MICHAEL P. MANNS, M.D.

Professor of Gastroenterology, and Director, Department of Gastroenterology and Hepatology, Medical School of Hannover, Hannover, Germany

Chronic Hepatitis

GIANNI MARONE, M.D.

Professor of Medicine, and Director, Division of Clinical Immunology and Allergy, University of Naples Federico II, Naples, Italy

Acute Rheumatic Fever

GAILEN D. MARSHALL Jr., M.D., Ph.D.

Assistant Professor of Medicine and Pathology, and Director, Division of Allergy and Clinical Immunology, University of Texas Medical School at Houston; Chief, Division of Allergy and Clinical Immunology, Medicine Service, Hermann Hospital, Houston, Texas

Idiopathic Anaphylaxis

JOSÉ M. MASCARÓ , Jr., M.D.

Postdoctoral Research Fellow, Department of Dermatology, Medical College of Wisconsin, Milwaukee, Wisconsin

Pemphigus

DAVID A. MATHISON, M.D.

Senior Consultant, Division of Allergy and Immunology, Scripps Clinic and Research Foundation, La Jolla, California

Aspirin Sensitivity in Rhinosinusitis and Asthma

REX M. McCALLUM, M.D.

Assistant Professor of Medicine, Division of Rheumatology, Allergy and Clinical Immunology, Duke University Medical Center; Director of Clinical Services, Duke University Arthritis Center, and Medical Director, Department of Medicine, The Medical Private Diagnostic Clinic, Durham, North Carolina

Systemic Necrotizing Vasculitis
Cogan's Syndrome

THOMAS C. MERIGAN, M.D.

Becker Professor of Medicine, and Director, Center for AIDS Research at Stanford, Stanford University School of Medicine, Stanford, California

Human Immunodeficiency Virus Infection: Potential Therapies for Immunologic Reconstruction

DEAN D. METCALFE, M.D.

Head, Allergic Disease Section, Laboratory of Clinical Investigation, National Institute of Allergy and Infectious Diseases, National Institutes of Health, Bethesda, Maryland

Food Allergy in Adults
Systemic Anaphylaxis

FRANÇOIS-B. MICHEL, M.D.

Professor, University of Montpellier; Head of Department, Montpellier Hospital, Montpellier, France

Asthma Provoked by Exposure to Allergens

BARTLY J. MONDINO, M.D.

Wasserman Professor and Chairman, Department of Ophthalmology; Director, Jules Stein Eye Institute, and Chief, Cornea-External Disease Division, University of California, Los Angeles, School of Medicine, Los Angeles, California

Immunologic Diseases of the External Eye

GABRIELLA MORONI, M.D.

Division of Nephrology and Dialysis, IRCCS Ospedale Maggiore di Milano, Milano, Italy

Lupus Nephritis

ERIC G. NEILSON, M.D.

C. Mahon Kline Professor of Medicine, Chief, Renal Electrolyte and Hypertension Division, and Director, Penn Center for Molecular Studies of Kidney Diseases, University of Pennsylvania School of Medicine, Philadelphia, Pennsylvania

Acute Hypersensitivity Interstitial Nephritis

PAUL M. O'BYRNE, M.B.

Professor of Medicine and Head, Division of Respirology, McMaster University School of Medicine, Hamilton, Ontario, Canada

Exercise-Induced Bronchoconstriction, Anaphylaxis, and Urticaria

JOHN L. OHMAN Jr., M.D.

Clinical Professor of Medicine, Tufts University School of Medicine; Associate Staff and Chief of Allergy, New England Medical Center, Boston, Massachusetts

Allergic Reactions Caused by Exposure to Animals

AMY S. PALLER, M.D.

Associate Professor of Pediatrics and Dermatology, Northwestern University Medical School; Head, Division of Dermatology, Children's Memorial Hospital, Chicago, Illinois

Atopic Dermatitis

JOSEPH E. PARRILLO, M.D.

James B. Herrick Professor of Medicine, Rush Medical College of Rush University; Chief, Sections of Cardiology and Critical Care Medicine, and Medical Director, Rush Heart Institute, Rush-Presbyterian-St. Luke's Medical Center, Chicago, Illinois

Postcardiac Injury Syndrome

MICHELLE PETRI, M.D., M.P.H.

Associate Professor of Medicine, Director, Hopkins Lupus Cohort, and Co-Director, Lupus Pregnancy Center, The Johns Hopkins University School of Medicine, Baltimore, Maryland

Systemic Lupus Erythematosus

THOMAS A.E. PLATTS-MILLS, M.D., Ph.D.

Professor of Medicine and Microbiology, Head, Division of Allergy, Asthma, and Immunology, and Director, Asthma and Allergic Diseases Center, University of Virginia School of Medicine, Charlottesville, Virginia

Allergic Rhinitis Caused by Dust Mite and Other Nonpollen Allergens

PAUL H. PLOTZ, M.D.

Chief, Arthritis and Rheumatism Branch, National Institute of Arthritis and Musculoskeletal and Skin Diseases, National Institutes of Health, Bethesda, Maryland

Dermatomyositis and Polymyositis

MICHAEL A. POLIS, M.D., M.P.H.

Associate Clinical Professor of Emergency Medicine, George Washington University Medical Center, Washington, DC; Senior Investigator, Laboratory of Immunoregulation, National Institute of Allergy and Infectious Diseases, National Institutes of Health, Bethesda, Maryland

Acquired Immunodeficiency Syndrome: Treatment of Opportunistic Infections

JOSEPH M. POLITO II, M.D.

Instructor in Medicine, Department of Gastroenterology-Hepatology, State University of New York at Stony Brook Health Sciences Center School of Medicine, Stony Brook, New York

Crohn's Disease

CLAUDIO PONTICELLI, M.D., F.R.C.P.(Edin)

Director, Division of Nephrology and Dialysis, Istituto Scientifico Ospedale Maggiore, Milano, Italy

Lupus Nephritis

ANDREW J. REES, M.B., Ch.B., M.Sc., F.R.C.P.

Reguis Professor of Medicine, University of Aberdeen; Honorary Consultant Physician and Nephrologist, Aberdeen Royal Infirmary, Aberdeen, United Kingdom

Goodpasture's Syndrome

DIANE M. REID, M.D.

Medical Officer, Clinical Hematology Branch, National Institute of Diabetes and Digestive and Kidney Diseases, National Institutes of Health, Bethesda, Maryland

Immunologic Thrombocytopenia

PETER J. RICHARDSON, M.D., F.R.C.P.

Consultant Cardiologist, King's College Hospital, London, United Kingdom

Inflammatory Myocarditis

ROBERT L. ROBERTS, M.D., Ph.D.

Assistant Professor, Division of Immunology/Allergy, Department of Pediatrics, University of California at Los Angeles Medical Center, Los Angeles, California

Hyperimmunoglobulin E Syndrome (Job's Syndrome)

JESSE ROTH, M.D.

Raymond and Anna Lublin Professor of Medicine, and Director, Division of Geriatric Medicine, The Johns Hopkins University School of Medicine; Scientist Emeritus, National Institute of Diabetes and Digestive and Kidney Diseases, National Institutes of Health, Bethesda, Maryland

Insulin Allergy and Insulin Resistance

HUGH A. SAMPSON, M.D.

Professor of Pediatrics, and Director, Pediatric Clinical Research Unit, The Johns Hopkins University School of Medicine, Baltimore, Maryland

Food Hypersensitivities in Children

DAVID D. SHERRY, M.D.

Associate Professor of Pediatrics, University of Washington School of Medicine; Director, Pediatric Rheumatology, Children's Hospital and Medical Center, Seattle, Washington

Juvenile Rheumatoid Arthritis

ALAN R. SHULDINER, M.D.

Associate Professor of Medicine, The Johns Hopkins University School of Medicine, Baltimore, Maryland

Insulin Allergy and Insulin Resistance

†N. RAPHAEL SHULMAN, M.D.

Chief, Clinical Hematology Branch, National Institute of Diabetes and Digestive and Kidney Diseases, National Institutes of Health, Bethesda, Maryland; Clinical Professor of Medicine, Georgetown University, Washington, DC

Immunologic Thrombocytopenia

KRISTI SILVER, M.D.

Instructor, Johns Hopkins Hospital, Baltimore, Maryland

Insulin Allergy and Insulin Resistance

F. ESTELLE R. SIMONS, M.D.

Bruce Chown Professor and Deputy Head, Department of Pediatrics and Child Health, University of Manitoba Faculty of Medicine; Head, Section of Allergy and Clinical Immunology, Children's Hospital, Winnipeg, Manitoba, Canada

Antihistamines (H_1-Receptor Antagonists)

KEITH J. SIMONS, Ph.D.

Professor and Head, Division of Pharmaceutical Sciences, Faculty of Pharmacy; Adjunct Professor, Department of Chemistry, Faculty of Science; Department of Pediatrics, Faculty of Medicine, University of Manitoba, Winnipeg, Manitoba, Canada

Antihistamines (H_1-Receptor Antagonists)

MARTHA SKINNER, M.D.

Professor of Medicine, Boston University School of Medicine; Director of Amyloid Research, Arthritis Center, Boston University Medical Center, Boston, Massachusetts

Amyloidosis

RAYMOND G. SLAVIN, M.D.

Professor of Internal Medicine and Microbiology, and Director, Division of Allergy and Immunology, St. Louis University School of Medicine, St. Louis, Missouri

Hypersensitivity Pneumonitis

DAVID L. SMITH, M.D.

Assistant Professor of Medicine and Pediatrics, Division of Allergy and Immunology, University of South Alabama College of Medicine, Mobile, Alabama

Drug Reactions

STEVEN SMITH, M.D.

Fellow in Nephrology, Columbia-Presbyterian Medical Center, New York, New York

Immunologically Mediated Nephritic Renal Disease

MICHAEL C. SNELLER, M.D.

Chief, Immunologic Diseases Section, Laboratory of Immunoregulation, National Institute of Allergy and Infectious Diseases, National Institutes of Health, Bethesda, Maryland

Takayasu's Arteritis

NICHOLAS A. SOTER, M.D.

Professor, Department of Dermatology, New York University School of Medicine; Medical Director, Charles C. Harris Skin and Cancer Pavilion, and Attending Physician, Tisch Hospital-The University Hospital of New York University, New York, New York

Physical Urticaria and Angioedema

KATHERINE M. SPOONER, M.D.

Medical Officer, Critical Care Medicine Department, National Institutes of Health, Bethesda, Maryland

Acquired Immunodeficiency Syndrome: Treatment of Opportunistic Infections

GORDON STARKEBAUM, M.D.

Professor of Medicine, University of Washington; Chief, Arthritis Section, Veterans Administration Medical Center, Seattle, Washington

Autoimmune Leukopenia

DONALD D. STEVENSON, M.D.

Clinical Member, Department of Molecular and Experimental Medicine; Senior Consultant, Division of Allergy, Asthma and Immunology, Scripps Clinic and Research Foundation, La Jolla, California

Aspirin Sensitivity in Rhinosinusitis and Asthma

E. RICHARD STIEHM, M.D.

Professor of Pediatrics, and Chief, Division of Immunology/Allergy, University of California, Los Angeles, School of Medicine; Attending Pediatrician, University of California at Los Angeles Center for Health Sciences, Los Angeles, California

Hyperimmunoglobulin E Syndrome (Job's Syndrome)

CHRISTIAN P. STRASSBURG, M.D.

Research Assistant and Fellow, Department of Gastroenterology and Hepatology, Medizinische Hochschule Hannover, Hannover, Germany

Chronic Hepatitis

TERRY B. STROM, M.D.

Professor of Medicine, Harvard Medical School; Director, Division of Immunology, Department of Medicine, Beth Israel Hospital, Boston, Massachusetts

Organ Transplant Recipients

†Deceased.

MANIKKAM SUTHANTHIRAN, M.D.

Professor of Medicine, Biochemistry and Surgery, Cornell University Medical College; Chairman, Department of Transplantation Medicine and Extracorporeal Therapy, The New York Hospital, New York, New York

Organ Transplant Recipients

ROBERT A. SWERLICK, M.D.

Associate Professor, Emory University School of Medicine, Atlanta, Georgia

Dermatitis Herpetiformis

NORMAN TALAL, M.D.

Professor of Medicine and Microbiology, and Chief, Division of Clinical Immunology, University of Texas Health Science Center at San Antonio; Chief of Rheumatology, Audie L. Murphy Memorial Veterans Hospital, San Antonio, Texas; Vice President, Medical Advisory Board, Sjögren's Syndrome Foundation, New York, New York

Sjögren's Syndrome

ABBA I. TERR, M.D.

Clinical Professor of Medicine, Stanford University School of Medicine, Stanford, California

Chemical Sensitivity

MARCIA G. TONNESEN, M.D.

Associate Professor of Medicine and Dermatology, State University of New York at Stony Brook Health Sciences Center School of Medicine; Attending Physician and Director of Phototherapy, University Hospital, State University of New York at Stony Brook, Stony Brook, and Chief, Dermatology, Medical Service, Northport Veterans Administration Medical Center, Northport, New York

Erythema Multiforme

MASSIMO TRIGGIANI, M.D., Ph.D.

Assistant Professor of Medicine, Division of Clinical Immunology and Allergy, University of Naples "Federico II", Naples, Italy

Acute Rheumatic Fever

ANTONIO UCCELLI, M.D.

Assistant Professor in Neurology, Department of Neurological Sciences, University of Genoa, Genoa, Italy

Multiple Sclerosis and Related Demyelinating Diseases

RADVAN URBANEK, M.D.

Professor of Pediatrics, and Head of the Department of Pediatrics, University Hospital, Vienna, Austria

Insect Sting Allergy in Children

ROBERT VOLPÉ, M.D., F.R.C.P.(C), F.A.C.P., F.R.C.P.(Edin. & Lond.)

Professor Emeritus, Department of Medicine, University of Toronto Faculty of Medicine; Director, Endocrinology Research Laboratory, Wellesley Hospital, Toronto, Ontario, Canada

Chronic Lymphocytic Thyroiditis

LISA M. WHEATLEY, M.D.

Associate Professor, University of Virginia School of Medicine, Charlottesville, Virginia

Allergic Rhinitis Caused by Dust Mite and Other Nonpollen Allergens

FREDRICK M. WIGLEY, M.D.

Associate Professor of Medicine, The Johns Hopkins University School of Medicine; Director, Division of Rheumatology, and Co-Director, Johns Hopkins and University of Maryland Scleroderma Center, Baltimore, Maryland

Scleroderma

RICHARD H. WINTERBAUER, M.D.

Head, Section of Pulmonary and Critical Care Medicine, Virginia Mason Clinic, Seattle, Washington

Sarcoidosis

DAVID T. WOODLEY, M.D.

Professor and Chairman, Department of Dermatology, Northwestern University Medical School; Dermatologist-in-Chief, Northwestern Memorial Hospital, Chicago, Illinois

Pemphigoid: Bullous and Cicatricial

ALEXANDRA S. WOROBEC, M.D.

Clinical Associate, Allergic Diseases Section, National Institute of Allergy and Infectious Diseases, National Institutes of Health, Bethesda, Maryland

Systemic Anaphylaxis

PREFACE

This, the fifth edition of *Current Therapy in Allergy, Immunology, and Rheumatology,* continues the tradition established in previous editions of providing timely information to clinicians on the therapy of allergic, immunologic, and rheumatologic diseases. Most textbooks of medicine are aimed at providing a comprehensive approach to pathogenesis, diagnosis, and clinical manifestations of disease with varying degrees of attention paid to therapy. In this volume, as in previous volumes, we have asked the authors to address pathogenic and diagnostic considerations only insofar as they pertain to therapy, to define the clinical problems clearly and succinctly, and to focus predominantly on the details of treating these diseases in all of their various manifestations.

We anticipate that this approach to the treatment of these diseases will be of particular interest and usefulness to practicing clinicians during this era of "managed care" when time constraints are a fact of life in the care of patients, and ready access to treatment guidelines and instructions pertaining to the initiation and followup of therapy are essential. In this regard, the availability of "expert opinion" on therapy of these diseases in a user friendly, concise format should prove to be extremely useful.

We have recruited a group of authors who are prominent clinical investigators and experts in the diseases in question, and who have extensive hands-on experience in the treatment of these diseases. We have provided no rigid guidelines to them; instead, we have asked them to draw from their own fund of knowledge, judgment, and clinical experience in the treatment of patients with the diseases on which they are writing. As a result, the reader will be exposed to the "personal" approach of these eminent experts from a variety of subspecialties. We are thankful to the authors for their willingness to share with us the fruits of their extensive experience in the treatment of these important classes of diseases.

Lawrence M. Lichtenstein, M.D., Ph.D.
Anthony S. Fauci, M.D.

CONTENTS

CONNECTIVE TISSUE DISEASE

VASCULITIS

HEART AND LUNG DISEASE

GASTROINTESTINAL DISEASE

HEMATOLOGIC DISEASE

RHINITIS

ALLERGIC RHINITIS

PETER S. CRETICOS, M.D.

The patient with allergic rhinitis experiences itchy and watery eyes, runny nose, sneezing, nasal congestion, and/or postnasal drainage with or without associated cough when exposed to a relevant aeroallergen. Perhaps the most important concept to grasp is that the problem is not simply an occasional or haphazard event; rather, because of repeated exposure to a seasonal or perennial allergen, the typical allergic patient's symptoms actually reflect an intense inflammatory component characterized by cellular recruitment, inflammatory mediator release, and heightened mucosal reactivity. The key to successful therapy of allergic rhinitis is therefore the suppression or prevention of the underlying inflammatory component of the disease.

PATHOPHYSIOLOGY

Our understanding of the allergic process has been advanced immeasurably by the tools of molecular biology. We now appreciate that the T cell is responsible for orchestrating the IgE-mediated allergic process. Initially, an antigen presenting cell (e.g., dendritic cell or langerhans cell) presents an appropriate peptide sequence to a CD4 positive T cell. In an allergic individual, processing of this peptide sequence results in the induction of a T helper cell subpopulation (termed TH2 positive lymphocytes), which induces an inflammatory (cytokine) cascade. These specific inflammatory cytokines (IL-3, IL-4, IL-5, GMCSF) have effects both on the immediate IgE-mediated allergic process through their interactions with mast cells and basophils and on the late-phase allergic process induced by basophils, eosinophils, and neutrophils that have been recruited into the inflammatory site.

RELEVANT ALLERGENS

Proteinaceous materials (i.e., allergenic proteins) from a variety of sources are capable of triggering the allergic process (Table 1). Allergic rhinitis can be precipitated by exposure to seasonal airborne allergens (e.g., pollens and mold spores) and/or to perennial allergens (house dust mite debris and fecal material, insect constituents, and animal dander and salivary protein).

Various tree pollens predominate during the early spring pollen season, whereas grass pollens are primarily responsible for late spring and summer symptomatology. Although ragweed is the dominant airborne allergen in North America during late summer and early fall, there are also other important weed pollens that are prominent in the spring (sheep sorrel) and the summer months (plantain). Mold spores can be prominent factors during damp periods of the year and, in particular, during the fall months when the leaves and corn stalks are decaying.

Perhaps even more important in respect to the allergic patient is the importance of persistent exposure to perennial allergens in inducing this smouldering clinical process. House dust mites, cockroaches, and other insect-related allergens and animal proteins comprise the bulk of the indoor allergen load. Dust mites, their decaying body parts, and their fecal particles represent a significant indoor allergen burden in the home. Dust mites feed off dried skin debris and accumulate in mattresses and boxsprings, feather pillows and comforters, carpeting, stuffed animals, upholstered furniture, and wool clothing. Although they have rather specific growth season requirements, which are dependent upon an optimal temperature (60° to 80° F) and humidity (55 to 85 percent), in our typical airtight homes with central heating and air conditioning systems that can easily circulate the allergen load through the indoor air, these dust mite particles represent a significant indoor burden. Furthermore, even during the drier periods of the year, the microenvironment in which the patient sleeps is conducive to continued mite survival because increased body temperature and perspiration create an appropriate microenvironment for their survival within the bedding and pillows.

Various indoor insects may also be important in inducing allergic disease. Cockroaches are most prominent in older dwellings and damp locations, especially those close to water. The allergic components of cockroaches again appear to be their decaying body

Table 1 Relevant Allergens

Seasonal
Tree pollens
Grass pollens
Weed pollens
Mold spores
Perennial
Dust mites
Insect debris
Animal dander/saliva/urinary proteins
Mold spores

parts, their fecal emanations, and interestingly, their salivary protein. Again the allergen smaller particle sizes are usually circulated through the indoor ventilation system and can induce both upper and lower respiratory problems. There are other insects (spiders, moths, centipedes) that need further characterization in terms of their allergenicity.

Domesticated animals represent another important source of allergen in the indoor environment. Approximately 70 percent of homes in North America have pets living within the household. The allergen load reflects protein from several different sources—the saliva, the urine, and, primarily, the dander of the animal. These protein particles easily become airborne and are circulated by the forced air heating or ventilation systems. It is important to recognize that a significant percentage of smaller particles (3 to 5 μm) will typically stay suspended in the air for up to 24 hours after being disturbed, as opposed to dust mite fecal particles, which tend to be heavier and to precipitate back to the floor within only 1 or 2 hours after disturbance.

Urinary protein is also the major allergen source from laboratory animals and various rodents such as mice, rats, guinea pigs, and hamsters. The nocturnal patterns of these animals and their frequent location in the bedrooms of homes can add considerably to the nocturnal allergen load to which the patient might be exposed.

Thus, it is apparent that a considerable allergen burden, reflective of both perennial as well as seasonal allergens, may impact upon an allergic patient's environment and result in the untoward clinical manifestations experienced by the patient during the appropriate "season." In fact, patients may experience seasonal rhinitis, perennial rhinitis, or perennial rhinitis with seasonal exacerbations.

DIAGNOSTIC APPROACH

The evaluation of the patient with rhinitis should include a thorough history, with particular attention to the home environment, the work setting, and hobbies that could induce or influence the allergic process. Appropriate laboratory tests, including skin testing and/or blood testing (radioallergosorbent test [RAST]) can help corroborate the clinical impression.

An important consideration is when to proceed with further diagnostic testing in the patient with rhinitis. Obviously, both the duration and the severity of the disease process help determine the clinical approach that should be undertaken. In patients with more persistent symptoms or symptoms reflective of exposure to multiple allergens, and in patients with inadequate response to simple pharmacotherapeutic measures, a further diagnostic evaluation is warranted.

A useful screen for the primary care physician is a multi-RAST screen, which incorporates five or six of the most important allergens for a geographic area onto a disc. If this multi-RAST screen is positive, it provides initial evidence for an allergic component to the patient's rhinitis and suggests that a more in-depth workup with carefully selected skin tests would be warranted.

Considerable discussion arises as to whether RAST testing to specific allergens is equivalent to or capable of providing as much information as skin testing. Studies have conclusively demonstrated that properly done RAST tests are the equivalent of a well-performed prick-puncture skin test. In either case, approximately 80 percent of patients with clinically relevant disease can be identified. However, in patients with a negative prick or puncture skin test, a secondary, intradermal skin test should be applied to the patient's arm. This will elicit positive skin test reactivity in an additional 15 percent of patients that would otherwise have been missed by the percutaneous (prick-puncture) test alone. There is no RAST equivalent of an intradermal skin test. However, the clinical relevance of this test must be determined based on the results of a careful history obtained from the patient.

Indeed, prick-puncture skin tests correlate strongly with challenge tests of the nose, eyes, or lungs. However, this close correlation observed with prick-puncture testing is not seen with challenges of intradermally sensitive patients.

Again, this points out the importance of corroborating any laboratory procedure with the clinical history. Obviously, a positive intradermal skin test to cat may point to a clinically relevant finding in a patient with a cat in the indoor environment. Whereas, a positive skin test to ragweed in a patient who lives on the West Coast, where no significant levels of ragweed are found, would be an irrelevant skin test finding.

THERAPEUTIC APPROACH

Based on an understanding of the pathophysiology of the allergic disease process, the management of allergic rhinitis reflects appropriate environmental control, judicious use of appropriate anti-inflammatory agents to suppress the underlying allergic inflammation with supplemental use of antihistamines and/or decongestants for "breakthrough" symptomatology, and consideration of immunotherapy in those patients who have not responded to these environmental and pharmacotherapeutic measures or who have had side effects with

Table 2 Management of Allergic Rhinitis

Allergen avoidance
Environmental control measures
Preventive "anti-inflammatory" therapy
Nasal corticosteroids
Cromolyn sodium
Supplemental "rescue" therapy
Antihistamines
Decongestants
Immunotherapy

From Creticos PS: Johns Hopkins Asthma and Allergy Center Press; with permission.

the medications or have persistent disease because of multiple exposure to allergens throughout the year (Table 2).

PATIENT EDUCATION

Of course, for this therapeutic approach to be effective a successful interaction with the patient is required. Indeed, the most crucial component of any patient therapeutic plan is the one that is most often neglected—patient education. The patient educator needs to work with the patient to review the plan of action, discuss the proper use of medications and their side effects, and provide access to the physician or staff when problems arise. This educational component is particularly important when dealing with a chronic or persistent disease process such as allergic rhinitis.

ENVIRONMENTAL CONTROL

Measures to reduce the indoor allergen burden can be particularly effective in dust mite or insect or animal allergic patients. Encasing mattresses and boxsprings, removing feather pillows or down-filled comforters and stuffed animals from a bedroom, removing carpeting from the bedroom or entire home, and minimizing upholstered furniture are all effective measures that should be considered in the dust mite allergic patient's home.

Decisions regarding animals often have a profound psychological component within the family structure. If possible, animals should be removed from the home of an animal-sensitive patient. At the least, the pet should be kept out of the patient's bedroom. Of course, the problem with this latter course of action is that the heating and ventilation systems will continue to circulate a significant component of the small-sized allergenic particles throughout the house. Consequently, a high efficiency particulate air filter (HEPA) filtration system may be a reasonable alternative in the bedroom of a patient unwilling to remove a pet from the premises.

Of course, in areas of the country where insects such as cockroaches are a factor, appropriate extermination should be considered. However, care should be exercised in choosing an insecticide. For example, pyrethrins are members of the chrysanthemum weed family and, as such, cross-react with ragweed. Hence, spraying this type insecticide would be the equivalent of spraying a liquid suspension of ragweed through the house. Alternate insecticide choices should be considered in a weed-sensitive patient.

PREVENTIVE ANTI-INFLAMMATORY THERAPY

A primary anti-inflammatory therapeutic agent should be used to prevent or suppress symptoms in those patients who experience persistent symptoms on a seasonal or perennial basis. Both glucocorticoid steroid preparations and nonsteroidal compounds have been developed, which can be safely applied topically to the nostrils.

Topical Nasal Steroid Preparations

Mechanisms

Topical nasal steroid preparations exert their anti-inflammatory effects through a number of different mechanisms. At a cellular level, these compounds penetrate the cell and bind to specific receptors within the cell to alter messenger RNA and subsequent protein expression. Their effects include inhibition of mediator synthesis of the arachidonic acid pathway, inhibition of leukocyte migration, and down-regulation of the effects of various inflammatory mediators on their target sites within the tissue.

Improvement in clinical symptoms is a direct measure of suppression of the underlying inflammatory process. In our laboratories, Pipkorn utilized a nasal challenge model to demonstrate that the topical application of a nasal steroid not only suppressed the late phase of the allergic response but also attenuated the acute allergic response. This is in contradistinction to oral prednisone, which ablated only the late phase of reactivity and had no effect on the immediate allergic response. Bascom and co-workers further characterized the effects of nasal steroids and showed that therapy resulted in a significant reduction in the influx of eosinophils and basophilic-type cells migrating into the nasal mucosa in response to an allergic stimulus (Fig. 1). Obviously, the importance of this is borne out in our approach to the management of the patient with allergic rhinitis. *It reiterates the importance of using a topical anti-inflammatory preparation on a regular daily basis to suppress the inflammatory component and emphasizes the particular benefit of using this type of medication prophylactically to prevent the evolution of the allergic process.*

Clinical Indications

Table 3 lists the topical steroid preparations that are currently available in the U.S. market. Efficacy has been demonstrated in seasonal allergic rhinitis, perennial allergic rhinitis, nonallergic rhinitis with eosinophilia

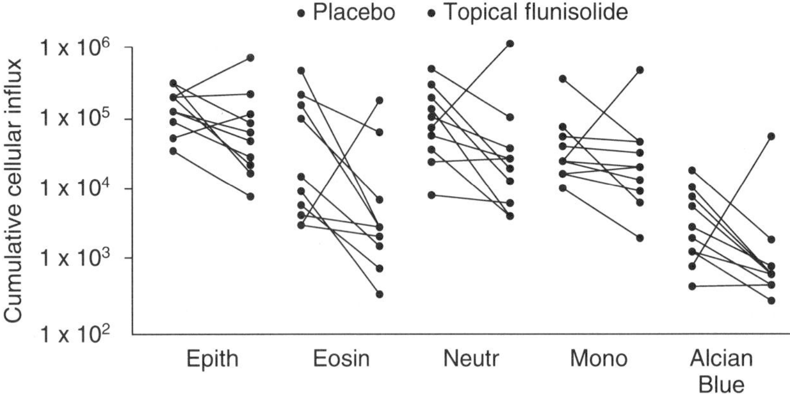

Figure 1 Topical flunisolide (TF) pretreatment (200 μg per day for 7 days) diminished the cumulative cellular influx between 3 and 11 hours after nasal antigen challenge, compared with placebo (P). (From Bascom R, Wachs M, Naclerio RM, et al. Basophil influx occurs after nasal antigen challenge: effects of topical corticosteroid pretreatment. J Allergy Clin Immunol 1988; 81:580–589; with permission.)

Table 3 Dosing Comparison of Intranasal Steroids

Drug	*Adult/Child >12 Dose/Day*	*Typical Dosing*
Beclomethasone*	168-336 μg/d† 42 μg/spray	One spray/nostril/q.i.d. or two sprays/nostril/b.i.d.
Budesonide*	128-256 μg/d† 32 μg/spray	One-two sprays/nostril/b.i.d. or two-four sprays/ nostril/q.d.
Dexamethasone*	672-1008 μg/d‡ 84 μg/spray	Two sprays/nostril/b.i.d.-t.i.d.
Flunisolide*	200-300 μg/d 50 μg/spray	Two sprays/nostril/b.i.d.-t.i.d.
Fluticasone§	100-200 μg/d 50 μg/spray	One spray/nostril/b.i.d. or one-two sprays/nostril/q.d.
Triamcinolone*	110-440 μg/d 55 μg/spray	One spray/nostril/q.d. up to two sprays/nostril/b.i.d.

*PDR, 1995.
†Adults and children over 6 years of age.
‡Possibility of systemic toxicity in extended normal dosing.
§PDR, 1995s.

(NARES), chronic rhinitis (presumably predominant nonallergic basis), and chronic rhinitis associated with nasal polyposis (Table 4). Clinical studies suggest that the majority (70 to 80 percent) of patients with allergic rhinitis will demonstrate very good to excellent symptom control with doses between 100 to 440 μg per day with somewhat less success in patients with chronic nonallergic problems. This dose can be delivered with most of the nasal steroid preparations by administering 1 to 2 sprays per nostril twice a day every day. The availability of both aqueous and dry formulations as well as the once or twice daily-dosing regimens should enhance patient compliance. *Therapy should be initiated at the maximally recommended dosage over the first 1 to 2 weeks of treatment in order to suppress the underlying inflammatory process. Once symptoms are brought under control, then the dosage should be adjusted to the lowest dose that still provides adequate therapeutic control.* The patient should be counseled in how to make appropriate incremental adjustments in dose based on fluctuations in clinical symptoms or period exacerbation. For example, an optimal dose of 2 sprays per nostril twice a day of a nasal steroid may be required during the brunt of the grass or ragweed seasons with a tapering to 1 to 2 sprays per nostril daily for maintenance control during the shoulder season in a patient with low-grade perennial rhinitis with seasonal exacerbations.

These points can be elucidated with several clinical studies that address efficacy. Norman, Creticos, and others studied 50 adult patients with seasonal spring pollenosis, who received either 200 μg of budesonide twice a day or placebo spray. The group receiving the nasal steroid preparation demonstrated a significant reduction (70 percent) in clinical symptoms within 3 days

Table 4 Intranasal Indications for Inhaled Corticosteroids

Drug	*SAR*	*PAR*	*NAR*	*NP*
Patients ≥6 yr old				
Beclomethasone*	✓	✓	✓	✓
Budesonide*	✓	✓	✓†	
Dexamethasone*	✓	✓	✓	✓
Flunisolide*	✓	✓		
Patients ≥12 yr old				
Fluticasone‡	✓	✓		
Triamcinolone*	✓	✓		

SAR, seasonal allergic rhinitis; *PAR,* perennial allergic rhinitis; *NAR,* nonallergic rhinitis; *NP,* nasal polyps.
**PDR,* 1995.
†≥12 yr old only.
‡*PDR,* 1995s.

of starting therapy, and this improvement was maintained through the duration of the spring grass pollen season (Fig. 2). Furthermore, a significant reduction in tame-esterase activity, a marker of nasal inflammation, was demonstrated in the nasal washings from the steroid-treated group only. This reaffirms the concept that topical nasal steroid therapy suppresses the nasal inflammatory process.

In a 12-week study by Turkeltaub and associates of perennial allergic rhinitis, those patients receiving the nasal steroid, flunisolide, had a 50 percent reduction in nasal symptoms as compared to the placebo group of patients. *However, in contrast to seasonal allergic rhinitis, it may take up to 1 week or longer to demonstrate clinically relevant improvement in symptoms in patients with perennial disease.*

Nasal polyposis can be a most troublesome development in patients with chronic rhinitis or rhinosinusitis. In certain instances, this requires close interaction with an ear, nose, and throat specialist. In more difficult or recalcitrant cases, endoscopic sinus surgery with polypectomy may be required. However, to prevent regrowth of the polypoid tissue, aggressive steroid therapy is necessary. Initially, this may necessitate a short course of oral prednisone therapy followed by transition to a topical nasal steroid for continued maintenance control. Several studies support this approach.

A study by Ruhno demonstrated that budesonide administered at a dose of 800 μg per day for 4 weeks significantly improved the severity of nasal symptoms and improved nasal peak expiratory flow rates in patients with nasal polyposis as compared to placebo-treated patients.

Maintenance Dosing

To be most effective, a topical nasal steroid needs to be administered on a regular daily basis. The importance of regular daily dosing has been alluded to in several studies. Juniper and co-workers addressed this issue in a double-blind, parallel, positive control study in which patients received either 200 μg of beclomethasone twice daily or 100 to 400 μg beclomethasone given on an as needed basis. This study demonstrated that not only were clinical symptoms much better controlled, quality of life parameters were also significantly improved in the group receiving daily maintenance therapy.

Equally important is the observation in several studies that a recrudescence of symptoms will occur within 3 to 5 days of discontinuation of therapy. This is cited in a double-blind placebo-controlled study of flunisolide by Turkeltaub and associates. Clinical efficacy with the topical nasal steroid preparation was demonstrated within 3 to 4 days of instituting therapy and was maintained over the 3-week treatment period. When flunisolide was discontinued during the latter part of the ragweed season, symptom diary scores worsened and became comparable to those of patients who were receiving placebo.

Safety Concerns

The issue of safety is a moot point with the newer synthetically derived nasal steroid preparations that provide efficacy in the overwhelming majority of patients at doses of less than or equal to 400 μg per day. Neither clinically significant changes in bone growth nor evidence of adrenal suppression have been observed in patients at these therapeutic doses.

Of interest is the observation that fluticasone has negligible absorption across the gastrointestinal tract (<1 to 2 percent) when it is delivered nasally. This makes it an excellent consideration in a patient who is already receiving an inhaled pulmonary steroid for control of asthma, and obviates any concern about gastrointestinal absorption of the swallowed nasally applied steroid and hence minimizes any additional total systemic steroid availability. Conversely, studies of bioavailability of budesonide suggest that a 30 percent higher therapeutic dose (≥1,600 μg) can be administered as compared to beclomethasone before equivalent effects on adrenal suppression can be observed. Obviously, these issues only pertain to therapy in asthmatic patients, but certainly they reiterate the safety of the doses employed for control of nasal symptoms with topical nasal steroids.

Oral Steroids

In some patients with severe nasal symptomatology, the use of topical nasal preparations will be unable to effect a beneficial resonse. In this instance, a short course of prednisone (a 30 mg dose tapered by 5 mg every 1 to 2 days) may significantly reduce the nasal edema and inflammation and hence allow the introduction of the topical nasal steroid on the third or fourth day of therapy with the resultant smooth transition to maintenance therapy with the nasal steroid preparation.

This may likewise be a critical issue in patients with nasal polyps where a more prolonged oral prednisone taper over 1 to 2 weeks may be necessitated to reduce the polypoid tissue to a point where the topical steroid preparation may provide effective maintenance control.

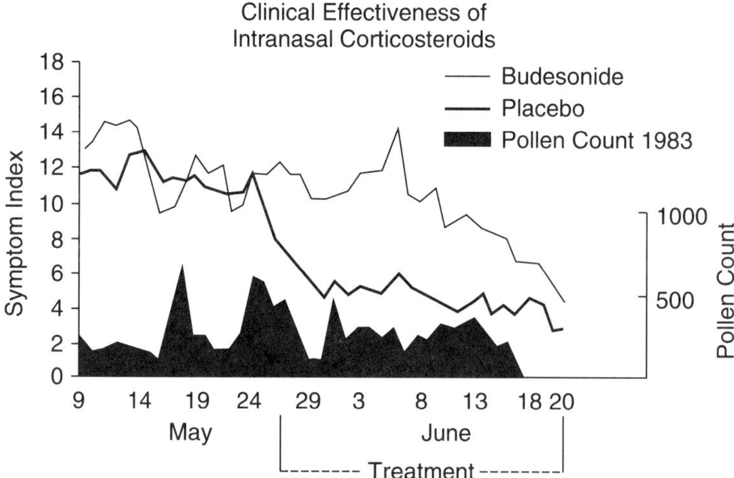

Figure 2 Daily mean (+SEM) combined nasal symptom scores (AM and PM recordings) during the baseline (May 9–23) and treatment (May 24-June 20) periods. Budesonide; placebo;--pollen count. (From Norman PS, Creticos PS, Tobey R, et al. Budesonide in grass pollen rhinitis. Ann Allergy 1992; 69:306–316; with permission.)

In patients with rhinitis medicamentosa caused by prolonged nasal decongestant therapy, a short course of oral prednisone (30 mg taper over 5 days) may allow sufficient reduction in nasal edema to allow a nasal steroid to be effectively applied. Alternatively, concomitant use of the nasal steroid in conjunction with the nasal decongestant for the first 5 to 7 days may then allow the nasal decongestant to be easily tapered and subsequently discontinued over the next 1 to 2 weeks. Otherwise, the patient is likely to experience equivocal results and discontinue the nasal steroid in favor of the continued use of the nasal decongestant, which provides "immediate" relief.

NONSTEROIDAL ANTI-INFLAMMATORY PREPARATIONS

Although the mechanisms of cromolyn's action are not completely understood, it appears that one of its actions may be to stabilize mast cell membranes and inhibit the subsequent release of inflammatory mediators associated with the allergic reaction.

Clinical studies have demonstrated the efficacy of nasal cromolyn for the treatment of both seasonal and perennial rhinitis. However, to be optimally effective, cromolyn requires judicious use by the patient on a regular daily basis. In the patient who is already symptomatic, an aggressive therapeutic regimen is mandated and it may take 1 to 2 weeks to achieve optimal results. In this situation, it would be advisable to start with two sprays in each nostril every 4 hours for the first 7 to 10 days. Once satisfactory control is achieved, it may be possible to taper the drug to 1 to 2 sprays per nostril three to four times a day for long-term control. Obviously, this reiterates the need to emphasize patient education to ensure patient compliance.

Perhaps the most successful therapeutic approach with cromolyn is to employ the drug prophylactically. When used prophylactically, the medication should be started as 1 to 2 sprays per nostril, four to six times a day for 1 to 2 weeks before the start of the allergen season. Again, with careful patient compliance, the therapeutic benefits of the drug should be achieved. Once symptom control is achieved, the drug can then be tapered to a more convenient regimen of two to four times per day to sustain relief.

Experience with cromolyn shows that 60 to 70 percent of patients who adhere to the prescribed dosage regimen will obtain very good to excellent results. This is best documented in pollen-induced seasonal rhinitis. In a double-blind randomized placebo-controlled comparative study, Handelman and coworkers divided 88 patients into two groups. Symptom diaries demonstrated that both groups of patients experienced similar symptoms during the 3-week baseline period of study. They were then randomized to therapy with either cromolyn, one spray per nostril six times a day, or a placebo spray. Through the course of the ragweed pollen season, patients maintained their symptom diaries on a regular daily basis. These diaries demonstrated that there was significantly less sneezing, rhinorrhea, nasal congestion, and eye irritation in the group treated with cromolyn as compared to the placebo group.

Adverse Effects

Cromolyn appears to act topically at or within the mucosal surface. Less than 7 percent of the dose is absorbed across the nasal mucosa and that which is absorbed is rapidly excreted unchanged in the bile and urine. It appears to be well tolerated by patients, with only mild nasal irritation or burning having been reported.

RESCUE THERAPY

Antihistamines, decongestants, and anticholinergic agents may be effective therapeutic agents for relief of mild or intermittent nasal symptoms. In the patients already on a primary anti-inflammatory therapeutic agent for control of persistent disease, adjunctive therapy with one of these respective agents may optimize control. In this regard, antihistamines should be employed for breakthrough symptoms of itchy, watery eyes; runny nose; and sneezing. Ipratropium may be particularly effective for control of rhinorrhea and/or postnasal drip. Decongestants may be helpful for control of nasal congestion and stuffiness.

Antihistamines

Antihistamines may be the primary agent for the relief of acute of intermittent symptoms of allergic rhinitis. Furthermore, they are an important adjunct to a primary anti-inflammatory agent in the long term management of persistent seasonal and perennial rhinitis.

The classic first-generation antihistamines are competitive antagonists to histamine for H_1-receptor sites on target cells on the nasal mucosa. However, they are highly lipophilic and easily penetrate the central nervous system resulting in significant drowsiness and sedation in 10 to 25 percent of patients. Perhaps more importantly, their use may interfere with the ability to perform tasks that require motor skills, such as driving a car or operating machinery. Unfortunately, this possibility cannot be predicted based on the sedating properties of the antihistamine. In some patients, especially the elderly, the traditional antihistamines may cause troublesome anticholinergic effects, such as difficulty with urination, impotence, or dryness of the mouth. A smaller number of patients may complain of gastrointestinal disturbances. These drugs should be used with caution in patients who have a history of epilepsy. Lastly, in higher dosages, adverse cardiovascular effects can also be induced by the first-generation antihistamines, ranging from palpitations to supraventricular tachycardia to ventricular disturbances.

In contrast, several of the new second- or third-generation antihistamines are nonsedating and most importantly do not interfere with the ability to perform motor tasks. Terfenadine, astemizole, and loratadine are examples of the newer nonsedating antihistamines. However, certain of these newer third-generation antihistamines (astemizole, terfenadine) have been associated with cardiac arrhythmias, which, although rare, have led to fatal or near-fatal outcomes. It is apparent that there are certain clinical settings that may predispose patients to the development of these adverse cardiovascular events—underlying hepatic disease, specific drug interactions, and certain cardiovascular settings (Table 5).

Obviously, with careful attention to a patient's clinical history, the clinician should feel comfortable in knowing when and for whom to prescribe one of these therapeutic agents.

Table 5 Clinical Settings Potentially Capable of Inducing Adverse Cardiac Events with the Use of Antihistamines

- Overdose
  - Accidental
  - Suicide attempt
- Underlying hepatic disease
  - Cirrhosis
  - Hepatitis
- Drug interactions
  - Macrolide antibiotics
    - Erythromycin, clarithromycin
  - Antifungals
    - Ketoconazole, itraconazole, troleandomycin
- Cardiovascular settings
  - Severe bradycardia
  - Congenital Q-T prolongation
  - Underlying ventricular tachyarrhythmias
  - Antiarrhythmias
    - Type 1A
      - Quinidine, procainamide, disopyramide
    - Type III
      - Sotalol, amiodarone

From Creticos PS: Johns Hopkins Asthma and Allergy Center Press; with permission.

In summary, antihistamines represent an effective therapeutic choice for the relief of mild or intermittent symptoms of allergic rhinoconjunctivitis. However, in more persistent or moderately severe seasonal or perennial allergic disease, their role is as an adjunctive medication in conjunction with a primary anti-inflammatory therapeutic agent for the most effective management of the allergic condition. The newer third-generation antihistamines are safe and effective nonsedating medications with once-and twice-a-day dosing regimens that should further enhance patient compliance.

Decongestant Preparations

Both topical and oral decongestant preparations are available for the relief of nasal congestion and edema. The topically applied nasal decongestant preparations effectively constrict mucosal blood vessels and can be very effective agents for the relief of nasal edema and the resultant nasal congestion. However, a significant number of patients who use this type medication on a more frequent daily basis are apt to develop a condition of rebound nasal congestion, rhinitis medicamentosa. They are most appropriately used acutely during an upper respiratory infection or for the occasional relief of bothersome nasal congestion.

The oral decongestant preparations have a somewhat limited therapeutic application because of their narrow therapeutic window. Higher doses of these agents can be associated with caffeine-like stimulatory side effects and may increase blood pressure, especially in patients with borderline hypertension. They should be avoided in patients with hyperthyroidism, diabetes, and in patients on antidepressant drugs.

Topical Anticholinergic Agents

Ipratropium is the newest nasal therapeutic agent approved for use in rhinitis. It is effective at a dosage of 1 to 2 sprays per nostril per day as needed for relief of persistent rhinorrhea or postnasal drainage. It may be used in conjunction with a topical steroid or cromolyn for optimal control of nasal symptoms.

COMPARATIVE STUDIES

Comparative studies have generally shown cromolyn to be comparable if not superior to antihistamines in the relief of allergic rhinitis. However, this conclusion should be balanced by the observation that nasal cromolyn more effectively controls nasal congestion, whereas antihistamines generally provide better relief of eye symptoms. Likewise, studies of nasal steroids show superior control of nasal symptoms when compared to antihistamines.

A study by Welsh and associates compared the effects of two different nasal steroid preparations to nasal cromolyn in the management of ragweed-induced fall pollenosis. Both aqueous nasal steroid preparations provided similar relief of nasal symptoms, which was significantly better than that seen with nasal cromolyn. Interestingly, this study also pointed out the importance of controlling upper airway symptomatology in patients with asthma. Indeed, those asthmatic patients treated with a nasal steroid preparation not only had improvement in their nasal symptoms but also a reduction in their need for inhaled bronchodilators to relieve their asthma symptoms.

IMMUNOTHERAPY

Multiple controlled studies have demonstrated the efficacy of immunotherapy in the management of allergic rhinitis caused by pollen, mold spore, dust mite, and animal sensitivity. These studies have shown that the effectiveness of immunotherapy is dependent on an optimal therapeutic dose being administered for an adequate length of time. In those patients with an inadequate response to pharmacotherapy, side effects to medication, or who experience persistent symptoms of rhinoconjunctivitis, a trial of immunotherapy may provide significant relief of allergic symptoms.

SUGGESTED READING

Bascom R, Wachs M, Naclerio RM, et al. Basophil influx occurs after nasal antigen challenge: effects of topical corticosteroid pretreatment. J Allergy Clin Immunol 1988; 81:580–589.

Creticos PS. Allergic rhinitis. In Busse W, Holgate T, eds. Asthma and rhinitis. London: Blackwell Scientific Publications, 1994:1394.

Creticos PS. Immunotherapy of allergic diseases. In Rich RR, Shearer WT, eds. Clinical immunology, principles and practice. St. Louis: Mosby, 1995:2002.

Handelman NI, Friday GA, Schwartz HJ, et al. Cromolyn sodium nasal solution in the prophylactic treatment of pollen-induced seasonal allergic rhinitis. J Allergy Clin Immunol 1977; 59:237–242.

Juniper EF, Guyatt GH, O'Byrne PM, et al. Aqueous beclomethasone dipropionate nasal spray: regular versus "as required" use in the treatment of seasonal allergic rhinitis. J Allergy Clin Immunol 1990; 86:380–386.

Naclerio RM, Proud D, Togias AG, et al. Inflammatory mediators in late antigen-induced rhinitis. N Engl J Med 1985; 313:65–70.

Norman PS, Creticos PS, Tobey R, et al. Budesonide in grass pollen rhinitis. Ann Allergy 1992; 69:309–316.

O'Hehir RE, Garman RD, Greenstein JL, et al. The specificity and regulation of T cell responsiveness to allergen. Annu Rev Immunol 1991; 9:676.

Pipkorn U, Proud D, Lichtenstein LM, et al. Inhibition of mediator release in allergic rhinitis by pretreatment with topical glucocorticoids. N Engl J Med 1987; 316:1506–1510.

Ruhno J, Andersson B, Denburg J, et al. A double-blind comparison of intranasal budesonide with placebo for nasal polyposis. J Allergy Clin Immunol 1990; 86:946–953.

Turkeltaub PC, Norman PS, Crepea S. Treatment of ragweed hay fever with an intranasal spray containing flunisolide, a new synthetic corticosteroid. J Allergy Clin Immunol 1976; 58:597–606.

Turkeltaub PC, Norman PS, Johnson JD, Crepea S. Treatment of seasonal and perennial rhinitis with intranasal flunisolide. Allergy 1982; 37:303–311.

Welsh PW, Stricker WE, Chu CP, et al. Efficacy of beclomethasone nasal solution, flunisolide, and cromolyn in relieving symptoms of ragweed allergy. Mayo Clinic Proc 1987; 62:125–134.

ALLERGIC REACTIONS CAUSED BY EXPOSURE TO ANIMALS

JOHN L. OHMAN Jr., M.D.

NATURE AND SOURCE OF MAMMALIAN ALLERGENS

Allergy to animals (restricted to mammals for the purposes of this chapter) represents a significant proportion of the inhalant allergies (allergic rhinoconjunctivitis and asthma) seen in clinical practice. In addition, touching animals can produce topical urticaria and more chronic eczematoid skin rashes. Environmental control is a primary modality of treatment of this kind of allergy because the source of the allergen can usually be identified and theoretically eliminated. Animal allergens, along with dust mite and cockroach allergens, are the primary sources of indoor allergen exposure for a large proportion of the urban population.

AEROBIOLOGY OF MAMMALIAN ALLERGENS

Animal allergens are particularly prone to cause asthma. When airborne particles that carry mammalian allergens have been studied, a significant proportion have been found to be small (<10 micron) and capable of penetrating to the peripheral airways. In contrast to dust mite allergens, mammalian allergen particles remain airborne for hours at a time following disturbance of dust, and they can be found on wall surfaces.

The major sources of mammalian allergen are the epithelium, saliva, and urine. For the cat and dog epithelial extracts contain relevant allergen. For rodents, however, the urine represents the major source of allergen and commercially available rodent epithelial extract may not have adequate amounts of allergen. Most mammalian extracts contain serum proteins including albumin, which do not represent major allergens but may cause some IgE binding in a proportion of patients who are allergic to animals. These serum components are highly cross-reactive between species and are responsible for a decreased specificity of mammalian-derived extracts when they are used as skin test reagents.

DIAGNOSIS

Effective treatment of animal allergy requires an accurate diagnosis (Fig. 1). When exposure to animals is intermittent, a history of symptoms on exposure is usually easy to obtain. The presence of multiple allergens within a particular indoor environment sometimes makes the diagnosis less certain. When the patient is living with an animal, the chronic nature of the symptoms can make diagnosis difficult. Some objective measure of sensitization is essential, and the easiest and most accurate test is the standard allergy skin test. The diagnostic sensitivity of this test is good when adequate quantities of relevant allergens are present. Currently in the United States only cat extracts are standardized for adequate quantities of the relevant major allergen, *Fel d* I. It is hoped that dog extracts will soon be standardized for the major dog allergen, *Can f* I. Adequate skin test reagents for rodent allergy will probably not be available for several years. The radioallergosorbent test (RAST) for circulating IgE antibody in serum is generally less sensitive and does not give more information than what is obtained with the skin test.

ENVIRONMENTAL CONTROL

Once a diagnosis has been made with reasonable certainty by combining the history with skin testing and a knowledge of the environment, environmental control becomes the first-line method of treatment.

Domestic

The cat and dog represent the primary sources of mammalian allergen exposure in most domestic settings. The occasional exposure to pet rodents usually does not represent a major problem because rodents are generally confined to cages and have small surface areas. Cats and dogs tend to roam throughout the house or apartment and distribute their allergen in many different places, including cushions, rugs, or bedding where the animal lays. Such reservoirs can contain a much larger quantity of allergen than exists on the surface of the animal at a given time. This represents an important source of exposure even when the animal is not present.

Removal of the animal is the preferable treatment. Over a number of years, surveys of allergists have indicated that a significant proportion of patients (usually about 50 percent) will not remove an animal because of a strong emotional attachment or for other personal reasons. Patients often doubt the connection between their asthma or rhinitis to the animal exposure. This places a burden on the physician to explain the nature of indoor allergen exposure and how constant low-level exposure can cause significant disease. Recent studies suggest that constant exposure to low levels of allergen may result in reactive airway disease, which can persist for long periods following allergen exposure. A trial period of separation can be helpful in convincing the patient that the animal is the cause of symptoms. Conclusions should be drawn with caution, however, because animal allergen levels may take many months to decline significantly after removal of the animal. Other allergens may also be important seasonally or nonseasonally in the production of symptoms.

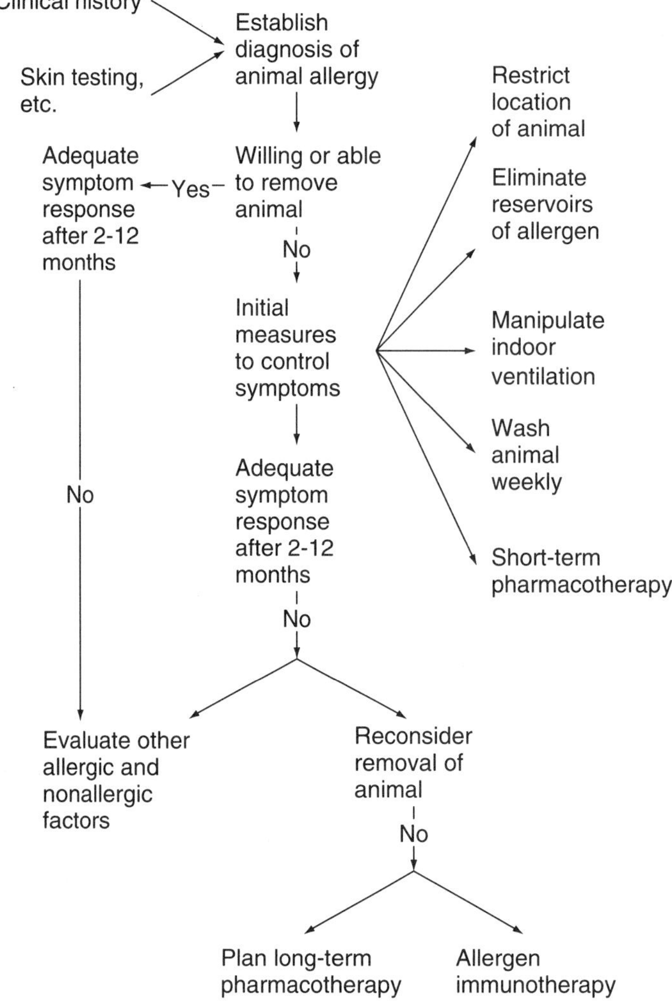

Figure 1 Algorithm for treatment of animal allergy.

Because of the strength of personal attachment to animals, it is usually wise to give the intransigent patient some time to fully consider the implications of keeping the animal. I usually wait a number of months before assuming that the animal will not be removed. During this time, the patient should be encouaraged repeatedly to reconsider the removal of the animal. If a fully informed decision is made to keep the animal then it is reasonable to proceed with treatment assuming the chronic presence of the animal.

Restriction of the animal within the environment is an alternative option when the animal cannot be removed. Elimination of bedroom exposure will greatly reduce the total allergen load. It is also important to keep the animal out of family living areas, especially where allergens can accumulate in reservoirs such as rugs and upholstered furniture.

Studies with the domestic cat suggest that washing the cat weekly will reduce the amount of allergen shed into the air. The rationale for this is based on studies that show deposition of the allergen at the base of hair follicles before it is shed into the environment, and other studies that show weekly washing of the animal results in progressive diminution in the amount of allergen that can be retrieved from the animal. Conclusive studies of the benefit of washing animals would require proof that the washing procedure significantly reduces the amount of human exposure, and these have not been done adequately. Therefore, weekly washing may be considered a reasonable measure pending conclusive demonstration of its benefit. A veterinarian should probably be consulted for advice about how to prevent excessive drying of the pelt.

Occupational

Occupational settings include laboratories and breeding facilities that house animals (frequently mice, rats, rabbits, and guinea pigs; less frequently cats, dogs, and primates,). Reduction in workday exposure requires attention to ventilation systems to ensure that at least 8 to 15 air changes per hour exist. Most exposure is in the zone of worker activity. Masks or respirators can significantly reduce exposure and symptoms. Patient compliance with the use of masks during a work shift is generally far below 100 percent. Lab coats and gloves significantly reduce topical exposure and frequent rinsing or washing of hands will prevent the deposition of allergen on the eyes when they are inadvertently rubbed. The use of ventilated hoods during procedures involving animals is often helpful. Each work setting needs to be investigated to try to determine the major source of the allergen. Unfortunately, a limited amount is known about the mechanism by which allergen becomes airborne.

PHARMACOLOGIC TREATMENT

There is no unique pharmacologic treatment for allergic reactions to animals. Pharmacologic treatment will inevitably be considered for symptoms resulting from domestic or work exposure that cannot be treated with avoidance alone.

Intermittent Exposure

Inadvertent exposure cannot be avoided in occupations such as law enforcement or social work where time must be spent in numerous domestic settings. There are many patients whose social contacts are extremely limited by the presence of animals in the homes of friends and relatives. The symptoms of asthma and rhinitis can occur rapidly with exposure and frequently become incapacitating. In some instances the symptoms of airway reactivity can persist for a number of days following the exposure. In these situations a variety of pretreatment regimens must be considered. For mild symptoms of rhinoconjunctivitis, pretreatment with an antihistamine might be considered with continued treatment during the exposure. Topical antihistamine and vasoconstrictor eye drops are sometimes helpful for allergic conjunctivitis. When asthmatic symptoms are bothersome, pretreatment with a beta-adrenergic spray and continued use as necessary during exposure may be required. The newer long-acting beta-adrenergic spray, salmeterol, might be very useful when exposure is anticipated to last a number of hours.

A history of severe asthma with exposure necessitates the consideration of a variety of other pretreatment regimens. Several inhalations of sodium cromolyn or nedocramil spray an hour before exposure can sometimes be helpful in conjunction with the use of a beta-adrenergic spray as needed. Topical corticosteroids can also be added as a pretreatment modality both nasally and by inhalation, but they must be used for at least 5 days before anticipated exposure and continued for several days following the exposure to prevent delayed symptoms. I have a number of patients whose holiday visits with relatives can only be handled in this way. Occasionally a backup supply of oral prednisone must be kept available.

Constant Exposure

Treating symptoms that are related to constant indoor exposure to an animal to which the patient is sensitized presents a different set of problems. It is often very difficult to determine exactly the role of the animal in chronic symptoms for reasons stated earlier. In addition, the use of potent and intensive treatment modalities may delay the decision to implement the most effective treatment—removing the animal. The result may be of no net benefit to the patient. There is no simple solution and the physician will frequently resort to the treatment of symptoms that are related to chronic, potentially avoidable, animal exposure. The principles of pharmacologic treatment are no different than with other forms of chronic asthma and will not be discussed further here.

IMMUNOTHERAPY

There have been a number of controlled studies of the effectiveness of immunotherapy in the treatment of cat and dog allergy; most studies show some benefit. This treatment has been shown to reduce bronchial sensitivity to inhaled allergen and also to reduce symptoms on exposure to cats and dogs. There is no evidence that the degree of effectiveness of immunotherapy in this disorder is any different than in pollen or dust mite allergy. Some have suggested that it is less effective when the exposure is constant versus intermittent as in pollen allergens. There may be some validity to this notion. However, immunotherapy in another situation where the exposure is more chronic (e.g., dust mite allergy) can be shown to be effective. The response to any kind of immunotherapy is not rapid and often a year is needed to demonstrate a beneficial response. Available studies do not provide accurate information about response rates or about how immunotherapy compares with other modalities of treatment. Based on uncontrolled clinical observation, I expect that some degree of beneficial response will occur in 50 to 70 percent of patients. Generally, immunotherapy should not be used in situations where symptoms are controllable with avoidance and/or modest doses of medication. The general indications for immunotherapy are summarized in Table 1.

With cat immunotherapy, potent extracts are available that are well standardized for the presence of the major cat allergen, *Fel d* I. Prick test concentrations of *Fel d* I that are diagnostic contain 5,000 BAU per milliliter (U.S. FDA Units) corresponding to 5 to 10 μg per milliliter of *Fel d* I. Immunotherapy is generally started with 0.1 cc of a 5 to 10 BAU per milliliter concentration with some allergists electing to start at lower doses in highly allergic patients. A variety of buildup schedules are used. Ten to 20 weekly shots are commonly used to build up to a maintenance dose of 0.2 to 0.5 cc of a 500 BAU per milliliter concentration every 2 to 4 weeks. This is the dose of allergen that is comparable to the dose that has been effective in controlled studies and to the dose of Antigen E that is effective in ragweed immunotherapy. Lower maintenance doses (down to 0.1 of a 50 BAU concentration) are sometimes required if large local or systemic

Table 1 Factors to Consider Before Starting Immunotherapy with Animal Dander Extracts

1. Presence of significant symptoms
2. Environmental control has been given reasonable effort
3. An adequate extract is available
4. Patient is not at high risk of a systemic reaction

reactions occur. I question whether benefit occurs at doses below this.

As in immunotherapy with other antigens, the degree of initial skin test reactivity is only weakly predictive, if at all, of the risk of systemic reactions. Systemic reactions occur in the following situations: (1) in unstable asthma, (2) with errors in dosage, (3) by not reducing the dose when the interval between shots is increased, and (4) by ignoring mild systemic reactions to previous shots that may have been misinterpreted by the patient or doctor. Unstable asthma with lowered pulmonary function should usually require the postponement of the shot. Further discussion of the technique or method of immunotherapy are beyond the scope of this chapter.

With other animal dander extracts that are less well standardized, the selection of dose is less precise and proceeds with certain assumptions. If a strong prick test reaction is produced with a dog epithelial extract, for example, then it can be assumed that adequate doses of allergen are present and that immunotherapy can be administered with comparable dilutions to that used with cat immunotherapy. Extracts of animal pelt should generally not be used because of the large quantity of serum components that is commonly present in these extracts and the likelihood that large amounts of irrelevant protein will be given. Even if a patient reacts to some of these serum components, the quantity of the serum allergen is out of proportion to the relevant epithelial allergen. In cat pelt extracts, for example, serum albumin concentrations frequently approach 1,000 μg per milliliter when *Fel d* I levels are in the 10 μg per ml range.

Epithelial extracts from animals in which the urine contains the major allergen (e.g., rats and mice) generally contain an unpredictable amount of relevant allergen. Some allergists assume that relevant allergen is present if prick test reactivity occurs on testing with these extracts. This is a conclusion that should be drawn with some caution because of the presence of cross reactivity of serum components between species. Immunotherapy with such rodent-derived epithelial extracts must be used with strong reservations.

As with potent pharmacologic therapy, the patient should not be led to believe that this treatment is a substitute for more effective measures such as removal of the animal.

SUGGESTED READING

Colloff MJ, Ayres J, Carswell F, et al. The control of allergens of dust mites and domestic pets: a position paper. Clin Exp Allergy 1992; 22(suppl):1–28.

Desjardins A, Benoit C, Ghezzo H, et al. Exposure to domestic animals and risk of immunologic sensitization in subjects with asthma. J Allergy Clin Immunol 1993; 91:979–986.

Ohman JL. Allergen immunotherapy: Review of efficacy and current practice. Med Clin North Am 1992; 76:977–991.

Ohman JL, Findlay SR, Leitermann KM. Immunotherapy in cat-induced asthma. Double-blind trial with evaluation of in vivo and in vitro responses. J Allergy Clin Immunol 1984; 74:230–239.

Schou C. Review: defining allergens of mammalian origin. Clin Exp Allergy 1993; 23:7–14.

CHRONIC RHINITIS CAUSED BY DUST MITE AND OTHER INDOOR ALLERGENS

THOMAS A.E. PLATTS-MILLS, M.D., Ph.D.
LISA M. WHEATLEY, M.D.

PERENNIAL ALLERGIC RHINITIS

Perennial allergic rhinitis (PAR) is caused predominantly by allergens to which the patient is exposed year round. Although some cases are related to occupational exposure, diet, or other allergens, the majority are caused by allergens inhaled in the patient's own home. Because symptoms are perennial, the inciting factors are generally not obvious and it is almost always necessary to establish that the condition is allergic. The major differential diagnoses include vasomotor rhinitis, nonallergic rhinitis with eosinophilia (NARES), and chronic rhinosinusitis with or without polyps. The symptoms of PAR can be attributed to the acute effects of mast cell mediator release as a result of IgE cross-linking (i.e., histamine), prolonged responses caused by mediators such as leukotrienes, and the delayed effect of a cellular influx that takes 6 to 24 hours. However, with daily indoor exposure these phases begin to overlap, superimposing histamine release on cellular or leukotriene effects, thus making acute responses to exposure less clear-cut. Consequently, many patients are not aware of the agents that cause their rhinitis. Once the contribution of immediate hypersensitivity to the patient symptoms is confirmed, treatment can be divided into (1) pharmacologic management, (2) avoidance of allergens

Supported by NIH Grants R37-AI-20565 and 1UO1-AI-34607.

to which the patient is specifically sensitive, and (3) immunotherapy.

Clinical Features

Patients with chronic allergic rhinitis present with a wide range of symptoms, including sneezing; watery or mucoid rhinorrhea; pruritus of the nose, palate or ears; as well as a variety of symptoms related to nasal obstruction. In addition, patients may report irritation, soreness, and pruritus of the eyes (conjunctivitis); pressure or pain in the nose, maxillary, or frontal areas; and/or systemic symptoms of fatigue, weakness, or malaise. Chronic rubbing of the nose may occur as well as dark circles under the eyes, especially in children. Nasal obstruction may give rise to chronic mouth breathing, thus bypassing the normal physiologic functions of the nose—humidification and warming and filtering the inhaled air. It is tempting to believe that mouth breathing leads to increased inhalation of allergen particles into the lung with a consequent increased risk of asthma; however, this has not been proved.

Distinction from Seasonal Rhinitis

Presumably the pathologic changes produced by exposure to pollen grains, mite feces, *Alternaria* spores, or cat dander should be very similar. However, there are some important clinical differences, with the most striking being that conjunctivitis is much more of a problem with outdoor exposure. It is unusual for conjunctivitis related to dust mites or cockroach or animal dander to require medical treatment, whereas it is a prominent symptom of many patients with pollen allergy. In addition, pruritus of the back of the throat, or palate, and itching in the ears are more commonly reported by patients with seasonal hay fever. The occurrence of conjunctivitis as part of hay fever but not PAR probably reflects the fact that particles the size of pollen grains (i.e., ~15 to 30 μm) would impact on the eye when blown by the wind, but not in still air indoors. It is reassuring to remember that symptoms related to pollen or fungal exposure outdoors are restricted to the relevant season, requiring no investigation for systemic disease or a local cause such as tumor or polyposis. In contrast, a more extensive differential diagnosis should always be considered in patients with perennial rhinitis.

Pathology

Allergen-carrying particles range from 2 to 30 μm in diameter; when inhaled through the nose the majority will impact on the nasal mucosa. The main proteins causing allergic reactions range from 5,000 to 60,000 kd molecular weight, are freely water soluble, and are released rapidly from the particles. Thus, although particles are cleared from the nose by ciliary action within 10 to 20 minutes, most of the protein content of the particles will already have been released within this time. On initial exposure it is assumed that the proteins interact with MHC Class II^+ dendritic cells and are transported with these cells to the local lymphoid tissue. Sensitization of a previously unexposed individual must take months or even years because it generally takes that long for individuals to develop symptoms when they are exposed to a new inhalant allergen such as rats (in an animal house) or guinea pigs (at home). The immune response is complex and includes IgE antibodies, IgG antibodies, and CD4 positive T cells (i.e., T helper cells).

Once a patient has made an IgE-antibody response, subsequent exposure can and does produce rapid symptoms. Thus, cat-allergic patients commonly report sneezing within minutes of exposure to a cat and dust mite–allergic patients will sneeze when they use a vacuum cleaner with an inadequate filtration system. These symptoms occur because of rapid release of histamine from mast cells in the epithelium or submucosa and/or from basophils, which migrate into the nose of allergic patients. However, the symptoms of perennial rhinitis are not explained by histamine alone. First, symptoms continue for hours or even days after complete cessation of exposure when there would be no further histamine release. Second, there are many other mediators present in the nose (e.g., leukotrienes, prostaglandins, tryptase, and cytokines). Third, the inflammation in the nose is characterized by the presence of eosinophils and/or eosinophil-derived proteins. (Previously, it was suggested that eosinophil recruitment might be predominantly the result of T-cell activation; however, it is now clear that mast cells and basophils are also important sources of several different cytokines. Thus, either the T cells [of T_H2 or T_H0 type] or mast cells could be the major source of the cytokines that bring eosinophils into the nose.)

Eosinophil production in the bone marrow is thought to be controlled by interleukin-5 (IL-5), IL-3, and granulocyte-macrophage colony–stimulating factor GM-CSF). IL-5 may be most important for prolonged eosinophil survival in the local tissue. On the other hand, selective recruitment of eosinophils via vascular cell adhesion molecules (VCAM) is influenced by many different cytokines, including IL-1, IL-4, IL-5, and (RANTES). The important conclusion for treatment is that pharmacologic management should be designed both to block the effects of histamine and to inhibit the effects of leukotrienes or cytokines. This latter effect is broadly and very loosely described as *anti-inflammatory.* The other important conclusion is that many, if not most, symptoms are delayed in time course, so that the patients are not sure what exposure produced the inflammation.

Management of Chronic Rhinitis

Chronic nasal symptoms of obstruction, excess secretions, sneezing, or pressure are extremely common; estimates range as high as 30 million cases in the United States. Many of these patients can be managed with over-the-counter antihistamines or antihistamine-decongestant mixtures. If these are effective, the patients may neither require nor seek further evaluation.

Routine health maintenance measures should be encouraged because oral decongestants can elevate blood pressure, which should therefore be monitored at least annually. Medical management thus starts with patients who have failed over-the-counter medicines and seek physician advice.

The differential diagnosis of perennial nasal symptoms can be divided into four major groups: (1) chronic rhinitis not caused by inhalant allergens, including vasomotor rhinitis and NARES; (2) sinusitis with or without nasal polyps; (3) anatomic abnormalities in the nose, or local pathology such as tumors; (4) rhinitis as part of systemic disease or as a complication of treatment of other diseases. It is simplest to think about these sequentially as part of management because the necessary level of investigation is dictated by the severity of symptoms and the response to treatment.

STAGE I: PERSISTENT SYMPTOMS

Evaluation by a Primary Care Physician or an Asthma and Allergic Disease Specialist

The patient history should document any variations in symptoms related to specific exposures, (e.g., work, animals, different houses, vacations, activities, or seasons). It is important to explain to the patient at an early stage that chronic symptoms can be caused by persistent exposure without clear exacerbation on exposure. The history should also cover general health issues and medications. Physical examination should include the ears, throat, and neck, as well as the nose. Anterior rhinoscopy before and after topical decongestant will identify swollen turbinates, excess mucus, erosion, and obvious polyps. The throat should be examined for large tonsils, "cobblestoning" of the posterior pharynx, ulceration, and thrush. Even if there is no history of wheezing or shortage of breath, it is useful to examine the chest and document a peak expiratory flow rate. Evidence of any breathing difficulty demands full examination of the chest, assessment of lung function (i.e., FEV_1 and FVC) and, in cases with abnormality, consideration of a chest radiograph. An IgE level is useful because a low level (i.e., 30 IU/ml) suggests that the patient's symptoms are not related to atopy.

Treatment

Antihistamines

Initial treatment consists of administration of antihistamines with or without decongestants. Patients who have problems with sedative effects of over-the-counter antihistamines will require the more expensive nonsedating antihistamines (loratadine 10 mg daily or terfenadine 60 mg twice a day). Astemizole may also be helpful in some cases, but it can cause weight gain and will suppress skin tests for up to 6 weeks, potentially hampering further investigation.

Anti-inflammatory

If response to antihistamines and/or decongestants is unsatisfactory, nasal treatment with steroids or cromolyn should be initiated. At this stage an allergy history is helpful. In selected cases examination of nasal eosinophils and serum IgE will help distinguish NARES and vasomotor rhinitis. Nasal steroids are supplied as aqueous sprays or pressurized aerosols, and patients will generally find one of these forms acceptable (Table 1). In cases in which secretions are watery and pruritus, sneezing, and eosinophils are not prominent, ipratropium bromide (Atrovent), a vasomotor treatment, can be tried. It can be used with or as a replacement for oral antihistamines. If response is still incomplete, the patient should be further evaluated. Also, if a patient continues to require regular nasal treatment to maintain control of symptoms, further evaluation of an allergic cause is indicated.

STAGE II: SEVERE SYMPTOMS

Local Treatment and Oral Treatment Unsuccessful – Referral to Specialist for Allergy Evaluation

In addition to the measures included in stage I, investigation should include skin testing with a range of common inhalant allergens, including dust mite, cat, dog, and cockroach, as well as common fungi (generally 8 to 16 fungi are tested) and the locally important pollens.

Blood tests should include a complete blood count (CBC) with differential cell count. If there is any question about the general health of the patient, a sedimentation rate, antinuclear antibodies (ANA), screening chemistries, and urinalysis should be performed to evaluate connective tissue and or metabolic disease. Thyroid function tests should be included if the history is suggestive.

In selected cases, particularly when there have been multiple courses of antibiotics or the symptoms suggest sinusitis, then computerized tomography (CT) of the sinuses should be conducted. In most centers it is possible to obtain a limited section coronal CT scan, which gives substantially more information than a sinus series without excessive cost or radiation. It is not clear that there are any indications for plain film sinus radiographs today. Further, if nasal polyps are seen on anterior rhinoscopy or rhinopharyngoscopy then CT is also appropriate. In children, the presence of polyps is an indication for a sweat test to rule out cystic fibrosis. Currently the indications for fiberoptic rhinopharyngoscopy are not well defined. Our view is that poorly responsive chronic rhinitis, unilateral bleeding or persistent bleeding, or unilateral obstruction should be investigated early. However, some centers recommend rhinopharyngoscopy in all cases not responsive to simple therapy.

Table 1 Treatment of Allergic Rhinitis

Over-the-counter treatments
Persistent nasal symptoms in an otherwise healthy patient
1. Sneezing, pruritus, rhinorrhea-oral antihistamines (see Table 2); adjust dosage or add oral decongestants
2. Predominant blockage—oral decongestants with antihistamine

Stage I
Persistent symptoms (>4 months)
1. Allergy assessment, history with or without skin testing, initiate allergen-avoidance measures
2. Topical nasal cromolyn or topical steroids (see Table 3), adjust dosage
3. Consider sinus computerized tomography (CT)
4. Consider oral antihistamines, using nonsedating antihistamines with or without oral decongestants

Stage II
Severe symptoms or local treatment inadequate or unacceptable
1. Full allergy history and skin testing obligatory—serum IgE and possible RAST testing
2. Explain allergen avoidance measures, outline implementation, visit home or workplace if possible
3. Continue local treatment, consistent use of increased topical steroid and cromolyn therapy
4. Immunotherapy in appropriate cases

Symptoms unrelenting
1. Reconsider diagnosis (e.g., chronic nasal infection, sinus infection, polyps, anatomic abnormalities, IgG or IgA deficiency, granulomatous disease, occupational allergy)
2. Consider emotional reasons for failure to recognize or accept treatment
3. Immunotherapy in appropriate cases
4. Sinus CT; consider surgery

Treatment for Suspected Allergic Rhinitis

Treatment for suspected allergic rhinitis is outlined below:

1. Continued treatment with optimal dose and preparation of local steroid with or without cromolyn *and* optimal dose of oral antihistamine and/or decongestants.
2. Detailed education and advice about avoidance of specific indoor allergens, based on the results of skin tests.
3. Short course of oral steroids in cases where symptoms remain severe.
4. Immunotherapy should be considered in cases where skin testing or radioallergosorbent test (RAST) indicates specific sensitivity, relevant exposure is likely, medical therapy is not effective, and the patient is able to comply both with regular injections and the measures necessary to ensure safety.

STAGE III: SYMPTOMS UNCONTROLLED

In patients who fail to respond to usual doses of pharmacologic therapy and appropriate allergen specific treatment, the diagnosis should be reconsidered. Chronic sinusitis should be excluded by sinus CT, and polyps/tumor or granulomatous disease should be excluded by rhinopharyngoscopy. Underlying immune deficiency should be evaluated through laboratory studies of serum IgG, IgA, and IgE, and CBC and differential. The possibility of unusual allergen exposure should be reconsidered (e.g., occupational exposure, a pet that has been ignored, extensive fungal contamination of the house). Diet should be discussed and, in selected cases, food skin testing, dietary restriction, or double blind oral challenges may be helpful.

Although emotional factors are difficult to evaluate, they should be considered in unremitting cases, for these may make the patient unwilling to recognize response to treatment, or to admit to an exacerbating factor (such as a pet).

In addition, substance abuse, particularly with cocaine, should be considered. However, persistent use of local decongestants (such as Afrin or Dristan), which can cause mucosal hypertrophy and/or side effects of antihypertensive drugs (e.g., propranalol) are a more common problem. Nasal congestion or increased secretion often complicates pregnancy and occasionally occurs with oral contraceptives. Hypothyroidism can also cause nasal congestion.

Further investigation may require nasal and or maxillary cultures for bacteria or fungi. In difficult cases it may be helpful to define nasal eosinophilia. Although NARES is now well recognized, in all cases it should carefully be considered whether there is a foreign antigen responsible for the nasal and peripheral blood eosinophilia. It is likely that further causes of chronic rhinitis with eosinophils will be identified. Some patients with *Trichophyton* colonization of their nails and immediate hypersensitivity present with chronic nasal symptoms; the majority of these patients have sinusitis.

Treatment

A clearly aggressive search for causation, including inhalants, diet, air pollution, and colonization should provide clues to appropriate specific management, including immunotherapy. In addition, all cases should receive aggressive local and oral treatment. Surgery for sinusitis or even relatively minor structural abnormalities in the nasal passages may also be helpful. Finally, short courses of oral steroids plus appropriate treatment for infection are indicated.

DETAILS OF MANAGEMENT

Allergen Avoidance

Effective allergen avoidance largely depends on accurate diagnoses. A careful history often suggests that the relevant allergens are domestic in origin. Exposure history requires careful questioning about the home, probing particularly about pets, carpeting, infestations, and dampness, which would predispose to molds and mites. There are good diagnostic skin test extracts for most of the allergens that contribute to the larger category of "house dust." This is certainly true for cat dander and house dust mites, although there is still some doubt about fungal allergen extracts. It is important to recognize that arthropods such as moths, beetles, and cockroaches also can contribute to house dust, and that patients are often skin-test positive to several allergens in the house. It is important not to give the impression that removing one item will indicate whether it is relevant or that increased vacuum cleaning for a few weeks will indicate whether mites are involved. If there are multiple allergens in the house, removal of one, even if it is important, may not give clear information because allergens that remain may be sufficient to perpetuate symptoms. The best approach is to consider the overall problem and, if necessary, visit the home. A progressive policy to reduce allergen exposure should then be outlined.

Domestic Animals

Most highly atopic patients who live with a cat, dog, guinea pig, mouse, or rabbit in the house will become allergic. Animals that live outside are much less of a problem. Any patient who has perennial rhinitis and positive results on immediate skin tests should be strongly urged to remove the relevant animal. It must be stressed that because it usually takes 6 weeks or more to remove cat or dog dander from a house, a short-term trial of removing the animal is useless. For cat allergen, it may be possible to reduce airborne levels by both removing reservoirs in the house (i.e., carpets, sofas) and using room air cleaners.

Dust Mites

Dust mites grow best at 65° to 80° F and with a relative humidity higher than 60 percent. They live on human skin scales or fungi on the skin scales, but they can eat a variety of different organic materials. The major allergens produced by dust mites accumulate and become airborne in the form of fecal particles.

Even before the discovery of the importance of dust mites by Spieksma and Voorhorst in 1964, it was common practice to advise patients about methods of reducing house dust. These included regular vacuum cleaning of the mattress, carpets, and curtains in the bedroom, together with regular washing of bedclothes. Some patients benefit from such practices but more often the results are poor. Furthermore, studies using measurements of dust mite allergen in dust suggest that this kind of protocol (even when followed) produces only modest reductions in allergen levels. Conversely, dust mite allergen levels in sanatoria or hospitals are often very low—less than 2 percent of the levels in houses—and dust mite allergic patients generally improve when they are kept away from their own home. The implication is that dust mite avoidance can work but requires fairly aggressive changes in a house.

Reduction of mite allergens can be achieved by removing the sites in which mites live (e.g., carpets in living rooms and bedrooms, feather pillows, upholstered furniture, nonwashable comforters, nonwashable clothes, soft toys); denaturing the allergen and killing the mites by washing items in hot water (130° F); and removing mite feces and other debris by regular vacuum cleaning or damp wiping of surfaces. There currently is no completely satisfactory acaricide. Acarosan is a moist powder containing the potent acaricide benzyl benzoate, which must be applied for at least 12 hours, and if applied aggressively, can be very effective; however, it, like all other acaricides, has difficulty penetrating carpets or sofas.

Our present policy is to recommend a complete change in the patient's bedroom—replace carpets with linoleum or wood, wash all bedding regularly in hot water (weekly or every 10 days), cover the mattress and pillows with an impervious or vapor-permeable cover, remove all soft toys and upholstered furniture, and keep clutter to a minimum. The rest of the house should be vacuumed regularly with a machine that has an effective filtration system; double thickness bags are generally the most effective. If patients do cleaning work, they should wear a mask. Soft furniture and curtains also should be vacuumed regularly. Polished floors are ideal, and in some climates carpets can be beaten in the sun. Mite- or fungus-allergic patients should avoid living in basements. For carpets and sofas that cannot be removed, it can be helpful to control humidity by using air conditioning in the summer and opening windows during a dry winter.

Fungi

Although fungi undoubtedly can cause allergic symptoms, it is difficult to assess their general importance as a cause of perennial rhinitis. Identifying viable fungal spores in a house with a culture plate or Burkhart spore trap is possible, but measuring allergen levels is not. It has been pointed out that the number of varieties of fungi is so great that it is difficult to exclude fungal allergy. Nonetheless, the quantities of fungal allergens in a house almost certainly can be reduced by some simple measures. Removal of house plants and other sources of humidity from all (or most) rooms in the house is essential. Increasing ventilation rates by opening windows is helpful. Most of the fungi implicated in allergy are fungi imperfecti, which appear as black or greenish stains. Obvious sites of fungal growth such as shower curtains, bathroom windows, damp walls, and areas with wood rot must be carefully cleaned or removed. Many of the measures taken to reduce the accumulation of dust mite allergens will also reduce both the production and accumulation of fungal allergens because both mites and fungi require humid conditions. However, many fungi flourish in colder conditions than mites; and fungal spores can survive prolonged periods of dryness, which would kill mites. Thus, fungi become established on basement walls, the tiles of a bathroom, and other surfaces that are not a suitable site for dust mite growth.

Cockroaches

Most patients who have problems with cockroaches in their home are already trying to eradicate them. They should be encouraged to persevere or to relocate themselves, and to use more effective strategies such as bait rather than traps.

Control of Airborne Allergens

Normal houses have dust particles in the air, but most are less than 5 μm in diameter. The allergens that we know most about are carried on large particles such as pollen grains (approximately 20 μm in diameter) and mite fecal particles (10 to 40 μm in diameter). In addition, many important fungal spores are large. In still air, particles of this size fall within 10 to 15 minutes. For dust mite allergens, the quantity of allergen that becomes airborne is a tiny fraction of the total amount present in carpets or bedding and is detectable only during domestic activity. Because of this, the major exposure to allergens probably occurs during activity; thus face masks, a good vacuum cleaner, and/or employing someone else to do the housework are useful avoidance techniques.

Filtering the air entering a house through an air handling unit may be helpful in preventing exposure to seasonal pollen or fungal allergens, but it is largely irrelevant for allergens produced within the house. Obviously, if an allergen falls within 10 to 15 minutes, filtering the inside air will have little effect on exposure to dust mite feces, for example. However, there is good evidence that cat allergen is airborne in the form of small particles (i.e., <2 μm in diameter), which do not fall rapidly. A high efficiency particulate air filter (HEPA) in the room can help some patients. However, the first approach with all house dust allergens is to reduce the sources and the reservoirs of dust in the house and thus reduce the amount that becomes airborne during domestic activity.

Antihistamines

In recent years many different second generation H_1 antagonists have been developed which produce dramatically less central nervous system (CNS) sedation. Three of these nonsedating antihistamines have been marketed for oral use in the United States – terfenadine, astemizole, and loratadine – and levocabastine a fourth, is available as eye drops. These antihistamines have little or no sedative effect and no anticholinergic effect. This difference is thought to result from the fact that they are not lipophilic and thus do not cross the blood-brain barrier easily. However, some patients still report quite marked alterations of mood. Both terfenadine and loratadine are available in combination with a decongestant (thus, Seldane and Seldane D; Claritin and Claritin D).

The new antihistamines are metabolized by a P_{450} enzyme in the liver that also acts on several other drugs, most notably erythromycin and ketoconazole. Thus taking erythromycin at the same time as a second-generation antihistamine will cause increased blood levels of the antihistamines terfenadine, loratadine, and astemizole. However, there is a specific problem with terfenadine because high blood levels can cause an elongation of the QTc interval demonstrable on electrocardiogram. Occasionally, this has resulted in a cardiac arrhythmia, usually torsades des pointes. A similar but smaller effect can occur with astemizole (Hismanal); no QTc effect has been seen with loratadine (Claritin).

The sedative effects of traditional antihistamines generally decrease with continued regular use. In general, antihistamines should be taken as soon as symptoms occur or on a regular basis. Individual patients respond differently to different antihistamines, and it is always worth trying several different types of both traditional and nonsedating antihistamines. Thus, it is neither unreasonable nor unusual to have to try Benadryl, Tavist, Dimetap, Seldane, and Claritin in difficult cases. Cyproheptadine (Periactin) and hydroxyzine (Atarax) are more commonly used for urticaria, but may be useful for occasional cases of rhinitis. Promethazine (Phenergan), because of its profound sedative and anticholinergic effects, is more widely used as an antitussive or as a sedative. The major side effect of traditional antihistamines is sedation, but many patients also complain of minor changes in mood or more marked psychotropic effects. These effects are very idiosyncratic and can be seen with all antihistamines. In addition, antihistamines occasionally give rise to insomnia, nervousness, tremors, or gastrointestinal disturbances. They should be used with caution in patients with a history of epilepsy, narrow angle glaucoma, stenosing peptic ulcer, or symptomatic prostatic hypertrophy (see Table 2).

Decongestants

Decongestants, which are alpha-adrenergic agonists, are available as local or oral formulations. As oral preparations, they are used both alone (e.g., Sudafed)

Table 2 Drugs with H_1 Receptor Activity

Class and Examples	*Trade Names**	*Usual Adult Dosage*	*CNS Sedation*	*Antihistaminic Activity*	*Anticholinergic Activity*	*Comments*
Ethanolamines						
Diphenhydramine	Benadryl	25-50 mg q6h	Marked	Moderate	Marked	Diphenhydramine also used in motion sickness; has local anesthetic effect
Clemastine	Tavist	1.34-2.68 mg b.i.d., t.i.d.				
Alkylamines						
Chlorpheniramine	Chlor-Trimeton	4 mg q4-6h	Mild	Marked	Moderate	Possibly some CNS stimulation; classic antihistamines to date
Brompheniramine	Dimetane	4 mg q4-6h				
Piperidines						
Azatadine (Rx)	Optimine	1-2 mg q12h	Mild to moderate	Moderate	Moderate	Cyproheptadine is a serotonin antagonist and used also in cold urticaria
Cyproheptadine (Rx)	Periactin	4 mg q6-8h				
Phenothiazines						
Promethazine (Rx)	Phenergan	12.5-50 mg q4-6h 2.5 mg q6h	Marked	Marked	Marked	Usually used for motion sickness, antiemetic, antitussive; promethazine has antiserotonin activity
Piperazines	Atarax	10-50 mg q6h	Mild	Moderate	Mild	Hydroxyzine also used as sedative and tranquilizer; antiemetic
Hydroxyzine (Rx)	Vistaril	50 mg q4-6h				
Second generation						
Terfenadine (Rx)	Seldane	60 mg b.i.d.§	Essentially none‡	Moderate to marked	None to very little	Not lipophilic; do not readily cross blood-brain barrier; longer duration; greater affinity to H_1 receptor
Astemizole (Rx)	Hismanal	10 mg q.d.§				
Loratadine (Rx)	Claritin	10 mg q.d.				
Cetirizine†						

CNS, Central nervous system; *Rx,* prescription required.
*Many of these drugs are available in sustained-action, delayed-release forms and in combination with decongestants.
†Not available in the United States.
‡CNS sedation is dose dependent.
§Higher dosage or combination with erythromycin may be associated with prolonged QTc interval on electrocardiogram and cardiac arrhythmias.

and in combination with antihistamines (e.g., Actifed). In general, antihistamines are not used locally with the exception of 4-way nasal spray, which contains pyrilamine. Furthermore, several new antihistamines (e.g., levocabastine) are in clinical trials as local preparations for the nose. Interestingly, the recent trials with local use of antihistamines in the nose and eyes have not confirmed the older (incorrect) view that local antihistamines were a potent cause of contact sensitization.

Topical decongestants can produce rebound vasodilation and lead to marked soreness of the nose with unremitting nasal congestion and nasal mucosal hypertrophy, often referred to as *rhinitis medicamentosa.* For this reason they are not useful in long-term management. However, short-term use of oxymetazoline sprays can be very helpful in relieving nasal obstruction. The general recommendation is never to use these sprays for more than 3 to 4 days at a time.

Local Nasal Steroids

Local nasal steroids are designed to be rapidly metabolized and thus to have minimal systemic side effects. There are local steroid preparations (e.g., Dexamethasone, Pred forte drops) that have systemic effects; however, the main preparations have minimal side effects (see Table 3). The activity of the various locally active steroids is not significantly different. Therefore the major distinctions relate to the solvents, methods of delivery, and rates of metabolism.

Currently beclomethasone, triamcinolone acetonide, and budesonide are available as pressurized nasal inhalers. The pressurized inhalers vary in the propellants, but in each case, exit velocity is very rapid so that sniffing at the time of use will have little effect on the pattern of deposition. In our experience all nasal steroids in pressurized inhalers can cause nasal irritation, soreness, and bleeding; however, this appears to be less of a problem with triamcinolone (Nasacort). The irritation can be decreased by pretreating the nose with saline. Steroids can also be delivered as a droplet spray using a pump (e.g., flunisolide [Nasalide]); beclomethasone [Beconase AQ, Vancenase AQ]. Although the preparations are different (flunisolide contains more propylene glycol and polyethelene glycol, which may explain the increased incidence of stinging), they have

Table 3 Inhaled Nasal Anti-Inflammatory Drugs

		Dose per Spray	*Initial Dose (in Sprays per Nostril)*	*Doses per Cannister*	*Irritant Effects*
Local steroids with minimal systemic effects					
Beclomethasone Diproprionate					
Beconase Vancenase	Pressurized	42 μg	>12 yr, 1 b.i.d. to q.i.d. 6-12 yr, 1 t.i.d.	200	+ +
Beconase AQ Vancenase AQ	Aqueous	42 μg	≥6 yr, 1-2 b.i.d.	200	+
Flunisolide					
Nasalide	Aqueous	25 μg	>6 yr, 2 b.i.d.	125	Stings
Triamcinolone acetonide					
Nasacort*	Pressurized	55 μg	2 q.d.	100	+
Fluticasone					
Flonase*	Aqueous	50 μg	1-2 q.d.	120	+
Budesonide					
Rhinocort	Pressurized	32 μg	≥6 yr, 2 b.i.d. or 4 q.d.	200	+
Cromolyn and nedocromil					
Nasalcrom Tilade†	Aqueous	5.2 mg	≥6 yr, 1 t.i.d. or q.i.d.	200	−
Steroids with systemic effect‡					
Dexamethasone					
Decadron Turbinaire	Pressurized	84 μg	>12 yr, 2 b.i.d. or t.i.d. 6-12 yr, 2 b.i.d.	170	+ +

*Not approved for use in children <12 years of age.
†The nasal form of Nedocromil is not yet available in the United States.
‡Dexamethasone and Prednisone are both available as ophthalmic solutions, which can be used for short-term treatment of severe nasal polyposis.

common properties. The sprays are designed to deliver droplets of approximately 8 microns diameter, which will impact on the nose; the velocity of the spray is such that it is better to give a slight sniff in when inhaling. The liquid has a tendency to run across the floor of the nasal passages and down the throat, thus reducing its activity. This latter problem can be helped by instructing the patient to turn their head upside down for about a minute after inhaling, which is most easily accomplished by lying on a bed and tipping the head over the edge. Finally, the liquid preparations have the advantage that they can be mixed with cromolyn (see below).

The individual steroids are labeled with specific dosage schedules (e.g., Beconase: 2 to 4 times a day; Nasacort: every other day). However, it is not clear that these recommended dosages are based on any pharmacologic differences and the ciliated nature of the nasal epithelium precludes development of a delayed-release preparation. Our experience is that any of the nasal steroids can be used daily or twice a day according to preference and side effects. The major side effects are soreness, crusting, and/or bleeding in the nose. In some cases bleeding can be reduced by less frequent use, by applying saline regularly, or by changing to an aqueous form or to cromolyn. Persistent bleeding is an indication for rhinopharyngoscopy. Erosions in the anterior vestibule can be helped by local application of petroleum jelly or 2.5 percent hydrocortisone ointment.

Many physicians have the impression that "local steroids" are metabolized in the mucosa and are thus only active locally. However, their key property is more likely to be first-pass metabolism in the liver, which dramatically decreases their systemic effects. However, in sufficient dose (i.e., ≥800 μg per day), these steroids can produce systemic effects. Current information about the relative activity of the breakdown products of local steroids is not very extensive. Thus, although experience has shown that local steroids are clearly very safe and patients can be reassured about their use, it should not be assumed that they cannot have side effects. Certainly patients on inhaled steroids, as well as nasal steroids, can easily exceed the doses that have been associated with systemic effects.

Steroids actually start acting within hours and many patients observe effects within a day. However, resolution of inflammation and therefore maximum effects may take a week or more and it is important to persuade patients to allow at least 2 weeks' trial for each new preparation. Our policy is to try patients with one of the newer pressurized inhalers first and if that does not produce a good result, to change to one of the liquid forms. In each case we start with two puffs to each nostril twice a day reducing to once daily if they achieve a good response.

Steroid nasal drops are the medical treatment of choice for nasal polyps whether or not they are associated with allergy. As with all nasal applications, the key problem with drops is their distribution. It is not possible to apply nasal drops by tilting the head backward when the patient is standing or sitting upright. To apply drops to the whole nose, patients should lie supine with their head completely upside down over the edge of a bed and stay in this position for at least 1 minute. As with all potent steroids applied topically, nasal drops may be effective on an alternate-day or even twice-weekly basis. Drops have less tendency to cause a sore nose, but have disadvantages because they are slightly less readily accepted than nasal sprays, and the dexamethasone or betamethasone is absorbed and can have systemic side effects.

Disodium Cromoglycate or Cromolyn Sodium

Disodium cromoglycate has been marketed as a 4 percent solution in nonpressurized spray form (Nasalcrom), which is effective but requires administration up to four to six times a day. This spray appears to be useful in hay fever, but in cases of perennial rhinitis the need for frequent application is a problem. Although patients tolerate frequently repeated sprays for the hay fever season, they are often unwilling to persist for the whole year. The dose of disodium cromoglycate spray is approximately 5.2 mg, and a higher concentration may well be more effective.

Cromolyn sodium may also be effective nasally in combination with local steroids. Nasalcrom can be directly mixed in equal volumes with Nasalide or Beconase AQ or Vancenase AQ. In addition, cromolyn as capsules can be added to the liquid steroids, either as five capsules of 20 mg or one 100 mg Gastrocrome capsule. Some patients respond very well to the mixture, which is apparently less irritating and is effective.

The mechanism of action of disodium cromoglycate has been widely discussed. It appears to have a definite mast cell–stabilizing effect that can reduce allergen-induced histamine release. However, there are good reasons for believing that it may have a more general effect in stabilizing membranes to reduce mediator release from macrophages, neutrophils, or both. The most important feature of the drug is the low incidence of local side effects and very rare systemic side effects.

Atropine and Ipratropium Bromide

Atropine and atropine-like drugs can dry mucosal surfaces but systemic use is not justified or effective for rhinitis. The atropine-like drug, ipratropium bromide, is available as a bronchodilator (Atrovent). Atrovent for lung use can be modified to be used in the nose by using the nasal nozzle from some nasal steroids. Ipratropium has been available for nasal use in Europe for some years and it is expected to be released in the United States for nasal use shortly. Ipratropium bromide may have a special role in cases of vasomotor rhinitis and may also be useful as an adjunct to nasal steroids.

Immunotherapy

Immunotherapy, or desensitization treatment, should be considered when the patient is definitely sensitive to a well-defined allergen, when there is good reason to believe that exposure to that allergen is responsible for symptoms, and when avoidance measures and pharmacologic treatment have not produced sufficient improvement. In addition, there are patients whose jobs require mental alertness and in whom antihistamines, cromolyn, or local steroid therapy are not appropriate or effective or cause unacceptable side effects.

House dust extracts were first used for desensitization in 1920 and appeared to be effective for both asthma and perennial rhinitis. The major constituents of house dust are now well recognized, and standardized extracts of both mite and cat allergens are available. In addition, it has been established that mite and cat extracts can be effective in immunotherapy for chronic rhinitis. In using aqueous mite extracts, the approach to desensitization is the same as that for pollen allergens. The extracts can be very potent, and fatal anaphylaxis has occurred with mite extracts. There is no justification for carrying out immunotherapy outside a clinic or office capable of resuscitation measures. Our experience with desensitization for allergic rhinitis has been similar to that for hay fever—about 80 percent of patients experience significant improvement in 1 to 2 years.

SUGGESTED READING

Barker LA. Histamine and antihistamines. In: Brody TM, Larner J, Minneman KP, Neu HC, eds. Human pharmacology: molecular to clinical, 2nd ed. St. Louis: Mosby, 1994; 787–800.

Platts-Mills TAE. Allergens. In: Frank MM, Austen KF, Claman HN, Unanue ER, eds. Samter's immunologic diseases, 5th ed. Vol 2. Boston: Little, Brown, 1994; 1231–1256.

Simons FER. New medications for rhinitis. In: Busse WW, Holgate ST, eds. Asthma and rhinitis. Cambridge, MA: Blackwell Scientific Publications, 1995; 1325–1336.

Van Cauwenberge PB, Ingels KJAO. Rhinitis: the spectrum of the disease. In: Busse WW, Holgate ST, eds. Asthma and rhinitis. Cambridge, MA: Blackwell Scientific Publications, 1995; 6–12.

PERENNIAL NONALLERGIC RHINITIS

VALERIE J. LUND, M.S., F.R.C.S., F.R.C.S.Ed.

Rhinitis in its broadest sense may be defined as inflammation of the lining of the nose, characterised by one or more of the following symptoms: nasal congestion, rhinorrhea, sneezing, itching, and disturbance of the sense of smell. The relative importance of each symptom depends upon the cause of the inflammation. However, the nose should not be considered in isolation and from a clinical perspective, "rhinosinusitis" better indicates the areas affected. Indeed, the entire respiratory tract should be regarded as a single organ and many forms of rhinitis are paralleled by lower respiratory tract diseases.

A classification of rhinitis is shown in Table 1, which also includes a number of conditions that must be considered in the differential diagnosis and that may coexist or contribute to the inflammation. It has been suggested that the term nonallergic rhinitis should be reserved for inflammation of the nasal mucosa that is unrelated to allergy, infection, structural lesions, or other systemic disease; nonallergic rhinitis is variously described as idiopathic, hyper-reactivity, intrinsic, or vasomotor rhinitis. This latter term is the least satisfactory because it implies that the cause is known. Since this is not the case, idiopathic is preferred, encompassing the provocation of watery rhinorrhea, nasal congestion, and sneezing in response to irritants such as tobacco smoke, strong smells, and changes in environmental temperature and humidity, all manifestations of an exaggerated defense response. Cold air–induced rhinitis may occur because of the release of mast cell mediators involving a non–IgE-dependent mechanism. Neurogenic mechanisms may be involved such as the watery rhinorrhea in response to temperature change, eating spicy foods (gustatory rhinorrhea), or the effect of emotion and stress. It should also be remembered that a variety of foods, alcohol, and drugs may produce hypersensitivity (e.g., aspirin), as well as specific allergic reactions. A subgroup, nonallergic rhinitis with eosinophilia syndrome (NARES), is characterised by the symptoms of rhinitis in the presence of nasal eosinophilia but in the absence of positive skin prick tests and raised IgE levels.

The diagnosis of perennial nonallergic rhinitis relies heavily upon a detailed history and a general ear, nose, and throat (ENT) examination, including, whenever possible, endoscopy of the nose. A considerable range of other investigations is available, only a small number of which are routinely employed (Table 2), but they may be applicable to individual cases. The most important thing to consider in the differential diagnosis is the possibility of rarer and more serious conditions such as malignancy and thereby eliminate them. Unilateral disease should always be regarded with suspicion. It is also important to consider factors that may contribute to the development of chronic inflammation of the nose (Table 3).

Table 1 Classification of Rhinitis

1. **Allergic**
   - Seasonal
   - Perennial
   - Occupational
2. **Infectious**
   - Acute
   - Chronic
     - Specific
     - Nonspecific
3. **Nonallergic, noninfectious**
   - Idiopathic
   - Occupational
   - NARES
   - Hormonal
   - Drug-induced
   - Irritants
   - Food
   - Emotional
   - Atrophic

Differential Diagnosis

1. **Polyps**
2. **Mechanical factors**
   - Deviated septum
   - Hypertrophic turbinates
   - Adenoidal hypertrophy
   - Anatomic variants in the ostiomeatal complex
   - Foreign bodies
   - Choanal atresia
3. **Tumors**
   - Benign
   - Malignant
4. **Granulomas**
   - Wegener's granulomatosis
   - Sarcoid
   - Infective
     - Tuberculosis
     - Leprosy
   - Malignant
     - Midline destructive granuloma
5. **Cerebrospinal rhinorrhea**

From International Rhinitis Management Working Group. International Consensus Report on Diagnosis and Management of Rhinitis. Eur J Allergy Clin Immunol 1994; 49(suppl 19):5; with permission.

PREFERRED APPROACH

Avoidance

In all cases of perennial nonallergic rhinitis, avoidance of irritants and provoking circumstances should be discussed. This can be a counsel of perfection, but requires patient acceptance and compliance to be effective. Recognition of the problem may allow them to reduce exposure to irritants such as cigarette smoke, either active or passive. Patients should be encouraged to stop the excessive long-term use of topical decongestants, which can result in rhinitis medicamentosa and should be offered alternative therapy such as topical steroids.

Table 2 Diagnostic Techniques

History
General ENT examination
In addition where appropriate and/or test is available:
Allergy Tests
- Skin tests
- Serum specific IgE
- Total serum IgE

Endoscopy
- Rigid
- Flexible

Nasal smear-cytology
Nasal swab-bacteriology
Radiology
- Plain sinus x-rays
- Computed tomography (CT)
- Magnetic resonance imaging (MRI)
- Chest radiograph

Mucociliary function
- Nasomucociliary clearance (NMCC)
- Ciliary beat frequency (CBF)
- Electron microscopy

Nasal airway assessment
- Nasal inspiratory peak flow (NIPF)
- Rhinomanometry (anterior and posterior)
- Acoustic rhinometry

Olfaction
- Quantitative suprathreshold and threshold testing
- Qualitative

Blood tests
- Full blood count and white cell differential
- Erythrocyte sedimentation rate
- Thyroid function tests
- Antineutrophil cytoplasmic antibody (ANCA)
- Immunoglobulins and IgG subclasses
- Antibody response to immunization with protein and carbohydrate antigens

From International Rhinitis Management Working Group. International Consensus Report on Diagnosis and Management of Rhinitis. Eur J Allergy Clin Immunol 1994; 49(suppl 19):13–18; with permission.

Topical Nasal Steroids

Timing of Therapy and Patient Selection

The availability of topical nasal steroids with a high therapeutic ratio attributable to first-pass deactivation in the liver and thus a negligible effect on the hypothalamic-pituitary-adrenal axis has significantly assisted our management of perennial nonallergic rhinitis. Since the introduction of beclomethasone dipropionate (BDP) in 1973, a range of preparations has become available, including budesonide, flunisolide, triamcinalone and, most recently, fluticasone propionate. In addition, topical formulations of betamethasone sodium phosphate and dexamethasone may be prescribed but may also have systemic effects. As soon as a working diagnosis is established, a topical steroid may be administered, and this applies even in the presence of other forms of rhinitis.

Table 3 Contributory Factors in the Development of Chronic Rhinosinusitis

Anatomic Variants
- Concha bullosa
- Enlarged ethmoidal bulla
- Everted uncinate process
- Paradoxical middle turbinate
- Agger nasi pneumatisation
- Haller cells
- Septal deflection

Mucociliary Abnormalities
- Congenital
- Acquired

Immune Deficiency
- Congenital
- Acquired

Allergy

Mechanisms of Action

Some aspects of steroid action are as yet unclear, but it is established that the steroid molecule penetrates the cell membrane and binds to hormone receptors in the cytoplasm. The steroid receptor complex is transferred to the nucleus where it binds to specific sites on the DNA molecule that have a regulatory influence on protein synthesis. The inflammatory cell infiltrate, in particular the number of mast cells and eosinophils, is reduced in the superficial mucosa, diminishing hyper-reactivity, vascular permeability, and release of mediators. Consequently intranasal steroids are effective against all symptoms of rhinitis, in particular nasal congestion and hyposmia.

Dosage, Routes, and Practical Considerations

Topical steroids are generally administered by freon-driven aerosols, by mechanical pump sprays in aqueous or glycol solutions, or as a dry powder given as two actuations to each side of the nose. Recommended frequency for BDP and flunisolide is twice daily; for budesonide, fluticasone, and triamcinalone, it is once daily. Recommended total daily dosage ranges from 200 to 400 μg.

Method of Instillation

Patients should be instructed to direct the spray superiorly and laterally avoiding contact with the nasal septum, while breathing in. Betamethasone sodium phosphate, which is available as aqueous drops and also in a form containing neomycin, may be instilled in the head-down and-forward position to enhance penetration into the middle meatus. This is particularly useful in chronic rhinosinusitis where mucopurulent secretion and obstruction of the ostiomeatal region is present.

Side Effects and Complications

Side effects and complications are minor and include dryness, crusting, slight spotting of blood, and occasional discomfort, which may be overcome by a change of delivery system such as to an aqueous form. Rarely, septal perforation has been reported with topical steroid use. However, the modern generation of topical steroids administered at the recommended dosage may be given with confidence to patients of all ages (≥ 4 years) and during pregnancy. In contrast, because both betamethasone sodium phosphate and dexamethasone are capable of producing minor systemic steroid effects, their use in the very young, during pregnancy, and in the long-term is not recommended, but they are useful as the initial therapeutic agent in uncomplicated perennial rhinitis.

Assessment of Therapeutic Response

It is important that patients have an adequate therapeutic trial of daily medication for at least 4 weeks before assessing clinical efficacy. Compliance will be significantly improved if patients understand that the clinical effect is not instantaneous and that it will only continue as long as the medication is administered. Once symptoms are controlled, the daily dosage may be reduced. Depending on the underlying cause of the condition, medication is usually required long term. Patients may be reassured that this poses no safety issues and should be advised to titrate dosages based on individual circumstance. The presence of eosinophils in nasal cytology specimens appears to be a particularly successful predictor of therapeutic efficacy for intranasal steroids.

THERAPEUTIC ALTERNATIVES

Systemic Corticosteroids

A short course of oral steroid such as prednisolone or dexamethasone can be useful in severe cases of rhinitis in emergency situations such as prior to an examination or job interview. They allow symptomatic control to be achieved rapidly, after which topical preparations may be used. The regimens for these agents follows: prednisolone 20 mg for 3 days, 15 mg for 3 days, 10 mg for 3 days, and 5 mg for 3 days; dexamethasone: 12 mg for 3 days, 8 mg for 3 days, and 4 mg for 3 days.

There are a number of contraindications to the use of systemic corticosteroids, including herpes keratitis, advanced osteoporosis, severe hypertension, diabetes mellitus, gastric ulceration, and chronic infection. They are not indicated in the treatment of rhinitis in children or in pregnant women.

Depot preparations of steroids (e.g., methylprednisolone) and ACTH analogues (e.g., Synacthen) are also available and although effective, they may produce severe side effects that cannot be reversed and may suppress adrenal cortex function for long periods. Consequently, their use in perennial nonallergic rhinitis is rarely warranted.

Anticholinergics

In some cases of perennial nonallergic rhinitis, watery rhinorrhea is the predominate symptom. Under these circumstances the anticholinergic agent, ipratropium bromide can be useful. It acts as an antagonist against the muscarinic receptors of the seromucinous glands. It has been shown to markedly inhibit methacholine-induced and cold air–induced nasal hypersecretion, but it has no effect on congestion, itching, or sneezing. It is administered as a topical spray and works rapidly if it is effective. The side effects are those of any nasal spray—dryness, crusting, irritation, and spotting of blood. In addition excessive dryness of the throat is sometimes experienced. Ipratropium bromide is not recommended in patients with glaucoma or prostatic hypertrophy.

Saline Douching

Saline douching can be most effective in cases of chronic rhinosinusitis, particularly when mucopurulent discharge is significant before instillation of active medication. Patients are asked to sniff or spray in a solution made of a pinch of table salt and a pinch of bicarbonate of soda dissolved in half a glass of warm water two to three times a day.

Decongestants

Systemic and topical decongestants remain popular with the general public, being readily available without prescription. Systemic decongestants are often sold in combination with antihistamines but evidence is lacking for their efficacy in nonallergic rhinitis. Long-term reliance on topical decongestants should be actively discouraged but the prior use of an agent such as oxymetazoline may facilitate instillation of an intranasal steroid for the first few days of treatment when congestion is severe, without fear of provoking rhinitis medicamentosa.

Antibiotics

Although the treatment of infectious rhinitis is beyond the scope of this chapter, broad spectrum antibiotics can be helpful in the presence of mucopurulent nasal secretion, which can occur in perennial nonallergic rhinitis. The choice of antibiotics is determined by microbiology, clinical severity, and patient factors. In chronic situations, those agents that inhibit *Haemophilus influenzae, Streptococcus pneumoniae,* and anaerobes will be most effective (e.g., amoxicillin clavulanate, cerfuroxime axetil with or without metronidazole).

Surgery

The majority of cases of simple perennial nonallergic noninfectious rhinitis can be managed medically. However, there are a number of contributory elements that may exacerbate the situation and may require surgical intervention, in particular, mechanical factors such as a deviated nasal septum, hypertrophied inferior turbinates, and anatomical variants within the middle meatus causing narrowing of the ostiomeatal complex (see Table 3). When considering surgery the following points should be borne in mind:

1. Surgical correction should be considered when medical treatment fails, but this will not necessarily obviate the need for long-term medication.
2. The sensation of nasal congestion may be due to many factors. It is advisable to exclude disease in the middle meatus by endoscopy and/or CT scanning before attacking the nasal septum and inferior turbinates.
3. Anatomic variants in the middle meatus should not be operated on per se as they occur in the normal population. Only do so if they are obstructing sinus outflow with associated infection.

There are many methods of inferior turbinate reduction producing varying periods of symptomatic relief (Table 4). Mucosal preservation is better achieved by submucous diathermy, submucous resection, and submucous outfracture (SMOFIT), but resection of variable amounts of the inferior turbinate remains popular. The effect of a decongestant spray may be helpful in deciding between reduction by shrinkage procedures and excision. When resecting the inferior turbinate, it should be remembered that it is the anterior turbinate that has the greatest effect on resistance to flow in the valve area. Techniques that produce fibrosis may also have an effect on local neuronal control of secretion as well as turbinate mass. However, any surgical interference with the turbinate can produce significant hemorrhage, adhesions, and crusting.

Vidian neurectomy represents a more direct surgical approach to secretion control by aiming to ablate the parasympathetic supply. A variety of routes to the Vidian nerve may be chosen, but results, especially in the long-term, are disappointing.

Table 4 shows the more common anatomic variants found in the middle meatus. The rationale and details of surgery in this area are beyond the scope of this chapter. Suffice it to say that based on pathophysiologic principles of disrupted mucociliary clearance from the sinuses, there has been a general move away from radical ablative surgery such as the Caldwell Luc approach to a more conservative and precise removal of diseased tissue within the critical drainage areas of the nose (i.e., the ostiomeatal complex). This has been facilitated by improved visualization, both diagnostically and therapeutically with rigid endoscopy and CT scanning. Nevertheless, patients still receive medication, in particular topical nasal steroids both before and after surgery. Indeed surgery is not generally undertaken unless the patient has had at least 3 months of medical therapy.

Table 4 Methods for Reduction of the Inferior Turbinate

Method
Submucous diathermy
Linear cautery
Submucous resection
Submucous outfracture
Laser cautery/reduction
Cryosurgery
Turbinectomy
Partial
Radical/subtotal

Table 5 Complications of Nasal Polypectomy

Complication
Death
Intracranial
Meningitis
Hemorrhage
Cerebrovascular accident
Orbital
Blindness
Diplopia
Epiphora
Hematoma
Nasal
Hemorrhage
Adhesions

NASAL POLYPS

The term nasal polyposis covers a wide spectrum of disease from the polypoid change often encountered in the middle meatus during chronic infection to the aggressive massive and recurrent polyps of cystic fibrosis or the aspirin sensitive asthma (ASA) triad. In between lie "ordinary" polyps, the cause of which remains obscure. A condition characterised by obstruction and anosmia, polyps behave like garden weeds, generally defying all medical and surgical efforts to eradicate them. Once diagnosed and differentiated from neoplasia (usually, though not exclusively, by their bilateral occurrence), corticosteroids in their many forms may be tried. Although allergy does not appear to cause polyp formation, mast cell reactions and eosinophil activation with subsequent inflammation appear to be important. For primary treatment betamethasone drops or parenteral steroids can be most useful. Surgery is frequently required and may take the form of conventional nasal polypectomy with snares up to and including total fronto-ethmo-sphenoidectomy. These procedures may be performed using a headlight, microscope, and fiberoptically illuminated speculum, or under endoscopic control. My preference is the latter, but such a procedure is always preceded by 6 to 8 weeks of medical treatment and CT scanning. Following surgery, any of the intranasal steroid sprays may be given ad infinitum. The complications of polypectomy, irrespective of the instrumentation and approach, are shown in Table 5.

PROS AND CONS OF TREATMENT

Perennial nonallergic rhinitis covers a considerable range of conditions affecting a large portion of the population. Although not life threatening, it has a significant effect on quality of life and carries a societal cost that should not be dismissed. Once the diagnosis has been made, careful consideration must be made of the various therapeutic options, which should be tailored to the individual patient.

SUGGESTED READING

International Rhinitis Management Working Group. International consensus report on the diagnosis and management of rhinitis. Eur J Allerg Clin Immunol 1994; 49(suppl19):1–34.

Mackay IS, ed. Rhinitis: mechanisms and management. London: Royal Society of Medicine Services, 1989.

Mackay IS, Lund VJ. Surgical management of sinusitis. In: Mackay IS, Bull TR, eds. Scott Brown's otolaryngology, 6th ed. Vol 4, Chap 12. London: Butterworths (in press).

Mygind N, Naclerio RM, eds. Allergic and non-allergic rhinitis: clinical aspects. Copenhagen: Munksgaard, 1993.

ANTIHISTAMINES (H_1-RECEPTOR ANTAGONISTS)

F. ESTELLE R. SIMONS, M.D.
KEITH J. SIMONS, Ph.D.

The newer, second-generation H_1-receptor antagonists, terfenadine, astemizole, loratadine, cetirizine, and acrivastine, although not significantly more effective than the older H_1-receptor antagonists, are relatively non-sedating and are gradually replacing their predecessors in the treatment of allergic rhinoconjunctivitis. They are safe for use in patients with rhinoconjunctivitis who have concurrent asthma, and they are effective in relieving pruritus, new wheal formation, and duration of whealing in patients with urticaria.

The second-generation H_1-receptor antagonists are more expensive than the least expensive first-generation H_1-receptor antagonists. In 1993, the average wholesale cost to the pharmacist of a 1-month supply of medication was $51.37 for terfenadine and $50.63 for astemizole, versus $46.60 for azatadine maleate (Optimine), $26.32 for dexchlorpheniramine maleate (Polaramine), $25.38 for clemastine fumarate (Tavist), and $2.45 for generic chlorpheniramine.

Formulations and recommended dosages of representative second-generation H_1-receptor antagonists are listed in Table 1.

ADVERSE EFFECTS

The major limitation of the first-generation H_1-receptor antagonists is their adverse effects, particularly central nervous system (CNS) effects. These medications are lipophilic, cross the blood-brain barrier readily, and bind readily to H_1-receptors, cholinergic receptors, serotonin receptors, and alpha-adrenergic receptors in the central nervous system. They produce sedation in 15 to 25 percent of users. Their effect is comparable to that produced by alcohol or by standard doses of antipsychotics (Fig. 1). In addition to depressive CNS effects, they may also cause neuropsychiatric effects or peripheral nervous system adverse effects, many of which are attributable to anticholinergic mechanisms (Table 2). In contrast, the second-generation H_1-receptor antagonists such as terfenadine, astemizole, loratadine, cetirizine, or acrivastine do not cross the blood-brain barrier readily and do not bind to cholinergic, serotonin, or alpha-adrenergic receptors.

The relative lack of sedation and other CNS effects produced by the newer H_1-receptor antagonists has been documented in many double-blind, placebo-controlled studies. Methods of assessment of sedation have been subjective, for example, the use of diary card scores to record daytime sleepiness, and objective, for example, multiple sleep-latency tests in which the investigator obtains an electroencephalographic record of the length of time a patient takes to fall asleep during the day under standardized conditions. It is important to note that investigators often report a poor correlation between subjective symptoms of sleepiness and objective measurements of CNS impairment, such as prolongation of reaction time, indicating that patients may not necessarily notice the reduction in alertness and functioning produced by the first-generation H_1-receptor antagonists. Some of the different tests used for comparative assessment of CNS adverse effects of first- and second-generation H_1-receptor antagonists are summarized in Table 3.

In contrast to first-generation H_1-receptor antagonists, second-generation H_1-receptor antagonists, in manufacturers' recommended doses, produce a low incidence of sedation. The incidence is not zero, however, particularly after cetirizine and acrivastine,

Table 1 Formulations and Dosages of Second-Generation H_1-Receptor Antagonists

Generic (Proprietary)	*Formulation*	*Recommended Dosage*
Terfenadine (Seldane)	Suspension, 30 mg/5 ml* Tablet, 60 mg, 120 mg*	*Pediatric*†: 3-6 yr, 15 mg b.i.d.; 7-12 yr, 30 mg b.i.d. *Adult:* 60 mg b.i.d. or 120 mg q.o.d.
Astemizole (Hismanal)	Suspension, 10 mg/5 ml* Tablet, 10 mg	*Pediatric**: <6 yr, 0.2 mg/kg/24 hr; 6-12 yr, 5 mg q.o.d. *Adult:* 10 mg q.o.d.
Loratadine (Claritin)	Tablet, 10 mg	*Adult:* 10 mg q.o.d.
Cetirizine (Reactine)	Tablet, 10 mg	*Adult:* 5-10 mg q.o.d.
Acrivastine (Semprex)	Tablet, 8 mg††	*Adult:* 8 mg t.i.d.
Levocabastine (Livostin)	Microsuspension, 50 μg per spray or 15 μg per drop	Topical, 2 sprays in each nostril b.i.d.-q.i.d. Topical, 1 drop in each eye b.i.d.-q.i.d.

*Not available in the United States at the time of publication.
†For patients weighing less than or equal to 40 kg.
††Available only in combination with pseudoephedrine 60 mg.

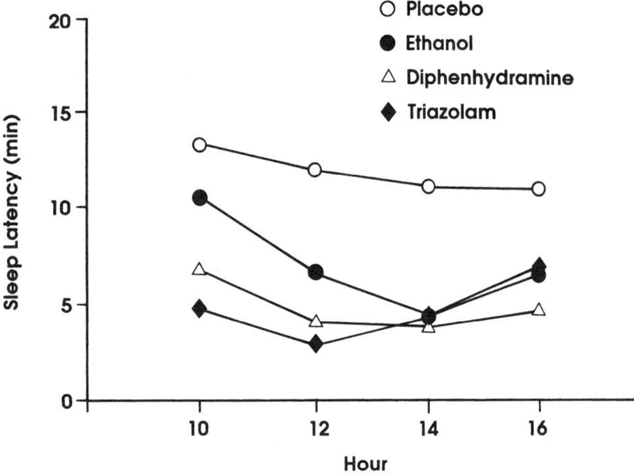

Figure 1 Sleep latency was measured at 1, 3, 5, and 7 hours after participants ingested a placebo, triazolam 0.25 mg, diphenhydramine 50 mg, or ethanol 0.6 g/kg at 0900 hours, in a double-blind, crossover study in 12 healthy young men. The sedative effects of diphenhydramine were similar to those of triazolam and alcohol and were significantly greater than those produced by placebo. (From Roehrs T, Zwyghuizen-Doorenbos A, Roth T. Sedative effects and plasma concentrations following single doses of triazolam, diphenhydramine, ethanol and placebo. Sleep 1993; 16:301–305; with permission).

and physicians may occasionally encounter patients who complain of sedation after ingestion of a second-generation H_1-receptor antagonist. Also, when manufacturers' recommended doses of any of these medications are exceeded, the incidence of sedation increases.

Interaction of Second-Generation H_1-Receptor Antagonists with CNS-Active Substances

In recommended doses, the second-generation H_1-receptor antagonists, in contrast to their predecessors, do not potentiate the adverse CNS effects of ethanol, diazepam, or other CNS-active chemicals.

Table 2 Possible Neurologic Adverse Effects of First-Generation H_1-Receptor Antagonists

Depressive	**Neuropsychiatric**
Ataxia	Anxiety
Coma	Confusion
Delirium	Depression
Drowsiness	Impaired mental efficiency
Lassitude	Impaired judgment
Sedation	Hallucinations
Dizziness	
Fatigue	
Stimulatory	**Peripheral**
Dystonia	Areflexia
Hyper-reflexia	Blurred vision
Insomnia	Dilated pupils
Tachycardia	Impotence
Irritability	Paresthesias
Headaches	Urinary retention
Seizures	

Other Adverse Effects

Other adverse effects of second-generation H_1-receptor antagonists have been reported. Rarely, patients develop a prolonged QTc interval and the ventricular arrhythmia known as torsades de pointes, accompanied by syncope and cardiac arrest after astemizole or terfenadine overdose or when these medications are ingested in usual doses under certain conditions (Table 4). Most patients using these H_1-receptor antagonists in recommended doses are apparently not at any increased risk for adverse cardiovascular system (CVS) effects, as confirmed in epidemiologic studies in which the risk of CVS effects from terfenadine was lower than the risk of CVS effects from first-generation H_1-receptor antagonists (Fig. 2).

Astemizole may cause appetite stimulation and inappropriate weight gain in some patients.

Safety in Pregnancy and Lactation

Embryo toxicity, fetal wastage, fetal anomalies, or other problems in pregnancy in humans have not

Table 3 Some Tests Used for Assessment of CNS Adverse Effects of H_1-Receptor Antagonists

Subjective Somnolence
Diary cards to record daytime sleepiness
Visual analogue scales to record daytime sleepiness
Stanford Sleepiness Questionnaire
Profile-of-Moods questionnaire for self-rating of sleepiness, impairment, and fatigue
Objective
Electroencephalogram
Multiple sleep-latency test
Latency of P300-evoked electroencephalographic potentials (measure of sustained attention and cerebral processing speed)
Performance
Dynamic visual acuity
Pupillary light responses
Critical flicker fusion
Simple reaction time
Choice reaction time
Digit-symbol substitution
Monitoring of computer-simulated driving errors
Monitoring of actual driving errors

Table 4 Risk Factors Associated with H_1-Receptor Antagonist–Induced QTc Prolongation, Torsades De Pointes and Other Adverse Cardiovascular (CVS) Effects

Risk Factors for CVS Effects	*H_1-Receptor Antagonist† Dosage Associated with CVS Effects*	*Comments*
Overdose or large dose	Astemizole up to 200 mg/day or 2.5-16.7 mg/kg/day (child) Terfenadine 120-360 mg/day	Many patients with CVS effects had no CNS effects; seizures and lethargy were rarely reported
Cardiac abnormalities, e.g., congenital increased QTc; ischemic heart disease	Astemizole 10-20 mg/day Terfenadine 120-180 mg/day	Multiple risk factors were noted in some patients, e.g., concomitant ingestion of CYP3A4 inhibitors or electrolyte imbalance
Hepatic dysfunction (cirrhosis)	Terfenadine 240 mg/day	—
Concomitant administration of other CYP3A4 inhibitors*	Terfenadine 120 mg/day	Medications ingested included: ketoconazole 200-400 mg, itraconazole 200-400 mg, or macrolide antibiotics; some patients also had a history of ischemic heart disease or prior prolonged QTc interval
Severe hypokalemia, hypomagnesemia, or hypocalcemia	Terfenadine 120-900 mg/day	Some patients also had ischemic heart disease, congestive heart failure, history of ethanol abuse, or concomitant ketoconazole ingestion

Modified from Simons FER. The therapeutic index of newer H_1-receptor antagonists. Clin Exp Allergy 1994;24:707–723; with permission.
*Medications that prolong the QTc interval may also be implicated.
†Acrivastine, cetirizine, and loratadine have not been documented to cause these effects.

been attributed to any of the second-generation H_1-receptor antagonists to date. The number of pregnant patients who have received these medications is small, however, and some of these agents are classified as Schedule C drugs to be used only if expected benefits outweigh the unknown potential risks of toxicity. H_1-receptor antagonists are excreted in breast milk; thus, when first-generation antihistamines are ingested by nursing mothers, they can cause sedation or irritability in infants.

CLINICAL PHARMACOLOGY

The second-generation H_1-receptor antagonists are reasonably well absorbed when given by mouth, with peak serum concentrations occurring approximately 2 hours after administration. Absolute bioavailability is unknown since no intravenous formulations are available for comparison with oral formulations. Terfenadine, astemizole, and loratadine are metabolized by the hepatic cytochrome P-450 system. Serum elimination half-life values range from less than 1 day for terfenadine and loratadine and their active metabolites, to 9.5 days for astemizole and its active metabolite desmethylastemizole. Serum concentrations of these medications are extremely low.

Cetirizine, the biologically active carboxylic acid metabolite of hydroxyzine, has a serum elimination half-life of 7 to 11 hours. Fifty percent of a dose is excreted in the urine as unchanged drug. Acrivastine and levocabastine are also excreted largely unchanged.

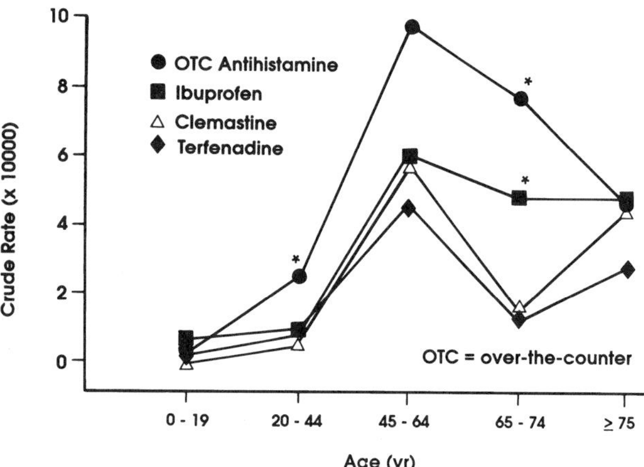

Figure 2 The hypothesis that terfenadine exposure increased the risk of cardiac arrhythmias was tested using an observational historical cohort study design and a drug-exposure period of 30 days in patients receiving terfenadine (n = 181,672), diphenhydramine, and other over-the-counter (OTC) antihistamines (n = 156,689), clemastine (n = 83,156), or ibuprofen (negative control, n = 181,672). The incidence of ventricular arrhythmias and cardiac arrest was higher in the OTC antihistamine group than in the terfenadine, ibuprofen, or clemastine groups. *An increased relative risk ($p < 0.001$) was identified when terfenadine and ketoconazole were coadministered. There was a trend towards an increased relative risk (not significant) when terfenadine and erythromycin were coadministered* (From Pratt CM, Hertz RP, Ellis BE, et al. Risk of developing life-threatening ventricular arrhythmias associated with terfenadine in comparison with over-the-counter antihistamines, ibuprofen, and clemastine. Am J Cardiol 1994;73:346–352; with permission).

Despite the differences in half-life values, a once-daily dosage is possible using astemizole 10 mg, loratadine 10 mg, or cetirizine 10 mg. Terfenadine is usually administered in a dosage of 60 mg twice daily, although terfenadine 120 mg once daily is recommended in some countries. Acrivastine is administered in a dosage of 2 mg three times daily and is only available in combination with pseudoephedrine 60 mg.

Many of the second-generation H_1-receptor antagonists, in addition to being pharmacologic antagonists of histamine, have antiallergic and anti-inflammatory effects. They should be given, if possible, before the anticipated exposure to allergen and subsequent allergic reaction, in order to bind preferentially to H_1-receptors in the tissue before agonist, histamine, does. Maximum antihistaminic effects of H_1-receptor antagonists occur several hours after peak serum concentrations have been achieved.

Lack of Subsensitivity

Long-term administration of *first*-generation H_1-receptor antagonists may be associated with an *apparent* decrease in efficacy; however, autoinduction of hepatic metabolism and increased hepatic clearance of the H_1-receptor antagonist, with consequent lower serum concentrations, does not occur.

The second-generation H_1-receptor antagonists terfenadine, loratadine, or cetirizine also are not eliminated more rapidly in long-term versus short-term use, and the efficacy of these medications in suppressing the histamine- or antigen-induced skin wheal and flare and in suppressing allergic rhinoconjunctivitis or chronic urticaria symptoms does not diminish during administration over 4 to 8 weeks, as demonstrated in most studies in which compliance has been monitored rigorously.

The apparent subsensitivity reported years ago with the first-generation H_1-receptor antagonists may have been due, at least partly, to poor compliance because of sedation and lack of efficacy. Additional studies of the subsensitivity phenomenon in humans are necessary since long-term treatment with H_1-receptor antagonists is often required.

EFFICACY OF NEWER H_1-RECEPTOR ANTAGONISTS IN TREATMENT OF ALLERGIC DISORDERS

Allergic Rhinoconjunctivitis

In patients with allergic rhinoconjunctivitis, the histamine released in the immediate hypersensitivity response accounts for most of the symptoms directly via stimulation of H_1-receptors on sensory nerve endings and vascular smooth muscle, and indirectly via muscarinic discharge. The second-generation H_1-receptor antagonists effectively relieve sneezing, itching, and nasal discharge in this condition, but they are not very effective in relieving congestion. Therefore, in patients with moderate or severe rhinitis, they seldom control symptoms completely. Sustained-release decongestants such as pseudoephedrine 60 to 240 mg are sometimes added to second-generation H_1-receptor antagonists such as terfenadine, astemizole, loratadine, cetirizine, and acrivastine to provide relief of congestion. Interestingly, these fixed–dose combination products are associated with a higher incidence of insomnia and other adverse CNS effects than those produced by the second-generation H_1-receptor antagonists alone or by first-generation H_1-receptor antagonist and decongestant combinations in which the sedative effect of the antihistamine is counteracted by the stimulant effect of the decongestant.

In randomized, prospective, double-blind studies in patients with seasonal or perennial rhinitis, the second-generation H_1-receptor antagonists have been found to be superior to placebo and comparable to a first-generation H_1-receptor antagonist such as chlorpheniramine. The newer medications seem to have similar efficacy to each other in patients with allergic rhinitis, although they have not all been compared directly. Currently, there is some interest in topical application of H_1-receptor antagonists such as levocabastine to the nasal mucosa and conjunctivae.

The second-generation H_1-receptor antagonists, although not significantly more effective than intranasal cromolyn in the treatment of allergic rhinitis, offer the advantage of less frequent dosing. They are not as effective as intranasal glucocorticoids in the treatment of allergic rhinitis symptoms, but they give better relief of associated allergic conjunctivitis symptoms.

Asthma

Concerns about potential adverse effects of H_1-receptor antagonists in asthma have been greatly exaggerated in the past. Patients with asthma who require an H_1-receptor antagonist such as terfenadine, astemizole, loratadine, or cetirizine for the treatment of concurrent allergic rhinoconjunctivitis will *not* be harmed by H_1-receptor antagonist treatment and may benefit from the modest anti-asthma effect of the H_1-receptor antagonist.

Chronic Urticaria

In prospective, controlled, double-blind studies in adults with chronic idiopathic urticaria, the second-generation H_1-receptor antagonists, terfenadine, astemizole, cetirizine, and loratadine, have been well tolerated and have resulted in significant remission of symptoms compared to the relief provided by placebo. They reduce pruritus and the number, size, and duration of urticarial lesions. No direct overall comparison of the efficacy of terfenadine, astemizole, loratadine, and cetirizine has yet been performed in patients with chronic urticaria.

Anaphylaxis

In patients with anaphylaxis, the treatment of first choice is epinephrine, but H_1-receptor antagonists are useful for adjunctive treatment of pruritus, urticaria, and rhinoconjunctivitis. There are no published studies of the second-generation H_1-receptor antagonists in anaphylaxis in humans. No intravenous formulations of these medications are available. The first-generation H_1-receptor antagonists chlorpheniramine and diphenhydramine, which can be administered intravenously, are therefore still used for adjunctive symptom relief in anaphylaxis.

Atopic Dermatitis

Histamine concentrations are increased in the skin and in the plasma of patients with active atopic dermatitis. In this disorder, second-generation H_1-receptor antagonists have not been optimally studied yet, and some investigators believe they should not replace hydroxyzine or other first-generation H_1-receptor antagonists for the treatment of itching until their efficacy has been confirmed in additional clinical trials.

Other

H_1-receptor antagonists are widely used for symptomatic treatment of upper respiratory tract infections, although there is limited evidence from double-blind, placebo-controlled studies to support this practice. Similarly, H_1-receptor antagonists have been widely prescribed for patients with acute otitis media, and for those with chronic otitis media with effusion, despite studies demonstrating that these medications do not significantly hasten the resolution of otitis media.

SUGGESTED READING

Meltzer ED. Antihistamine- and decongestant-induced performance decrements. J Occup Med 1990; 32:327–334.

Pratt CM, Hertz RP, Ellis BE, et al. Risk of developing life-threatening ventricular arrhythmia associated with terfenadine in comparison with over-the-counter antihistamines, ibuprofen and clemastine. Am J Cardiol 1994; 73:346–352.

Roehrs T, Zwyghuizen-Doorenbos A, Roth T. Sedative effects and plasma concentrations following single doses of triazolam, diphenhydramine, ethanol and placebo. Sleep 1993; 16:301–305.

Simons FER. The therapeutic index of newer H_1-receptor antagonists. Clin Exp Allergy 1994; 24:707–723.

Simons FER, Simons KJ. The pharmacology and use of H_1-receptor antagonist drugs. N Engl J Med 1994; 330:1663–1670.

ASTHMA

ASTHMA PROVOKED BY EXPOSURE TO ALLERGENS

JEAN BOUSQUET, M.D., Ph.D.
PHILIPPE GODARD, M.D.
FRANÇOIS-B. MICHEL, M.D.

Allergic diseases are mediated by allergens that trigger IgE-bound mast cells to release vasoactive mediators, resulting in an ongoing inflammatory reaction causing nonspecific hyper-reactivity that may persist for several days. Repeated allergen challenges lead to a complex inflammatory state that eventually results in the remodeling of airways.

The treatment of allergic asthma is based on allergen avoidance, which is always recommended and may be associated with pharmacologic treatment and specific immunotherapy (SIT). A complete allergy evaluation is therefore required to identify the allergens to which the patient is sensitive and to better control allergic asthma. Treatment objectives of allergic asthma are as follows:

1. The reduction of symptoms caused by allergen exposure, nonspecific hyper-reactivity, and inflammation.
2. Improved quality of life. Patients with severe asthma often experience school or work absenteeism, have difficulty exercising, and their social life is altered. Treatment should help patients maintain normal activity.
3. Alteration of the natural course of the disease, although there is no data to indicate that any treatment may have such properties.
4. Avoidance of side effects induced by treatments.
5. Patient education to improve an understanding of the disease and compliance with treatment.

MECHANISMS OF ALLERGIC ASTHMA

Asthma is a multifactorial and complex disease in which allergic factors and nonallergic triggers (viral infections, irritants, exercise, drugs, aspirin, occupational factors, stress, air pollution) interact and result in bronchial obstruction and inflammation. Although the role of inhalant allergens in asthma has been debated for some time, their efficacy has now been established. Bronchial challenge with allergens can induce a bronchoconstrictive response in airways. The occurrence of allergic asthma and exacerbations of the condition have been clearly associated with high levels of indoor allergens such as house dust mites, animal danders, or insect dusts, as well as with seasonal allergens such as grass pollens or molds. Allergen avoidance has been shown to reduce asthma symptoms and nonspecific bronchial hyper-reactivity. On the other hand, food allergy is only rarely involved in asthma.

The inhalation of allergens leads to a complex activation of various cell types and the release of inflammatory and neurogenic mediators; however, two different situations seem to exist. Although very few pollen grains can reach the lower airways, these allergens borne on submicroscopic particles frequently elicit asthma by an IgE-mediated mechanism. Pollen-induced allergic reactions that are prolonged over several days almost always lead to nonspecific bronchial hyper-reactivity, which is usually transient in patients only allergic to pollens, lasting from a few weeks to a few months until the end of the pollen season.

On the other hand, house dust mites and other perennial allergens induce a sustained inflammation of the bronchi, leading to a variable degree of nonspecific bronchial hyper-reactivity. In the long term, inflammation leads to a permanent remodeling of the airways, which is involved in an accelerated decline of pulmonary function and is characterized by a poorly reversible bronchial obstruction that appears after some decades of chronic asthma. It is therefore proposed that immunologic and anti-inflammatory treatments should be used in combination, but after a long course of the disease, inflammation and remodeling are the major cause of symptoms, implying that the immunologic treatment is less effective (Fig. 1).

OVERALL MANAGEMENT OF ASTHMA

Epidemiologic studies show that there is an increase in prevalence and severity of asthma. The reasons for

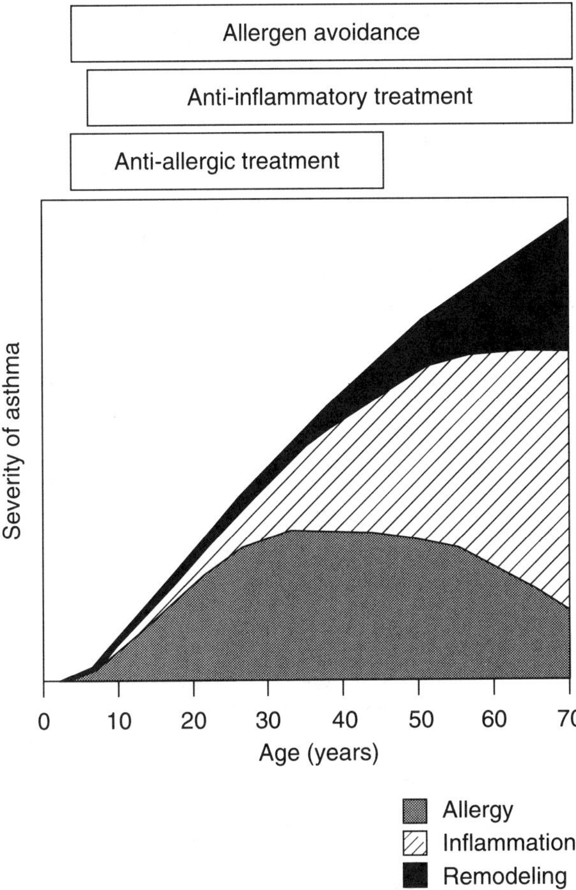

Figure 1 Evolution of allergic asthma and treatment consequences. Allergic asthma usually begins early in life triggered by allergens and eventually results in inflammation and remodeling of airways. Until inflammation and remodeling are extensive, antiallergic treatment may be effective, though later, such treatment is likely to be less effective. Anti-inflammatory treatment should be started early in the course of allergic asthma since inflammation always follows allergy. Allergic triggers can induce asthma throughout life; therefore, allergen avoidance should be continued lifelong.

these unsatisfactory trends are not completely understood, but at least two major factors have been identified. Obstruction of airways in asthma is directly linked to inflammation, but the majority of patients are treated only with bronchodilators. A second major factor is the patients' (and even some doctors') poor understanding of asthma and its treatment. These considerations indicate that the management of asthma should be improved both by using anti-inflammatory drugs early in the course of the disease and by education programs.

Within the past 5 years several attempts have been made to establish a consensus on the management of asthma. The International Consensus on the Diagnosis and Management of Asthma was published in March 1992 in an attempt to propose a unified approach. The panel of experts devised a six-part program for effective management of asthma, which forms the basis of the consensus and is outlined.

1. *Educate patients to develop a partnership.* Educating asthmatic patients is very important so that they can alter their treatment as needed without consulting their physician. Education also leads to an improved control of asthma and a reduced number of attacks, particularly the life-threatening ones. This may be achieved by a permanent and coordinated relationship among specialists (pneumologist, allergist, physical medicine), general practitioners, medical co-workers (nurses, physiotherapists, health education teachers, psychologists), and the asthmatic patient.
2. *Assess and monitor severity with objective measures of lung function.* Spirometry should be used for the initial assessment and periodic re-evaluations should be scheduled. Regular use of home peak flow monitoring is recommended for patients who use medications daily.
3. *Avoid and control asthma triggers.* Environmental control measures are an important prevention strategy that should always be attempted, although they are rarely completely effective. Immunotherapy may be used in carefully selected patients with mild to moderately severe asthma using standardized high quality extracts.
4. *Establish plans for chronic management.* Inhalation therapy is the preferred route of administration of antiasthma drugs. The early and prolonged use of anti-inflammatory drugs appears to be beneficial for the patient although more data are needed to assess the long-term effects of these drugs. Because asthma is both a dynamic and a chronic condition, planning medication needs requires taking the variability of airflow obstruction into consideration; therefore, a "step-up" and "step-down" approach is proposed in which the number and frequency of medications are increased or decreased according to symptoms. A color-coded asthma zone management system has been developed to help patients better understand and monitor the variable nature of this chronic disease and take appropriate action to maintain control of asthma. Written plans for each zone are essential to improve patient adherence.
5. *Establish management plans for exacerbations.* Exacerbations usually reflect either a failure of chronic management or exposure to a noxious agent, including allergens. The early introduction of corticosteroids and frequent administration of inhaled $beta_2$-agonists are required to manage exacerbations.
6. *Provide regular follow-up care.* Patients need regular supervision and support by a clinician who has knowledge of asthma. Continuous monitoring is essential to ensure the therapeutic goals.

Allergen Avoidance

In industrialized countries, most time is spent indoors where the environment is an important asthma trigger. Environmental controls to reduce exposure to indoor and outdoor allergens is essential but rarely complete. Furthermore, even when an allergen is largely removed from a patient's environment the benefit of such measures may take several weeks or months to be perceived. When possible, environmental control measures should always be applied, even if their efficacy is incomplete, because they may improve the patient's condition and reduce the need for immunologic or pharmacologic treatments.

Indoor Allergens

Among the wide variety of indoor allergens, mites, animal allergens (furred animals), cockroaches, and fungi are the most important. Reducing mite populations is difficult, but it has been demonstrated that mite avoidance measures result in the improvement of asthma. However, not all studies have been conclusive and there are no data on the long-term effects. Measures such as replacing bedding, using mattress covers, washing bedding and textiles, and removing floor coverings can lead to a lower concentration of mites and mite allergens in mattresses and house dust. Frequent vacuum-cleaning is less effective. Regulating the humidity by means of ventilation and heating is important, but the efficacy of these measures is not known. Acaricides, including benzyl benzoate, pyrethrins, pirimiphos methyl, and liquid nitrogen are being used but currently have little or no proven effect. Both benzyl benzoate and tannic acid can effectively reduce mite numbers but the difficulty of applying them so that they reach deep into the furniture reduces their effectiveness. Moreover, long-term exposure of acaricides requires investigation of their toxic effect. All these measures are expensive and no cost-benefit study has been undertaken.

Removal of pets from the home environment is highly effective, but it may take several weeks before efficacy can be demonstrated. Removal of pets may present difficult emotional problems. Washing cats every week reduces airborne levels of allergens, whereas keeping cats isolated is not effective.

Cockroaches are controlled by regular thorough cleaning of infested homes and by the use of pesticides, which may irritate the airways of asthmatic patients.

Molds can be reduced by removing or cleaning mold-laden objects or foods and maintaining a low humidity (<50 percent). Molds can grow in heating or cooling systems, which should be inspected regularly.

Outdoor Allergens

Pollens and molds represent the major classes of outdoor allergens. It is almost impossible to completely avoid outdoor allergens, but exposure may be reduced by remaining indoors when pollen and mold counts are highest and by closing windows and using filters in homes and cars.

Occupational Sensitizers

Over a thousand substances have been identified as occupational allergens and irritants that cause asthma. Controls for these allergen levels above which the sensitization occurs frequently have been proposed for many chemicals. However, when a patient has been sensitized, the level of allergen inducing symptoms may be extremely low. Taking prompt measures to avoid further exposure to occupational sensitizers as soon as a patient's occupational asthma is recognized helps to prevent the development of irreversible airflow limitation. Attempts to reduce occupational exposure have been successful, especially in industrial settings, and some potent sensitizers such as castor bean have been replaced by less allergenic substances.

Food Allergens

Although food allergy is less prevalent than inhalant allergy in asthma, when a patient is allergic to a given food, strict avoidance is highly recommended.

Pollutants

The avoidance of indoor irritants such as tobacco smoke, wood smoke, sprays, and air pollutants is also of importance since these components may worsen asthma. Several studies have shown that peaks of outdoor pollutants exacerbate asthma, and it is recommended that patients with severe asthma avoid air pollution episodes.

Specific Immunotherapy

The efficacy of SIT in treating inhalant allergy was contested some years ago. Significant improvements have been made, but allergen injections that used potent extracts resulted in a greater number of severe systemic reactions. It is therefore essential to consider the following factors when evaluating the respective value of SIT in comparison with other available therapeutic methods:

1. Potential severity of the condition to be treated
2. Availability of standardized high quality extracts
3. Efficacy of available treatments
4. Cost and duration of each type of treatment
5. Risk incurred by the patient as a result of the allergic disease and the treatments

To minimize risk and improve efficacy, SIT needs to be prescribed by specialists and administered by physicians who are trained to manage acute systemic reactions if anaphylaxis occurs (Table 1).

The major short-term objectives of SIT are to

Table 1 Recommendations to Minimize Risk and Improve Efficacy of SIT in Allergic Asthma

1. Specific immunotherapy needs to be prescribed by specialists and administered by physicians trained to manage systemic reactions if anaphylaxis occurs
2. Patients with multiple sensitivities and/or nonallergic triggers may not benefit from specific immunotherapy
3. Specific immunotherapy is more effective in children and young adults than older patients
4. For safety reasons it is essential that patients be asymptomatic at the time of the injections because lethal adverse reactions occur more often in asthma patients with severe airways obstruction
5. FEV_1 with pharmacologic treatment should reach at least 70 percent of the predicted values for both efficacy and safety reasons

From National Institutes of Health. International Consensus Report on the Diagnosis and Management of Asthma (NIH publication #92-3091). Bethesda, Md: US Department of Health and Human Services, 1992.

reduce the allergic triggers and precipitating symptoms and, in the long term, to decrease bronchial inflammation and nonspecific bronchial hyper-reactivity when bronchial damage is not prominent. Moreover, at present SIT appears to be the only treatment that might modify the course of the disease either by preventing the development of new sensitivities or by altering the natural history of asthma.

The selection of the allergic asthmatic patient is critical for successful SIT (Table 2).

Pollen Allergy

Controlled studies have shown that with an appropriate extract and schedule, SIT is effective in asthma caused by grass, ragweed, *Parietaria,* and birch pollen. However, the safety of SIT depends on the extract used. With highly effective standardized extracts, up to 20 percent of patients may experience systemic side effects. The duration of SIT is still a matter of debate, but it has been suggested that after a 3-year course, the effect of the treatment lasts for several years. SIT is therefore indicated when an adequate pharmacologic treatment is unable to control symptoms, when the pharmacologic treatment induces side effects, and/or when the pollen season is extended.

House Dust Mite Allergy

House dust immunotherapy should not be used any more. The efficacy of mite SIT in asthma has been assessed in many controlled studies. Standardized extracts are effective, but 5 to 30 percent of patients exposed to such treatment experience systemic reactions according to the protocol. With other extracts the results are more disparate. The duration of SIT with mite extracts is still a subject of debate but may require life-long treatment.

Allergy to Animal Proteins

Although it has been recommended by the Position Papers of the European Academy of Allergy and Clinical Immunology and World Health Organization-International Union of Immunological Societies (IUIS) that allergen avoidance is preferred to SIT in treating animal dander allergy, SIT may be an option, especially for occupational exposure, since it has been shown to be effective.

Allergy to Molds

Molds are major allergens in asthma, but most patients are polysensitized. Most extracts are not standardized yet. SIT using standardized extracts of *Alternaria* and *Cladosporium* has been shown to be effective. However, SIT with many mold species or with extracts of unknown quality should not be administered.

Immunotherapy with Other Extracts or Other Routes

Although SIT may be administered by oral or sublingual routes, more data are needed to confirm that these forms of administration are effective in asthma and to determine the candidates for SIT. Specific immunotherapy with extracts of undefined allergens (bacteria, foods, *Candida albicans,* insect dusts) should not be used any more.

Promising new developments of immunotherapy are currently being tested. They include the use of recombinant allergens, peptides derived from purified allergens, or nonspecific approaches such as anti-IgE monoclonal antibodies.

Pharmacotherapy

Classification of Antiasthma Medications

Medications for asthma are used to reverse and prevent symptoms and airflow limitation and have been classified by the World Health Organization/National Heart, Lung, and Blood Institute (WHO/NHLBI) technical report on asthma in controllers and relievers (Table 3).

Controllers. Controllers are medications shown to help keep persistent asthma under control. They include anti-inflammatory agents, which are the most effective controllers, and long-acting bronchodilators.

Corticosteroids are currently the most effective anti-inflammatory agents. When administered by the inhaled route for extended periods of time they can reduce the frequency of exacerbations, chronic symptoms, or bronchial hyper-responsiveness, and improve lung function. Systemic side effects may be observed, but

Table 2 Considerations for Initiating Immunotherapy in Allergic Asthma

1. Presence of a demonstrated IgE-mediated disease
   Positive skin tests and/or serum specific IgE
2. Documentation that specific sensitivity is involved in asthma symptoms
   Exposure to the allergen(s) determined by allergy testing based on symptoms
   If required, bronchial challenge with the relevant allergen(s)
3. Characterization of other triggers that may be involved in asthma symptoms
4. Severity and duration of asthma symptoms
   Subjective symptoms
   Objective parameters (e.g., work loss, school absenteeism)
   Pulmonary function (*essential*); EXCLUDE patients with severe asthma
   Monitoring of the pulmonary function by peak flow
5. Response of asthma symptoms to nonimmunologic treatment
   Response to allergen avoidance
   Response to pharmacotherapy
6. Availability of standardized or high quality extracts
7. Age of the patient
   Consider other treatment in
   Children >5 yr old
   Adults <50 yr old
8. Contraindications
   Treatment with β-blocker
   Other immunologic disease
   Inability of patients to comply
9. Sociologic factors
   Cost
   Occupation of candidate
   Asthma impairing quality of life despite adequate pharmacologic treatment
10. Objective evidence of efficacy of immunotherapy for the selected patient (availability of controlled clinical studies)

Table 3 Classification of Antiasthma Drugs

	Control of Chronic Asthma Symptoms Over Weeks to Months	*Relieve Exacerbations Over Minutes or Hours*	*Serious Side Effects*
Inhaled corticosteroids	+ + +	−	+†
Oral corticosteroids	+ +	+ + (over hrs)	+ + + (long term)
Cromoglycate	+	−	−
Nedocromil	+	−	−
Inhaled β_2-agonists			
Short-acting	±	+ + +	?
Long-acting	+ +	+ + +	?
Oral β_2-agonists	±	+ +	+
Theophylline			
Sustained released	+	+ +	+ + (short term)
Short acting	−	+ +	+ + (short term)
Inhaled anticholinergic	−	+ +	−
Ketotifen	+*	−	sedation
Immunotherapy	+	−	+ + (short term)

Modified from WHO/NHLBI. Global Strategy Management of Asthma; with permission.
*Applicable to children.
†Applicable to high doses.

their clinical relevance is still not established for daily doses under 1 mg of beclomethasone or budesonide or equivalent amounts of other agents. However, the risks of uncontrolled asthma appear to be more important than the likely limited risk of this form of treatment. Oral or systemic corticosteroids are highly effective but expose patients to serious side effects when administered for a long period of time. They are, however, needed in severe cases to control asthma symptoms.

Cromolyns (disodium cromoglycate and nedocromil sodium) are less potent as anti-inflammatory agents than corticosteroids but they have been shown to be effective in children with allergic asthma and in adults with mild persistent asthma. These drugs are sometimes called "antiallergic" agents but they also act on nonallergic asthma.

Long-acting beta$_2$-agonists and sustained-release theophylline are classified as controllers although their

	Intermittent	Mild persistent	Moderate persistent	Severe persistent
"Controllers"		• One daily anti-inflammatory medication (e.g.) low dose ICS or nedocromil or DSCG • Possibly add LA bronchodilator (especially if night symptoms)	• Daily anti-inflammatory medication: high dose ICS • And LA bronchodilator (especially if night symptoms)	• Multiple daily anti-inflammatory medication: high dose ICS • And LA bronchodilator (especially if night symptoms) • If necessary add oral CS
"Relievers"	• Intermittent reliever medication taken as needed: inhaled short-acting β_2-agonist • Intensity of treatment depends on severity of exacerbation: oral CS may be required	• Short-acting bronchodilator: inhaled β_2-agonist as needed for symptoms, do not exceed 3-4 times in one day • Intensity of treatment depends on severity of exacerbation: oral CS may be required	• Short-acting bronchodilator: inhaled β_2-agonist as needed for symptoms, do not exceed 3-4 times in one day • Intensity of treatment depends on severity of exacerbation: oral CS may be required	• Short-acting bronchodilator: inhaled β_2-agonist as needed for symptoms • Intensity of treatment depends on severity of exacerbation: oral CS may be required
Environmental control	Allergen avoidance + environmental control			
Specific immunotherapy	• Consider immunotherapy in seasonal asthma uncontrolled by medications	• Consider immunotherapy in perennial asthma depending on guidelines		• Usually DO NOT consider immunotherapy

Figure 2 Stepwise treatment of allergic asthma. *CS,* corticosteroids; *DSCG,* disodium cromoglycate; *ICS,* inhaled corticosteroids. (Modified from WHO/NHLBI. Global strategy management of asthma: World Health Organization. Publication number 95-3656, Jan 1995).

effect on inflammation appears to be weak (theophylline) or minimal (beta$_2$-agonists). Ketotifen has been found to have some efficacy in controlling childhood asthma. H_1-blockers are not recommended in the treatment of allergic asthma.

Relievers. Relievers are short-acting bronchodilating medications that act quickly to relieve bronchoconstriction and its accompanying acute symptoms such as cough, chest tightness, and wheezing. Bronchodilators principally act to dilate the airways by relaxing smooth muscle, but they do not reverse airways inflammation and hyper-responsiveness. Inhaled short-acting beta$_2$-agonists represent the treatment of choice for acute exacerbations of asthma. They are used as required to control episodic bronchoconstriction. Other relievers include inhaled anticholinergics, short-acting theophylline, and oral short-acting beta$_2$-agonists.

Route of Administration of Drugs

Medications for asthma can be administered by different routes but the inhaled route is preferred because the drug is directly delivered to the target organ, allowing for smaller doses to be administered. It has been observed that 200 μg of inhaled salbutamol are equivalent to an oral dose of 4,000 μg. The lower doses make it possible to reduce side effects and the first-pass hepatic metabolism of inhaled corticosteroids further increases the safety of this treatment. In addition, it appears that inhaled corticosteroids reduce bronchial hyper-responsiveness more than oral ones.

Stepwise Pharmacologic Treatment of Asthma

Although no cure for asthma has yet been found, it is reasonable to expect that in most patients with asthma, control of the disease should be achieved and maintained using a stepwise approach. The selection of pharmacologic treatment options should be based on asthma severity and the patient's current treatment (Fig. 2). Because asthma is a dynamic and chronic condition, medication plans need to accomodate variability among and within patients. An essential aspect of any treatment plan is the need to monitor the effect of the treatment and to adapt it as needed. Allergic asthma is exacerbated during allergen exposure; thus it is recommended that patients modify their treatment before the expected allergen exposure to better control asthma.

SUGGESTED READING

Bousquet J, Michel FB. Specific immunotherapy in asthma: Is it effective? J Allergy Clin Immunol 1994; 94:1–11.

Global strategy for asthma management and prevention. NHLBI/WHO workshop report. National Institute of Health. National Heart, Lung, and Blood Institute. Publication number 95-3656, Jan 1995.

Malling H. Position paper of the EAACI: Allergen standardization and skin tests. Methods of skin testing. Allergy 1993; 48(suppl 14):55–56.

National Institutes of Health. International Consensus Report on Diagnosis and Treatment of Asthma (Publication #92–3091). Bethesda, Md: US Department of Health and Human Services, 1992.

Platts-Mills TA, Thomas WR, Aalberse RC, et al. Dust mite allergens and asthma: Report of a second international workshop. J Allergy Clin Immunol 1992; 89:1046–1060.

Pope AM, Patterson R, Burge H. Indoor allergens. Assessing and controlling adverse health effects. Washington DC: National Academic Press, 1993.

ASTHMA IN ADULTS

PETER S. CRETICOS, M.D.

Asthma is a heterogeneous disease process in which both hereditary and environmental factors contribute to the development and expression of the clinical symptoms experienced by the patient. A variety of triggering factors can incite exacerbations of symptoms. Our perception of the disease is one with a spectrum of intermittent but mild symptoms to that of persistent symptoms with chronicity.

The National Heart, Lung, and Blood Institute (NHLBI) and World Health Organization (WHO) Global Initiatives for Asthma Workshop report defines asthma as "a chronic inflammatory disorder of the airways in which many cells play a role, in particular mast cells, eosinophils, and T lymphocytes. In susceptible individuals this inflammation causes recurrent episodes of wheezing, breathlessness, chest tightness, and cough particularly at night and/or in the early morning. These symptoms are usually associated with widespread but variable airflow limitation that is at least partly reversible either spontaneously or with treatment. The inflammation also causes an associated increase in airway responsiveness to a variety of stimuli."

The key to successful management of the asthmatic disease process is to treat the acute symptomatology and, most importantly, to suppress the underlying inflammatory component, resulting in a reduction in bronchial hyper-responsiveness, attenuation of diurnal variability with improvement in lung functions, and a reduction in the chronic symptoms of asthma.

DIAGNOSTIC APPROACH

The work-up of the asthmatic patient should include a thorough history, physical exam, and appropriate laboratory tests to corroborate the physician's clinical impression. Particular emphasis should center on the home setting, work site, occupational exposures, avocational interests, and other possible environmental influences. Asthma is one disease in which identification of the specific (allergic) triggering factor(s) and subsequent appropriate environmental manipulation to reduce exposure to the allergen burden can have a dramatic impact on the patient's disease process.

The strong association of allergy with asthma mandates an allergic evaluation of all patients with other than mild and intermittent symptoms. Skin testing to a panel of inhalant allergens relevant to the patient's geographic region provides immediate confirmation of (IgE-mediated) allergic sensitization, which correlates both with the frequency and the severity of the asthmatic's disease. An alternative to skin tests is blood testing (radioallergosorbent [RAST] testing) for specific IgE against appropriate allergens. As with any laboratory test, the findings need to be correlated with the clinical history to determine their clinical relevance.

THERAPEUTIC APPROACH

Successful management of the patient with allergic asthma requires an integrated approach that incorporates environmental control, the judicious use of an appropriate anti-inflammatory therapeutic agent to suppress the underlying inflammatory component, and supplemental use of a bronchodilator to treat "breakthrough" symptoms. Immunotherapy should be considered in those patients who have not responded to environmental and pharmacotherapeutic measures, who have had side effects with the medications, or who have persistent disease because of continuous exposure to allergens throughout the year (Table 1).

PATIENT EDUCATION

Indeed, a successful strategy for management of asthma necessitates a partnership between the patient and the health care team. Integral to this therapeutic approach is the "empowerment" of the patient in the development and implementation of any treatment strategy, which requires an appreciation of patient education as more than simple role memorization. Rather, it is a learning process in which the patient is an active participant in the management of his or her disease (Table 2). This involves helping the patient understand asthma, having the patient learn and practice the skills necessary to manage asthma, establishing an open communication channel for the patient with members of the health care team, and developing a joint treatment plan. This latter point cannot be overemphasized, since a disinterested or uninformed patient is apt to spell failure for any long-term management plan.

Table 1 Concepts in Preventive Therapy

Environmental control
"Primary" anti-inflammatory agent
Cromolyn/nedocromil
Inhaled corticosteroids
"Maintenance" bronchodilator
Long-acting β_2-agonists
Methylxanthines/theophyllines
"Rescue" bronchodilator
Short-acting β_2-agonists
Anticholinergics
Immunotherapy

From Creticos PS: Johns Hopkins Asthma and Allergy Center Press; with permission.

ENVIRONMENTAL CONTROL

Cigarette smoke, aerosol sprays, and cooking odors are important irritants capable of triggering an asthmatic's symptoms in the indoor environment. Even more critical to the asthmatic patient is the role of persistent exposure to perennial indoor allergens in inducing a smoldering asthmatic process (Table 3).

House dust mites, molds, cockroaches and other insects, and animals are the primary sources contributing to the indoor allergen burden. Proteinaceous particles from decaying body parts (dust mites, roaches), fecal emanations (dust mites, roaches), dander (animals), saliva (cats, roaches), and urinary protein (rodents, cats) represent the major allergen "load."

Those particles smaller than 10 μm in diameter can easily reach the lower respiratory tract and induce asthma symptoms. Our airtight homes with wall-to-wall carpeting, indoor pets, and central heating and ventilation systems are conducive to creating an indoor environment that ensures a patient is exposed to a constant allergen burden.

Table 2 Objectives of Patient Education

Helping patients understand their asthma
Learning and practicing the skills necessary to manage asthma
Positive feedback-imaging-behavior modification
Adherence to treatment plan

Table 3 Primary Allergens in Asthma

Perennial Allergens
Dust mites
Animals (e.g., cat)
Insects (e.g., cockroach)
Mold spores
Seasonal Allergens
Pollens
Trees
Grasses
Weeds
Molds

Measures to reduce the allergen burden in the indoor environment have been addressed in the chapter *Allergic Rhinitis*. To reiterate, the importance of dust mite control, animal avoidance, and insect eradication cannot be overstressed because the asthmatic's disease process can be significantly attenuated or even ablated through these measures.

Not to be overlooked is the importance of pollen allergens in inducing asthmatic symptoms. Intact pollen grains (e.g., ragweed pollen, 23 μm diameter) are too large to reach the lower airways. However, a significant amount of their "total allergenic activity" is not only attributable to intact pollen but also to pollen fragments (< 10 μm diameter) and microaerosol suspensions (3 to 7 μm diameter). The relevance of this is observed during the pollen season as millions of pollen grains settle to the ground; whereupon dew, rainfall, and humidity extract the relevant protein from the pollen grains, which then becomes airborne as microaerosol particles. A similar phenomenon occurs with mold in which soluble protein from the mold spores and mycelial elements is dispersed into the atmosphere.

PREVENTIVE ANTI-INFLAMMATORY THERAPY

Our recognition and understanding of the importance of inflammation in the asthmatic's disease process underscores the importance of employing a compound with anti-inflammatory properties as a primary therapeutic agent in the management of asthma. In this context, early therapeutic intervention should be aimed at suppressing mild but persistent symptoms with this primary anti-inflammatory agent in an attempt to prevent their escalation into a more moderate to severe disease process. Presently, nonsteroidal anti-inflammatory compounds (e.g., cromolyn, nedocromil) and synthetic glucocorticosteroids are choices to be considered by the physician.

Cromolyn

The compound, cromolyn, is a derivative of a naturally occurring antispasmodic extracted from a mediterranean weed. Cromolyn sodium has been demonstrated to be clinically efficacious in the management of seasonal allergic asthma, perennial allergic asthma, exercise-induced asthma, occupational asthma, and certain types of irritant-induced asthma. Its mechanisms are not completely understood, but it appears that one of its actions may be to stabilize mast cell membranes, inhibiting the subsequent release of inflammatory mediators. It also has been shown to interfere with the migration of eosinophils into the inflammatory site and to decrease the number of eosinophils and the concentration of eosinophilic inflammatory mediators (e.g., eosinophil cationic protein) in bronchial lavage fluids of treated asthmatics.

The most successful therapeutic approach with cromolyn is to employ the drug prophylactically, beginning 7 to 10 days prior to the allergen season. Because of cromolyn's safety profile, an aggressive approach to treatment can be ascribed to with an initial inhaled dose of two puffs (6,400 μg) four times daily being recommended (Table 4). Obviously, this necessitates patient compliance, but with a motivated patient instructed in the necessity of using the drug diligently in this early treatment phase, it may be possible to reduce this dosage to a regimen of two to three times a day for sustaining control of the patient's symptoms.

Table 4 Cromolyn: Recommended Dosages for Asthma Treatment

Route	*Dose/Actuation*	*Typical Dose*	*Total Dose*
MDI	800 μg	2-4 puffs q.i.d.	6.4-12.8 mg
Spinhaler	20 mg/cap	1 cap q.i.d.	80 mg
Nebulized	10 mg/ml	20 mg q.i.d.	80 mg

In symptomatic patients it is even more important to emphasize aggressive dosing of the drug, since it may be necessary to double the dose to two to four puffs four times daily during the first week or two of therapy to effect control. Furthermore, it may be necessary to extend treatment to 2 to 4 weeks before optimal efficacy occurs. Once control is achieved, it may be possible to taper the dosage to a more "user friendly" regimen that ensures patient compliance.

Clinical studies demonstrate that cromolyn-treated patients receiving 6,400 μg per day (two puffs four times daily) show improvement in daytime-nocturnal asthma, cough, peak expiratory flow, overall asthma symptoms, pulmonary function, and the need for supplemental bronchodilators. Comparative studies show cromolyn to be as efficacious as a bronchodilator in the management of asthma. However, the combination of cromolyn with a beta$_2$-agonist has been shown to result in better symptom control than cromolyn alone. Although theophylline provides similar clinical benefit, the low frequency of adverse effects associated with cromolyn represents a significant advantage in therapy.

The use of a spacer can further improve both drug delivery and clinical response in patients and a strong case can be made to employ a spacer in all cases in which inhaled cromolyn is prescribed. Likewise, the nebulized formulation of cromolyn can be employed to maintain therapeutic levels when and if a metered dose inhaler (MDI) cannot be continued. This is particularly useful in cases involving young children who cannot learn correct MDI technique, instances of severe lower airway inflammation (bronchitis, respiratory infection) that make an aerosol intolerable, or when intolerance to the aerosol propellent is a factor.

Nedocromil

Nedocromil is a nonsteroidal anti-inflammatory compound termed a pyronoquinoline (Table 5). It is a synthetically derived dicarbocylic acid with a tricyclic

Table 5 Nedocromil

Chemical class:
Pyranoquinoline
Mechanism of action:
Effects on activation of and mediator release from a variety of cells activity on neurogenic pathways
Clinical indication:
Mild to moderate asthma
Dosage:
2 puffs q.i.d. until symptoms under control; then, reduce to a maintenance dosage of 2 puffs b.i.d.

From Creticos PS: Johns Hopkins Asthma and Allergy Center Press; with permission.

ring backbone. These synthetic alterations have resulted in a compound with a broader spectrum of anti-inflammatory activity as compared to cromolyn. Studies have demonstrated that nedocromil has activity on a variety of cell types involved in the asthmatic cascade (eosinophils, neutrophils, epithelial cells, mast cells), inhibits inflammatory mediator release, and has a modulatory effect on neural pathways with implications on both the immediate and late phases of the asthmatic's clinical response. Clinical studies have demonstrated efficacy in seasonal and perennial asthma, cold air–induced, SO_2-induced, exercise-induced, and cough variant asthma.

In studies employing bronchoprovocation, nedocromil appears comparable to beclomethasone dipropionate (BDP) in reducing the underlying bronchial hyper-responsiveness of patients with mild to moderate asthma (Fig. 1). In this context, one of the more clinically relevant features of airway inflammation is a heightened diurnal variability in peak expiratory flow (PEF). Nedocromil has been shown to both attenuate this diurnal flux and improve overall lung function (FEV_1, PEF) when used on a regular daily basis.

In contrast, maintenance therapy with a short-acting beta$_2$-agonist (e.g., albuterol) neither results in a sustained improvement in PEF nor a reduction in the diurnal variability in peak flow. The relevance of this may be correlated with bronchoalveolar lavage studies showing that nedocromil inhibits the influx of inflammatory cells (e.g., eosinophils) into the lungs, whereas a bronchodilator (albuterol) does not.

In contrast to cromolyn, nedocromil given in a dose of two puffs (4 mg) four times daily results in improvement in asthma symptoms within days of initiating therapy (Fig. 2). For optimal control, the drug should be initiated at a dose of two puffs four times daily for the first 1 to 2 weeks of therapy to ensure suppression of the bronchial hyper-responsiveness, improve lung function, and reduce symptoms. Once control is established, then the drug should be reduced to a twice-a-day maintenance regimen of two to four puffs for sustaining control.

For chronic maintenance therapy, studies show nedocromil, 4 mg four times daily, to be comparable to low-dose inhaled corticosteroids (BDP $\leq$ 400 μg per day) and superior to maintenance bronchodilator therapy (albuterol, two puffs four times daily) in reducing daytime-nocturnal asthma, wheezing, shortness of breath, and/or cough. When added to maintenance theophylline (400 to 800 μg per day) nedocromil has been shown to result in further improvement in clinical symptoms and an ability to reduce and/or replace theophylline, with no loss of therapeutic effectiveness. Various studies have shown an added benefit when nedocromil has been added to a maintenance regimen of theophylline, beta$_2$-agonists, and inhaled corticosteroids. This may be particularly beneficial in allowing patients with moderate to severe asthma to reduce their total inhaled steroid requirements and yet maintain sustained control.

In direct comparison studies, nedocromil appears comparable to cromolyn in improving the asthmatic symptoms of patients with predominantly allergic asthma, but superior to cromolyn in treating predominantly nonallergic asthmatics.

In summary, nedocromil appears to represent a therapeutic agent with a broader spectrum of activity than cromolyn and, most importantly, a compound that can be reduced to a twice-a-day maintenance dosage for effective control. Its ease of administration and safety make it a reasonable choice for use in patients with mild to moderate asthma.

Inhaled Corticosteroids

Synthetic corticosteroids adapted for inhalation into the lungs have dramatically altered our approach to the treatment of asthma. Their ease of administration and their favorable risk-benefit ratio compared to oral steroids has made them the drug of choice for suppressing asthmatic inflammation.

Corticosteroids may act through several different mechanisms, including inhibition of cellular recruitment, arachidonic acid metabolism, mediator synthesis, restoration of beta$_2$-receptor responsivity, and down regulation of the effects of various inflammatory mediators on their target sites. The clinical relevance of these findings is demonstrated in properly performed provocation studies, which show that inhaled corticosteroids given for an adequate length of time block both the immediate and late phases of a (specific) allergen-induced challenge, reduce airway inflammation, and inhibit development of nonspecific airway reactivity (Fig. 3). Chronic administration results in a decrease in hyper-responsiveness to both specific (allergen) and nonspecific (irritant) stimuli.

As with the nonsteroidal anti-inflammatory preparations, prophylactic use of an inhaled steroid provides the best opportunity to prevent or disrupt the inflammatory cascade of asthma. In this context, therapy should be started 5 to 7 days prior to allergen exposure and maintained through the ensuing season. Adjustments in dosage can be made based on assessment of clinical symptoms and peak expiratory flow rates.

In symptomatic patients, judicious adherence to the treatment regimen is necessary starting with an initial dose adequate to bring symptoms under control and then tapered as tolerated to the lowest effective dose that

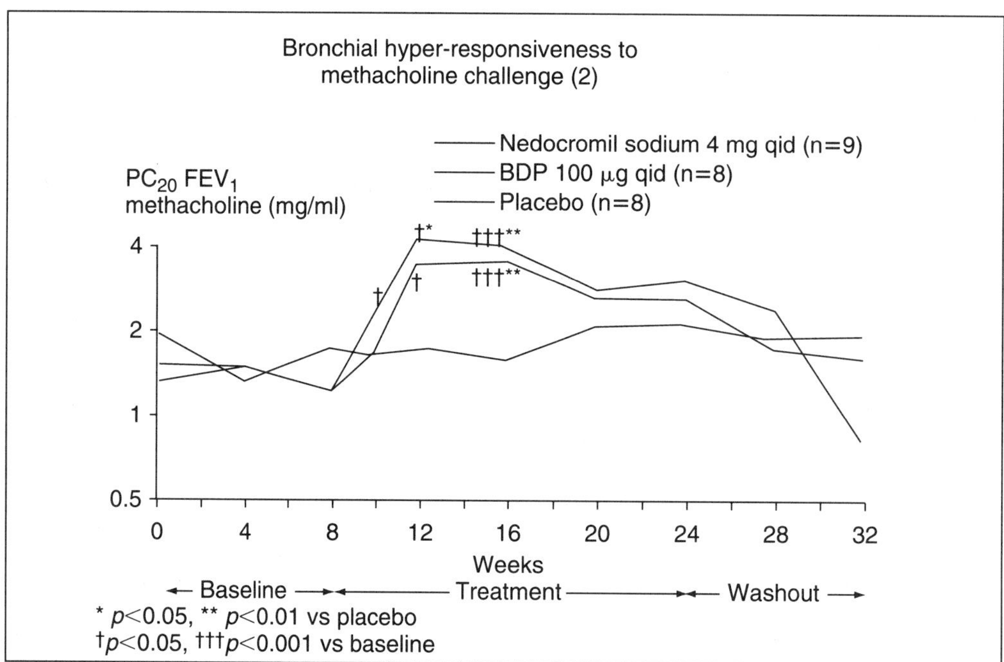

Figure 1 A second study carried out by Bel and Sterk in Holland showed a comparable reduction in bronchial hyper-responsiveness (BHR) (methacholine $PC_{20}FEV_1$) with nedocromil sodium (4 mg q.i.d.) and BDP (100 μg q.i.d.) during 16 weeks' treatment in 25 patients with intrinsic asthma previously controlled on inhaled bronchodilators. BHR decreased significantly after 4 ($p < 0.05$) and 8 ($p < 0.01$) weeks' treatment. (From Bel EH, et al. The long term effects of nedocromil sodium and beclomethasone diproprionate on bronchial responsiveness to methacholine in nonatopic asthmatic subjects. Am Rev Respir Dis 1990; 141:21–28; with permission.)

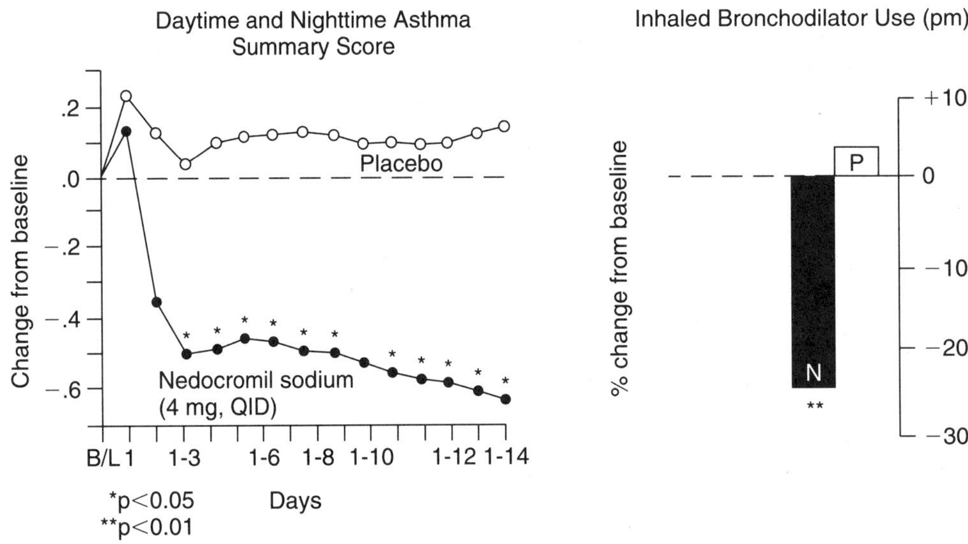

Figure 2 Change from baseline of cumulative mean asthma symptom summary scores and, as required, inhaled bronchodilator use for treatment weeks 1 and 2 (when nedocromil sodium was added to maintenance bronchodilator therapy). After a 2-week baseline period, patients maintained on sustained-release theophylline or oral β_2-agonist bronchodilators were randomized to receive 4 mg nedocromil sodium (n = 60) or placebo (n = 61) four times a day, for 16 weeks. *Closed circles* indicate nedocromil sodium *(N); open circles* indicate placebo *(P)*. Statistically significant differences (*$p < 0.05$, **$p < 0.01$) favoring nedocromil sodium were determined from days 1 to 3 onward. The use of as-required inhaled bronchodilator decreased in the nedocromil sodium group and increased slightly in the placebo group during the 2-week analysis period. (Modified from Cherniack RM, et al. A double blind multicenter group comparative study of the efficacy and safety of nedocromil sodium in the management of asthma. Chest 1990; 97:1299–1306.)

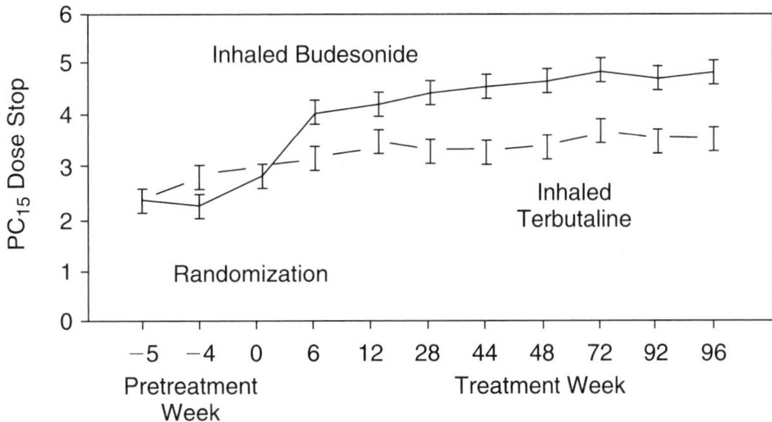

Figure 3 β_2-agonists and bronchial hyper-responsiveness. (From Haahtela T, et al. Comparison of a beta$_2$-agonist terbutaline, with an inhaled corticosteroid, budesonide, in newly detected asthma. N Engl J Med 1991; 325:388–392; with permission.)

Table 6 Inhaled Corticosteroid Preparations

Compound	*Dose/Actuation*	*Typical Dosage*	*Total Dose*
Beclomethasone (Vanceril/ Beclovent)	50 μg	2-4 p q.i.d.	400 μg-800 μg
Flunisolide (AeroBid)	250 μg	2-4 p b.i.d.	1,000 μg-2,000 μg
Triamcinolone (Azmacort)	[200] 100 μg	2-4 p q.i.d.	800 μg-1,600 μg
Budesonide* (Pulmicort)	200 μg	2-4 p b.i.d.	200 μg-1,600 μg
Fluticasone* (Flovent)	100/200 μg	1-2 p b.i.d.	200 μg-1,000 μg

*Not yet approved in the U.S.; *p*, Puff.

sustains symptom control during the maintenance phase of therapy. This dose must be adequate to suppress the underlying inflammatory component, improve pulmonary function, and reduce the frequency and severity of symptoms.

Table 6 lists the topical inhaled corticosteroid preparations available in the U.S. market along with their dosing schedule. The NHLBI guidelines have given us a handle on the therapeutic approach to patients based on the severity of their disease. With this in mind, a reasonable approach for control of mild (200 to 400 μg per day), moderate (400 to 800 μg per day), and severe asthma (>800 μg per day) can be constructed.

Implicit in these suggestions is the importance of beginning therapy with a maximally recommended dose over the first 1 to 2 weeks in order to bring the inflammatory process under control quickly (800 to 1,500 μg per day), and then to reduce this to the lowest dose that still provides adequate therapeutic control (≈200 to 800 μg per day).

As with cromolyn, the key to success with inhaled corticosteroid therapy is patient compliance. Thus, dosing frequency and the number of doses (puffs) required to achieve effective control become important factors. Toogood's early studies of BDP suggested that dosing four times daily was the most efficient approach. Once control is achieved, twice-daily dosing may provide equal therapeutic benefit, especially with inhanced patient compliance. However, therapy needs to be individualized based on the patient's appreciation of symptom control, PEF readings, and periodic spirometric measurements.

A difficult issue in the United States has been the relationship of dosage among the various inhaled corticosteroid preparations. No direct clinical comparisons have been done between the three preparations presently available in the United States. However, two inhaled steroid preparations, budesonide and fluticasone, neither yet commercially available in the United States, have been extensively studied. Comparative studies of budesonide with beclomethasone have shown comparable efficacy of the two compounds at lower (400 μg per day) and higher (1,500 μg per day) dosage comparisons. The improved risk:benefit ratio of budesonide suggests that it may allow up to a 30 percent higher dosing before comparable effects on adrenal suppression are observed. Likewise, fluticasone should also improve our therapeutic armamentarium, since it appears that 30 to 40 percent less of a dose may confer a similar degree of clinical response.

The importance of this finding is in the treatment of more moderate to severe asthma where dosages of greater than or equal to 800 μg per day may be frequently necessitated. The difficulty with BDP (50 μg per puff) is that patients are unlikely to administer 20 to 30 puffs per day (1,000 to 1,500 μg per day) for any reasonable period of time. Therefore, formulations that can deliver 200 to 250 μg per puff and provide reasonable assurance of comparability on a microgram-to-microgram basis will dramatically improve our ability to manage the more difficult asthmatic.

The question of the safety of topical steroids becomes a relevant issue, especially if higher dosage therapy is required. Systemic toxicity with adrenal axis suppression, growth retardation, osteoporosis, and cataracts have all been reported with daily oral prednisone and alternate-day oral prednisone. At issue is whether these effects are likely to be seen with higher dosages of inhaled corticosteroids. Studies now provide a reasonable level of comfort in both children and adults with respect to these adverse events. The data suggest that adrenal suppression is not likely to be encountered in children until a dosage of greater than 800 μg per day is administered, and in adults at a dose greater than 1,200 μg per day. Likewise, short-term studies of growth in asthmatic children suggest that a dosage of greater than or equal to 800 μg per day of budesonide would be required before any evidence of clinically relevant growth retardation may appear (Fig. 4). Further studies are required to address the issue of whether clinically relevant findings are observed at doses of 400 to 800 μg per day of beclomethasone.

A few reported cases of posterior, subcapsular cataracts have been reported in patients taking inhaled steroids, but this risk appears to be directly related to the previous use of oral corticosteroids in these patients and not to the specific use of the inhaled steroid preparation. Local side effects attributable to topical steroid therapy include oral candidiasis, hoarseness, and dysphonia. Simply instructing the patient to rinse out the mouth after use of the inhaled steroid can minimize fungal overgrowth. Use of a spacer device with the inhaler can also obviate this concern.

As previously mentioned, the use of a spacer can further improve both drug delivery and clinical response in patients. Thus, the use of a spacer should be the first manipulation attempted in patients not demonstrating satisfactory results before considering the addition of an additional therapeutic agent. In fact, a strong case can be made for the use of a spacer device in any patient placed on a primary anti-inflammatory therapeutic agent. In this regard, further studies that address spacer design, optimal particle size, and respirable fraction delivered to the lungs would further our progress in this area.

Bronchodilator Therapy

Preventive therapy is the desirable approach to the management of asthma. However, sympathomimetic bronchodilators are important adjunctive medicines for relief of acute symptoms or for the treatment of breakthrough symptoms in a patient already on a maintenance primary anti-inflammatory drug.

In essence, the need for bronchodilator use should be considered as an "early warning signal" for the asthmatic. That is, if a patient's asthma symptoms begin to increase in frequency or if the patient begins to note the need for a bronchodilator on a more frequent basis (>3 days in a week), then that should be an indication of worsening asthma. Steps should then be taken to identify the basis for the worsening of the asthmatic condition. In a patient who is not already on a primary anti-inflammatory agent, this would be an indication that such a drug should be started. If a patient is already on a primary anti-inflammatory agent, then the dosage of that compound should be doubled. Subsequent adjustment to the medication regimen should be based on the therapeutic response to these initial manipulations.

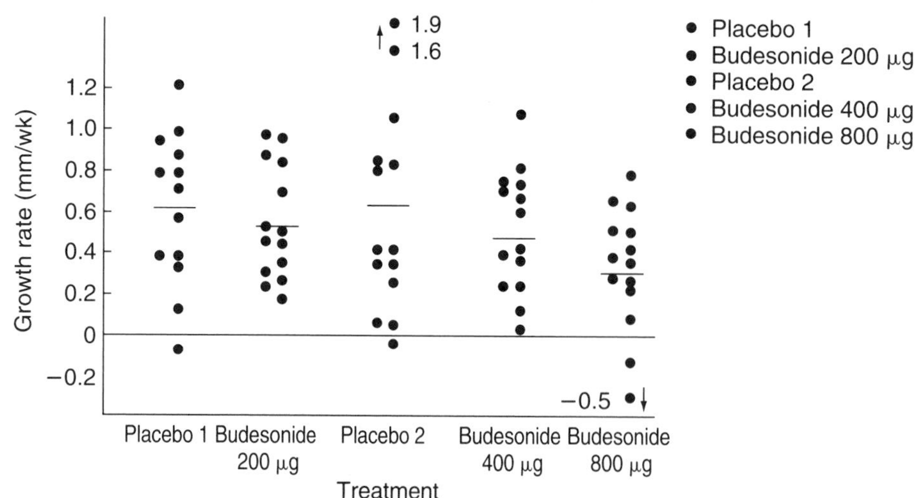

Figure 4 Effects of inhaled steroids on linear growth. (Modified from Wolthers DH, et al. Growth of asthmatic children during treatment with budesonide: A double blind trial. BMJ 1991; 303:163–165.)

Maintenance Bronchodilators

Salmeterol

The recent introduction of salmeterol has provided the option of employing this long-acting, inhaled $beta_2$ sympathomimetic drug for maintenance control of asthma and prevention of bronchospasm, control of nocturnal asthma, and prevention of exercise-induced asthma (Table 7). The primary place for this therapeutic agent is in patients already maintained on a primary anti-inflammatory drug for whom addition of a "maintenance bronchodilator" would optimize control. In this context, the addition of salmeterol could obviate the need for increasing the corticosteroid dose in a less than optimally controlled patient, thus improving the risk: benefit ratio of the total drug therapy regimen.

This drug is also an appropriate therapeutic choice for control of nocturnal asthma, where the longer duration of action would provide reasonable control for a majority of patients. In contrast, short-acting bronchodilators (3- to 4-hour duration) would not be expected to provide an adequate duration of coverage through the evening hours. This would also be a superior choice in patients with gastroesophageal reflux where use of theophylline would further aggravate lower esophageal sphincter pressure and result in worsening reflux.

The final indication for this agent is in exercise-induced asthma. Indeed, because of its longer duration of action, it may provide protection against several different exercise events during a 10- to 12-hour period.

The normal dosage range is one to two puffs (42 μg per puff) twice a day. Patients should be cautioned not to exceed a twice-daily dosing frequency because the prolonged half-life of the drug may result in an exaggerated pharmacologic response with tremor, muscle cramps, headache, or adverse cardiovascular events. Furthermore, the drug should never be used to relieve acute symptoms of bronchospasm. In that regard, a short-acting selective $beta_2$ agent should be used for relief of breakthrough symptoms in a patient already on maintenance therapy with salbutamol.

Long-Acting Theophylline Preparations

Theophylline therapy has been a cornerstone of asthma therapy through the years. As with beta-adrenergic sympathomimetic agents, theophylline appears to exert its primary influence through relaxation of smooth muscle of the bronchial tree by inhibiting the breakdown of the enzyme phosphodiesterase with a resultant increase in cAMP concentrations, which results in smooth muscle cell relaxation.

As emphasized, our current approach to the treatment of asthma involves the aggressive use of an inhaled preventive therapeutic agent. As a result, theophylline is now viewed as an adjunctive, albeit important, therapeutic agent in those asthmatic patients whose condition is not easily controlled by the use of inhaled nedocromil or inhaled corticosteroids supplemented by an inhaled $beta_2$-selective sympathomimetic agent. This current strategy reflects not only the appreciated superior anti-inflammatory properties of these preventive inhaled agents but also the toxic effects associated with theophylline therapy.

In view of the small margin between therapeutic effects and toxicity, individualization of dose is mandatory with theophylline therapy (Table 8). The use of sustained-release long-acting (once or twice daily) preparations has improved this aspect of care because of the more consistent theophylline-release characteristics, which provide more consistent plasma concentration with less-marked peak-trough variation. In this regard, it is important not to switch among various preparations because significant differences in serum blood levels may result because of the differences in absorption characteristics among preparations from different manufacturers.

The new once-a-day sustained-release products may

Table 7 Salmeterol

Entity
Long-acting β-agonist
Dosage
2 puffs (42 μg) b.i.d.
CX Uses
Maintenance treatment of asthma and prevention of bronchospasm
Prevention of nocturnal asthma
Prophylaxis against exercise-induced asthma
Contraindications
Not for relief of acute asthma symptoms
Do not exceed 2 puffs b.i.d. dosage

Table 8 Factors Affecting Theophylline Blood Levels

Conditions Increasing Theophylline Blood Levels
Older age (>50 years)
Obesity
Liver disease
Congestive heart failure
Chronic obstructive pulmonary disease
Acute viral infections
High-carbohydrate, low-protein diet
Influenza A vaccine
Drug use
Troleandomycin
Erythromycin preparations
Allopurinol
Cimetidine
Propranolol hydrochloride
Conditions Decreasing Theophylline Blood Levels
Young age (1-16 years)
Cigarette smoking
Eating charcoal-broiled meat
Low-carbohydrate, high-protein diet
Drug use
Phenobarbital
Phenytoins
Isoproterenol hydrochloride

From Kaliner M, Eggleston PA, Mathews KP. Primer on allergic and immunologic diseases, Ch 3: Rhinitis and asthma. JAMA 1987; 258:2851-2873. Copyright 1987, American Medical Association; with permission.

be most useful in the subset of asthmatics with nocturnal symptoms who otherwise find it difficult to sleep through the night because of the short duration of activity of classic sympathomimetic agents.

Rescue Bronchodilators

Short-Acting Selective Beta$_2$-Agonists

Sympathomimetic bronchodilators have become a mainstay in the therapeutic approach to the treatment of asthma. These agents are the drug of choice for relief of acute bronchospasm. They are used effectively alone for the treatment of mild or intermittent asthma symptoms, and they are also effective in preventing or reversing exercise-induced asthma. Table 9 lists the various catecholamine and noncatecholamine compounds that are available. Improved beta$_2$-selectivity and increased duration of action are seen with the majority of the noncatecholamine derivatives.

The therapeutic effects of beta-adrenergic agents include bronchodilatation as a result of activation of a cell membrane's adenylate cyclase enzyme, which converts ATP to cAMP, resulting in sequestration of intracellular calcium. This leads to relaxation of smooth muscle; increased ciliary movement, which should improve clearance of secretions; and stabilizing effects on the mast cell to decrease mediator release. However, in regard to this last action, provocation studies demonstrate that beta-adrenergic agents can effectively ablate the immediate asthmatic response but have no demonstrable clinical effect on the late phase of airway reactivity.

Selective beta$_2$-agonists provide better bronchodilation than do the theophylline products in both the acute and chronic state. Furthermore, the addition of aminophylline to maximum-dose inhaled beta-agonist therapy provides no further improvement in the bronchodilator response. However, in chronic therapy, receptor subsensitivity may develop. This has led to considerable discussion as to whether these agents should be administered on a regular (four times daily) maintenance dosage schedule, which again reinforces the approach that a short-acting beta$_2$ agent should be used on an as-needed basis for relief of acute symptoms. Typical dosing is one to two puffs every 4 to 6 hours because it is needed for relief of breakthrough asthma symptoms. However, it should again be reiterated that these drugs should not be overused. Their increased need should signal the need to address the underlying trigger of the asthmatic exacerbation and to make appropriate adjustments in the patient's primary anti-inflammatory regimen.

Another important point to emphasize is the proper administration of the aerosol. Careful demonstration of inhaler technique by the physician, nurse, or patient educator is mandatory and often requires repeated reinforcement. Several techniques for delivery are satisfactory, but most investigators would suggest discharging the inhaler when it is 1 to 1½ inches (two fingers) away from the open mouth (open-mouth technique). The patient should then take a slow, deep inspiration (from functional residual capacity to total lung capacity) and then hold the breath for 8 to 10 seconds. This technique improves deposition and can result in nearly doubling the amount of medication reaching the lower respiratory tract. In patients with poor technique, delivery can be improved by employing a spacer. Typically, 2 to 3 minutes should lapse between the first and second puffs from an aerosol bronchodilator, so that the maximal bronchodilating effect of the first puff can allow better penetration of the second puff.

Certainly, with the environmental concerns related to ozone depletion as a result of extensive industrial use of CFCs, the development of non-CFC and powder formulations of selected beta$_2$-agonist preparations has resulted in several new formulations that should be available soon. These may also be advantageous for patients prone to irritant effects of a freon-metered device.

Table 9 β-Adrenergic Agonists for Inhalation

*Drug**	*Selectivity†*	*Onset of Action (minutes)*	*Peak Action (minutes)*	*Duration (hours)*
Catecholamines				
Epinephrine (Primatene, 0.2 mg/p)	α_1, β_1, β_2	2-7	15-20	0.5
Isoproterenol (Isuprel, 0.125 mg/p)	β_1, β_2	2-5	5	1.5-2
Isoetharine (Bronkometer, 0.34 mg/p)	β_2	2-5	15	1.5-2
Noncatecholamines				
Bitolterol (Tornalate, 0.37 mg/p)	β_2+	3-5	30-60	4-8
Metaproterenol (Alupent, 0.65 mg/p)	β_2+ +	5-10	120-180	3-4
Terbutaline (Brethaire, 0.25 mg/p)	β_2+ + +	5-10	90-120	3-4
Albuterol (Proventil, Ventolin, 0.09 mg/p)	β_2+ + +	5-15	60-90	4-6
Pirbuterol (Maxair, 0.2 mg/p)	β_2+ + +	3-5	30-60	4-6

**p*, Puff; Usual doses are 1-2 p every 4-6 hours; bitolterol, 2-3 p every 6-8 hours; metaproterenol, 2-3 p every 4 hours.
†+ = low selectivity; + + = moderate selectivity; + + + = high selectivity.
Adapted from P.S. Creticos. In Smith and Reynard: Drug Therapy of Asthma, Textbook of Pharmacology, Philadelphia: WB Saunders.

Oral beta-agonist preparations are available, but inhalation delivers more of the active drug directly to the mucosal surface and, at the same time, minimizes side effects. Oral therapy may be useful in certain situations (e.g., acute viral infection) in which airway irritation prevents the comfortable use of an inhaled therapeutic agent. Side effects associated with beta-agonist therapy include tremor; nervousness; and, with higher doses of even the selective $beta_2$-agents, palpitations or tachycardia.

Anticholinergic Agents

The parasympathetic nervous system appears to play a prominent role in cold air–induced asthma, SO_2-induced asthma, and cough-variant asthma. This may be a reflection of direct neural (parasympathetic) activity, reflex cholinergic bronchoconstriction, or the interplay between neural mechanisms and inflammatory mediators.

Ipratropium has been shown to be effective in reducing the cholinergic hyper-reactivity present in many patients with chronic bronchitis, emphysema, and asthma. It is administered as a metered dose inhalation of two puffs every 6 hours as needed. Although the therapeutic response obtained with ipratropium is comparable to albuterol in terms of its bronchodilating effect (increase in FEV_1), its onset of action is considerably slower (15 to 30 minutes).

Immunotherapy

Numerous studies with pollens (weeds, grasses, trees), animal allergens, and dust mites support the efficacy of immunotherapy in treating allergic rhinitis. However, only a few well-controlled studies evaluating the role of immunotherapy in treating patients with allergic asthma have been carried out.

Studies employing bronchial provocation with specific allergens (e.g., cat and/or dust mites) have demonstrated the ability to significantly shift the $PD_{20}FEV_1$ (ten-fold to 100-fold) in patients immunized with an optimal dose of standardized extract. Most recently, a major study of the role of immunotherapy in adults with seasonal ragweed-induced asthma demonstrated improvement in the ragweed-immunized patients both in clinical endpoints (fewer symptoms, decreased medication usage, increased PEF readings) and in objective parameters (a reduction in skin test sensitivity, decreased bronchial responsivity to ragweed upon bronchial provocation, a rise in specific IgG ragweed antibodies, and a blunting of the usual seasonal rise in IgE ragweed antibodies). As in ragweed-induced allergic rhinitis, this study of ragweed allergic asthmatics again demonstrates that clinical success hinges upon the use of an appropriate therapeutic dose.

SUGGESTED READING

Barnes PJ. A new approach to the treatment of asthma. N Engl J Med 1989; 321:1517–1526.

Barnes PJ. Inhaled glucocorticoids for asthma. In: Wood AJJ, ed. Drug therapy. N Engl J Med 1995; 332(13):868–875.

Bel EH, et al. The long term effects of nedocromil sodium and beclomethasone dipropionate on bronchial responsiveness to methacholine in nonatopic asthmatic subjects. Am Rev Respir Dis 1990; 141:21–28.

Cherniack RM. A double blind multicenter group comparative study of the efficacy and safety of nedocromil sodium in the management of asthma. Chest 1990; 97:1299–1306.

Djukanovic, et al. Effect of an inhaled corticosteroid on airway symptoms in asthma. Am Rev Respir Dis 1992; 145:669–674.

Haahtela T, et al. Comparison of a B_2-agonist, terbutaline, with an inhaled corticosteroid, budesonide, in newly detected asthma. N Engl J Med 1991; 325(6):388–392.

National Institutes of Health. Global Initiative for Asthma. Global strategy for asthma management and prevention NHLBI/WHO workshop report (NIH publication # 95–3659). Bethesda, Md: US Department of Health and Human Services, Jan 1995.

National Institutes of Health. National Asthma Education Program Expert Panel Report. Executive summary: Guidelines for the diagnosis and management of asthma (NIH publication # 91–3042A). Bethesda, Md: US Department of Health and Human Services, June 1991.

Pearlman DS, et al. A comparison of salmeterol with albuterol in the treatment of mild-to-moderate asthma. N Engl J Med 1992; 327(20):1420–1425.

Petty TL. Cromolyn sodium is effective in adult chronic asthmatics. Am Rev Respir Dis 1989; 694–701.

Sears, et al. Regular inhaled beta-agonist treatment in bronchial asthma. Lancet 1990; 336:1391–1396.

Wolthers OH, et al. Growth of asthmatic children during treatment with budesonide: A double blind trial. BMJ 1991; 303:163–165.

CHILDHOOD ASTHMA

ROBERT F. LEMANSKE Jr., M.D.
JAMES E. GERN, M.D.

EPIDEMIOLOGY

Asthma is the most common chronic lower respiratory tract illness in children. The prevalence of morbidity and mortality associated with asthma appears to be increasing throughout the world, and these trends appear to be particularly notable for children and young adults. In the United States, minority populations tend to be at highest risk of adverse outcomes potentially related to poverty, poor access to health care, and environmental factors (e.g., allergen [mite and cockroach] and smoke exposure, viral infections). Therefore, the combination of minority status and youth obviously forms a high-risk group. The morbidity related to asthma in children involves not only the traumatic experiences associated with emergency department visits and hospitalizations, but school absenteeism and the stigmata inherent with chronic disease in this age group as well. It is important to realize that asthma-related mortality is increasing, particularly in the high-risk groups mentioned above, and that these deaths are occurring despite the availability of medications that should attenuate these alarming trends.

DEFINITION

Asthma is more of a syndrome than a specific disease entity and involves the following characteristics: *airway obstruction* (or airway narrowing) that is reversible (but not completely so in some patients) either spontaneously or with treatment, *airway inflammation,* and *airway hyper-responsiveness* to a variety of different stimuli (Fig. 1). The airway obstruction in asthma is related to both bronchial smooth muscle constriction as well as airway edema, mucous secretion, and inflammation. Extensive histopathologic changes, including airway mucous plugging, epithelial cell disruption, eosinophil infiltration, and smooth muscle hypertrophy or hyperplasia are demonstrable in patients dying in status asthmaticus; interestingly, similar, albeit less intensive changes, can be seen in patients whose symptoms are acceptably controlled with intermittent bronchodilator therapy. The relationship of these inflammatory changes to age, triggering factors, and drug therapy are currently under intense study.

An important physiologic feature of asthma is the presence of airway hyper-responsiveness or so-called twitchy airways. This feature can be demonstrated following bronchoprovocation with exercise or methacholine. Patients with a variety of other conditions such as allergic rhinitis, cystic fibrosis, or chronic bronchitis, and relatives of asthmatics can also exhibit airway hyper-responsiveness but, in general, patients with asthma appear to be the most sensitive to these types of challenges.

The main symptoms of asthma include wheezing, coughing, and shortness of breath related to one or a combination of various triggering factors, including allergen exposure, exercise, respiratory tract infections, irritant exposure (e.g., changes in temperature or humidity, strong odors, tobacco smoke), certain drugs (e.g., aspirin and other nonsteroidal anti-inflammatory agents), strong emotions (e.g., laughing or crying), and gastroesophageal reflux. It should be emphasized that not all patients with asthma wheeze; many children may present only with a troublesome chronic cough, usually worse at night.

THERAPY OVERVIEW

As one might anticipate, therapy for asthma is directed towards relieving bronchial smooth muscle constriction with the use of bronchodilators, attenuating the inflammatory component with anti-inflammatory agents, and decreasing airway hyper-responsiveness. Appropriate therapeutic strategies should employ education (patient, family, teachers, co-workers), environmental control, medications, and a means of monitoring disease activity to gauge either the severity of an acute exacerbation or the response to therapy over time (e.g., home peak flow monitoring). Thus, whenever possible, a partnership arrangement among physician, nurse, pharmacist, patient, family, school, and work personnel should be formed to optimize chronic therapy and to develop and administer acute intervention strategies. The overall goals of therapy are listed in Table 1.

THERAPEUTIC OPTIONS

Environmental Control

Allergen or irritant exposure can produce acute problems, and chronic exposure can diminish overall disease control. Indoor pollutants such as tobacco smoke and wood burning stoves increase asthmatic symptoms in children, and maternal smoking during infancy is a risk factor for the persistence of asthmatic symptoms and attenuation of pulmonary function into childhood. In genetically predisposed individuals, chronic exposure to allergens such as house dust mites and pets can augment airway hyper-responsiveness and, depending on the level of exposure, induce acute asthmatic episodes as well. Thus, an allergy consultation should be part of the evaluation of any child over 2 to 3 years of age with chronic asthma. Once specific identification of important allergens has been established, environmental control measures should be instituted (Table 2).

Supported by NIH Grants #AI34891, AI00995, HL51843, M01 RR03186.

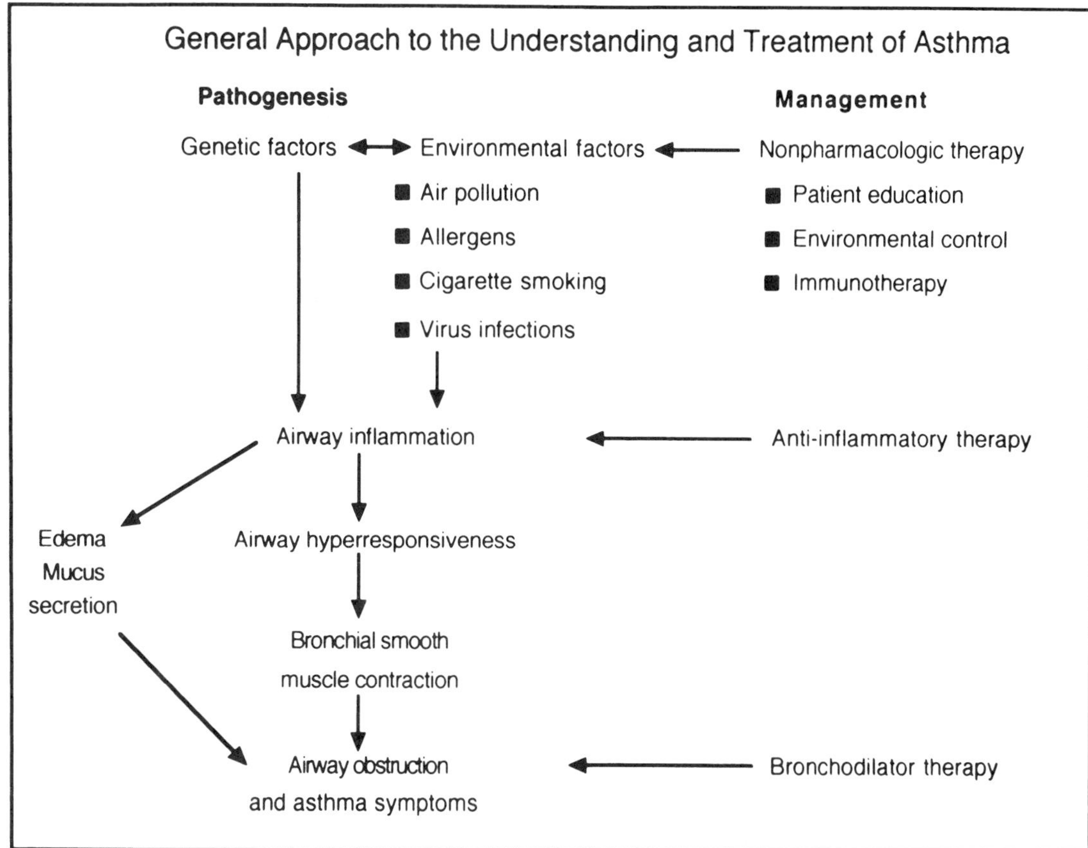

Figure 1 Pathogenesis of asthma symptoms. (Modified from National Asthma Education Program [NAEP], National Institutes of Health. Guidelines for the diagnosis and management of asthma [NIH publication #91–3042]. Bethesda, Md: US Department and Human Services, 1991.)

Table 1 Goals of Asthma Therapy

Maintain normal activity levels (including exercise)
Maintain (near) "normal" pulmonary function rates
Prevent chronic and troublesome symptoms (e.g., coughing or breathlessness in the night, in the early morning, or after exertion)
Prevent recurrent exacerbations of asthma
Avoid adverse effects from asthma medications

From National Asthma Education Program. Guidelines for the diagnosis and management of asthma (NIH publication #91-3042). Bethesda, Md, US Dept. of Health and Human Services, 1991; with permission.

Table 2 Control Measures for Indoor Allergens

Pets
Find pets a new home, or keep them outdoors
If pets "cannot" be removed from the home,
Wash cats or dogs weekly
Keep them out of the bedroom
House Dust Mites
Encase the mattress in an airtight cover
Either encase the pillow or wash it weekly
Wash the bedding in water of 130° F weekly
Avoid sleeping or lying on upholstered furniture
If possible, remove carpets from bedroom and play areas
Maintain relative humidity <50%
Molds
Remove carpets laid over cement slab
Ensure adequate ventilation for bathroom areas
Use dehumidifiers in basement areas to reduce humidity <50%
Encase pillows or wash weekly to discourage mold growth

MEDICATIONS

Overall Approach

The selection of medications for asthma treatment are influenced by a number of factors. First, some patients develop asthma symptoms only in response to well-defined triggers. For example, children who develop wheezing and coughing exclusively with viral infections may only need to be treated during these isolated episodes. Bronchospasm only related to certain running sports could be treated with premedication alone. Second, the age of the patient influences the choice of a drug delivery system, as well as compliance with prescribed therapy. In children, the taste of medication is an obvious important consideration. Children under 5 years of age may not be able to use a metered dose inhaler

Table 3 Dosage for Maintenance Therapy in Childhood Asthma

Bronchodilators
Beta agonists
Inhaled
Examples albuterol, metaproterenol, terbutaline, pirbuterol, bitolterol
Mode of Administration
Metered dose inhaler, 2 puffs q4-6h
Powder inhaler device, 1 capsule q4-6h (albuterol)
Nebulizer solution
Albuterol 5 mg/ml, 0.1-0.15 mg/kg in 2 ml saline q4-6h maximum 5.0 mg
Metaproterenol 50 mg/ml, 0.25-0.50 mg/kg in 2 ml of saline q4-6h maximum 15.0 mg
Oral
Liquids
Albuterol 0.1-0.15 mg/kg q4-6h (maximum 4 mg)
Metaproterenol 0.3-0.5 mg/kg q4-6h (maximum 10 mg)
Tablets
Albuterol 2-4 mg q4-6h; 4 or 8 mg sustained-release albuterol q12h
Metaproterenol 10-20 mg q4-6h
Terbutaline 2.5-5.0 mg q4-6h
Theophylline
(Dosage is based on serum level. Dosage to achieve serum concentration of 5-15 μg/ml)
Liquids
Tablets, capsules (caution: pharmacokinetics of different brands may vary considerably)
Sustained release tablets, capsules (dosing interval [q/d vs b.i.d. vs t.i.d.] will depend on product formulation and rate of metabolism)
Ipratropium bromide
Metered dose inhaler (18 μg/puff), 2 puffs q.i.d.
Nebulizer solution (250 μg/ml)
Ages 3-12 yrs 100-500 μg q8h
>12 yrs 250-500 μg q8h

Anti-inflammatory Agents
Anti-allergic compounds
Cromolyn sodium
MDI, 1 mg/puff 2 puffs b.i.d. to q.i.d.
Nebulizer solution 20 mg/2 ml ampule; 1 ampule b.i.d. to q.i.d.
Nedocromil sodium
MDI, 1.75 mg/puff 2 puffs b.i.d. to q.i.d.
Glucocorticoids
Inhaled Preparations

Glucocorticoid	*μg per Inhalation*	*Usual Starting Dose and Interval*	*Maximum Dose (puff/day)*	
			Ages 6-12	*Ages >12*
Beclomethasone dipropionate	42	2-4 puffs b.i.d. to q.i.d.	10	20
Triamcinolone acetonide	100*	2-4 puffs b.i.d. to q.i.d.	12	16
Flunisolide	250	2-4 puffs b.i.d.	4	8

*200 μg per actuation, but 100 μg retained in spacer

Oral Preparations*†
Liquids
Prednisone 5 mg/5 ml
Prednisolone
5 mg/5 ml
15 mg/5 ml
Tablets
Prednisone 1, 5, 10, 20, 50 mg
Methylprednisolone 2, 4, 8, 16, 24, 32 mg

*Burst therapy 1-2 mg/kg/day split b.i.d. to t.i.d. for 5-7 days.
†Maintenance therapy, lowest daily dose, alternate day whenever possible.

(MDI) correctly, even with a spacing device. In this age group, medications may be delivered using a home nebulizer; however, not all medications (e.g., inhaled corticosteroids) can be delivered in this manner. Convincing adolescent patients to use preventative medications can be a challenging problem. Third, the symptom pattern (intermittent versus chronic) and disease severity (e.g., mild, moderate, and severe) influence the type and number of medications used in attempt to achieve adequate disease control.

Beta-Agonists

Beta-adrenergic agonists are the most effective bronchodilators. They are potent, rapid-acting, and come in a variety of different delivery systems (Table 3) that can accommodate most adult and pediatric patients. Although beta-agonists may be administered orally, the inhaled route is preferred in most circumstances because of greater efficacy and fewer side effects. For these reasons, most patients with asthma are prescribed a beta-agonist to use as both rescue medication for acute bronchospasm or for prophylaxis prior to exercise or allergen exposure (see Table 3). Adrenergic receptors in the lung are predominantly of the beta-$_2$ subtype, and agents with beta-$_2$ greater than beta$_1$ specificity should be used whenever possible. Intermediate acting beta-$_2$ agonists (e.g., albuterol, metaproterenol, terbutaline, pirbuterol) have their onset of action within 5 to 10 minutes following inhalation (longer if taken orally), and usually have a 4 to 6 hour duration of action. The long-acting beta-agonist, salmeterol, has an onset of action within 20 to 30 minutes following administration and can produce bronchodilation as long as 12 to 18 hours in the majority of patients. Because of this delayed onset of action, salmeterol should be used ***only*** as a maintenance and ***not*** as a rescue medication.

Recent studies suggest that the regular use of intermediate acting beta-agonists in asthma may be associated with adverse effects over time. Other studies, including evaluations using salmeterol, have not documented these claims. However, until this controversy can be definitively resolved, patients using more than eight puffs of an intermediate beta-agonist per day, or more than 1.5 metered dose inhalers (MDI) per month, should be evaluated promptly so that the underlying disease process rather than its manifested symptoms can become the major focus of therapy.

Theophylline

Theophylline is a dimethylated xanthine that is similar in structure to the common dietary xanthines, caffeine (coffee and carbonated beverages), and theobromine (tea). It is an effective bronchodilator when used orally, rectally, or intravenously. Theophylline attenuates the airway obstructive response to both allergen exposure and exercise and may have some anti-inflammatory properties as well. Its primary use is in the management of chronic asthmatic symptoms rather than in acute exacerbations.

The efficacy and toxicity of theophylline in treating asthma are directly related to its serum concentration. Approximately 75 percent of the maximal effect in relieving airway obstruction can be achieved when serum concentrations approach 10 μg per milliliter; in patients with inadequate symptom control with this serum level, cautious increases in dosages could potentially alleviate symptoms without producing adverse effects (usually nausea, headache, tremor, insomnia, hyperactivity). Thus, most children will show an acceptable risk-benefit ratio with theophylline usage when serum concentrations are between 5 and 15 μg per milliliter. Serum theophylline levels should be monitored periodically because theophylline metabolism may vary greatly, even in individual patients. In particular, both viral infections and certain medications (e.g., erythromycin) may decrease theophylline clearance, increasing the potential for theophylline toxicity.

With the development of sustained-release (SR) oral theophylline preparations, the concerns regarding large peak-trough variations have been minimized. These preparations are available in tablets and beaded capsules, the latter of which can be sprinkled on food to facilitate compliance in small children. Dosage is based on age and weight (Fig. 2). The dosing interval will be dictated by the formulation used and the individual metabolism of the patient. As a general rule, children under 8 years of age should be started on a three-times-a-day schedule, whereas older children and adolescents may achieve acceptable symptom control by taking the medication twice daily. SR theophylline is particularly helpful in the management of nocturnal asthma.

When prescribing theophylline, one should be aware of the assortment of behavioral and learning problems sometimes attributed to its use. For the majority of children, these effects are not clinically significant; however, it may be prudent to avoid theophylline in children who already have psychological or school problems and in whom the drug could be another potential confounding variable.

Ipratropium Bromide

Ipratropium bromide is a bronchodilator that acts by blocking the binding of acetylcholine at muscarinic receptors in bronchial smooth muscle. The safety margin of ipratropium is very wide compared to that of atropine, and inhalation does not produce significant cardiovascular or central nervous system (CNS) effects. Because ipratropium bromide is generally a less potent bronchodilator than currently available intermediate acting beta-agonists and has a slower onset of action (approximately 1 hour), it is beneficial in only a small subset of children with asthma. Ipratropium may be more useful in the treatment of chronic obstructive pulmonary disease. It is available in both an MDI (18 μg per puff) and a nebulizer unit dose solution (250 μg per milliliter).

Cromolyn and Nedocromil Sodium

Cromolyn (all ages) and nedocromil ($\geq$12 years) sodium are two structurally distinct compounds which have both anti-allergic and anti-inflammatory effects. Both compounds are administered via the inhaled route, with cromolyn currently available in both an MDI and a nebulizer solution and nedocromil as an MDI only. When administered 5 minutes before challenge, both compounds are effective for the prevention of both the

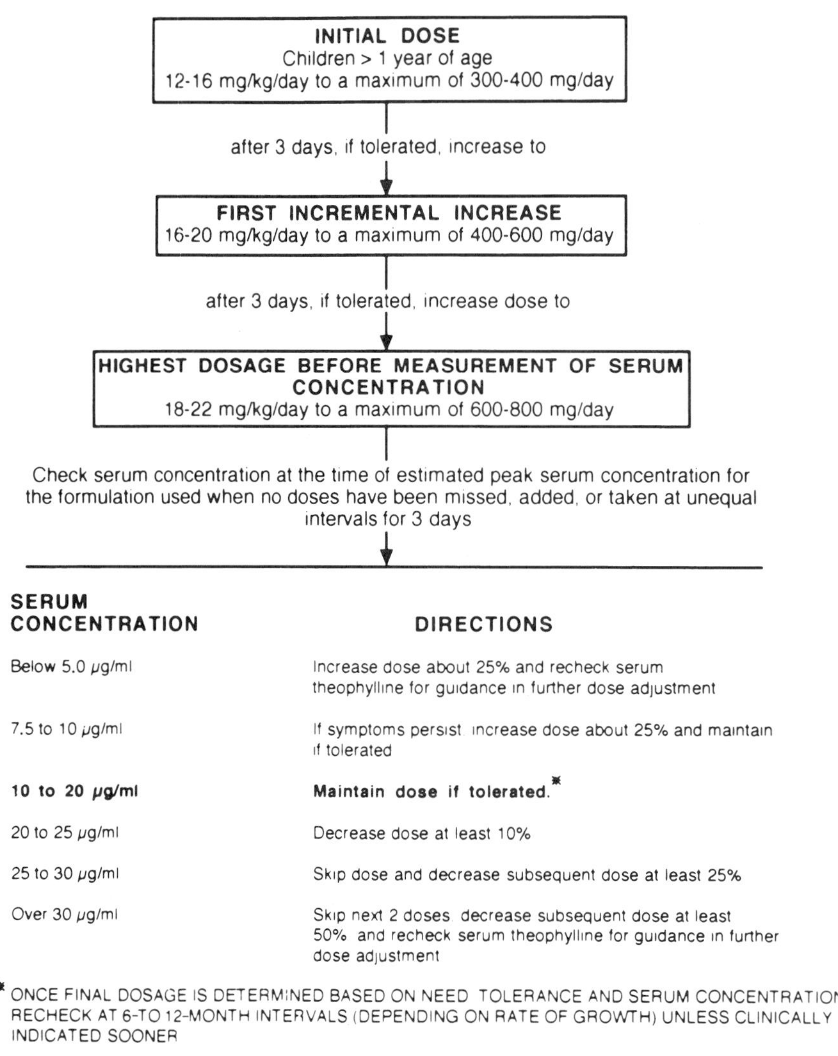

Figure 2 Guidelines for dosing with theophylline. (Modified from National Asthma Education Program [NAEP], National Institutes of Health. Bethesda, Md: Guidelines for the diagnosis and management of asthma [NIH publication #91–3042]. US Department of Health and Human Services, 1991.)

early and late response to allergen challenge, and both attenuate exercise-induced bronchospasm. The rapidity of this prophylactic response (minutes) is at odds with the slow onset of efficacy of cromolyn (weeks) and nedocromil (days) in the management of chronic asthmatic symptoms. The improvement in asthma symptoms is accompanied by a decrease in airway hyper-responsiveness. These medications are remarkably safe, and are thus the preferred first-line anti-inflammatory agents in the management of chronic asthmatic symptoms in children.

Glucocorticosteroids

At present, glucocorticosteroids (CS) are the most effective and consistent medications in improving airway obstruction and hyper-responsiveness. Unfortunately, CS have multiple adverse effects, which are related to dose, frequency of administration (months more than days; every day more than alternate day) and route of administration (oral more than inhaled). Inhaled CS (ICS) should be used in the management of chronic childhood asthmatic symptoms that are unresponsive to initial treatment with cromolyn or nedocromil sodium or in children receiving daily or alternate day oral CS in an attempt to improve asthma control using a less toxic mode of CS delivery. A list of the currently available ICS in the United States is provided in Table 3. At present, on a microgram per microgram basis, there is no convincing data that any one formulation is ***clinically*** more potent or less likely to produce side effects.

As a general rule, doses below 400 μg per day are

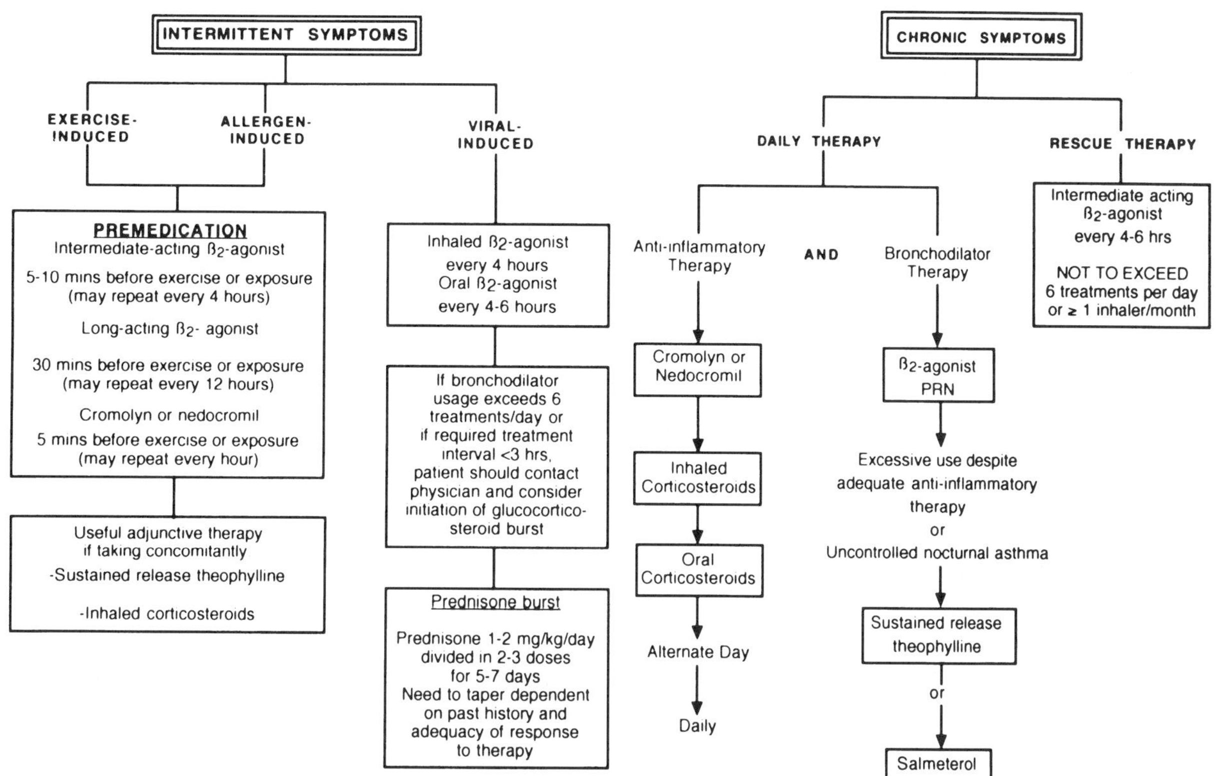

Figure 3 Guide to pharmacologic therapy of asthma based on triggering event and frequency of symptoms. (Modified from National Asthma Education Program [NAEP], National Institutes of Health. Bethesda, Md: Guidelines for the diagnosis and management of asthma [NIH publication #91–3042]. US Department of Health and Human Services, 1991.)

usually safe, and doses of 400 to 800 µg per day are reasonably safe for use in children. Once dosages greater than 800 µg per day are needed, the potential for significant effects on linear bone growth and adrenal suppression are substantially increased. It should be emphasized, however, that individual tolerances of CS doses vary considerably; therefore, all children requiring ICS at dosages greater than 400 µg per day or prolonged oral CS at any dosage should have growth measurements accurately assessed routinely. These children may also benefit from consultation with an asthma specialist.

The most frequent side effects seen with conventional doses of ICS are oral candidiasis and hoarseness. These problems can be substantially reduced by the use of spacer devices alone or in combination with rinsing of the mouth following use.

At present, no preparation of CS is available for nebulizer use. Therefore, in children unable to use an MDI effectively even with the use of a spacer device, oral corticosteroids may have to be utilized. As indicated previously, the lowest possible dose, preferably administered on alternate days, should be prescribed.

TREATMENT OF CHRONIC ASTHMA

At the outset, it should be recognized that asthma is a heterogenous disease or syndrome. Therefore, multiple treatment approaches are possible. Although this chapter highlights the pharmacologic management of both acute and chronic asthma, control of environmental triggers and patient education deserve equal emphasis.

The pharmacologic treatment of asthma can be viewed in terms of both the frequency (intermittent versus chronic) (Fig. 3) and intensity (mild, moderate, and severe) of symptoms. A classification by frequency will involve the identification of various triggering factors (exercise, allergen, infection), while stratification by disease intensity will further influence the types of medications initially prescribed, as well as guide adjustments in maintenance asthma therapy depending on each patient's fluctuations in symptoms over time.

Intermittent Therapy

Exercise-Induced Asthma

Exercise is a common triggering factor for asthma; in many patients, it may be the only one. The propensity to develop exercise-induced asthma (EIA) is related to the intensity of exercise, the climatic conditions (cold, dry air is most likely to trigger bronchospasm), and the degree of airway hyper-responsiveness. Inhalation of an intermediate beta-agonist 5 to 10 minutes prior to exercise will significantly attenuate the response to exercise in approximately 80 percent of patients. If a patient forgets

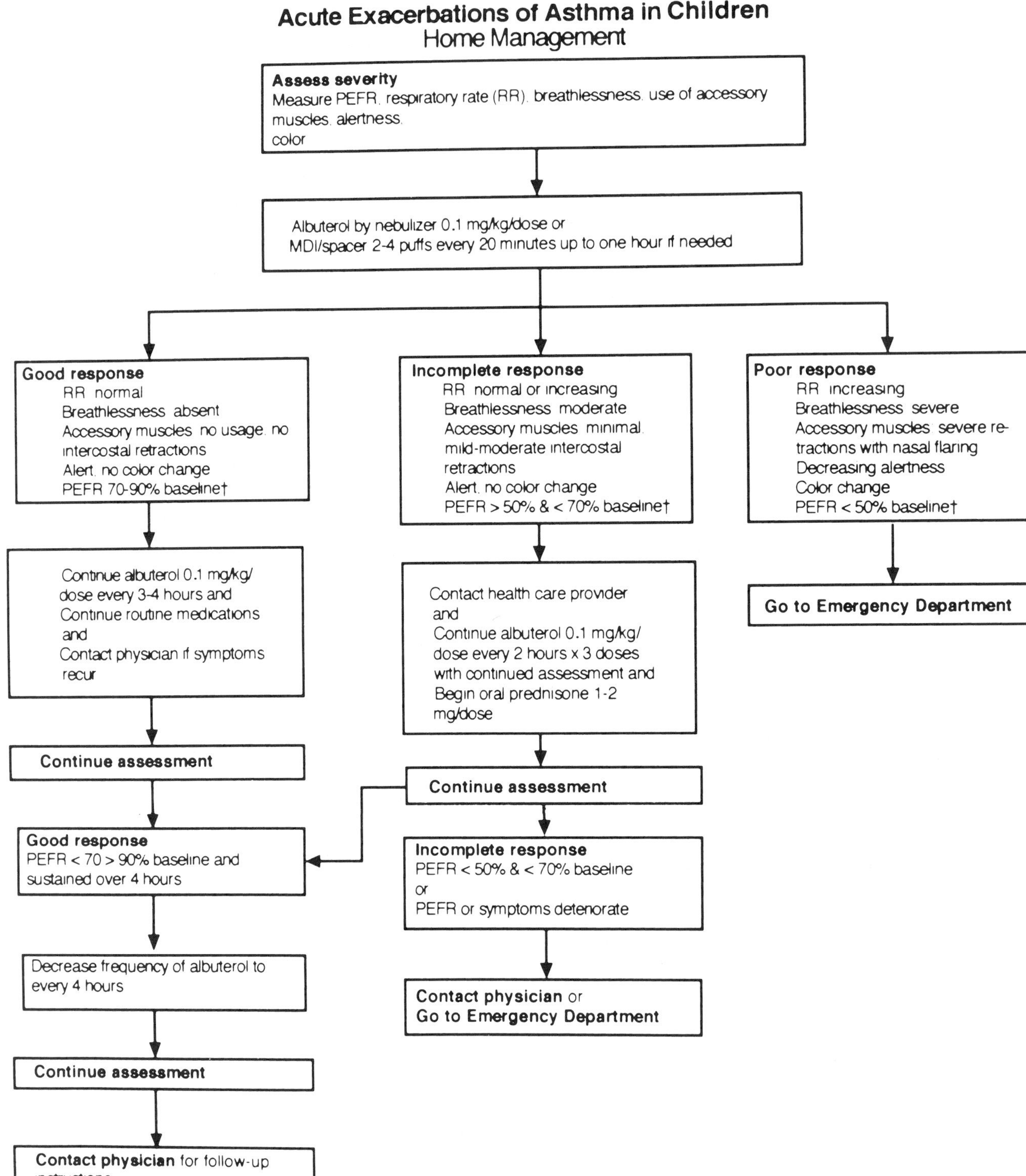

Figure 4 Home management of acute asthma symptoms in children. (Modified from National Asthma Education Program [NAEP], National Institutes of Health. Bethesda, Md: Guidelines for the diagnosis and management of asthma [NIH publication #91–3042]. US Department of Health and Human Services, 1991.)

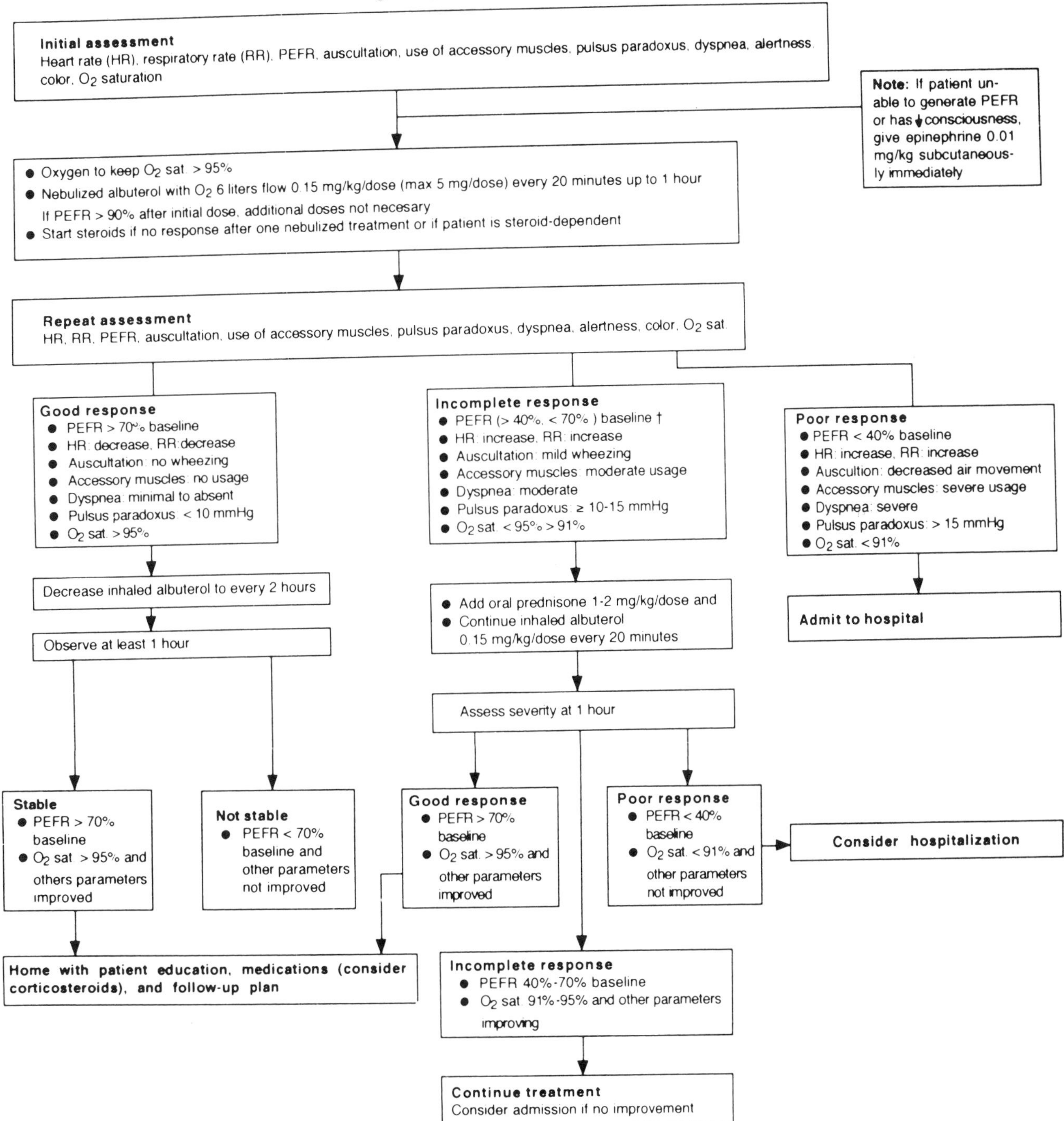

* Therapies are often available in a physician's office. However, most acutely severe exacerbations of asthma require a complete course of therapy in a Emergency Department.

† PEFR % baseline refers to the norm for the individual, established by the clinician. This may be % predicted based on standardized norms or patient's personal best.

Figure 5 Emergency room management of acute asthma in children. (Modified from National Asthma Education Program [NAEP], National Institutes of Health. Bethesda, Md: Guidelines for the diagnosis and management of asthma [NIH publication #91–3042]. US Department of Health and Human Services, 1991.)

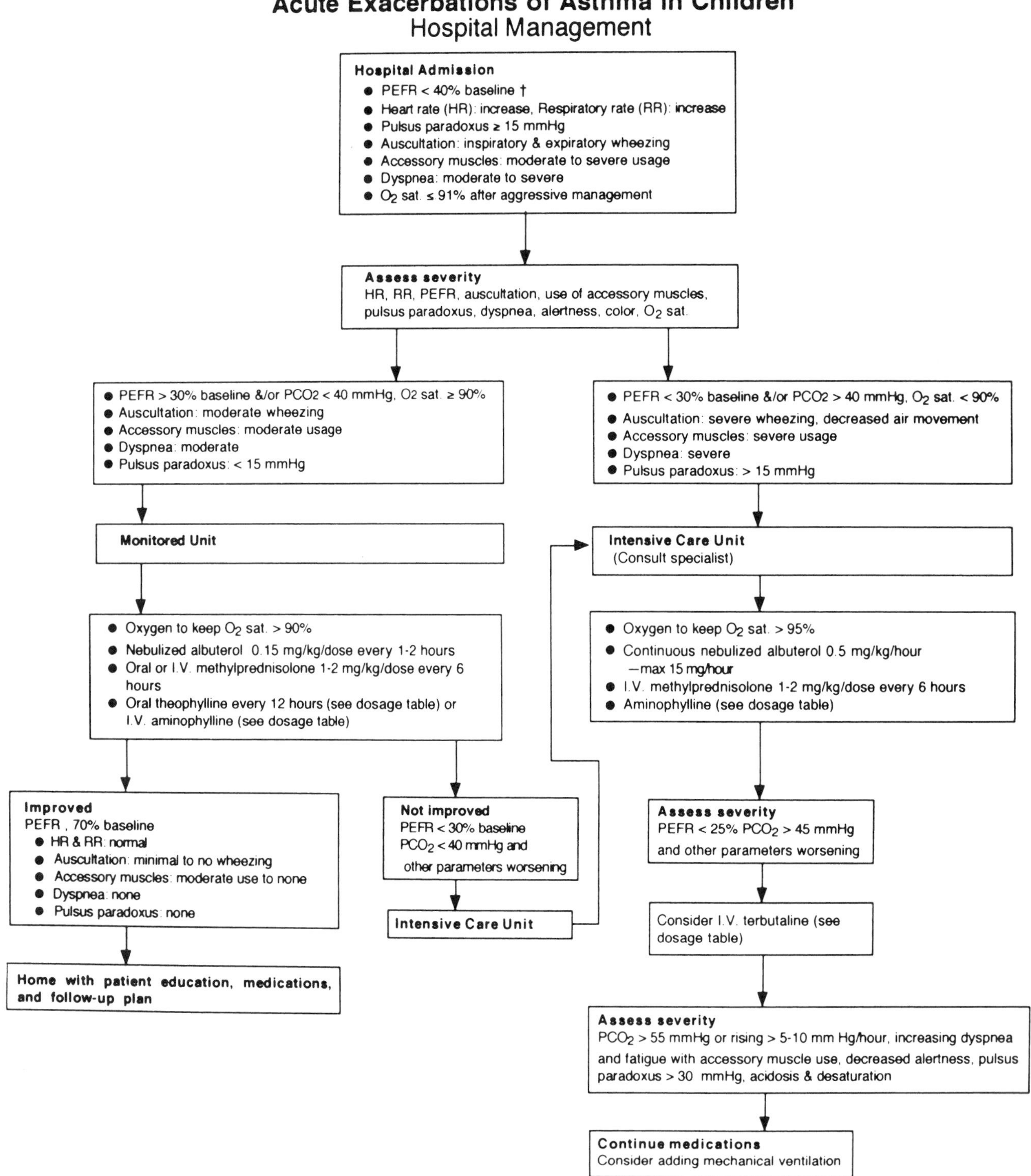

Figure 6 Inpatient management of acute asthma in children. (Modified from National Asthma Education Program [NAEP], National Institutes of Health. Bethesda, Md: Guidelines for the diagnosis and management of asthma [NIH publication #91–3042]. US Department of Health and Human Services, 1991.)

to premedicate, beta-agonists may also be used as a rescue medication. Cromolyn or nedocromil sodium are also effective if taken 5 minutes before exercise, but are ineffective for rescue. The combination of a beta-agonist and either cromolyn or nedocromil should be tried in patients not responding sufficiently to either medication alone. The long-acting beta-agonist, salmeterol, is also effective but needs to be administered 20 to 30 minutes prior to exercise and should not be viewed as a rescue medication. Patients receiving chronic theophylline therapy will also notice some benefit with regard to EIA. In patients not responding satisfactorily to these medications, a more careful evaluation of overall disease activity is warranted.

Virus-Induced Asthma

Infections are a common precipitant of asthma in children. Since viruses are the predominant etiologic agents, treatment with antibiotics is not usually helpful unless the asthmatic episode is accompanied by otitis media and/or sinusitis. In mild cases of wheezing and/or cough associated with rhinorrhea and low-grade fever, initial treatment with a beta-agonist may be tried. The response will vary depending on the virus (respiratory syncytial virus, rhinovirus, and parainfluenza virus are problematic in children) and the airway geometry of the patient (smaller airways in infants will be more affected by edema, inflammation, and mucous secretion). Symptoms unresponsive to bronchodilator therapy should be treated with oral prednisone for a period of 5 to 7 days.

Allergen-Induced Asthma

The development of asthmatic symptoms resulting from exposure to relevant allergens in sensitized patients can best be treated by avoidance. In the case of animal sensitivity, the issues pertaining to avoidance and/or removal are challenging once patients and/or other family members have bonded to their pets. When situations arise in which avoidance cannot be accomplished (holiday visitations to relatives), premedication with a beta-agonist and/or cromolyn and nedocromil can be useful; both treatments would need to be administered every 2 (cromolyn and nedocromil) to 4 (beta-agonists) hours during exposure.

Chronic Therapy

Once asthma symptoms occur on a daily basis, patients should receive maintenance scheduled therapy that controls symptoms with the least number of side effects. As outlined by the National Asthma Education Panel, the initial and progressive selection of therapy will depend on disease severity. Once bronchodilator therapy is being used for more than prophylaxis for exercise, allergen exposure, or for 5 to 7 days during a viral upper respiratory infection, the introduction of anti-inflammatory therapy should be considered. However, it should be emphasized that the appropriate treatment of acute symptoms in addition to and/or concomitant with chronic therapy will depend on the triggering factor involved (see Fig. 3).

TREATMENT OF ACUTE ASTHMA

The treatment of acute exacerbations of asthma will depend on their severity as assessed by the initial response to bronchodilator therapy and objective measurements of airflow obstruction (peak flow rates, spirometry, pulse oximetry, physical exam findings, and vital signs). Algorithms for appropriate management in the home (Fig. 4), emergency department (Fig. 5), and hospital (Fig. 6) have been developed by the National Asthma Education Panel.

It should be emphasized that the overall goal of asthma therapy should be to eliminate, or at least significantly reduce, acute asthmatic exacerbations that require emergency room treatment or hospitalizations. Written treatment plans for chronic management as well as acute intervention strategies for mild, moderate, and severe exacerbations should be developed for all patients and reviewed at each visit. One potentially useful approach is to calculate "zones" based on home peak flow measurements. The first goal is to ascertain the patient's personal best peak flow rate, which requires the appropriate use of medications to maximize pulmonary function. Once this value has been established, the calculation of green (80 percent to 100 percent of personal best), yellow (50 percent to 80 percent of personal best), and red (<50 percent of personal best) zones can be accomplished. Peak flow rates in the green zone should indicate stable disease activity, provided no other warning signs are present (nocturnal awakenings caused by asthma, exercise intolerance, and so on). If the patient's peak flow rate is in the yellow zone and the administration of a beta-agonist does not result in bringing the peak flow rate back into the green zone, many asthma specialists would recommend doubling the maintenance dose of anti-inflammatory therapy until peak flow rates are consistently back in the green zone. If peak flow rates continue to deteriorate while in the yellow zone or are in the red zone, oral corticosteroid therapy should be initiated and the patient should contact a physician as soon as possible. In children too young to perform peak flow measurements, signs and symptoms that would be present if peak flow rates were in each zone can be developed and used by parents to gauge the severity of any asthmatic exacerbation.

SUGGESTED READING

Cypcar D, Busse WW. Role of viral infections in asthma. Immunol Allergy Clin N Am 1993; 13:745.

Cypcar D, Lemanske Jr RF. Asthma and exercise. Clin Chest Med 1994; 15:351.

Duff AL, Platts-Mills TAE. Allergens and asthma. Pediatr Clin N Am 1992; 39(6):1277.

Gern JE, Lemanske Jr RF. Beta adrenergic agonist therapy. Immunol Allergy 1993; Clin N Am 13:839.
Larsen GL. Current concepts—asthma in children. N Engl J Med 1992; 326:1540.
National Asthma Education Program, National Institutes of Health. Guidelines for the diagnosis and management of asthma (NIH publication #91–3042). Bethesda, MD,: US Department of Health and Human Services, 1991.
National Asthma Education Program, National Institutes of Health. Teach your patients about asthma: a clinician's guide (NIH publication #92–2737). Bethesda, MD: US Department of Health and Human Services, 1992.

ASPIRIN SENSITIVITY IN RHINOSINUSITIS AND ASTHMA

DAVID A. MATHISON, M.D.
DONALD D. STEVENSON, M.D.

Aspirin has been used for over 90 years in the United States as an anti-inflammatory, antipyretic, and analgesic agent, and in recent decades as a platelet-inhibiting agent to prevent thrombotic and embolic disease. The average per capita consumption is more than 60 tablets per year. Idiosyncratic reactions to aspirin may be anaphylactoid or manifest by exacerbation of rhinosinusitis and asthma or urticaria-angioedema; only a very few individuals have both respiratory and cutaneous response to aspirin.

The typical aspirin-sensitive respiratory syndrome usually begins in adulthood. The disease begins with a perennial vasomotor-irritant-aggravated type of rhinitis and evolves over decades. Half of these patients also have IgE-mediated cutaneous reactions to aeroallergen extracts. An eosinophilic hyperplastic rhinosinusitis with nasal polyps progresses, and not infrequently is complicated by bouts of purulent bacterial sinusitis. Asthma then appears and progresses, frequently requiring treatment with systemic corticosteroids. The hallmark of aspirin sensitivity is the appearance of facial or generalized flush, ocular and nasal congestion, and watering, and acute, often severe, asthmatic attack within 30 minutes to 3 hours after ingesting an ordinary dose of aspirin or aspirin-like nonsteroidal anti-inflammatory drugs (NSAIDs). Even though the patient usually learns to avoid aspirin and similar drugs, the underlying respiratory disease progresses.

The prevalence of aspirin sensitivity in patients with rhinosinusitis and asthma varies according to the population studied and methods used to detect the sensitivity. Less than 2 percent of asthmatic children report a history of reaction to aspirin; 3 to 5 percent of hospitalized adult asthmatic patients give a history of reactions to aspirin. At Scripps Clinic and Research Foundation, an asthma and allergic diseases center, we found that about 10 percent of our asthmatic population was aspirin-sensitive. Among asthmatic patients with pansinusitis and nasal polyps, 30 to 40 percent were aspirin-sensitive.

One mechanism of action of aspirin is inhibition of prostaglandin synthesis via acetylation of cyclooxygenase. Aspirin-like NSAIDs cross-react in aspirin-sensitive patients in proportion to their individual ability to inhibit cyclooxygenase (as shown in Table 1). Nonacetylated salicylates, analgesics, and inhibitors of platelet aggregation that do not act through cyclooxygenase inhibition have not been shown to be cross-reactive. NSAIDs administered in opthalmic drops (indomethacin, ketorolac [Acular], diclofenac [Voltaren], suprofen [Profenal], and flurbiprofen [Ocufen]) and by injection (ketorolac [Toradol]) provoke reactions in aspirin-sensitive patients. The mechanism of respiratory reaction to aspirin is likely related to a shift in arachidonic metabolites from the cyclooxygenase-prostaglandins to 5-lipoxygenase–leukotrienes pathway with a surge of production of leukotrienes, which in turn stimulate airways in sensitive individuals.

The diagnosis of aspirin-sensitive rhinosinusitis and/or asthma is presumed when the history of reaction to aspirin is typical; is probable for the patient with the typical syndrome of eosinophilic rhinosinusitis with polyps and/or asthma; is possible even in the patient who has recently taken aspirin; and can be confirmed/denied only by cautious oral challenges with aspirin (see below). There is no proven in vitro laboratory test to confirm sensitivity to acetylsalicylic acid (ASA) or NSAIDs.

PREVENTION

Since aspirin sensitivity may appear only after years of progression of rhinosinusitic-asthmatic respiratory disorder and may vary in its expression, and since many asthmatic patients can avoid aspirin and NSAIDs, the most conservative approach is to advise avoidance of these drugs by substituting 325 to 500 mg (but not 1,000 mg) doses of acetaminophen or use of other analgesic, anti-inflammatory, or platelet-inhibitor drugs that do not cross-react with aspirin (see Table 1).

TREATMENT OF REACTION TO ASPIRIN

Acute unexpected asthmatic reaction after aspirin or NSAID ingestion in the unsuspectedly sensitive

Table 1 Cross-Reactivity Between Aspirin and Nonsteroidal Anti-Inflammatory Drugs in Aspirin-Sensitive Rhinosinusitis and Asthma

Cyclooxygenase Inhibition	*Cross-Reactivity*
Strong inhibitors, even at low doses	High (99%)
Indomethacin (Indocin)	
Meclofenamate (Meclomen)	
Mefenamic acid (Ponstel)	
Naproxen (Aleve, Anaprox, Naprosyn)	
Ibuprofen (Advil, Haltran, Medipren, Motrin, Nuprin, Rufen)	
Fenoprofen (Nalfon)	
Diflunisal (Dolobid)	
Ketoprofen (Orudis, Oruvail)	
Piroxicam (Feldene)	
Sulindac (Clinoril)	
Tolmetin (Tolectin)	
Diclofenac (Voltaren)	
Flurbiprofen (Ansaid)	
Ketorolac (Toradol)	
Etodolac (Lodine)	
Nabumetone (Relafen)	
Oxaprozin (Daypro)	
Weak inhibitors, even at high doses	Low (<35%)
Acetaminophen (Datril, Tylenol)	
Phenylbutazone (Butazolidin)	
Salicylic acid (Disalcid, Salflex) Salsalate	
Noninhibitors/Analgesics/Platelet-Inhibitors	None or rare case reported
Propoxyphene (Darvon)	
Dipyridamole (Persantine)	
Hydroxychloroquine (Plaquenil)	
Ticlopidine (Ticlid)	
Choline, Magnesium (Trilisate, Doan's, Magan) Sodium salicylate	

individual or after unintended or mistaken ingestion of aspirin or an NSAID in the known sensitive individual may have a fatal outcome and therefore should be treated as an emergency. Unlike an allergen-provoked asthmatic attack, which may respond over minutes to inhaled bronchodilator, aspirin-provoked bronchospasm, once started, usually progresses, even while an inhaled bronchodilator is used. The attack of bronchospasm diminishes only gradually over hours. Treatment consists of continuous (>30 to 120 minutes) of nebulized bronchodilator (albuterol 0.083 percent solution 2.5 mg unit does every 30 minutes), epinephrine 200 to 300 μg by subcutaneous injection, oxygen (3 to 5 liter flow through nasal clips or via 34 percent Venturi mask), intravenous corticosteroid (bolus of 125 mg of methylprednisolone sodium succinate for injection) and aminophylline (loading dose if no prior methylxanthine of 5 mg per kilogram over 30 minutes followed by 1 mg per kilogram per hour adjusted according to serum levels of theophylline). Should respiratory failure, evidenced by patient exhaustion, hypoxemia despite oxygen and/or carbon dioxide retention (arterial Pco_2 greater than 60 mm Hg) ensue, then intubation and mechanical ventilation are indicated.

TREATMENT OF ONGOING RESPIRATORY DISEASE

The aspirin-sensitive respiratory syndrome is a progressive eosinophilic inflammation of the mucosal lining of the respiratory tract, often to the point of polyp formation and pansinusitis and/or asthma incompletely responsive to nonsteroidal therapies. Systemic corticosteroid, such as prednisone 40 to 60 mg daily, if tolerated without serious side effects, for 10 to 20 days followed by 20 mg on alternate mornings for several months may be required to control advanced disease. For polypoid pansinusitis with chronic purulent aerobic and/or anaerobic bacterial or fungal infection unresponsive to systemic corticosteroid and antibiotics (such as clarithromycin 500 mg twice daily and metronidazole 500 mg four times daily for 10 to 20 days), endoscopic polypectomy and sinusoidal surgery by an experienced surgeon are indicated. Once the mass of inflamed tissue obstructing the respiratory tracts has been relieved with medical and/or surgical therapy, twice daily topical insufflated nasal and/or inhaled corticosteroid (beclomethasone, budesonide, flunisolide, or triamcinolone) may prevent further inflammation. Occasionally, alternate morning prednisone 10 to 20 mg doses are required to control ongoing inflammation. Aspirin desensitization followed by daily aspirin or NSAID treatment is an additional modality that may be offered to the individual with intractable inflammatory mucosal disease, intolerable side effects from corticosteroid treatments, and/or another indication for aspirin or NSAID desensitization-treatment (discussed at the end of this chapter).

CHALLENGES WITH ASPIRIN

Rhinosinusitic-asthmatic patients who have recently tolerated aspirin or NSAIDs and for whom aspirin or NSAIDs are indicated may elect to use these drugs but should be made aware of potential risk of developing sensitivity. However, patients who have a high potential for aspirin sensitivity (i.e., pansinusitis with polyps and asthma necessitating corticosteroid treatment) or have a history of aspirin-sensitive respiratory reactions and who also have headache, rheumatic, cardiovascular, or diabetic disease for which aspirin is indicated, or for whom aspirin desensitization followed by continued treatment with aspirin for the respiratory disease per se (see the following section) has been recommended, can safely undergo oral ASA or NSAID challenges or desensitization followed by daily administration of aspirin.

Currently there is no standardized protocol for oral challenges with aspirin or NSAIDs. Challenges with bronchial inhalation and nasal insufflation of lysine acetylsalicylate and intravenous indomethacin have also been reported. Oral ASA challenges and desensitizations must be performed using a number of safety practices. At Green Hospital of Scripps Clinic and Research Foundation, we perform challenges within the hospital, where emergency resuscitative equipment, an intensive care unit, and trained personnel are readily available. Challenges are always started in the morning so that optimal time and staff for treatment are available to ensure ease of recovery from the expected respiratory reaction. Patients are challenged at a time when their asthma is in remission; if need be, we administer additional corticosteroid for several days to a week prior to challenge to insure that there is full remission. To proceed with the challenge, the patient must have a forced expiratory volume (FEV_1) greater than 70 percent of predicted or his or her best previously recorded, and in absolute numbers, this must be greater than 1.5 L.

Patients are instructed to continue theophylline and corticosteroid medications and to suspend anticholinergics, antihistamines, cromolyn and nedocromil, acetaminophen, nonaspirin salicylates, and inhaled adrenergic bronchodilator medications for 24 hours prior to challenge. We recognize that continuation of medications may prevent a mild reaction and thereby lead to a false-negative result. However, withholding medications may allow spontaneous deterioration of bronchial patency during the challenge, which could lead to a false conclusion of bronchospasm. Blinded challenge with placebo over 1 day with repeated spirometric measurements as planned during aspirin challenge is essential to identifying subjects likely to have false-positive responses during the oral ASA challenge.

Patients with mild asthma for whom the history does not suggest likelihood of aspirin reactivity (no rhinosinusitis or nasal polyps and previous recent ingestion of aspirin without apparent reaction) can be challenged over one-half of a day with 30, 150, 325, and 650 mg doses of aspirin (or 5 percent, 10 percent, 50 percent, 100 percent of the usual therapeutic dose of another NSAID) administered at hourly intervals with spirometric measurements also performed hourly and continued for 2 hours after the last dose. This is equivalent to the "test dose" method used for other medications when risk of adverse reaction is judged to be unlikely. However, if a truly ASA-sensitive patient is challenged with ASA during only one-half of a day, the cumulative doses of ASA are likely to induce very severe and intractable bronchospasm that will be difficult to treat and may require intubation and ventilation.

Asthmatic patients with moderate asthma but without rhinosinusitis polyps who have not ingested aspirin or an NSAID for months or years may undergo a 1-day challenge. Aspirin doses of 30, 60, and 150 mg are administered hourly and then 325 and 650 mg at 2-hour intervals (5 percent, 10 percent, 20 percent, then 50 percent and 100 percent of the usual dose for another NSAID) with spirometry measurements at hourly intervals continued for 3 hours after the last dose. This is a more conservative test dose method for use when an adverse response is not expected. The same disclaimer applies to this 1-day challenge if a truly ASA-sensitive patient is challenged.

Asthmatic patients with history of adverse respiratory response to aspirin or NSAIDs or those with severe disease, including rhinosinusitis with nasal polyps and remote history of aspirin ingestion, should undergo challenges over a 2-day interval with a 3, 15, or 30 mg initial dose followed by 60 and 100 mg on the first day at 3-hour intervals and then 150, 325, 650 mg at 3-hour intervals on the second day (1.5 percent or 5 percent, 10 percent, 20 percent, then 30 percent, 50 percent, 100 percent of the usual dose for other NSAIDs) with spirometric measurements recorded hourly and continued for 3 hours after the last dose on both days. A two-day challenge is not initiated unless or until a full-day placebo challenge has confirmed stable lung function.

For any patient, if ocular, nasal, or asthmatic symptoms appear, or if there is fall in FEV_1 of greater than 20 percent, no additional doses of ASA are administered and the patient is treated with inhalations of adrenergic (albuterol 0.083 percent solution 2.5 mg unit dose) bronchodilator delivered by nebulized aerosol and repeated at 10- to 30-minute intervals until improvement occurs. If no response appears after the initial treatment, 200–300 μg of epinephrine is administered subcutaneously; and, if there is no response, intravenous corticosteroid and aminophylline and oxygen are initiated and preparations for transfer to intensive care for intubation and mechanical ventilation are made. Ordinarily, there is gradual recovery from the reaction over hours coincident with treatment, with a mean recovery time of 7 hours, and slower recovery over 24 hours is not unusual.

Challenge response is interpreted to be "negative" if no symptoms and less than a 15 percent fall in FEV_1 occur during the entire period of observation. Patients with negative challenge are instructed to proceed with the indicated drug in ordinary therapeutic dosages. However, if there is a history suggestive of previous reaction, they are also cautioned that they may redevelop reactivity to aspirin or NSAIDs if they omit the treatment for a day or more and must continue to be cautious regarding the use of aspirin or NSAIDs.

Challenge response is interpreted to be "asthmatic" if the fall in FEV_1 exceeds 20 percent and, if on another day, blinded similar challenge with a placebo or non–aspirin-like drug produces a fall in FEV_1 of less than 15 percent and no symptoms. Asthmatic reactions are judged as "purely asthmatic" if no nasal-ocular symptoms occur. Response is judged to be "partial-asthmatic" if FEV_1 falls 15 to 20 percent or "nasal-ocular" if nasal-ocular symptoms occur without asthmatic symptoms or signs. A "classic" reaction is nasal-ocular and bronchospastic (>20 percent fall in FEV_1).

TREATMENT WITH ASPIRIN AFTER DESENSITIZATION

Patients with aspirin-sensitive respiratory disease for whom aspirin or an NSAID drug is indicated for concomitant disease or ongoing treatment of the respiratory disease per se may be desensitized and continued on daily dose(s) of ASA or NSAIDs. Desensitization is accomplished by repeated daily challenges, providing the criteria for initial challenge are met, beginning with the dose that provoked reaction on the previous day, and continuing upward until 650 mg (100 percent of the usual dose of another NSAID) is achieved without reaction. Figure 1 shows an example of desensitization. We have successfully desensitized over 150 aspirin-sensitive rhinosinusitic-asthmatic patients by repeated incremental oral aspirin challenges, as noted previously, until each patient was able to ingest 650 mg of aspirin without response. In some patients, up to eight or more aspirin-provoked asthmatic attacks were required before a desensitized state was achieved. Sensitization will

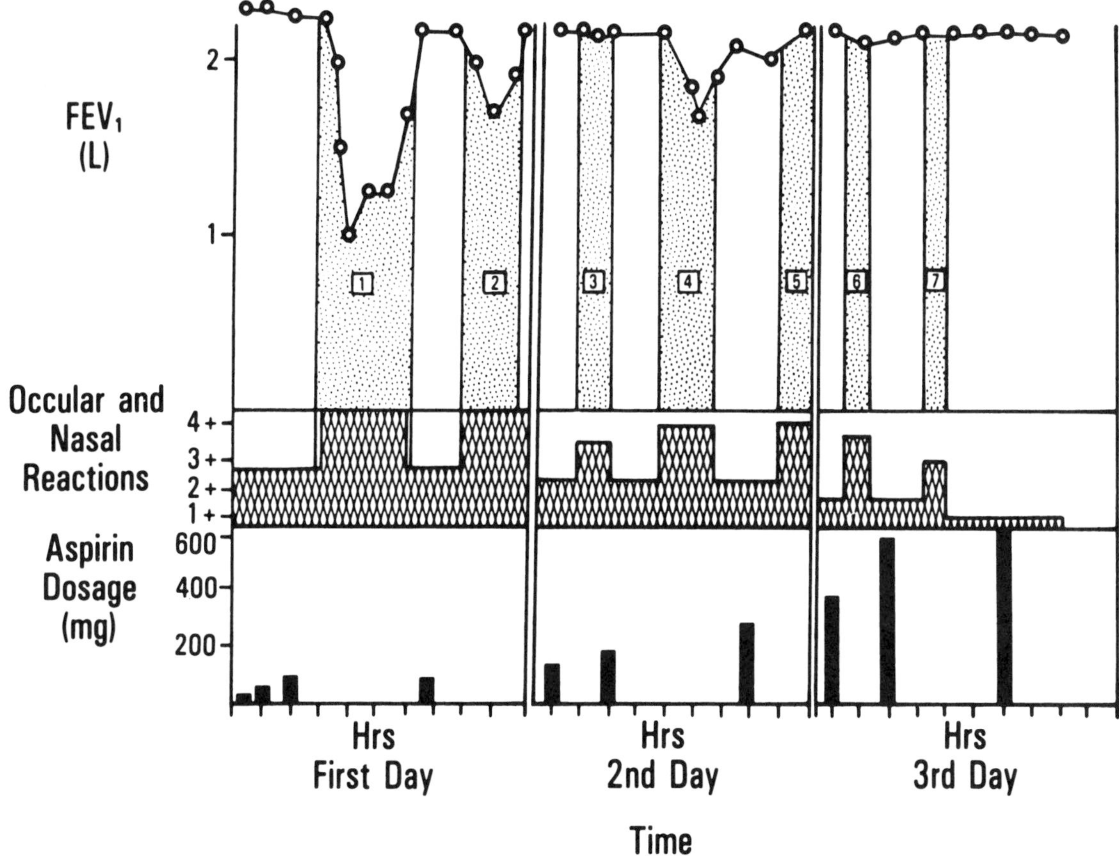

Figure 1 Aspirin challenges – desensitization in an aspirin-sensitive asthmatic patient; seven (numbers in boxes, stippled and hatched areas) nasal-ocular reactions, some (1, 2, 4) with asthmatic reaction as well, occurred before 650 mg dose on third day was tolerated without reaction, indicating desensitized state.

recur from 1 to 5 days after the interruption of aspirin therapy; for this reason, it is imperative that the patient continue taking aspirin or an NSAID on a daily basis if continuous treatment with aspirin is the objective.

As of 1990, 65 asthmatic patients, from over 100 asthmatic patients with aspirin sensitivity confirmed at Scripps Clinic by oral aspirin challenge, elected to be desensitized and continue open trials of aspirin treatment, 320 mg daily up to 650 mg four times daily, for periods of up to 8 years. Half of these patients continued aspirin treatment and had significant improvement in symptom scores, reduced emergency visits or hospitalizations, and decrease of systemic and inhaled (but not nasal-insufflated) steroid dose as compared to pretreatment and to a control group of aspirin-sensitive patients not treated with aspirin. The half who discontinued treatment did so primarily because of alimentary side effects; respiratory disease, though improved during aspirin treatment, tended to revert toward pretreatment status after discontinuation of aspirin. In separate studies, we have desensitized-treated aspirin-sensitive patients with chronic rhinosinusitis without asthma and have shown favorable response in blinded studies in the majority of these individuals. Other reports of aspirin desensitization and treatment in both aspirin-sensitive and tolerant asthmatic patients have been published and generally support the efficacy of this treatment regimen.

SUGGESTED READING

Brooks PM, Day RO. Nonsteroidal anti-inflammatory drugs—differences and similarities. N Engl J Med 1991; 324:1716–1725.

Mathison DA, Simon RA, Stevenson DD. Aspirin, SO_2/sulfite and other chemical sensitivities in asthmatic patients. In: Spector SC, ed. Provocative challenge procedures: background and methodology. New York: Marcel Decker 1995; 599–622.

Stevenson DD, Simon RA. Sensitivity to aspirin and nonsteroidal anti-inflammatory drugs. In: Middleton E, Adkinson NF, Busse WW, et al, eds. Allergy principles and practice, 4th ed. St Louis: Mosby, 1993; 1747–1765.

Sweet JM, Stevenson DD, Simon RA, Mathison DA. Long-term effects of aspirin desensitization—treatment for aspirin-sensitive rhinosinusitis asthma. J Allergy Clin Immunol 1990; 85:59–65.

EXERCISE-INDUCED BRONCHOCONSTRICTION, ANAPHYLAXIS, AND URTICARIA

PAUL M. O'BYRNE, M.B.
MARK D. INMAN, M.D., Ph.D.

EXERCISE-INDUCED BRONCHOCONSTRICTION

Exercise is a common cause of bronchoconstriction in patients with asthma. The term "exercise-induced asthma" has often been used to describe this phenomenon; however, this is a misnomer, because exercise, unlike allergen inhalation, is not known to cause asthma, but rather causes bronchoconstriction in patients with asthma. Thus, the term exercise-induced bronchoconstriction is preferred, because it may help to alleviate the confusion, often held by parents of asthmatic children, that exercise is to be avoided because it is a cause of the child's asthma.

Exercise-induced bronchoconstriction is likely caused by the airways' efforts to condition to body temperature and to fully humidify the increased volumes of air inhaled during exercise. In some asthmatics, this results in the release of bronchoconstrictor mediators (most likely from airway mast cells), of which the most important are the cysteinyl leukotrienes (LT),LTC_4 and LTD_4, and histamine. The closer to body temperature and fully humidified the inspired air is during exercise, the less likely bronchoconstriction is to occur.

Exercise-induced bronchoconstriction occurs in 70 to 80 percent of patients with current symptomatic asthma, and it is more likely to occur in patients with moderate to severely increased airway responsiveness. Indeed, for any given exercise challenge, the magnitude of the resulting bronchoconstriction is correlated with the degree of airway hyper-responsiveness. This means that in many patients with mild, episodic asthma, who generally have mildly increased airway responsiveness, even strenuous exercise does not cause bronchoconstriction. This has important practical implications in treating exercise-induced bronchoconstriction, and these are considered in the following discussion. Occasionally, exercise-induced bronchoconstriction is the only manifestation of asthma, and the management of this clinical entity is different from that of patients in whom exercise-induced bronchoconstriction is only one part of regular daily symptoms.

The degree and intensity of exercise needed to cause bronchoconstriction varies among asthmatics. Conventionally when exercise-induced bronchoconstriction is being tested for in a laboratory, 5 to 8 minutes of exercise sufficient to raise the heart rate to 80 percent of the predicted maximum is performed on a bicycle ergometer or a treadmill. Exercise-induced bronchoconstriction rarely occurs during the exercise itself. Much more commonly, bronchodilation occurs during exercise, and this lasts for 1 to 3 minutes following exercise. This is followed by the onset of bronchoconstriction, beginning by 3 minutes, generally peaking by 10 to 15 minutes and is resolved by 60 minutes. At one time this acute, transient bronchoconstriction was believed to be occasionally followed by a late-phase bronchoconstriction. However, more recent studies with appropriate controls have not confirmed exercise-induced late-phase bronchoconstrictor responses.

In most patients with exercise-induced bronchoconstriction, the episode of bronchoconstriction is followed by a period during which exercise causes less bronchoconstriction. This has been called the refractory period after exercise. The refractory period is caused by the release of inhibitory prostaglandins (likely prostaglandin E_2) in the airways, which partially protects the airways against repeated episodes of exercise-induced bronchoconstriction. The refractory period after exercise generally lasts less than 4 hours.

MANAGEMENT OF EXERCISE-INDUCED BRONCHOCONSTRICTION

General Measures

Although exercise is a common cause of bronchoconstriction in asthmatics, the combination of general measures and pharmacologic interventions can prevent exercise-induced bronchoconstriction from occurring in almost all asthmatics. The aim of management must be to ensure that exercise is not avoided by asthmatics. Indeed, asthmatics should exercise as much as they wish, and they should be encouraged by the fact that many athletes have won Olympic medals despite having symptomatic asthma.

Improved understanding of the pathophysiology of exercise-induced bronchoconstriction has resulted in the recommendation of general management measures that reduce its severity. The measures are based on the observed relationships between the severity of the bronchoconstriction and the magnitude of the minute ventilation and the temperature and humidity of the inspired air. Therefore, improving the patient's level of physical fitness with a regular exercise program reduces the minute ventilation for any given exercise workrate and thereby the severity of the bronchoconstriction. Also, the warmer and more humid the inspired air, the less bronchoconstriction occurs. Thus, when exercising in cold, dry conditions, patients should be instructed to breathe through a loosely fitting scarf or mask. Lastly, ensuring that patients know how and when to use a metered dose inhaler or spinhaler correctly will greatly enhance the chance that the pharmacologic measures described below will be effective.

Pharmacologic Measures

If exercise-induced bronchoconstriction is occurring on a daily basis as part of poorly controlled asthma, the most important treatment strategy is to improve asthma control. The most effective way to do this is with inhaled corticosteroids, which will not improve exercise-induced bronchoconstriction in the short term, but over weeks to months as airway hyper-responsiveness improves, the magnitude of bronchoconstriction after a given workload will lessen. At the same time, patients should be instructed to use prophylactic treatment prior to exercise. The most usual approach is to advise patients to take two puffs of an inhaled beta$_2$-agonist, 5 to 10 minutes before exercise, which will prevent exercise-induced bronchoconstriction in most patients. An alternative approach is to inhale cromoglycate (20 mg spincap or 2 to 4 puffs from a metered dose inhaler is usually sufficient) 15 to 20 minutes before exercise. Occasionally in patients with more severe asthma, higher inhaled doses of beta$_2$-agonists, such as four puffs, are needed. In exceptional situations, most often in very high performance athletes or in patients exercising in extreme conditions such as very cold, dry air, the combination of four puffs of an inhaled beta$_2$-agonist and cromoglycate has been demonstrated to be significantly better than either drug used alone. A difficult clinical situation exists with children who often exercise vigorously on and off through the day without thinking to pretreat themselves prior to exercise. The long-acting inhaled beta$_2$-agonist, Formoterol, has been demonstrated to provide protection against exercise-induced bronchoconstriction for most of the day and may have a role in this particular situation.

Other types of antiasthma treatments are not very effective in protecting against exercise-induced bronchoconstriction. For example, oral beta$_2$-agonists and methylxanthines are marginally effective or ineffective in almost all patients. Ketotifen does not provide adequate protection in children. As already described, long-acting inhaled beta$_2$-agonists have been demonstrated to provide prolonged protection against exercise-induced bronchoconstriction, but this type of prolonged protection is not usually needed for the exercise requirements of most patients. Nedocromil sodium does not appear to have any advantage in protecting against exercise-induced bronchoconstriction when compared to cromoglycate.

If patients either forget to take prophylactic treatment for exercise-induced bronchoconstriction, or experience breakthrough symptoms despite treatment, the bronchoconstriction should be treated with two to four puffs of an inhaled beta$_2$-agonist. Cromoglycate is not effective in this situation.

Several new drugs are being tested as possible prophylactic agents against exercise-induced bronchoconstriction, including leukotriene antagonists, which do protect patients, and in some this protection is complete. Also, one of these compounds under clinical development, can provide protection for up to 8 hours. Inhaled furosemide and inhaled prostaglandin E_2 also can significantly protect against exercise-induced bronchoconstriction. None of these compounds have been directly compared to inhaled beta$_2$-agonists, which would need to be done before their use can be recommended.

EXERCISE-INDUCED ANAPHYLAXIS AND URTICARIA

Fortunately, exercise-induced anaphylaxis is a much less common clinical entity than exercise-induced bronchoconstriction. It is independent of the presence of asthma, although it is associated with atopy and presents clinically as the manifestations of generalized anaphylaxis after a bout of exercise, which is usually, but not always, vigorous exercise. The anaphylactic reaction begins as a sensation of warmth in the skin, progressing to pruritus and erythema and sometimes to urticaria and angioedema, which can involve the face and upper airways, leading to respiratory distress, stridor, and potentially respiratory arrest. Patients also often complain of abdominal symptoms of cramping, vomiting, and diarrhea and can have hypotension and cardiovascular collapse.

The mechanism of exercise-induced anaphylaxis involves mast cell degranulation with the release of mediators such as histamine and possibly leukotrienes. The reason for exercise causing widespread mast cell activation is not known. A family history of exercise-induced anaphylaxis has been identified in some patients. In addition, the development of symptoms after exercise can be inconsistent, occurring on one occasion and not on another, despite similiar exercise conditions. In a subset of patients, exercise-induced anaphylaxis occurs only after the ingestion of certain foods. The foods most often implicated are shellfish, wheat, and nuts. The food itself does not cause anaphylactic reactions, unless exercise occurs within 4 to 6 hours. Interestingly, many of these patients do not appear to have IgE-mediated hypersensitivity reactions against the food alone.

Exercise may also cause cholinergic urticaria in some patients. This manifests as a pruritic rash in some patients or may result in confluent urticaria in others and the development of anaphylaxis. Patients with cold urticaria have usually recognised the development of similar symptoms in other conditions where body temperature is increased such as during a hot bath, which is not the case with patients with exercise-induced anaphylaxis.

MANAGEMENT OF EXERCISE-INDUCED ANAPHYLAXIS AND URTICARIA

General Measures

Every effort should be made to prevent the development of exercise-induced anaphylaxis in patients who have previously experienced the phenomenon. As anaphylaxis is most likely to occur after vigorous exercise, patients should be advised to perform moderate levels of exercise and to desist if any of the prodromal symptoms develop. It is also unwise for the patient to exercise alone. Exercise should be performed with a partner who understands the possibility of anaphylaxis developing and what to do should it occur. If the patient has recognised the association between the ingestion of certain foods and the development of exercise anaphylaxis, he or she should be advised on food avoidance, and particularly on the need to avoid exercise for more than 6 hours after ingesting the food.

Pharmacologic Measures

The management of exercise-induced anaphylaxis is similar to anaphylaxis to any other agent. The mainstay is the immediate use of epinephrine and antihistamines and the maintenance of a patent airway. All patients with known exercise-induced anaphylaxis must carry an epinephrine autoinjector (Epi-Pen) with them, and they should have an antihistamine readily available and know how to use these medications. Patients experiencing anaphylaxis should also be brought to medical attention as soon as possible because occasionally intubation is necessary to protect the airways. Fully developed exercise-induced anaphylaxis must be treated as an acute medical emergency and ideally should be treated in a hospital emergency department. Other measures that are needed include the insertion of an intravenous line and the delivery of intravenous solutions to maintain blood pressure and the administration of intravenous hydrocortisone, inhaled bronchodilators, and antihistamines. Rarely, the use of pressor agents is needed if the systemic blood pressure cannot be maintained any other way. Unfortunately there is no effective prophylactic treatment for exercise-induced anaphylaxis.

In contrast to exercise-induced anaphylaxis, exercise-induced cold urticaria can be helped by the prophylactic use of ingested antihistamines 1 to 2 hours prior to exercise. The development of full-blown urticaria and anaphylaxis should be treated as previously described.

SUGGESTED READING

Anderson SD. Exercise-induced asthma. The state of the art. Chest 1985; 87S:191.

Casale TB, Keahey TM, Kaliner M, et al. Exercise-induced anaphylactic syndromes. JAMA 1986; 255:2049.

Kidd JM, Cohen SH, Sosman AJ, et al. Food-dependent exercise-induced anaphylaxis. J Allergy Clin Immunol 1983; 71:407.

Latimer KM, O'Byrne PM, Morris MM, et al. Bronchoconstriction stimulated by airway cooling: Better protection with combined inhalation of terbutaline sulphate and cromolyn sodium than with either alone. Am Rev Respir Dis 1983; 128:440.

Manning PJ, Watson RM, Morgolskee DJ, et al. Inhibition of exercise-induced bronchoconstriction by MK-571, a potent leukotriene D_4 receptor antagonist. N Engl J Med 1990; 323:1736.

Manning PJ, Watson RM, O'Byrne PM, et al. Exercise-induced refractoriness in asthmatic subjects involves leukotriene and prostaglandin interdependent mechanisms. Am Rev Respir Dis 1993; 148:950.

STATUS ASTHMATICUS

J. MARK FITZGERALD, M.B., F.R.C.P.C.
ANTON GRUNFELD, M.D., F.R.C.P.C.

Status asthmaticus or acute life-threatening asthma is usually defined as a severe asthma attack necessitating care in the emergency department (ED) or hospitalization. It is a common medical emergency that in the past has been shown to be poorly managed. Its immediate optimal management is of importance, but it is also important to recognize that subjects who visit the ED are at risk for further life-threatening attacks. Therefore the opportunity should be taken not only to manage the current attack optimally, but also to initiate appropriate specialist referral and follow-up to reduce the subsequent risk for life-threatening events.

PATIENT EVALUATION

Certain historical features should alert the physician to be more cautious in evaluating a patient with acute asthma, and these are discussed further in the context of discharge planning. Monosyllabic speech and difficulty in completing a full sentence represent clear evidence of a severe attack. The patient's and caregivers' responses are important to document, particularly with a view to the subsequent prevention of future life-threatening events. For example, was the patient on appropriate anti-inflammatory treatment, did he or she increase medication with the first sign of deteriorating asthma, especially the use of greater than usual doses of beta-agonist?

A previous history of a life-threatening episode or current use of prednisone should also alert the examining physician to be more cautious, particularly with regard to the decision on discharge or admission.

Clinical Examination

Signs of severe life-threatening attacks of asthma include tachycardia, tachypnea, hyperinflation, wheeze, accessory muscle use, and pulsus paradoxicus, all of which should alert the physician to greater caution. Various attempts have been made to formulate a scoring index based on clinical parameters and level of airflow obstruction, but all have generally been unsuccessful in subsequent prospective validation studies. The poor correlation between these indices and subsequent need for admission highlight the fact that the assessment of the patient in the ED should be multifactorial.

Investigations

After the history, the most important investigation is the objective measurement of airflow obstruction. It not only gives the clinician information with regard to the severity of the attack at presentation, but also allows response to therapy to be monitored. Failure to use objective measurements will lead to patients with suboptimal management being discharged from the ED. Many patients poorly perceive the level of airflow obstruction and therapeutic discussions based on clinical examination, or a patient's perception of symptoms may lead patients to unacceptable risk of relapse.

Arterial Blood Gases

Routine use of arterial blood gases is not warranted, particularly with the ready availability of pulse oximetry. In patients who have very severe airflow obstruction, and in particular if the FEV_1 is less than 40 percent of predicted values, arterial blood gases are indicated. In addition, arterial blood gases should be measured if there is concern with regard to whether a patient's clinical status is deteriorating. A normal or rising PCO_2 should alert the physician to the possible need for intubation and mechanical ventilation.

Chest Radiograph

Similar to arterial blood gases, routine chest radiographs are not required, particularly if the patient has only a moderately severe attack and is responding appropriately to bronchodilator therapy. A chest radiograph should be ordered if there is a failure to respond, so that an unrecognized pneumothorax or pneumomediastinum is not present. Patients with airflow obstruction severe enough to require hospitalization should also receive a chest radiograph.

Electrocardiogram

In general, routine use of an electrocardiogram (ECG) is not required unless the patient is in an age group where ischemic heart disease is a possible differential diagnosis, particularly if there is some question of chest tightness that may have some features suggestive of ischemia. Previous studies have shown that during an acute attack of asthma, signs of right ventricular strain may be present on ECG, including T-wave inversion, but these promptly revert in a matter of hours, once the acute attack is under control.

Sputum Examination

The routine use of sputum examination for Gram stain and culture and sensitivity is not warranted. If the exacerbation is associated with a respiratory tract infection, it will usually be viral in origin.

THERAPY

Treatment of patients with severe asthma must be initiated early and aggressively and should continue while the assessment of the patient is in progress.

Table 1 First-Line Drugs for Treatment of Acute Asthma

Agent	*Recommended Dosage*
Oxygen	High flow, to maintain an SaO_2 >92%-95%. Can be delivered by nasal prongs, mask, or an endotracheal tube
beta$_2$-agonists	**MDI:** Initial dose is 4-8 puffs (albuterol 100 μg/puff). Can be repeated every 15-20 min up to 3 times. In severe disease the dose can be increased by one puff every 30-60 sec up to 20 puffs, as needed **Wet nebulizers:** Initial dose is 5-10 mg of albuterol (1-2 ml plus 3 ml of saline) every 15-20 min. For patients with severe attacks, wet nebulization can run continuously
Corticosteroids	Prednisone: 40-60 mg orally stat, then daily for 1 to 2 wk *or* Methylprednisolone: 125 mg IV. Repeat every 8 hr for 24 hr *or* Hydrocortisone: 500 mg IV. Repeat every 8 hr for 24 hr Parenteral therapy to be followed by 1 to 2 wk of oral prednisone

First-Line Drugs

The first line of treatment of patients with severe asthma consists of routine supplemental oxygen, aggressive use of bronchodilators, and, importantly, corticosteroids.

Oxygen

Oxygen should be given to all patients in status asthmaticus. In severely ill patients, extreme hypoxemia and hypercapnia are frequently seen and must be addressed urgently. Oxygen can be delivered by nasal prongs, mask, or an endotracheal tube to maintain an SaO_2 > 92 to 95 percent (Table 1). Oxygen will not suppress the respiratory drive in acute asthma.

Bronchodilators

Sympathomimetic drugs have been used in the management of life-threatening asthma since the 1950s. Adrenaline, the original agent, has gradually been replaced by selective beta$_2$-agonists. There is little disagreement that aerosol forms of beta$_2$-agonists are the agents of first choice to relieve bronchoconstriction in acute asthma. They provide more significant bronchodilation, the most prompt relief, and they are cheaper and have fewer side effects than other agents. Aerosolized beta$_2$-agonists have also been shown to be at least equal to and often superior to parenteral therapy with the same agent, with fewer side effects. Beta$_2$-agonists have also been shown convincingly to be effective even for those patients who have pretreated themselves unsuccessfully with the same medications prior to their arrival at the ED. The reason for self-administered beta$_2$-agonists not being effective prior to arrival in the ED may be due to underdosing or improper use of metered dose inhalers. Equally effective delivery of aerosolized beta$_2$-agonists can be achieved by using nebulized medication or metered dose inhalers, preferably with a spacer device. Most physicians are accustomed to using wet nebulizers for treatment of severe asthma. These devices are also well accepted by patients. Metered dose inhalers, on the other hand, have several advantages: the medication given this way can be administered and repeated very quickly (2 minutes versus 10 to 20 minutes for the wet nebulizers). Using metered dose inhalers is cheaper, offers an opportunity to demonstrate their effectiveness, and helps physicians to educate the patient in their proper use. The dosage of beta$_2$-agonists is empirical and is titrated to patient response (see Table 1). If aerosolized therapy is used aggressively, intravenous forms of beta$_2$-agonists are usually not needed.

Corticosteroids

Corticosteroids have become a first-line drug in the treatment of acute exacerbations of asthma because of the recognition of the pivotal role of inflammation in the pathogenesis of this disease. There continues to be controversy regarding the optimum dose, route, and frequency of administration and the type of preparation used. Corticosteroids are now recommended for all but the mildest attacks of asthma. Unquestionably, the administration of steroids favorably influences the outcome of both admitted and discharged patients. What remains in doubt, in spite of a recent meta-analysis by Rowe and colleagues supporting this view, is whether or not corticosteroids, if administered early and in high doses, can prevent hospital admissions. The onset of action of corticosteroids is slow and not expected to be substantial in the first 2 hours of treatment. In addition, the decision to admit or discharge a patient is complex, involving medical and nonmedical considerations. Oral administration is cheaper and has been found to be equally effective even in severe asthmatic exacerbations. The parenteral preparations should probably be reserved for patients unable to take oral medications (see Table 1).

Second-Line Drugs

Most patients will respond to first-line drugs with significant relief of bronchoconstriction; however, for those who do not improve, there are other agents. These include anticholinergics, adrenaline, intravenous salbutamol, and methylxanthines.

Table 2 Second-Line Drugs for Treatment of Acute Asthma

Agent	*Recommended Dosage*
Anticholinergics	Ipratropium bromide should be given to patients with severe and near-death asthma **MDI:** Initial dose is 4-8 puffs (20 μg/puff) every 15-20 min, to be repeated 3 times. The dose can be increased by one puff every 30-60 sec to a maximum of 20 puffs, as needed **Wet nebulization:** Initial dose is 0.25 to 0.5 mg (1-2 ml in 2 to 3 ml of saline) every 15-20 min or continuous if necessary. It may be mixed with the beta$_2$-agonists
Adrenaline	Adrenaline: 0.3-0.5 ml (1:1,000) subcutaneously every 15-20 min, as required Adrenaline infusion: 4-8 μg/min (1 ml of 1:1,000 adrenaline in 250 ml of D5W gives 4 μg/ml solution. The infusion is started at 1-2 ml/min)
Intravenous beta$_2$-agonists	Albuterol: 4 μg/kg, over 2 to 5 minutes. Albuterol can subsequently be given as an infusion at 0.1-0.2 μg/kg/min
Aminophylline	Aminophylline loading dose: 3-6 mg/kg intravenously over ½ hr. The dose should be halved if the patient is already on theophylline. Followed by an infusion at 0.2-1 mg/kg/hr. Blood level monitoring is recommended

Anticholinergic Agents

Ipratropium bromide, the anticholinergic agent most commonly used, has been shown to have a slower onset of action and to produce less bronchodilation when used alone than beta$_2$-agonists. There is good evidence of an additive effect of ipratropium when used in combination with aerosol beta$_2$-agonist, but this effect although statistically significant, has generally been small, and its clinical relevance is uncertain. Because of concerns regarding the cost of ipratropium solution, all patients presenting with acute asthma should not routinely receive this agent, and it should be reserved for patients failing to respond to beta-agonists. The recommended dosages are empirical (Table 2).

Adrenaline

Adrenaline has been used in the treatment of acute asthma since 1951. With the current, more specific beta$_2$-agonists, adrenaline is seldom needed. In certain circumstances such as anaphylaxis with a prominent bronchospastic component, adrenaline is the drug of choice. Equally, in circumstances where inhaled bronchodilators are not available, subcutaneous adrenaline can be lifesaving (see Table 2).

Intravenous Albuterol

Aggressive treatment with inhaled albuterol eliminates the need to use intravenous albuterol. However, in severely ill patients, prior to endotracheal intubation and ventilation, or in patients responding poorly to inhaled albuterol, the intravenous preparation can be tried.

Methylxanthines

Aminophylline has been used for many years in the treatment of acute asthma. It has been shown, however, that aminophylline confers no additional benefit to the use of beta$_2$-agonists alone. A recent analysis by Littenberg of 13 adequately designed studies in patients with acute, severe asthma showed that the evidence for supporting its use was inconclusive. Aminophylline has a narrow therapeutic margin and can cause significant toxicity, especially in hypoxic patients. The metabolism of theophylline is affected by multiple factors, making close monitoring of its levels during therapy imperative. The combination of the above factors has led to recent recommendations that methylxanthines should not be used during the first 4 hours of treatment of the patient in the ED. If one chooses to use aminophylline, recommended dosages are shown in Table 2.

Intubation and Mechanical Ventilation

Most patients will respond promptly to bronchodilator and corticosteroid treatment. Attention should be paid to patients who do not respond and timely preparations for intubation and mechanical ventilation should be made for the few patients who require it. The decision to intubate an asthmatic patient is ultimately made on clinical grounds. For patients in respiratory arrest, or for patients with decreased sensorium or coma who cannot protect their airways, endotracheal intubation is mandatory. Otherwise, the decision usually evolves over minutes or hours, based on the ongoing clinical observations of the patient's response to treatment. Patients who deteriorate in spite of aggressive bronchodilator therapy and become exhausted and/or confused, whose respiratory effort is decreasing, who are diaphoretic, cyanotic, or whose vital signs are unstable are not likely to improve without a period of respiratory support. These patients need endotracheal intubation and mechanical ventilation. Correctable conditions such as deterioration attributable to a pneumothorax should be sought and rapidly corrected. Arterial blood gases can be obtained to strengthen the clinical decision; their values may show hypoxia, increasing hypercapnia, and acidosis. However, the decision to intubate the patient should not be delayed while waiting to obtain arterial blood gases.

A physician experienced with airway management should proceed with the intubation, while an anaesthetist should be contacted early if the attending physician is not comfortable intubating the patient. It is important to decide which patients are likely to deteriorate and to proceed expeditiously with a rapid-sequence intubation for them, thereby avoiding "crash intubations." Patients should be preoxygenated with 100 percent oxygen.

Ketamine, the induction agent of choice in asthma, is a phencyclidine analog that induces a state of dissociative anesthesia, putting the patient in a trance-like, cataleptic state. The patient maintains muscle tone, pharyngeal and laryngeal reflexes, and respiratory drive. In addition, ketamine is a bronchodilator, acting both directly and indirectly through catecholamine release. It is as effective as halothane or enflurane in preventing bronchconstriction. One-quarter to one-third of adult patients receiving ketamine experience a postanesthesia emergence reaction, during which the patient experiences vividly dysphoric dreams and unpleasant experiences. The emergence reaction can be controlled with the use of benzodiazepines, particularly midazolam. The recommended dosage of ketamine is 1.5 mg per kilogram administered intravenously over 1 minute. The ketamine bolus can be repeated as the bronchodilating effect wears off in 20 to 30 minutes. An infusion can also be started.

Succinylcholine, a depolarizing paralytic agent, is the agent of choice for paralysing to facilitate endotracheal intubation. It is the fastest acting agent, and it is effective and safe used in conjunction with ketamine for intubation of asthmatic patients. The recommended dosage of succinylcholine is 1.5 mg per kilogram administered intravenously as a bolus.

Vecuronium, a nondepolarizing paralytic agent, should only be used for maintenance of paralysis. Although the rate of complications for intubated asthmatic patients is high, the mortality rate is usually low. Strict attention should be paid to maintaining adequate paralysis and low flow rates or tidal volumes to reduce peak airway pressures and associated barotrauma in intubated patients. Admission and treatment in the intensive care unit is mandatory.

CRITERIA FOR ADMISSION OR DISCHARGE

Most patients presenting with exacerbations of asthma respond well to treatment and are discharged safely home. Hospital admission rates vary between 10 to 25 percent and, depending on a variety of factors, between 5 and 25 percent of patients discharged suffer a relapse. Attempts have been made to predict the need for hospital admission from the initial patient evaluation. Although not entirely successful, some broad guidelines are emerging. However, in no situation is the discharge of patients with treated asthma entirely free of risk.

Spirometry

Spirometric measurements have limitations and should not be relied upon in isolation for decision-making regarding the admission or discharge of asthmatic patients. However, data from several studies indicate that patients fall within discernible groups (Table 3).

Table 3 Spirometric Admission and Discharge Criteria in Acute Asthma

Prebronchodilator Treatment

FEV_1 <1.0 L or PEFR <100 L/min or <25% predicted or best will usually require admission

Postbronchodilator Treatment

FEV_1 <1.6 L or PEFR <200 L/min or <40% predicted or best, admission is recommended

FEV_1 1.6-2.1 L or PEFR 200-300 L/min, or between 40%-60% predicted or best, discharge may be possible after consideration of risk factors and follow-up care

FEV_1 >2.1 L or PEFR >300 L/min, or >60% predicted or best, discharge is likely after consideration of risk factors and follow-up care

Historical Risk Factors

The majority of patients who die in status asthmaticus do so prior to reaching the hospital. The best way to identify asthma patients at risk of death is to identify those who have had a recent hospital admission and in particular those who have had one or more life-threatening attacks requiring mechanical ventilation. There are at least two distinctive high risk groups:

1. **Patients with a history of near fatal episode** regardless of the underlying severity of the disease and other risk factors, and
2. **Patients with underlying severe disease** judged by chronic severe symptoms, systemic steroid requirement, frequent regular use of bronchodilators, frequent ED visits, or hospitalization. Patients in this group also may have one or more of the following problems: recent discharge from the hospital for severe asthma, poor self-care or noncompliance with medications, depression or severe emotional disturbance, other significant psychological factors, or shortcomings in education or supervision. Patients with these characteristics (Table 4) will clearly require careful consideration and close follow-up if discharged.

DISCHARGE PLANNING AND FOLLOW-UP

The goal of asthma therapy is the return of the patient to full function. With rare exceptions, disability is not acceptable. Patients should function with minimal or no symptoms and their asthma should not affect their school, work, or exercise. With a physician's help, each patient should have a plan on discharge from the ED and instructions on how to deal with exacerbations.

Regular use of $beta_2$-agonists is often required for at least 48 hours after discharge and patients should be

Table 4 Patient Characteristics for Potentially Fatal Asthma

Near fatal episode of asthma
Sudden precipitous attack
Recent ED visit
Frequent hospitalization
Recent use or dependence on systemic steroids
Recent attack of prolonged duration
Poor compliance or knowledge of asthma
Return to the same environmental triggers

advised on how to modify treatment according to symptoms. If the patient is unable to control symptoms, he should return to the ED. Patients should know the results of their pulmonary function tests, thus facilitating treatment decisions at the time of their next presentation to the ED. Prior to discharging a patient, the physician should verify that the patient knows how to use the metered dose inhaler.

Corticosteroids are indicated, upon discharge from the ED, for most patients. The treatment should be individualized, based on responses to past treatment and recent symptoms. The recommended dosage of prednisone is 30–60 mg per day for 7 to 14 days.

Steroids can usually be stopped rather than tapered as long as patients are taking maintenance inhaled corticosteroids. Patients discharged from the ED should be re-evaluated within a week by their family physician and decisions regarding maintenance anti-inflammatory therapy should be made at this time. There is also evidence that patients discharged from the ED benefit from facilitated referrals to specialists.

In summary, many acute exacerbations of asthma can be prevented with appropriate maintenance anti-inflammatory therapy and its prompt increase with the first signs of deteriorating asthma. When these acute attacks do occur, frequent bronchodilator therapy, primarily with beta-agonists, systemic corticosteroids, and supplemental oxygen, should form the mainstay of treatment.

SUGGESTED READING

Littenberg B. Aminophylline treatment in severe acute asthma. JAMA 1988; 259:1670–1684.

Rowe BH, Keller JL, Oxman AD. Effectiveness of steroid therapy in acute exacerbation of asthma: A meta-analysis. Am J Emerg Med 1992; 10:301–310.

Zimmerman JL, Dellinger RP, Shah AN, Taylor RW. Endotracheal intubation and mechanical ventilation in severe asthma. Crit Care Med 1993; 21:1727–1730.

SKIN DISEASE

CHRONIC URTICARIA

FRANCES LAWLOR, M.D., F.R.C.P.I., D.C.H.
MALCOLM W. GREAVES, M.D., Ph.D., F.R.C.P.

The characteristic skin lesion in urticaria is the wheal, an edematous pale papule, which frequently itches. Since the lesions of urticaria are continually evolving and disappearing, wheals are not invariably seen and when present are associated with a blotchy macular, papular, and annular erythema. In approximately 45 percent of patients with urticaria subcutaneous swelling occurs either at the same time, before, or after the urticarial episode. This frequently affects the mucous membranes and is known as angioedema. Currently when urticaria and angioedema occur together, they are considered part of the same disease. Each urticarial wheal generally lasts less than 24 hours and angioedema swellings less than 72 hours. Both fade to leave normal-appearing skin.

Urticaria can be arbitrarily divided into acute urticaria, which is present less than 12 weeks, and chronic urticaria, which lasts longer than 12 weeks and may last years. In the patients who present with chronic urticaria, a physical urticaria must be considered either as the sole condition or as an associated disease since chronic idiopathic urticaria and the physical urticarias frequently coexist. The diagnosis and treatment of the physical urticarias are considered elsewhere.

Apart from those patients with physical urticaria, the cause of chronic urticaria is unknown, hence its synonym, chronic "idiopathic" urticaria. Allergy or infection do not play a significant role in the pathogenesis of the condition. Thyroid autoantibodies are present more frequently than in the general population but are only occasionally associated with overt thyroid disease. Recently a histamine-releasing IgG autoantibody reacting with the high affinity IgE receptor or with IgE itself has been found in patients' serum, supporting the view that chronic urticaria is an autoimmune disease in some patients. In 75 percent of patients, aspirin worsens the disorder. In a very small number, preservatives, dyes, and colorings can be reproducibly shown to aggravate the condition, possibly through a nonimmunologic mechanism. Drugs such as morphine, codeine, and tubocurarine, which induce mast–cell histamine release, may also augment chronic urticaria.

A careful history (Table 1) taken from a patient suffering from chronic urticaria will generally reveal all the diagnostic information obtainable. A physical examination, including physical urticaria provocation testing where necessary, should confirm the diagnosis.

THERAPY OF CHRONIC IDIOPATHIC URTICARIA

The treatment of chronic idiopathic urticaria can be divided into nondrug management and drug treatment for both the urticaria and for the treatment of acute superimposed severe episodes of angioedema, which may have associated systemic symptoms. These are considered separately.

Nondrug Management

Explanation

Chronic idiopathic urticaria is a distressing condition, both because of the itching and the alarming symptoms attributable to involvement of the skin and mucous membranes. It is helpful to explain the nature of the condition with its remissions and exacerbations and to explain that it is unlikely that a direct cause will be found. More than 50 percent of patients remit within 6 months. Although the condition cannot be cured its symptoms can usually be controlled. Treatment is more effective at reducing pruritus and wealing than reducing erythema, and a certain amount of erythema may be expected unless control is complete. Measures to cool the affected skin invariably cause welcome, though temporary, relief. These include wearing light, loose clothes, working and sleeping in a cool room, and frequent showering or bathing with tepid water. Cooling creams or lotion, including calamine lotion, are also useful.

It is important to avoid aspirin and aspirin-containing drugs. Other nonsteroidal anti-inflammatory drugs should be avoided if possible. Paracetamol is safe. Angiotensin converting enzyme inhibitors should be

Table 1 Chronic Urticaria: Taking a History

Lesions on the skin	How long have the symptoms been present? What do they look like? How long do individual lesions last? Is the skin normal after they have gone away? How often do they occur? Are they provoked by exercise, hot baths, emotion, friction, sustained physical pressure, cold, sunlight, or water?
Eyes, lips, face, throat and tongue	Do they swell? How often does this happen? How long does the swelling last?
Generally	When you have swelling or rash is there any difficulty breathing or swallowing? Any pain in the abdomen or vomiting? Any associated joint pain?

avoided if a suitable alternative drug is available because these have caused severe angioedema in some people, and their relationship to chronic idiopathic urticaria is unclear.

Avoidance of food additives and antioxidants is controversial, since not all believe that these substances play a part. However, if the patient and the physician wish, a placebo-controlled drug and diet challenge test schedule may be undertaken (Table 2). This can be conducted on an outpatient basis, with the patient keeping a daily diary of the severity of the urticaria. A positive reaction would need to be confirmed by rechallenge before any specific dietary restriction is advised.

Alternatively (and less satisfactorily) the patient could embark (without challenge testing) on a restricted diet avoiding the colorings, E102-E180; the benzoate preservatives, E210–219; and the antioxidants, E300-E322. This diet could be continued for 4 to 6 weeks and if there is no major improvement, the diet could be abandoned.

Table 2 Drug and Diet Challenge Test Schedule Used at St. John's Institute of Dermatology

1. Control
2. Tartrazine 10 mg
3. Control
4. Sodium benzoate 500 mg*
5. Control
6. Hydroxybenzoic acid 200 mg
7. Control
8. Yeast extract 0.6 g
9. Control
10. Penicillin 0.5 mg (not to be given if history of asthma or severe penicillin reaction)
11. Control
12. Aspirin 100 mg (not to be given if history of asthma or severe aspirin reaction)
13. Control
14. New coccine 10 mg*
15. Control
16. Canthaxathine 100 mg*
17. Control
18. Sunset yellow 10 mg*
19. Control
20. Annatto 10 mg
21. Control
22. Butylhydroxytoluene 50 mg
23. Butylhydroxytoluene 50 mg
24. Control
25. Butylhydroxyanisol 50 mg
26. Control
27. Ascorbic acid 600 mg
28. Control
29. Sodium nitrate 100 mg
30. Control
31. Quinoline yellow 10 mg
32. Control
33. Sodium glutamate 200 mg

*One-tenth of the dose is to be given if a patient is under 10 years of age or if there is a history of asthma.

Drug Treatment Using Antihistamine Therapy

The mainstay of drug treatment in chronic idiopathic urticaria is H_1-antihistamine therapy in adequate dosage. The antihistamines block the combination of histamine with its receptors. Generally the half-life of the antihistamines is more prolonged in the elderly than in children. The half-lives of some of the active metabolites are longer than that of the parent compound. There is very little information about the use of antihistamines during pregnancy, although there have been no confirmed reports of teratogenicity. Antihistamine treatment in pregnant women should be avoided if possible, but if it is necessary, the agents of choice are chlorpheniramine and tripelennamine.

The timing of antihistamine ingestion in relation to food is generally not important. Since many patients' urticaria is worse at a particular time of the day, it is wise to take the antihistamine approximately 1 to 2 hours before itching and wealing are maximal. Since each individual responds differently to each antihistamine it is usually necessary to be flexible both in dosage and in the antihistamine used and to be ready to change the antihistamine prescribed until control is optimal and adverse effects are minimal.

The "classic" H_1-antihistamines, apart from hydroxyzine, are generally less effective and cause more unwanted effects than the newer minimally sedating antihistamines. However, the older H_1-antihistamines are useful if night sedation is required. These include chlorpheniramine maleate, diphenhydramine hydrochloride, and hydroxyzine hydrochloride (Table 3). The tricyclic antidepressant doxepin has additional H_2-receptor antagonist properties. It is very useful in depressed and agitated adult patients as a single nighttime dose of 25 to 50 mg. It should not be combined with terfenadine or monoamine oxidase inhibitors.

The Newer H_1-Receptor Antagonists

The newer "second-generation" H_1-receptor antagonists seem to have similar efficacy to each other.

Table 3 First-Generation Antihistamines

Drug	*Trade Name*	*Form/Strength*	*Usual Adult Dosage*	*Children's Dosage*	*Time to Peak Level After Oral Intake (hours)*	*Half-Life (hours)*	*Side Effects Common to All*	*Other Rare Effects Common to All*
Chlorpheniramine maleate	Piriton	Tablets, 4 mg, 8 mg, 12 mg	8 mg-12 mg b.i.d. or t.i.d.	0.35 mg/kg/24 hr	2.8 ± 0.8	27.9 ± 8.7	Drowsiness, decreased alertness, GI upset, appetite stimulation, anticholinergic effects, i.e., dry mouth, blurred vision, urinary retention, impotence, abnormalities of liver function	Tachycardia, prolongation of QT interval, heart block, and arrhythmias
Chlorpheniramine maleate	Chlor-Trimeton	Syrup, 2.5 mg/5 ml; Parenteral, 10 mg/ml						
Hydroxyzine hydrochloride	Atarax Ucerax	Capsules, 10 mg, 25 mg, 50 mg; Syrup	10 mg/5 mg 10, 25, 50 mg b.i.d. or t.i.d.	5 mg/kg/24 hr	2.1 ± 0.4	20.0 ± 4.1		
Diphenhydramine hydrochloride	Benadryl	Capsules, 25 mg, 50 mg; Elixir, 12.5 mg/5 ml; Parenteral, 50 mg/ml	25 mg-50 mg t.i.d.	50 mg/kg/24 hr	1.7 ± 1.0	9.2 ± 2.5		
Tripelennamine hydrochloride	PBZ PBZ-SR Pyribenzamine	25 mg, 50 mg; Timed-release, 50 mg, 100 mg	Tablets, 25 mg-50 mg q4-6h	5 mg/kg/24 hr in 4-6 divided doses or if > 5 years, 50 mg b.i.d. or t.i.d.				
Doxepin		10 mg, 25 mg	10 mg-25 mg b.i.d. or 50 mg at night					

Table 4 Properties of Second-Generation Antihistamines

Drug	*Trade Name*	*Form/Strength*	*Usual Adult Dosage*	*Children's Dosage*	*Onset of Action (hours)*	*Duration of Action (hours)*	*Precautions*	*Drug Interactions*	*Side-Effects*	*Other Effects*
Terfenadine	Triludan	60 mg, 120 mg tablets; 30 mg 35 ml suspension	60 mg b.i.d., 120 mg q.d.; do not exceed	3-6 yr, 15 mg b.i.d.; 7-12 yr, 30 mg b.i.d.	1-2	24	Hepatic impairment, QT prolongation, electrolyte disturbance	Macrolide antibiotics, imidazole antifungals, neuroleptics, tricyclics, diuretics	Ventricular arrhythmias	
Astemizole	Hismanal	10 mg tablets; 5 mg/1 ml suspension	10 mg q.d.; do not exceed	6-12 yr, 5 mg q.d.	Very slow	Up to 4 weeks	Same as for terfenadine; use adequate contraception	Same as for terfenadine	Weight gain, ventricular arrhythmias	
Cetirizine	Zirtek	10 mg tablets, 5 mg/5 ml solution	10 mg q.d.; increase to 10 mg b.i.d., if necessary	6-12 yr; 10 mg q.d.	0.5	24	Renal insufficiency		May cause drowsiness in higher dosage	May inhibit mast cell activation; inhibits leukocyte migration; inhibits vascular adhesion molecule expression
Loratadine	Claritin	10 mg q.d.; 5 mg/5 ml syrup	10 mg q.d.; increase to 10 mg b.i.d., if necessary	2-7 yr, 5 mg q.d.; 7-12 yr, 10 mg q.d.	2	12-24			May cause drowsiness in higher dosage	
Acrivastine	Semprex	8 mg capsules	8 mg t.i.d.	None	0.5	< 12	Renal failure			

Their main advantage is that they do not produce atropine-like anticholinergic effects and generally cause little or no drowsiness in the dosage suggested by the manufacturer. However, since it is sometimes necessary to increase the dosage, drowsiness may be a problem at higher dosages (Table 4).

The forerunner of the second-generation antihistamines was terfenadine. All antihistamines have the potential to worsen urticaria for reasons that remain obscure. Occasionally patients taking terfenadine have suffered erythematous rashes, worsening of their urticaria with angioedema, photosensitivity, and peeling of the skin on the hands and feet. The most potentially serious adverse effect of terfenadine is the development of a prolonged QT interval, which may lead to a polymorphic ventricular tachycardia (torsades de pointes). This uncommon problem can be avoided if the adult dosage of terfenadine does not exceed 120 mg per day and if it is not concurrently used with the macrolide antibiotics (e.g., erythromycin), imidazole antifungals (e.g., itraconazole and fluconazole), or the tricyclic antidepressants (e.g., doxepin). Terfenadine should also be avoided in patients with hepatic dysfunction or those with electrolyte imbalance. The exact mechanism of this not known, although abnormalities in the cytochrome P-450 activity have been postulated.

Astemizole has three properties of note:

1. Its duration of action is prolonged to 4 weeks and its active metabolite is present in the body for 6 weeks.
2. It has been associated with the development of torsades de pointes as described previously, and it should be prescribed using the same precautions as apply to terfenadine. Furthermore a daily dosage of 10 mg should not be exceeded.
3. Almost all patients who take astemizole gain weight, and if astemizole is used, the patient should be advised to restrict food intake at the same time.

Loratadine has not been associated with adverse cardiac reactions and has been used safely without any reported drowsiness in a dosage of up to 40 mg twice daily. Cetirizine is claimed to have action in addition to its H_1-antihistamine activity, including inhibition of leukocyte activity, especially eosinophil adhesion to the endothelium and eosinophil migration. It is excreted unchanged in the urine, and the dosage should be decreased in those with renal impairment.

The antihistamine ketotifen has mast cell stabilizing properties and has been administered in a dose of 1 to 2 mg twice daily. In practice this drug seems to be no more effective than one would expect from its antihistaminic properties. There is evidence that the addition of the H_2-blocker, cimetidine, may confer additional therapeutic benefit but the clinical value of adding H_2- to H_1-antagonists is difficult to demonstrate in clinical practice.

Acrivastine is a short-acting antihistamine that may be most suitable for those who suffer from intermittent symptoms only and is probably best used on demand or possibly added to give extra control in those already taking a longer-acting second-generation antihistamine. It is also excreted unchanged in the urine.

If it proves difficult to achieve control it is often helpful to combine antihistamines (e.g., cetirizine and loratadine) and to take the drugs to coincide with the time of greatest symptoms. Besides antihistamines, other types of drugs have been proposed to suppress the whealing and itching of chronic idiopathic urticaria. These include the calcium channel antagonist, nifedipine, and beta-adrenergic drugs such as terbutaline. These have been disappointing in our experience. Short courses of systemic steroids may rarely have a place in the management of acute crisis during the course of chronic urticaria, but it is unwise to embark on long-term steroid treatment because of development of tolerance and side effects. The recent realization that in some patients with chronic urticaria the disease is attributable to a functional anti–high-affinity IgE receptor on anti-IgE autoantibodies is prompting exploration of nonspecific immunotherapy (cyclosporin, intravenous immunoglobulin), but these are experimental measures at the present time.

Drug Treatment of Nonhereditary Angioedema

Mild to moderate angioedema occurring regularly may often respond to an H_1-antihistamine in adequate dosage taken regularly. Dosages used are similar to those for chronic urticaria. Any of the previously listed drugs that may worsen the condition should be stopped. If the attacks of angioedema are intermittent or unpredictable (i.e., once fortnightly or less frequently) an antihistamine can be taken as soon as symptoms occur and continued until the episode remits.

In moderate angioedema affecting the buccal mucosa or throat, other measures are required as necessary in addition to antihistamine treatment (Table 5). Severe oropharyngeal edema with or without anaphylaxis may require introduction of an airway and administration of oxygen. In such patients admission for at least 24 hours for monitoring may be necessary.

Table 5 Emergency Treatment of Angioedema

Moderately severe affecting the buccal mucosa:
Medihaler-Epi 4-8 puffs onto the oral mucosa
Severe angioedema:
Adrenaline 1 : 1,000 (1 mg/ml) subcutaneously to a maximum of 1 ml in divided dosage
IV chlorpheniramine 10-20 mg (max 40 mg/24 hr)
IV hydrocortisone succinate (100-300 mg)
Self-administration of adrenaline:
Adrenaline Min-1-Jet 0.5 ml
Adrenaline Epi-Pen 0.3 ml (adult)
0.15 ml (pediatric)

In patients with severe oropharyngeal obstruction, with or without anaphylactic symptoms and ventilation, oxygen use may be necessary

In severe angioedema or when systemic symptoms of shortness of breath, wheezing, or difficulty in breathing are present or if there is evidence of systemic anaphylaxis, subcutaneous adrenaline 1:1,000 should be administered. An antihistamine may be administered intravenously in addition to the adrenaline, and intravenous hydrocortisone is usually given at the same time. Patients who experience frequent or severe episodes of angioedema with or without anaphylactic symptoms and those who frequently attend the emergency department can be taught the self-administration of adrenaline. Adrenaline is available for this purpose as the Adrenaline Min-1-Jet or the adrenaline Epi-pen and should be administered at the onset of an attack.

SUGGESTED READING

Simons FER. The therapeutic index of newer H_1-receptor antagonists. Clin Exp Allergy 1994; 24:707.

Simons FER, Simons KS. The pharmacology and use of H_1-receptor-antagonist drugs. N Engl J Med 1994; 330(23):1663.

Sullivan TJ. Pharmacology modulation of the whealing response to histamine in human skin identification of doxepin as a potent in vivo inhibitor. J Allergy Clin Immunol 1982; 69:260.

PHYSICAL URTICARIA-ANGIOEDEMA

NICHOLAS A. SOTER, M.D.

Urticaria occurs as circumscribed, raised, erythematous, usually pruritic, evanescent areas of edema that involve the superficial portions of the dermis. When the edematous process extends into the deep dermis and subcutaneous tissue, it is known as angioedema. In humans, reactions occurring in the skin and mucous membranes after the activation of mast cells by various physical stimuli are known as physical urticaria-angioedema.

The immunoglobulin E (IgE)-dependent nature of certain acquired forms of physical urticaria-angioedema has been demonstrated by the passive transfer of the cutaneous reaction to the skin of normal individuals with serum (Prausnitz-Küstner reaction). In addition, the experimental challenge of patients with various forms of physical urticaria-angioedema has provided *in vivo* human models to study its pathogenesis. These experimental models synthesize observations of the evolution of the clinical manifestations, histologic analysis of lesional tissue alterations, measurement of mediators released into the circulation, alterations of plasma effector systems, and assessment of function of peripheral blood leukocytes. Such experimental studies also have implicated the mast cell as a prominent effector cell in various forms of physical urticaria-angioedema.

These are genetic and acquired forms of physical urticaria-angioedema. The eliciting stimuli can be divided into those related to mechanical trauma, temperature, light, stress, water, and exercise (Table 1).

PREFERRED THERAPEUTIC APPROACH

The evaluation of a patient with physical urticaria begins with a thorough history and physical examination.

H_1-antihistamines are the major class of therapeutic agents used in the management of physical urticaria-angioedema. The original agents are now known as traditional, classic, or first-generation H_1-antihistamines. These H_1-antagonists have been divided into subgroups based on their chemical structure (Table 2). In recent years, low-sedating or second-generation H_1-antihistamines have been developed (Table 3).

H_1-antihistamines are absorbed from the gastrointestinal tract after oral administration. Their effects

Table 1 Physical Urticaria-Angioedema

Stimulus and Type of Response	*Clinical Presentation*
Mechanical trauma	
Dermographism	
Immediate	Erythema, wheal
Delayed	Erythema, wheal, nodules
Pressure	
Immediate	Erythema, deep local swelling
Delayed	Erythema, deep local swelling, fever, chills, arthralgia
Vibration	Angioedema
Temperature	
Cold	
Immediate	Erythema, wheal, angioedema, headache, hypotension, syncope, wheezing, nausea, vomiting, diarrhea
Delayed	Erythema, deep local swelling
Familial	Erythema, fever, arthralgia, leukocytosis
Heat	
Cholinergic	Erythema, small wheal, dizziness, headache, syncope, wheezing, nausea, vomiting, diarrhea
Local	Erythema, wheal
Light	
Solar	Erythema, wheal, angioedema, syncope, wheezing
Stress	
Adrenergic	Erythema, wheal with halo
Water	
Aquagenic	Erythema, small wheal
Exercise	Erythema, wheal, hoarseness, difficulty swallowing, syncope

can be observed within 30 minutes of administration, are maximal within 1 to 2 hours, and usually persist for 4 to 6 hours. Some of these therapeutic agents may have a longer duration of action.

The metabolism of H_1-antihistamines takes place by the hepatic cytochrome *P*-450 system, in which they are conjugated to form glucuronides. The H_1-antihistamines also induce hepatic microsomal enzymes and thus may facilitate their own metabolism. Excretion of these compounds in the urine is almost complete by 24 hours after administration.

Approximately 25 percent of patients receiving first-generation H_1-antihistamines experience an adverse reaction. However, there are considerable variations in the responses of individual subjects. Sedation is the most common problem associated with these therapeutic agents. This sedative effect is pronounced with the aminoalkyl ether and the phenothiazine subgroups. The soporific effect of other subgroups is less marked, especially the alkylamine subgroup. The sedative effect ameliorates in most individuals within a few days of continual administration of H_1-antihistamines. If tolerance to the sedative manifestations does not occur, a trial of an agent from another subgroup should be undertaken. Other central nervous system (CNS) effects include dizziness, tinnitus, incoordination, blurred vision, and diplopia. The CNS effects at times may be stimulatory, especially with the alkylamine group; these effects include nervousness, irritability, insomnia, and tremor.

Table 2 First-Generation, H_1-Antihistamine Drugs Available in the United States

Chemical Class	*Generic Name*
Alkylamine (propylamine)	Brompheniramine maleate Chlorpheniramine maleate Dexchlorpheniramine maleate Triprolidine hydrochloride
Aminoalkyl ether (ethanolamine)	Clemastine fumarate Diphenhydramine hydrochloride Doxylamine succinate
Ethylenediamine	Pyrilamine maleate Tripelennamine citrate Tripelennamine hydrochloride
Phenothiazine	Methdilazine hydrochloride Promethazine hydrochloride Trimeprazine tartrate
Piperidine	Azatadine maleate Cyproheptadine hydrochloride Phenindamine tartrate
Piperazine	Hydroxyzine hydrochloride Hydroxyzine pamoate

Gastrointestinal complaints are the second most frequent side effect and are noted especially with the ethylenediamine group. Anorexia, nausea, vomiting, epigastric distress, diarrhea, and constipation have been reported.

Traditional H_1-antihistamines have anticholinergic effects, including dry mucous membranes, difficulty in micturition, urinary retention, dysuria, urinary frequency, and impotence. These clinical manifestations are prominent with therapeutic agents from the aminoalkyl ether, the phenothiazine, and the piperazine subgroups.

When H_1-antihistamines are consumed in combination with alcohol or other therapeutic agents with CNS depressant effects such as diazepam, there may be an accentuation of the central depressive effects. Agents of the phenothiazine subgroup may block the vasopressor effect of epinephrine. H_1-antihistamines are contraindicated in patients receiving monoamine oxidase inhibitors.

The low-sedating or second-generation H_1-antihistamines currently available in the United States are terfenadine, astemizole, loratadine, and cetirizine. Low-sedating H_1-antihistamines have become popular therapeutic agents because of their lack of both sedative and anticholinergic side effects. These agents minimally cross the blood-brain barrier and preferentially bind to peripheral H_1-receptors.

The administration of first-generation H_1-antihistamines should be initiated at a low dosage level at defined regular intervals and increased to tolerance. For example, 4 mg of chlorpheniramine maleate can be administered every 4 to 6 hours with a 4 mg increase in dosage every 48 to 72 hours to a maximum level of 16 mg at each time point. Moreover, some of the preparations, including chlorpheniramine maleate, are available in long-acting forms that can be administered every 12 hours. If the H_1-antihistamine chosen is not effective or tolerated, therapy with another H_1-drug from a different chemical class should be instituted. Empiric trials of drugs from different classes may be carried out, and combinations of H_1-antihistamines also can be used.

Table 3 Low-Sedating or Second-Generation H_1-Antihistamines

Drug	*Chemical Class*	*Dosage*	*Onset of Action*	*Restrictions*	*Side Effects*
Terfenadine	Piperidine	60 mg b.i.d.	Hours	Concomitant imidazole antifungals or macrolide antibiotics	Torsades de pointes; prolongation of QT interval
Astemizole	Piperidine	10 mg/day	Days	Empty stomach; concomitant imidazole antifungals or macrolide antibiotics	Torsades de pointes; prolongation of QT interval; increased appetite
Loratadine	Piperidine	10 mg/day	Hours	None	None
Cetirizine	Piperazine	5-10 mg/day	Hours	None	None

Once control of physical urticaria-angioedema has been achieved, antihistamine dosage should be tapered rather than stopped abruptly, inasmuch as flares may occur. The low-sedating H_1-antihistamines are administered at specified doses and not increased in amount (Table 3).

H_2-antihistamines possess an imidazole ring and lack the aryl ring of H_1-antihistamines. These therapeutic agents are less lipophilic, which presumably accounts for their lack of CNS effects. Although these therapeutic agents were originally developed for use in peptic ulcer disease, they have been used in dermatology because of the H_2-receptors of the cutaneous microvasculature.

Empiric trials of traditional H_1-antihistamines are used in the treatment of both acute and recurrent episodes of physical urticaria-angioedema. In double-blind, placebo-controlled studies, traditional H_1-antihistamines were shown to be statistically superior to placebos in the treatment of urticaria and angioedema. However, comparative studies of the subgroups of traditional H_1-antihistamines have shown them to be of equal efficacy. If an agent from one therapeutic subgroup of H_1-antihistamine proves ineffective, then an agent from another subgroup should be administered. At times, H_1-antihistamines from different subgroups may be combined. Hydroxyzine hydrochloride has been reported to be of particular efficacy in cholinergic urticaria. The combination of H_1- and H_2-antihistamines is of benefit in few patients with dermographism. During hypothermic cardiopulmonary bypass, cold urticaria was successfully managed after the administration of H_1- and H_2-antihistamines.

Other Therapeutic Approaches

Induction of tolerance by repeated exposure to the appropriate physical stimulus has been achieved in some patients with certain forms of physical urticaria-angioedema. In one study, the oral administration of the impeded androgen danazol was of benefit in cholinergic urticaria. The administration of propranolol hydrochloride prevents attacks of adrenergic urticaria. A few patients with various forms of physical urticaria have responded to treatment with ultraviolet B phototherapy.

The tricyclic antidepressant doxepin hydrochloride, which has activity against both H_1- and H_2-histamine receptors, may be of value. Topical preparations of doxepin hydrochloride are now available, but have not been studied in patients with physical urticaria-angioedema.

Systemic corticosteroid therapy has no place in the management of physical urticaria-angioedema except in some patients with delayed pressure urticaria. The side effects of corticosteroids outweigh the therapeutic benefits in most patients.

Epinephrine injections are widely employed, particularly in hospital emergency units, but their use is rarely required or indicated in physical urticaria-angioedema unless laryngeal edema or respiratory tract compromise complicates attacks.

The role of dietary manipulation has been suggested in one study of delayed pressure urticaria.

Antipruritic lotions containing menthol may provide temporary relief.

PROS AND CONS OF TREATMENT

The decision to treat physical urticaria-angioedema depends on the frequency and severity of the symptoms and signs and focuses on empiric trials of H_1-antihistamines. Combinations of H_1- and H_2-antihistamines may be used. It is desirable to avoid repeated injections of epinephrine and the systemic administration of corticosteroids. Urticaria has a capricious course, may respond to the administration of placebos, and may resolve spontaneously.

SUGGESTED READING

Champion RH, Greaves MW, Kobza Black A, et al, eds. The urticarias. Edinburgh: Churchill Livingstone, 1985.

Czarnetzki BM. Urticaria. Berlin: Springer-Verlag, 1986.

Juhlin L. Recurrent urticaria: Clinical investigation of 330 patients. Br J Dermatol 1981; 104:369–381.

Soter NA. Physical urticaria/angioedema as an experimental model of acute and chronic inflammation in human skin. Springer Semin Immunopathol 1981; 4:73–81.

HEREDITARY ANGIONEUROTIC EDEMA

VIRGINIA H. DONALDSON, M.D.

Persons with hereditary angioneurotic edema (HANE) are deficient in $C\bar{1}$-inhibitor function because of various structural alterations of the $C\bar{1}$-inhibitor gene. This disorder is transmitted as an autosomal dominant trait, and all affected persons are heterozygous. Patients have recurrent attacks of bland, nonpitting, circumscribed swellings of the skin and mucous membranes, particularly of the respiratory and gastrointestinal (GI) tracts. The swellings are often mild but may be incapacitating when the GI tract is involved, and they occur at irregular intervals. The incidence of fatal edema of the respiratory tract has been reported to be as high as 25 percent, but we have not found it to be this high. Affected young children may have subcutaneous swellings or unexplained episodes of abdominal pain that may be due to this disease, but more typical and severe symptoms usually do not occur until adolescence. Typical crises of disabling abdominal pain, usually with vomiting and sometimes diarrhea, last for 1 to 3 days and may occur without subcutaneous swellings so that the patient may not relate the abdominal symptoms to peripheral edema. There are numerous reports of the need for tracheostomy during such episodes, but we have not had to resort to this procedure.

PATHOPHYSIOLOGY

To satisfactorily manage patients with HANE, one must appreciate the pathophysiology of the disease. $C\bar{1}$-inhibitor regulates several enzymes in plasma that may release vasoactive polypeptides, which increase vascular permeability. It is a major inhibitor of the kinin-releasing enzyme, plasma kallikrein, and of activated Hageman factor (factor XIIa), which can activate plasma prekallikrein. It is the only plasma inhibitor of the activated first component of complement, $C\bar{1}$, and its $C\bar{1}r$ and $C\bar{1}s$ subunits, and is critical to the control of the activation and action of the classical pathway of complement. In its absence, $C\bar{1}$ becomes spontaneously active and then cleaves and inactivates the fourth, C4, and sometimes the second, C2, components of complement, probably releasing vasoactive polypeptides in the process. This creates a secondary deficiency of C4 and sometimes of C2. Other plasma inhibitors can control the kinin releasing mechanism by inhibiting activated Hageman factor, kallikrein and the fibrinolytic enzyme, plasmin, thereby restricting the release of polypeptides that enhance vascular permeability.

PREVENTIVE MEASURES

Ideally, episodes of swelling should be prevented either with long-term prophylaxis or short-term prophylaxis when an attack may be initiated by predicted events such as surgery or dental extractions.

Once an episode of edema is underway, mediators of the increased vascular permeability have already been released, and one can only hope to reduce the severity or duration of the attack. Therefore, treatment is aimed at preventing these attacks. Successful pharmacologic approaches have included prevention of the activation of kinin-releasing enzymes or increasing the blood levels of normal $C\bar{1}$-inhibitor.

Androgens

Oral androgens have provided the most successful preventive therapy. Synthetic attenuated androgens such as danazol or stanozolol taken prophylactically increase the serum concentrations of $C\bar{1}$-inhibitor, presumably by enhancing the function of the normal $C\bar{1}$-inhibitor gene, which each patient has. These are well-tolerated by females, even though their use is usually associated with a weight gain of about 8 pounds in the beginning of treatment, which is troublesome to some. Hypomenorrhea, but not usually amenorrhea, and occasionally mild hirsutism may occur. These side effects are usually accepted by women whose lives have been impaired by disabling episodes of edema. We do not usually administer androgenic substances or other prophylactic therapy to patients who have mild, infrequent episodes of swelling, (e.g. less than one per month).

Oxymetholone, which can provide long-term protection from edema with relatively few side affects, may be given in doses of 15 mg daily. Danazol in daily doses of 200 mg, or stanozolol, 2 mg daily, will usually prevent symptoms. Stanozolol is the less expensive of the two. If abdominal discomfort recurs, the dose of danazol is increased to 400 mg daily for 1 to 2 months. Once symptoms are clearly controlled, the dose is reduced to 200 mg again, with the aim of finding the minimum dose that will control the patient's symptoms. Many patients ultimately take only 100 or 50 mg daily or even every other day. Patients are warned that at times of planned surgery, especially dental surgery, they may require additional coverage with an increased dose of danazol (twice the daily dose) for 4 to 5 days before the event and for several days afterwards. Patients are advised to increase their doses at times of emotional stress because they are likely to have bouts of edema at such times. The goal of treatment is to keep them free of symptoms. We do not treat the biochemical alterations associated with HANE, but when therapy is adequate, the plasma levels of C4 and $C\bar{1}$-inhibitor may be increased above pretreatment levels, although not necessarily to the normal range. These observations do indicate the adequacy of treatment and are helpful in estimating the degree of protection a patient has.

Symptoms of HANE have been said to remit during pregnancy, but we have not found this to be usual, and instead, they often worsen. Androgens should be avoided during pregnancy. A somewhat masculinized female infant was reported to have been born to a patient receiving an attenuated androgen.

It is important to note that women with HANE who take oral contraceptives usually suffer increasingly frequent and severe bouts of HANE. This occurs because the minimal levels of $C\bar{1}$-inhibitor in their plasma provided by their normal $C\bar{1}$-inhibitor gene are depressed by oral contraceptives; the mechanism is unknown.

When treating males with hereditary angioneurotic edema, it would seem logical to use less expensive androgens (e.g., methyl testosterone). We have observed significant polycythemia in one such patient. When danazol was substituted for testosterone, the polycythemia cleared.

Undesirable effects of attenuated androgens may include altered libido, weight gain and some hirsutism, myalgias, and muscle cramps. Myalgias may occur even without this treatment. Infrequently, some of our patients have had elevated serum CPK levels even before treatment. We do not know the reasons for this. Some develop hematuria, probably reflecting bladder inflammation. Occasionally a patient receiving danazol will complain of tremulousness, anxiety, or dizziness, but the causes are unclear. Some have had elevated plasma levels of SGOT or SGPT, but none have had jaundice to our knowledge.

Antifibrinolytic Agents

Antifibrinolytic agents have been successful as preventive therapy. Their effect may depend on the physiologic or pathologic enhancement of plasminogen activation in blood that may then promote the activation of $C\bar{1}$. It is not clear that the ameliorating effect of these agents is due to their antifibrinolytic action. Amicar (epsilon aminocaproic acid, or 6-aminohexanoic acid) has been used in a wide range of dosages, depending on the degree of control of symptoms. One report described muscle necrosis apparently caused by a prolonged high dose (30 g per day) of epsilon aminocaproic acid. We have observed this complication at a lower dosage on one occasion. It is possible that one or more unidentified host factors may predispose certain individuals to this complication. Another antifibrinolytic compound called tranexamic acid (trans-4-[aminomethyl]cyclohexanecarboxyl acid) has been beneficial in dosages of 2 g per day for adults and 1.5 g per day for children, without notable toxicity. One must be alert to the risk of thromboembolic disease, particularly in patients with a history of thrombosis, when using antifibrinolytic drugs. Intravenous tranexamic acid or Amicar has been used for immediate short-term treatment. Antifibrinolytic agents probably prevent extensive edema formation in some way after the onset of an attack, for patients are aware that they are having a bout of intestinal edema, for example, but the symptoms are markedly ameliorated.

It has become clear that one should avoid giving angiotensin converting enzyme (ACE) inhibitors such as Captopril to patients with HANE. Polypeptide kinins, which mediate edema formation in these patients, are inactivated by cleavage by these enzymes, and when they are inhibited, symptoms may worsen. Indeed, brisk bouts of edema and even shock have occurred when patients with HANE have been given ACE inhibitors. Similarly, patients with acquired deficiencies of $C\bar{1}$-inhibitor (vide infra) should not be given such a drug.

TREATMENT OF AN EPISODE OF ACUTE EDEMA

Minor episodes of subepithelial swelling need no treatment, but the patient with edema of the face and neck should be closely observed for spread of edema and signs of airway involvement. When hoarseness or other signs of a compromised airway occur, one must consult an otolaryngologist in case tracheostomy becomes imperative. This procedure is usually not needed, but some reports have indicated it to be a lifesaving measure. Airway involvement can be a true medical emergency in this disorder. Other treatment that may be beneficial includes an oropharyngeal spray of a 1:1,000 dilution of recemic epinephrine (0.2 to 0.3 ml). Cautious sedation with antihistamines may be beneficial. These patients may be badly frightened when airway symptoms or difficulty in swallowing occurs during an attack because they have seen affected relatives die during such episodes.

When an episode of abdominal colic occurs, symptomatic treatment with narcotics may be required to relieve pain. These patients run the risk of becoming addicted. When there is a major loss of fluid from the vascular compartment, replacement with physiologic intravenous fluids may aid in the recovery. In one instance, the hematocrit of a patient sustaining such a crisis rose to 75 percent. The leukocyte count is usually elevated only in proportion to the degree of hemoconcentration, unless some complicating factor is present, and the patient is usually afebrile.

It is logical to think of replacement therapy in the case of an ongoing attack. A number of reports indicate that fresh frozen plasma may relieve the patient of an episode of edema. Physicians are reluctant to report less favorable events, but instances of worsening of an episode of swelling are known to have occurred during infusion of fresh frozen plasma. The discrepancies in response to this treatment probably result from the differences in the times from the onset of an attack at which treatment was administered, but this is difficult to judge from published reports. By the time a patient comes to a physician or an emergency department, the attack has probably been underway for a number of hours or more than a day. At this time, the inciting events have probably been removed by one or another physiologic mechanism, and the enzymatic activity (e.g., $C\bar{1}$-esterase activity, orkallikrein) that can be found in plasma during an attack is decreasing. Thus, replacement therapy may appear to have been helpful but may have been unnecessary because the attack would have abated in a short time.

Fresh frozen plasma contains an excess of substrates from which vasoactive peptides can be released by active enzymes in the patient's plasma that are normally controlled by $C\bar{1}$-inhibitor, and if it is given early during an attack, it could theoretically worsen the edema. Therefore, we do not advise early administration of fresh frozen plasma, but purified preparations of $C\bar{1}$-inhibitor can be safe and effective at this time (see below).

When surgery is planned, on the other hand, and the patient is clearly in remission, fresh frozen plasma given before and on the day of surgery has appeared to prevent edema. In addition, increased plasma concentrations of $C\bar{1}$-inhibitor and C4 may be found after this treatment.

A partially purified preparation of human $C\bar{1}$-inhibitor has been available in Europe for several years and is under investigation in the United States. The material has been safe from the risk of transmission of hepatitis or immunodeficiency viruses. Earlier preparations frequently induced hepatitis. It does not worsen symptoms. When given promptly at the onset of an attack, symptoms will regress in 30 to 90 minutes.

PEDIATRIC MANAGEMENT: SHORT-TERM THERAPY

When a child must have surgery that might be predicted to induce a bout of edema, antifibrinolytic therapy for several days before the event and for 4 to 5 days after has been reported to prevent bouts of edema. We have given danazol to preadolescent or adolescent children, not yet physically mature, for a week before surgery and continued it for 4 to 5 days afterwards. The drug is withdrawn gradually. This time schedule is used because we have found that after 6 to 7 days of danazol treatment (200 mg daily) the concentrations of $C\bar{1}$-inhibitor and C4 are increased in the plasma of patients treated in this manner.

ACQUIRED $C\bar{1}$-INHIBITOR DEFICIENCY

Numerous instances of severe bouts of swellings essentially identical to those of patients with HANE have been reported in patients who are deficient in $C\bar{1}$-inhibitor on the basis of an acquired disorder, including (1) lymphomas or other syndromes with expanded B-cell populations and (2) autoimmune deficiency because of an autoantibody directed against $C\bar{1}$-inhibitor. Clues to the acquired nature of the disease are found in the complement component levels in serum because although patients with HANE have normal serum concentrations of antigenic properties of the C1q subcomponent of $C\bar{1}$, this protein has been reduced in the acquired form with only one unexplained exception. Functional levels of $C\bar{1}$-inhibitor are markedly reduced in the autoimmune form but antigen levels may be disproportionately high, probably because the inhibitor is complexed with antibody in the circulation.

Treatment must depend in part on the underlying disease when associated with a lymphoma. In the autoimmune form, the cause is unlikely to be apparent. Treatment with danazol may not be helpful or may be disadvantageous, but some have reported benefit. In our own experience, a severe and nearly fatal bout of airway edema in a patient occurred when he had a high titer of antibody to $C\bar{1}$-inhibitor. When relieved of antibody load by plasmapheresis, he improved remarkably. Others have not always found this to be a helpful approach. Although we have identified no pathologic cells responsible for this antibody and do not know the reason for its occurrence, intermittent therapy with a cytotoxic agent has prevented a recurrence. Autoimmune $C\bar{1}$-inhibitor deficiency is difficult to manage largely because its cause is likely to be obscure.

SUGGESTED READING

Agostoni A, Cicardi M. Hereditary and acquired $C\bar{1}$-inhibitor deficiency: Biological and clinical characteristics in 235 patients. Medicine 1992; 71(4):206–215.

Atkinson JC, Frank MM. Oral manifestations and dental management of patients with hereditary angioedema. J Oral Pathol Med 1991; 20:139–142.

Cicardi M, Bergamaschini L, Cugno M, et al. Long-term treatment of hereditary angioedema with attenuated androgens: A survey of a 13-year experience. J Allergy Clin Immunol 1991; 87:768–773.

Cicardi M, Bisiani G, Cugno M, et al. Autoimmune $C\bar{1}$-inhibitor deficiency: Report of eight patients. Am J Med 1993; 95:169–175.

Donaldson VH, Bernstein DI, Wagner CJ, et al. Angioneurotic edema with acquired $C\bar{1}$-inhibitor deficiency and autoantibody to $C\bar{1}$-inhibitor: Response to plasmapheresis and cytotoxic therapy. J Lab Clin Med 1992; 119:397–406.

Marasini B, Cicardi M, Martignoni GC, Agostoni A: Treatment of hereditary angioedema. Klin Wochenschr 1978; 56:819–823.

DERMATITIS HERPETIFORMIS

JENS GILLE, M.D.
ROBERT A. SWERLICK, M.D.

Dematitis herpetiformis (DH) is a chronic, intensely pruritic, papulovesicular skin eruption typically distributed in a symmetrical fashion on extensor surfaces. DH may present at any age; however, it usually starts in the second or third decade. Characteristically, patients feel localized burning, stinging, or itching about 12 to 24 hours before the appearance of the lesions. Essentially all patients with DH have a gluten-sensitive enteropathy (GSE) that most commonly is asymptomatic. If gastrointestinal symptoms do occur, they clinically resemble celiac sprue. In addition to GSE, DH can be associated with a number of other internal abnormalities (Table 1).

The ability of DH patients to both normalize the morphologic changes of the intestine and to improve their skin lesions by strictly adhering to a gluten-free diet has provided strong evidence that associated GSE plays a fundamental role in the pathogenesis of DH. The high occurrence of certain major histocompatibility complex antigens such as HLA-B8, HLA-DRw17, HLA-DQw2 in DH patients is viewed as a major immunogenic factor contributing to a relative immune susceptibility. Granular deposits of polyclonal IgA found in both involved and uninvolved dermal skin are a universal phenomen in DH patients; however, their role in the pathophysiology of DH is still unknown.

Even if the clinical presentation is not classic and straightforward, DH can usually be diagnosed by direct immunofluorescence of perilesional skin. Typically, in

Table 1 Selected Disorders Associated with Dermatitis Herpetiformis

Gluten-sensitive enteropathy (GSE)
Gastric abnormalities (atrophy, hypochlorhydria)
Thyroid abnormalities (autoimmune thyroiditis, hypothyroidism, hyperthyroidism, thyroid nodules, and malignancy)
Gastrointestinal lymphoma
Autoimmune diseases (systemic lupus erythematosus, dermatomyositis, Sjögren's syndrome, rheumatoid arthritis, myasthenia gravis, and others)

vivo-bound granular IgA deposits are found in the papillary dermis, which by definition distinguish the entity DH from other subepidermal blistering eruptions.

THERAPY

There are two therapeutic strategies to treat patients with DH—pharmacologic therapy and a gluten-free diet. The choice of therapy depends on a variety of factors, including the knowledge of the benefits and the risks that accompany both drug and dietary treatment. Sulfones are the pharmacologic agents of choice in the therapy of DH. Three drugs within this class, diaminodiphenylsulfone (dapsone, DDS), sulfapyridine, and sulfamethoxypyridazine, are used to treat DH, although only dapsone is freely available in the United States. Drug therapy typically results in rapid relief of severe itching and burning, and the appearance of new lesions ceases within 24 to 48 hours. Sulfones are usually well tolerated, yet they do not improve the associated GSE and have a small risk of severe side effects. In contrast, a gluten-free diet treats both bowel and skin disease and is essentially devoid of significant risks. However, a gluten-free diet is difficult for the patient to manage, and effective control of the skin eruption with strict dietary treatment may take many months to years. Therefore, sulfones are generally the initial treatment of choice in order to rapidly control the rash, while a gluten-free diet should be offered to patients with associated symptomatic GSE or those desiring drug-free treatment.

Diaminodiphenylsulfone

Diaminodiphenylsulfone (dapsone) is a remarkably effective agent for DH treatment. The responsiveness to dapsone has almost become an additional criterion for the diagnosis of DH. A variety of other skin disorders that are characterized histologically by infiltration with polymorphonuclear leukocytes may also respond to dapsone, but a presumptive diagnosis of DH in patients who fail to respond to dapsone should suggest an alternative diagnosis.

The initial dose for an average adult patient is usually 50 to 100 mg daily, depending on the severity of the disease and the expected risks of dapsone therapy. Approximately two-thirds of all DH patients will sufficiently respond to 100 mg per day of dapsone. Since many side effects (Table 2) are dose dependent, it is critical to establish the minimum dose that is required to suppress symptoms for each patient. However, few patients without other medical problems will experience side effects at daily doses of 100 mg or lower.

If the skin rash is adequately controlled, the daily dose should be reduced every 2 to 4 weeks by 25 to 50 mg until the daily dose is 25 to 50 mg. Subsequently, the dosage should be administered every second day, reviewed in 2 to 4 weeks, and then every third day until skin lesions reappear. In DH patients, who have not responded to 100 mg daily after 2 to 4 weeks, the dose can be increased in 25 to 50 mg increments every 2 to 4 weeks. Patients generally tolerate dosages up to 150 or 200 mg daily. Occasionally, initial dosage of 300 to 400 mg per day may be required, though side effects usually do not allow dapsone treatment at such high doses.

The use of dapsone in the treatment of DH is limited by its side effects and contraindications (see Tables 2 and 3). Two categories of toxicity are appreciated: dose-dependent and idiosyncratic reactions. Dose-dependent side effects include the well-documented hematologic effects of dapsone therapy, such as hemolysis and methemoglobinemia. A dose of 100 mg daily will transiently decrease hemoglobin levels by 1 to 2 g per deciliter. In particular, this will affect the elderly population and patients with ischemic heart disease, peripheral vascular disease, or cerebrovascular insufficiency. Concomitant administration of vitamin E can effectively blunt dose-dependent decreases in hemoglobin levels at daily doses of 800 U.

Methemoglobinemia is regularly seen in patients treated with dapsone, although it is uncommonly symptomatic at doses below 150 mg per day. If methemoglobin concentrations reach critical levels, related symptoms, such as headache, nausea, fatigue, and cyanosis, can occur. Both methylene blue (Urolene blue, Star Pharmaceuticals) and cimetidine (400 mg three times daily) can reduce dose-dependent methemoglobinemia. Levels of methemoglobin can be measured, yet the dose of dapsone and concomitant methylene blue or cimetidine treatment can usually be adjusted on a clinical basis. Although the initial dose of methylene blue is 65 mg twice daily, it can be escalated up to as much as 130 mg four times daily. Methylene blue is well tolerated except for occasional bladder irritation, particularly if it is not administered in divided doses. Patients need to know that this therapy will turn their urine blue.

Dapsone may also cause a variety of other adverse reactions on an idiosyncratic or allergic basis. These reactions include agranulocytosis, infectious mononucleosis-like hepatitis, various cutaneous eruptions, psychosis, and peripheral neuropathy (see Table 2). The severe cases of agranulocytosis almost invariably occur within the first 8 to 12 weeks of therapy. The risk has been estimated to be as high as 1:240 to as rare as 1:20,000.

Because of its potential and pharmacologic side effects, dapsone therapy requires close laboratory monitoring before and during treatment. Complete blood cell

Table 2 Selected Side Effects of Dapsone Therapy

Hemolytic anemia
Methemoglobinemia
Headache
Nausea
Fatigue
Cyanosis
Gastrointestinal irritation
Psychosis
Skin eruption
Hepatitis, infectious mononucleosis-like with lymphadenopathy
Hypalbuminemia
Peripheral neuropathy
Leukopenia-agranulocytosis

Table 3 Absolute and Relative Contraindications of Dapsone Therapy

Sulfa allergy
History of adverse reactions to sulfones
G-6-PD deficiency
Anemia
History of hemoglobulin abnormalities
Ischemic heart disease
Peripheral vascular disease
Cerebrovascular insufficiency
Liver, lung, and kidney disorders

counts, differential white blood cell counts, hemoglobin, and renal and liver parameters should be obtained before starting dapsone therapy. Since hemolysis may be life threatening in patients with glucose-6-phosphate dehydrogenase (G-6-PD) deficiency, this condition represents a rigid contraindication for dapsone therapy. Although the incidence of G-6-PD deficiency is considered low in northern European populations who are at greatest risk for DH, we routinely screen all patients prior to treatment. Complete blood counts with differential are checked weekly during the first 2 weeks of therapy and then twice monthly during the next 3 months of therapy to monitor for leukocytopenia or agranulocytosis. Thereafter, complete blood parameters and liver and renal function are periodically determined at 2- to 3-month intervals. Thyroid abnormalities are frequently associated with DH and may affect dapsone metabolism. It may be prudent to obtain functional thyroid parameters if clinical hyperthyroidism or hypothyroidism is suspected.

Sulfapyridine and Sulfamethoxypyridazine

Sulfapyridine and sulfamethoxypyridazine are almost exclusively used as alternative drugs in DH patients who do not tolerate dapsone or in whom its hemolytic potential makes it unsuitable, such as in patients with cardiopulmonary problems. In part, their limited use is also caused by their unavailability in many countries. Sulfapyridine appears to be less effective in controlling DH symptoms than dapsone. The initial dose is 500 mg twice daily, but it may require up to 2 to 3 g daily in order to completely alleviate cutaneous lesions. Sulfamethoxypyridazine, however, is a very effective drug in patients who are at risk under dapsone treatment or who have been unable to tolerate dapsone. An adequate response is seen in most patients at daily doses of 0.5 to 1.0 g.

As with dapsone management, the initial dose of both drugs should be reviewed after 2 to 4 weeks and adjusted to the minimum dose necessary to prevent symptoms. Side effects include morbilliform skin rashes, nausea, depression, and severe bone marrow suppression that requires close monitoring of complete blood counts.

Gluten-Free Diet

Since it has been demonstrated that both skin eruption and associated GSE improve and normalize with strict avoidance of dietary gluten in DH patients, it is commonly accepted that gluten is central to the pathophysiology and development of DH. Strict adherence to a gluten-free diet can substantially reduce the dose of sulfone therapy or even enable the patient to discontinue drug treatment completely. In addition, since sulfone therapy does not affect the enteropathy in DH patients, there are compelling reasons to encourage patients with DH to try the gluten-free diet, particularly those individuals with symptomatic GSE.

Although dietary treatment appears to be an attractive alternative to medication for many patients, it is very difficult to maintain. The gluten-free diet requires a life-long avoidance of gluten, specifically, the gliadin fraction of gluten found in common grains (wheat, rye, oats, barley, and in some patients also soy, millet, and buckwheat). Even the intake of trivial amounts of gluten may prevent improvement of clinical symptoms. In addition, dietary treatment may need several months to years in order to alleviate cutaneous lesions in DH patients. This is particularly true in patients who have been treated with sulfones for an extended period of time. Nevertheless, a gluten-free diet should be offered as an appropriate and sufficient therapeutic approach for motivated patients who wish to avoid life-long drug therapy. Additional candidates for a gluten-free diet are patients with any of the disorders listed in Table 3. The patients should be supervised by experienced dietitians who are well versed in a gluten-free diet. Additional information and support are provided by the Celiac Sprue Association, U.S.A. (2313 Rocklyn Drive #1, Des Moines, IA 50322) and by the Gluten Intolerance Group of North America (P.O. Box 23063, Seattle, WA 98102–0353).

Topical Therapy of DH Skin Lesions

Topical treatment of cutaneous lesions may not only decrease the duration of healing and the subjective discomfort caused by severe itching and burning, but it can also aid the patient to better tolerate skin symptoms under a given dose of sulfone therapy or dietary treatment. The occasional development of new lesions in DH patients can usually be managed by topical application of a medium-strength (e.g., triamcinolone 0.1 percent) or high-potency (e.g., betamethasone 0.05 percent) glucocorticoid cream or ointment. Since most patients can predict the sites of newly developing skin lesions because of the localized burning and itching that occurs 12 to 24 hours in advance, the eruption can be repressed by immediate use of topical steroids. DH patients need to be advised on the considerable side effects of topically applied corticosteroids. Their use should be restricted to the minimum possible and has to be avoided in critical areas such as facial and intertriginous skin.

AVOIDANCE OF EXACERBATING FACTORS

Halogens may provoke and exacerbate DH lesions in selected patients. Both the external application through patch testing (10 to 25 percent potassium iodide in petrolatum) and the internal administration (e.g., iodine or potassium periodide) can produce DH symptoms or may result in exacerbation of pre-existing skin lesions. The influence of both medical and dietary treatment on the susceptibility to halogens in DH patients has not been intensively studied. Therefore, it is difficult to precisely determine the dose of exposure required for inducing DH symptoms in a given individual. Our impression is that dietary iodides usually do not affect the clinical course of DH. Nonetheless, patients with DH should be counseled on the exacerbating potential of halogens, especially with regard to diagnostic procedures involving high quantities of iodides.

Furthermore, a subgroup of DH patients is susceptible to induction of DH symptoms by nonsteroidal anti-inflammatory drugs (e.g., indomethacin, ibuprofen). The susceptibility appears to be increased in patients with dapsone therapy. Clinically, the exacerbation can present as a rapid development of new skin lesions that may mimic drug-induced skin eruptions. Since similar reactions have not been reported after administration of acetaminophen, this antianalgesic drug can serve as an alternative medication for temporary relief of minor pains.

SUGGESTED READING

Coleman MD. Dapsone: Modes of action, toxicity and possible strategies for increasing patient tolerance. Br J Dermatol 1993; 129:507.

Hall RP III. Dermatitis herpetiformis. J Invest Dermatol 1992; 99:873.

Katz SI. Dapsone. In: Fitzpatrick TB, et al, eds. Dermatology in general medicine. 4th ed. New York: McGraw-Hill, 1993; 2865.

Leonard JN, Fry L. Treatment and management of dermatitis herpetiformis. Clin Dermtol 1992; 9:403.

McFadden JP, Leonard JN, Powles AV, et al. Sulfamethoxypyridazine for dermatitis herpetiformis, linear IgA disease and cicatricial pemphigoid. Br J Dermatol 1989; 121:759.

HERPES GESTATIONIS

RUSSELL P. HALL III, M.D.

Herpes gestationis (HG) is a rare, autoimmune, blistering disease of pregnancy and the puerperium. It is important to note that herpes gestationis is not related to herpes virus infection, but rather was named because of the clinical appearance of the lesions. This confusion has led some authors to propose the name pemphigoid gestationis. Herpes gestationis is an extremely pruritic eruption, which most often begins in the third trimester of pregnancy. However, it can present earlier in the pregnancy, in the postpartum period, or occasionally with the use of oral contraceptives.

CLINICAL CHARACTERISTICS OF HERPES GESTATIONIS

The characteristic presentation of a patient with HG is an intensely itchy, erythematous papulovesicular eruption over the abdomen. Often the initial lesions are localized to the umbilicus. Lesions may coalesce to form plaques or may present as an urticarial eruption or frank bullae. Eruptions may also occur on the extremities, back, palms and soles, but mucous membrane lesions are rarely noted. A characteristic feature of herpes gestationis is severe pruritus. This itching is oftentimes the initial presenting symptom. Patients often experience significant flares of their disease within 24 to 48 hours after delivery, even in the face of previously well-controlled or inactive disease.

HG often, but not always, recurs in subsequent pregnancies; when it does recur it often presents earlier. In addition, it can flare with use of oral contraceptives or with the onset of menses after delivery.

DIAGNOSIS

HG is thought to be an immunologically mediated blistering skin disease. Its diagnosis is based on the examination of normal appearing, perilesional skin by direct immunofluorescence. These studies of the skin of patients with herpes gestationis reveals a linear band of C3 (the third component of complement) at the basement membrane. In addition, approximately 50 percent of patients with herpes gestationis will also have a linear band of IgG at the basement membrane. Only a minority of patients with HG will have evidence of circulating IgG, which can bind to normal skin using indirect immunofluorescence, limiting the diagnostic utility of this test. Other immunoreactants are infrequently seen.

Examination of the sera of patients with herpes gestationis reveals the presence of a low titer, complement-fixing IgG, which is directed against a 180 kD protein of the hemidesmosome. Antibodies against this protein are also found in the sera of patients with the autoimmune blistering disease bullous pemphigoid, which is predominantly a disease of the elderly. The relationship of these two diseases as well as the role of pregnancy and the associated endocrinologic changes seen in patients with herpes gestationis is not known. The importance of the IgG antibody has been confirmed by the observation that the skin of the newborn also has evidence of linear deposits of C3 and can occasionally develop blisters that spontaneously disappear along with the maternal IgG.

FETAL RISK

The risk to the fetus of patients with HG is controversial. Initial reports suggested a slight increased risk of still births and small-for-gestational-age infants. Recent reports, however, have not documented an increased risk of fetal mortality, although a trend towards low-birth-weight infants has been noted. Occasionally infants born of mothers with HG are born with blisters or other cutaneous lesions. These lesions are transient and are thought to be the result of maternal IgG crossing the placenta and binding to the fetal skin. Although the risk to the fetus of patients with herpes gestationis is most likely quite low, it is important that all physicians involved in the care of the mother and child be made aware of the diagnosis of HG and of the implications of that diagnosis.

TREATMENT

The goals of treatment of patients with HG are to relieve the intense pruritus, stop the appearance of new skin lesions, and treat the erosions that occur as the result of the blisters. These goals can be achieved through the use of systemic or topical corticosteroids.

Systemic Corticosteroids

The majority of patients with HG will require treatment with systemic corticosteroids. A single morning dose of 20 to 40 mg of prednisone per day is effective in controlling both pruritus and new lesion formation in most patients. In patients with extensive disease or who fail to clear in 3 to 5 days, dividing the dose of prednisone into morning and evening doses is often helpful in achieving control. Rarely patients may require up to 60 to 80 mg of prednisone per day to achieve control of their eruption. Once the new lesions have stopped appearing and the pruritus is controlled, the prednisone should be slowly tapered by 5 mg every 7 to 14 days until new blisters or symptoms develop.

Patients that experience flares of the disease postpartum should be treated in a similar manner to the initial therapy. Severe postpartum disease in which blisters continue to develop despite 40 to 60 mg per day of prednisone is occasionally seen. When this occurs immunosuppressive therapy may be necessary. All patients that require any postpartum therapy should be advised regarding appropriate nursing practice. Flares of HG that occur with menses or oral contraceptives are most often mild and can be treated with a short course of 20 to 40 mg of prednisone per day for 5 to 10 days or aggressive topical therapy (see following section).

Patients with HG usually respond quickly to therapy with systemic corticosteroids. In addition, there is little data to suggest that the administration of systemic corticosteroids during pregnancy to patients with HG results in a worse prognosis for the fetus.

Topical Therapy

The recent advent of high potency topical steroids has offered some patients with mild disease an alternative treatment. High-potency topical corticosteroids such as 0.05 percent clobetasol propionate (Temovate) or 0.05 percent diflorasone diacetate (Psorcon) can be used two to three times a day in patients with limited disease to help control itching and new lesion formation. Alternatively more frequent application (six times per day) of less potent topical corticosteroids such as 0.05 percent fluocinonide (Lidex) can be used in patients with limited disease. Although some systemic absorption of corticosteroids does undoubtedly occur with this therapy, patients may be able to avoid higher doses of systemic corticosteroids. In these patients the strength of the topical steroid should be tapered gradually to the lowest strength, clinically effective topical corticosteroid.

Systemic antihistamines are only minimally effective in managing the itching associated with herpes gestationis. Cool, open compresses with either tap water or saline are useful in treating the weeping lesions that develop as a result of blister formation. These erosions should be observed closely for signs of secondary infection.

Whether systemic or topical corticosteroids are

used, it is important to always use the minimal effective dose of either preparation. In addition, the patient should be made aware that the development of a few vesicles or urticarial plaques every 1 to 2 weeks should not result in an increase of the dose of systemic corticosteroids. Finally, the treatment of patients with HG must be undertaken in close consultation with the patient's obstetrician and the prospective pediatrician so that the therapy and any potential complications of either HG or the treatment can be anticipated and managed appropriately.

SUGGESTED READING

Holmes RC, Black MM. The fetal prognosis in pemphigoid gestationis (herpes gestationis). Br J Dermatol 1984; 110:67–72.

Lawley TJ, Stingl G, Katz SI. Fetal and maternal risk factors in herpes gestationis. Arch Dermatol 1978; 114:552–555.

Morrison LH, Labib RS, Zone JJ, et al. Herpes gestationis autoantibodies recognize a 180-kD human epidermal antigen. J Clin Invest 1988; 81:2023–2026.

Shornick JK, Bangert JL, Freeman RG, et al. Herpes gestationis: Clinical and histologic features of twenty-eight cases. J Am Acad Dermatol 1983; 814:214–224.

Yancey KB. Herpes gestationis. Dermatol Clin 1990; 8:727–735.

ATOPIC DERMATITIS

AMY S. PALLER, M.D.

Atopic dermatitis is a chronic, severely pruritic disorder characterized by dry skin, eczematous patches, lichenification, and a predisposition to staphylococcal pyodermas. The term "atopic" refers to the fact that affected children frequently have elevated IgE levels and a family or personal history of other atopic disorders, especially allergic rhinitis or asthma. The disorder usually begins in infancy but occasionally occurs later in childhood or even in adulthood. The incidence of atopic dermatitis has been rapidly increasing, particularly in urban areas, and the disorder is now thought to occur in 10 percent of 1-year-old infants. The diagnosis is made by the characteristic distribution and clinical features of the rash.

Treatment of atopic dermatitis must be individualized, and based upon several clinical and historical criteria (Table 1). For most patients, atopic dermatitis is a condition that flares readily when therapy is discontinued. Therefore, the regimen must be amenable to long-term patient compliance and safety. For patients with mild atopic dermatitis, the application of emollients and low-strength corticosteroid preparations suffices. For more severely affected patients, the use of stronger corticosteroid preparations and, occasionally, systemic medication may be necessary. Education of patients and parents, including discussions about the chronicity of the disorder and the suppressive, but not curative, effect of medication, is critical for successful therapy. Patients should be reassured, however, that therapy can result in dramatic improvement and that disfiguring pigmentary changes and lichenification can be prevented. Physicians should discuss expected features and complications, exacerbating factors, handling of acute flares, and the choice of reasonable maintenance therapy. The Eczema Association for Science and Education (1221 S.W. Yamhill, Suite 303, Portland, OR, 97205, 503–228–4430) provides educational brochures in English and Spanish. In the United Kingdom, the National Eczema Society also has educational materials.

Table 1 Clinical Features That Determine Therapy

Age of patient
Age of onset and course of the dermatitis
Location of involvement, degree of lichenification
Previous response to therapy
Seasonal variation
Occupational history if relevant
Presence of secondary infection
Prior diagnostic studies

FACTORS TO CONSIDER IN CHOOSING THERAPY

Initial evaluation should consider the possibility of other diagnostic possibilities, particularly seborrheic dermatitis, juvenile plantar dermatosis, allergic or irritant contact dermatitis, scabies, psoriasis, mycosis fungoides, and rarely, immunodeficiency such as Wiskott-Aldrich syndrome or hyperimmunoglobulinemia E syndrome.

Criteria for the diagnosis of atopic dermatitis have been well established (Table 2). In addition to the history and examination, the presence of an elevated serum IgE level and eosinophilia may provide further evidence of atopy. Specific tests may be indicated to consider alternative diagnoses, such as mineral oil scrapings to show the scabies mite. Questions regarding the time of onset (usually after the first 2 months of age), degree of pruritus, sensitivity to irritants, and seasonal variations may help to establish the diagnosis. Determining the bathing habits and past experiences with trials of topical corticosteroid preparations and antibiotics will help in management. Attention should be paid to the distribution and character of lesions on physical examination and to the coexistence of secondary infection or other abnormalities that may suggest a systemic abnormality. No routine laboratory testing is necessary.

Table 2 Criteria for Atopic Dermatitis

Major Features (need three or more)
1. Pruritus
2. Typical appearance and distribution of lesions
   Facial and extensor involvement in infancy and early childhood
   Flexural involvement and lichenification by adolescence
3. Chronic or frequently relapsing dermatitis
4. Personal or family history of atopy (atopic dermatitis, allergic rhinoconjunctivitis, asthma, urticaria)

Minor, Less Specific Features
1. Xerosis
2. IgE reactivity (High serum IgE, prick test or RAST tests positive)
3. Ichthyosis; keratosis pilaris; hyperlinearity of palms
4. Hand/foot dermatitis
5. Periauricular fissures
6. Cheilitis
7. Scalp dermatitis (i.e., cradle cap)
8. Perifollicular accentuation, especially in dark-skinned patients
9. Increased tendency towards cutaneous infections, especially *Staphylococcus aureus* and *Herpes simplex*

Modified from Hanifin JM, Rajka G. Diagnostic features of atopic dermatitis. Acta Dermatol Venereol 1980; 92(suppl):44.

Table 3 Exacerbating Factors in Atopic Dermatitis

Dry skin
Sensitivity to irritants (wool, sweat, saliva)
Sensitivity to allergens (foods, airborne, contact allergens)
Infection (*S. aureus,* molluscum, H. simplex)
Coexisting pruritic disease, such as chickenpox
Emotional stress

The rash of atopic dermatitis is aggravated by a number of factors (Table 3). Patients with the disorder have extremely dry skin attributable to increased transepidermal water loss and epidermal hyperproliferation induced by inflammation. The decreased efficiency of the stratum corneum as a protective barrier perpetuates inflammation by increasing the access of allergens and irritants. The dermatitis often becomes aggravated by the low humidity of winter and irritants such as detergents and soaps, wool, and saliva. Dermatitis may be exacerbated during summer months because of the irritant reaction to sweat and sweat retention. Soaking in water and frequent handwashing may result in extensive evaporative loss from skin; however, such actions can actually increase the hydration of skin if good emollients are subsequently applied. In general, patients should avoid choosing occupations with frequent handwashing or exposure to irritating chemicals.

The process of rubbing or scratching leads to more rash and more pruritus ("itch-scratch cycle"), so that any cause of pruritus tends to aggravate the dermatitis. Cutaneous infections and superimposed allergic contact dermatitis (see following discussion) may also exacerbate the dermatitis by increasing local inflammation, dryness, and pruritus. Many patients also note a flare of the atopic dermatitis when noncutaneous infections occur such as viral infections or streptococcal pharyngitis.

Emotional stress can impact tremendously on the severity of atopic dermatitis. Familial discord, often triggered by the increased demands of a child with atopic dermatitis, and interpersonal problems with other children at school, including teasing or exclusion of the child, are common problems for the patient with atopic dermatitis. Likewise, major stress such as death of a family member or separation from parents by divorce is also associated with eczematous flares. These psychological problems should be explored and dealt with by the family and personal counseling should be sought, if appropriate.

COMPLICATIONS OF ATOPIC DERMATITIS

The most common complication of atopic dermatitis is secondary bacterial infection of affected areas of skin, especially at excoriated sites. The usual organism is *Staphylococcus aureus,* and the lesions of impetigo usually appear as superficial yellow crusting overlying erythema, although small superficial pustules are sometimes seen. Patients with secondary infection will often not respond to appropriate therapy for the underlying eczema unless the infection is cleared with systemic antibiotics.

Eczema herpeticum (Kaposi's varicelliform eruption) is a complication of atopic dermatitis that is characterized by the abrupt development and rapid spread of the vesicles of Herpes simplex. The lesions are usually groups of intact or umbilicated vesicles and pustules overlying erythema. Screening tests, such as Tzanck smear or immunodetection with anti–herpes simplex antibodies should be performed, and viral culture is confirmatory. Children with atopic dermatitis also have an increased risk of the development and spread of molluscum contagiosum, particularly at sites of xerosis and inflammation.

Contact urticaria may manifest as hives or lead to the development of dermatitis such as on the cheeks and perioral area of infants. Older patients may develop contact urticaria from occupational exposure. The reaction usually occurs within 30 minutes at the site of direct contact.

Allergic contact dermatitis may be an important exacerbating factor, and may be difficult to distinguish from the atopic dermatitis itself. Nickel and agents in topical medications are the most important causes in patients with atopic dermatitis. For example, a patch of recalcitrant dermatitis near the umbilical area may be caused by nickel contact from the snap on pants or a belt buckle, rather than the atopic condition.

Neomycin and lanolin frequently cause reactions in patients with atopic dermatitis, since these agents may be present in topical antibiotic preparations and emollients, respectively. Patch testing allows confirmation of the suspected allergen, but false-positive reactions are common in patients with atopic dermatitis.

POSSIBLE ALLERGIC TRIGGERS

The significance of food-induced atopic dermatitis remains controversial. Prick tests and radioallergosorbent test results do not correlate well with response to avoidance and challenge and are most useful if negative. Challenge studies have shown that the ingestion of certain foods, particularly eggs, milk, soy, wheat, and peanuts, can initiate reactions in patients with atopic dermatitis within 2 hours after challenge. However, the unclear relationship between these studies and the occurrence of the dermatitis itself and the fact that removal of these offending allergens does not control the dermatitis suggest that dietary therapy is not of much value for most patients with atopic dermatitis. Furthermore, dietary manipulation may be difficult to implement, particularly in children. Most dermatologists consider food allergies to be of little significance and reserve dietary manipulation for patients with severe eczema who do not respond to more traditional measures.

Airborne allergens have also been implicated as triggers for atopic dermatitis, based largely upon the distribution of lesions at exposed body areas and supporting evidence by positive patch testing. Airborne allergens, such as dust mites, pets, and molds, are probably more significant for older children and adults, but the allergens are difficult to remove from the environment. Highly motivated patients may take measures to limit dust, such as frequent vacuuming (by another person), encasing mattresses and pillows in occlusive materials, and removing of dust-entrapping curtains, drapes, and stuffed animals.

MANAGEMENT OF ATOPIC DERMATITIS

After the pattern of the dermatitis, aggravating factors, and response to previous therapy are assessed, a therapeutic plan with reasonable goals may be initiated. The regimen usually includes avoidance of exacerbating agents, improved lubrication of skin, and application of anti-inflammatory agents (Table 4).

Table 4 Therapy of Atopic Dermatitis

1. Education and reassurance of patient and family
2. Lubrication: Lukewarm baths or compresses at least once daily, followed by the application of a moisturizing cream or ointment such as petrolatum to the wet skin; moisturizers may be applied more frequently if needed
3. Application twice daily of anti-inflammatory topical corticosteroid preparations, preferably in a moisturizing base. The selection of corticosteroid should be based on the age of the patient, location of lesions, and response to previous therapy
4. Administration of oral antibiotics if eroded, crusted, or pustular lesions are present (e.g., course of cephalexin for 2 weeks)
5. Trial of antihistamines, such as hydroxyzine or combination of H_1- and H_2-blockers. Topical doxepin is now available
6. Alternative agents for more severely involved patients—tar preparations, ultraviolet light therapy, systemic corticosteroids, interferon-gamma, or cyclosporin
7. Avoidance of irritants and specific allergens, such as food or aeroallergens, as appropriate for the individual

General Measures

Many patients with atopic dermatitis benefit from a daily bath or shower, which adds water to the outer layer of skin, followed immediately by the application of emollient creams or ointments. Harsh soaps should be substituted with mild or superfatted soaps. The bathwater should be lukewarm since hot water increases skin dryness. Bubble baths are best avoided since they are irritating, but bath oils may be beneficial. Humidifiers are also helpful during dry winter months, but they must be cleaned at least weekly to avoid the dissemination of molds.

Although most patients are troubled by dryness and pruritus in winter, some patients experience more difficulty in the summer, and irritation from sweat may be a major problem. These patients may complain of pruritus with the application of thicker lubricants and benefit from lubricating lotions, which are less occlusive. Such patients are also helped by the use of air conditioners in summer months. Similarly, most patients improve with a regimen of daily baths followed immediately by lubrication. Others cannot tolerate water at all, especially if there are many excoriated or infected sites, and benefit from temporary avoidance of water.

Corticosteroids

Anti-inflammatory topical corticosteroid preparations are usually necessary to clear the inflammatory lesions. The strength and base of the chosen topical preparation depends on the location and severity of the rash and on the age and tolerance of the patient. Fluorinated corticosteroids should never be used for more than a few days on the face or intertriginous areas because of the risk of skin atrophy. Milder eruptions or eruptions on younger children may clear with the use of weak, nonfluorinated agents only such as hydrocortisone or a nonfluorinated medium-strength corticosteroid, whereas patients who are older or with more severe pruritus and inflammation may require a fluorinated moderate or high-strength corticosteroid. Most patients with dry skin prefer ointment or emollient based preparations, especially during winter months, while others prefer to use cream based preparations covered with lubricating agents. Corticosteroid gels and lotions are usually too drying for patients with atopic dermatitis.

Systemic corticosteroids are indicated only for patients with severe involvement who do not respond adequately to topical agents, and short courses are often included for patients who require hospitalization to reverse an acute flare. Exacerbations following discontinuation of systemic corticosteroid therapy are a further disadvantage of this therapeutic approach.

Antipruritics

Oral antihistamine preparations, especially hydroxyzine, doxepin, and diphenhydramine, may be valuable, especially for their sedative effects at night when scratching is most intense. Nonsedating antihistamines usually provide little relief. The addition of the H_2-blocker, cimetidine, has been useful in many patients with atopic dermatitis. The newly released topical doxepin may diminish cutaneous pruritus, but it may also cause sedation if large amounts are applied.

Other Therapy

Weeping dermatitis is often due to secondary infection and requires compresses to dry the areas and to remove crusts and debris. Burow's solution or cool saline compresses should be applied two to three times daily for 20 to 30 minutes using a thin cloth, such as a handkerchief, to allow for evaporative loss. Topical corticosteroid or lubrication may be applied after the compressing.

If bacterial infection is suspected and involves more than a small area, the patient should be treated with systemic antistaphylococcal antibiotics. The choice of systemic therapy should be based upon the local resistance patterns of *S. aureus,* since many staphylococcal organisms are now resistant to erythromycin. Cephalosporins and dicloxacillin are frequently used alternatives. If herpetic infections develop and show a predisposition towards spread, systemic acyclovir therapy is indicated.

Other topical agents that have been helpful for patients with atopic dermatitis include ultraviolet light, mild tar preparations that are applied directly to the skin (e.g., T-derm oil, Estargel or Psorigel) or added to bathwater (e.g., Balnetar), and keratolytics such as urea or salicylic acid for lichenified plaques. For patients with severe, recalcitrant atopic dermatitis, systemic administration of daily subcutaneous interferon-gamma or oral cyclosporin by a specialist familiar with these medications is an alternative possibility.

Indications for Referral and Admission

Patients who are difficult to manage or who require more than moderate-strength topical corticosteroid preparations should be referred to a dermatologist for management. Patients with severe atopic dermatitis who cannot be managed effectively as outpatients may respond to the intensive topical or systemic management of brief hospitalization. Patients with significant eczema herpeticum or severe secondary bacterial infections may also require observation and treatment in the hospital.

SUGGESTED READING

Cooper KD. New therapeutic approaches in atopic dermatitis. Clin Rev Allergy 1993; 11:543.

Dahl MV. Atopic dermatitis: the concept of flare factors. South Med J 1977; 70:453.

Hanifin JM. Atopic dermatitis in infants and children. Pediatr Clin N Am 1991; 38:763.

Hanifin JM, Rajka G. Diagnostic features of atopic dermatitis. Acta Dermatol Venereol 1980; 92(suppl):44.

Sampson HA. Atopic dermatitis. Ann Allergy 1992; 69:469.

CONTACT DERMATITIS

VINCENT A. DeLEO, M.D.

The term contact dermatitis is used to describe adverse reactions in the skin that occur secondary to direct contact with chemicals in the environment. The response is one of dermatitis or eczema, which are morphologic responses of the skin, representing inflammation of the epidermis with edema between the keratinocytes. Therefore the process does not include reactions such as contact urticaria, which result from chemical contact and are not dermatitic. The reaction can be a manifestation of direct damage by the chemical or it can be mediated by immune mechanisms. In the case of the former, the response is referred to as *irritant contact dermatitis,* whereas the immune-mediated response is called *allergic contact dermatitis.* The mechanism of the irritant response is variable and is specific to the chemical structure of the irritant. The mechanism of the allergic reaction is a T-cell mediated, Type IV response.

Irritant contact dermatitis is one of the most common of all dermatologic maladies and can be caused by an almost infinite number of naturally occurring and man-made agents. The most common of these are surfactants and solvents. Allergic contact dermatitis, on

Table 1 The Most Common Agents Causing Allergic Contact Dermatitis

- *Plants*
  - Toxicodendrum
    - Poison Ivy, Oak, Sumac
- *Rubber*
  - Mercaptobenzothiazole
  - Thiurams
  - Carbamates
  - Black Rubber Paraphenylene diamine
- *Medicaments*
  - Benzocaine
  - Thimerosal
  - Neomycin sulfate
  - Quinolones
- *Cosmetics*
  - Fragrances
    - Cinnamic Aldehyde
    - Balsam of Peru
  - Vehicles, preservatives and additives
    - Lanolin alcohol
    - Imidazolidinyl urea
    - Quarternium-15
    - Formaldehyde
    - Ethylenediamine dihydrocholoride
    - Cl + Me-isothiazolinone
    - Parabens
  - Hair dyes
    - p-Phenylenediamine
- *Metals*
  - Nickel sulfate
  - Potassium dichromate
  - Cobalt dichloride
- *Resins*
  - Colophony
  - Epoxy resin
  - p-tert-Butylphenol formaldehyde resin

the other hand, is thought to be related to a finite number of chemicals capable of eliciting the immune response. The number usually quoted is 3,000 different substances (Table 1). Irritant contact dermatitis accounts for approximately 70 to 80 percent of all cases of contact dermatitis, while allergic reactions cause the remainder.

DIAGNOSIS

Although the mechanism of the response to the exogenous chemical is different for allergic and irritant contact dermatitis, the response in the clinical setting is very similar. This is probably because the mechanism of both responses ultimately involves many of the same cells, inflammatory mediators, and cytokines. The response is an eczematous dermatitis and can be either *acute* with erythema, edema, and vesicles; *subacute* with erythema, edema, scale, and oozing; or *chronic* with erythema, scale, and lichenification.

The diagnosis of irritant contact dermatitis is based on the appearance of an eczema in a localized distribution combined with a history of exposure to irritating substances. While the diagnosis of allergic contact dermatitis is also suggested by history and physical findings, it is dependent on positive response to patch testing.

The distribution of contact dermatitis is key to the diagnosis of this condition. Most irritant dermatitis involves the hands. This is obviously because the hands are usually the first part of the skin surface to contact the environment, at home and in the workplace. Irritant contact dermatitis of the hands is the most common occupational skin disease. Allergic reactions frequently involve the hands, face, and feet. Other areas can also be involved with specific antigens. Nickel dermatitis, for example, frequently presents in a "jewelry distribution," involving the earlobes, neck, and wrist; medicament allergy involves those areas where topical medication has been applied, as for example, the lower legs in individuals with stasis dermatitis.

TREATMENT

Treatment of contact dermatitis depends on the morphology of the eczema involved, the distribution and extent of the skin surface involved, the chronicity of the reaction, and the history of chemical exposure. ***Treatment consists of identification and avoidance of the offending agent(s) and amelioration of the inflammatory response.***

Reduction of inflammation is based on cool water soaks, which help to dry and cool acute eczema and can be used to help emolliate dry, chronic eczematous skin, and administration of topical or systemic corticosteroids. The strength of the topical steroid used depends on the severity of the dermatitis, the area of the body involved, and the age of the patient (Table 2).

Side effects of topical steroid usage include atrophy, systemic absorption with attendant side effects, and acneform eruptions, especially of the face. Recently even contact allergy has been reported, especially to hydrocortisone. With the exception of contact allergy, the risk of all side effects are increased with increasing potency and when the steroid is used in children, on large surface areas, and in intertriginous areas.

The lowest potency steroids include hydrocortisone and desonide. ***Low-potency agents should be the only ones used in children and on the face and in intertriginous areas such as the groin and the axillae in adults. In fact, in very small children and on the face of adults, hydrocortisone is the only agent that can be used with absolute assurance of no significant side effects.***

Medium-range agents include triamcinolone acetonide (<0.1 percent) and betamethasone valerate; the high-potency agents include some products of betamethasone dipropionate and the very highest potency include clobetasol propionate. In addition, the product should be chosen according to the base that will most assist in the therapeutic process—cream, lotion, or ointment.

Systemic antihistamine therapy may be utilized if itching is severe. It should be remembered, however, that the itch of contact dermatitis is not histamine mediated to any great extent and the benefit of antihistamines is

Table 2 Topical Adrenocorticoid Strengths

Generic Name	*Strength (%)*	*Some Trade Names*
Low-Potency Adrenocorticoids		
Alclometasone dipropionate	0.05	Aclovate
Clocortolone pivalate	0.1	Cloderm
Desonide	0.05	Tridesilon
Dexamethasone	0.04-0.1	Decaderm
Dexamethasone sodium phosphate	0.1	Decadron
Flumethasone pivalate	0.03	Locacorten
Flurandrenolide	0.0125	Cordran, Drenison
Hydrocortisone acetate	0.1-1	Cortaid, Cortefete
Methylprednisolone	0.25-1	Medrol
Medium-Potency Adrenocorticoids		
Beclomethasone dipropionate	0.025	Propaderm
Betamethasone benzoate	0.025	Uticort, Beben
Betamethasone valerate	0.05-0.1	Valisone, Betnovate
Clobetasol butyrate	0.05	Eumovate
Desoximetasone	0.05	Topicort
Diflucortolone valerate	0.1	Nerisone
Fluocinolone acetonide	0.01-0.25	Synalar
Flurandrenolide	0.025-0.05	Cordran, Drenison
Hydrocortisone butyrate	0.1	Locoid
Hydrocortisone valerate	0.2	Westcort
Mometasone furoate	0.1	Elocon
Triamcinolone acetonide	0.015-0.1	Aristocort, Kenalog
High-Potency Adrenocorticoids		
Amcinonide	0.1	Cyclocort
Betamethasone dipropionate	0.05	Alphatrex, Diprosone
Desoximetasone	0.05-0.25	Topicort
Diflurasone diacetate	0.05	Florone, Maxiflor
Fluocinonide	0.05	Lidex
Halcinonide	0.025-0.1	Halog
Triamcinolone acetonide	0.5	Halciderm, Aristocort
Very High-Potency Adrenocorticoids		
Betamethasone dipropionate	0.05	Diprolene, Diprolene AF
Clobetasol proprionate	0.05	Dermovate, Temovate
Diflorasone diacetate	0.05	Psorcon

Modified from Maddin S. Dermatologic therapy. In: Moschella S., Hurley H. eds. *Dermatology.* 3rd edition, Vol 2, Philadelphia: Saunders, 1990: 2193.

based on their sedating qualities. Therefore soporiphic antihistamines, like diphenhydramine or hydroxyzine, should be used, and the chosen dosage should be sedating. Such agents should be used primarily before bedtime if the patient is to continue to work or drive an automobile.

Contact dermatitis of all types may become secondarily infected with bacteria, usually *Staphylococcus aureus.* When suspected, an antibiotic should be administered. The antibiotic should always be given systemically since topical antibiotics may only complicate the process of contact dermatitis. Erythromycins or cephalosporins are the drugs of choice and the dosage for both drugs, erythromycin and cephalexin, is 250 mg four times per day for 10 days.

With *acute eczema of short duration* (a few days or a week or two) the physician should take a detailed history of exposure of the body part involved. It should include exposure at the workplace, in the home, and in leisure activities. The history should include the topical agents applied by the patient before the visit, since in many cases the initial problem will have been complicated by the application of an irritant or allergen. The patient should be instructed to avoid those agents that may have caused or may be complicating the process. The inflamed skin areas should be soaked in cool water two to four times a day for approximately 10 to 15 minutes. The skin should be gently dried and a topical steroid in a cream base should be applied. In children and for the face, groin, and axillae of adults the mildest group of topical steroids should be used. For other areas of the body the moderate, high, or, less frequently, the most potent classes of agents should be used. The eruption should dry and become subacute within 3 to 4 days. At that point, the soaks can be decreased in frequency or discontinued, and the topical steroid can be maintained. If the skin becomes too dry the topical steroid can be changed to an ointment-based product. The reaction should be completely resolved within 1 to 2 weeks.

If the *acute eczema of short duration* is extensive or involves the face or genital areas with extensive edema, systemic steroids can be used. This usually occurs with allergic disease caused by poison ivy (or oak or sumac) or hair dye. The dosage for an adult is 40 to 60 mg per day of prednisone orally for the first day, with a gradual taper over a period of 14 days. Complications should always be considered before instituting therapy in individuals with other disease processes. The entire dosage should be given in the morning with milk or food and the taper should never be for less than 2 weeks. Shorter courses of steroids frequently result in a rebound flare of the disease. There is no place for systemic steroid therapy in irritant contact dermatitis.

In *subacute eczema of short duration* avoidance of irritants and allergens should be undertaken. Usually soaking of the skin will not be necessary. The patient should be treated with a steroid appropriate for the area of the body and the age of the patient as outlined earlier, but the agent must be in an ointment base.

In *subacute or chronic eczema of long duration,* that is more than 2 or 3 weeks, the same therapeutic maneuvers as just outlined should be undertaken, but patch testing to identify the allergen should be considered. Only such testing can identify the causative agent if allergic disease is present. Once the process has continued, especially in spite of therapy, allergy is more likely.

Only patch testing can identify the causative allergen in allergic contact dermatitis. Identification and instruction of the patient in avoidance of allergen exposure is the only way to "cure" the disease. The physician must keep a high index of suspicion when treating patients thought to have irritant contact dermatitis. If avoidance of irritants and topical steroids do not result in clearing after a few weeks then patch testing must be undertaken. The reader is referred to the references for a discussion of the techniques of patch testing.

In *chronic eczema* topical steroids in ointment bases should be used. Cool water soaks with application of the steroid ointment to moist skin will assist in emolliating the dry, lichenified skin.

In many cases of irritant contact dermatitis of the *subacute or chronic eczematous type of long duration,* irritants cannot be completely avoided. In such cases a strategy of treating chronic disease should be undertaken once contact allergy has been ruled out by adequate patch testing. This most commonly involves treatment of chronic dermatitis of the hand. Such patients should be encouraged to use emolliation, and topical steroids should be saved only for acute flares of disease. The best agents include petrolatum and hydrophilic ointment, but a multitude of over-the-counter moisturizers are available. Agents with fragrance, and when possible, preservatives should be avoided since these can cause allergy with long-term usage.

Finally, specialized procedures can be used to treat chronic dermatitis, including phototherapy and photochemotherapy, which are available through referral to dermatologists who specialize in those modalities.

The chronic use of systemic corticosteroids in the treatment of dermatitis is to be discouraged and only used with dermatologic consultation and under the direst circumstances. In such cases other diseases like psoriasis should always be considered and appropriate testing, including skin biopsies, may be necessary.

Avoidance Strategy

Instructing patients to avoid irritants or allergens is an essential part of the therapy of contact dermatitis. In the management of most patients this will necessitate an understanding of the patient's job and home environments, including skin care regimens.

As previously stated, if the dermatitis is recurrent or chronic, patch testing must be done to identify the offending allergen or to rule out allergy so that the patient can be treated for chronic dermatitis of the irritant or endogenous type with assurance.

If the patient encounters wet work on the job, such exposure should be minimized. In most cases of suspected occupational contact dermatitis, patch testing should be done initially or shortly after the beginning of therapy if such therapy does not resolve the dermatitis. If no allergy is found, protective gloves may be utilized, depending on the safety of using such protective garments.

In the home environment the patient should be instructed to use rubber gloves whenever wet work is anticipated. Since the hands perspire in such gloves, if the job lasts for more than a few minutes, the patient should be instructed to wear cotton gloves beneath the rubber gloves.

A growing problem is allergy to rubber gloves. The types of reactions caused by such gloves include allergic contact dermatitis of the delayed type, which is due to rubber accelerators and contact urticaria caused by the latex molecule itself, which is an immediate type of sensitivity and can even lead to anaphylaxis. The easiest way to avoid both reactions is to recommend vinyl rather than latex gloves. When such allergy is suspected proper testing (RAST and/or scratch-prick testing) should be carried out since allergy of the immediate type should be known to the patient so as to avoid serious consequences from future exposure.

It should also be remembered that gloves of either latex or vinyl do not prevent the penetration of some allergens. The reader is referred to the reference texts for a discussion of those antigens.

Patients should be instructed to decrease handwashing and to use only cream-based soaps. Antibacterial or deodorant soaps should be avoided and a moisturizer such as petrolatum should be applied immediately after each washing.

Patients with facial dermatitis should be instructed to avoid all cosmetics during acute disease flares. If the reaction recurs the patient should be patch tested. Simply changing from one product or cosmetic line to another is almost always futile since common agents are used in various products. One strategy that may be tried short of patch testing is to switch to fragrance-free cosmetic if fragranced agents were used at the time of the eruption. This may work since the most frequent cosmetic allergen is fragrance.

Frequently, agents used to treat dermatitis induce a secondary allergic contact dermatitis. These agents include topical antibiotics, especially neomycin and bacitracin; topical caines and diphenhydramine; fragrances and preservatives in moisturizers and body lotions; and even topical corticosteroids themselves. The safest agents to use are petrolatum-based ointments that do not contain the agents just listed. Two agents that seem to cause few problems are Synalar ointment and Diprosone ointment.

SUGGESTED READING

Adams RM. Occupational skin disease. Philadelphia: Saunders, 1990.
Cronin E. Contact Dermatitis. New York: Churchill Livingston, 1980.
Fisher AA. Contact Dermatitis. Philadelphia: Lea & Febiger, 1986.
Maddin S. Dermatologic Therapy. In: Moschella S, Hurley H, eds. *Dermatology.* 3rd ed, Vol 2. Philadelphia: Saunders, 1990: 2193.
Marks JG, DeLeo VA. Contact and occupational dermatitis. St. Louis: Mosby, 1987.

PEMPHIGUS

JOSÉ M. MASCARÓ Jr., M.D.
LUIS A. DIAZ, M.D.

The term *pemphigus* encompasses a group of chronic autoimmune blistering diseases of the skin characterized by cell-to-cell detachment (acantholysis). This loss of adhesion between keratinocytes induces the formation of intraepidermal blisters. Pressure applied to the edge of a bulla can cause extension of the epidermal separation and, if shearing forces are applied to normal-appearing skin, they produce denudation. These events are both termed Nikolsky's sign, a typical finding in pemphigus, although it can be seen in other dermatologic conditions. Pemphigus can be subdivided into four main disease processes: pemphigus foliaceus, pemphigus vulgaris, drug-induced pemphigus, and paraneoplastic pemphigus.

PEMPHIGUS VARIANTS

Pemphigus foliaceus is characterized by blister formation at the level of the stratum granulosum. These are fragile blisters that rupture easily. The disease usually manifests as large areas of desquamated erythematous dermatitis. It can occur all over the body, but it is usually most prominent on the face and trunk. In some cases the lesions can extend, and the disease may present as a generalized exfoliative dermatitis. Mucosal blisters or erosions are rarely observed. Pemphigus foliaceus is usually a benign disease except in older individuals with extensive lesions. In certain areas of Brazil and other South American countries, there is an endemic form of pemphigus foliaceus that is termed Fogo Selvagem (wild fire). The cause of Fogo Selvagem is unknown, but there is substantial epidemiologic evidence indicating that it may be precipitated by an environmental factor (probably an insect). Pemphigus erythematosus (Senear-Usher syndrome) represents a variant of pemphigus foliaceus with features of systemic lupus erythematosus occurring in the same patient.

Pemphigus vulgaris is the most common form of pemphigus on the North American continent and in other parts of the world. Blister formation occurs deeper in the epidermis, just above the basal cell layer. The majority of patients present with oral and/or scalp lesions, and only a few demonstrate glabrous skin lesions initially. In later stages of the disease the skin involvement can be widespread. Cutaneous lesions start as flaccid blisters arising on normal or erythematous skin. They rupture easily, resulting in large, denuded areas that show little tendency to spontaneous healing. Pemphigus vulgaris is a severe disease, and it had a high mortality (60 to 90 percent) before the introduction of glucocorticosteroids in therapy. Pemphigus vegetans, an uncommon variant of pemphigus vulgaris, is characterized by large, fungating lesions occurring predominantly in skin folds (groin and axilla).

Drugs may induce or trigger pemphigus. Penicillamine, captopril, and many other drugs have been implicated in drug-induced pemphigus. These patients usually present with morbilliform or urticarial eruptions, and then skin lesions more typical of pemphigus foliaceus than of pemphigus vulgaris appear. Most cases improve after discontinuation of the causative drug, but some patients will need systemic therapy to control their disease. The mechanism of acantholysis in drug-induced pemphigus is unknown. It is feasible that the drug may have a direct effect in the epidermis where it could unmask antigenic sites that sensitized the patient. The antiepidermal autoantibodies will then cause acantholysis.

Paraneoplastic pemphigus is a recently described autoimmune bullous disease. The clinical features are polymorphous, and the lesions can resemble those of erythema multiforme or lichen planus. Patients usually present with pruritic papulosquamous lesions that evolve to vesicles and blisters. Mucous membrane involvement is a prominent feature of paraneoplastic pemphigus.

Patients have persistent painful blisters or erosions of the oral mucosa. There is always an associated neoplasm in paraneoplastic pemphigus. The most frequent neoplasms have been hematologic malignancies (non-Hodgkin's lymphoma, chronic lymphocytic leukemia, Waldenström's macroglobulinemia), but association with thymoma, sarcomas, or squamous cell carcinomas has also been reported.

LABORATORY EVALUATION

Acantholysis is the histologic hallmark of all forms of pemphigus. Histopathologic examination in pemphigus foliaceus reveals the presence of acantholytic intraepidermal blisters located in the subcorneal region of the epidermis. Occasionally the presence of eosinophilic spongiosis can be seen, although this feature is also found in pemphigus vulgaris and bullous pemphigoid. In pemphigus vulgaris, cutaneous biopsies show acantholytic cells and suprabasal intraepidermal blisters. The appearance of basal cells in the floor of the blisters has been described as a "row of tombstones." Histologic findings in the prodromal eruption of drug-induced pemphigus are usually nonspecific. In later lesions the picture can be similar to pemphigus foliaceus or pemphigus vulgaris depending on the clinical appearance. In paraneoplastic pemphigus, light microscopy reveals the presence of suprabasilar acantholysis and intraepidermal clefts. In addition, vacuolar degeneration of the basal cell layer and the presence of necrotic keratinocytes have been described as characteristic findings.

All forms of pemphigus have circulating IgG autoantibodies directed against the cell surface of keratinocytes. Direct immunofluorescence (IF) demonstrates deposition of IgG with or without complement on the cell surfaces of the epidermis from lesional skin of almost all patients. In addition, immunoreactant deposition at the basement membrane zone has also been seen in some patients with paraneoplastic pemphigus. IgG autoantibodies directed against the cell surface of keratinocytes can be demonstrated by indirect IF in the sera of approximately 80 to 85 percent of pemphigus patients tested against stratified squamous epithelia. In general, antibody titers correlate with disease activity, and they can be used to monitor therapy. The antibodies in paraneoplastic pemphigus can also bind with the cell surface of simple, columnar, and transitional epithelia (rodent bladder epithelia), and they are occasionally associated with anti–basement membrane zone antibodies.

The serum of pemphigus foliaceus patients recognizes, by immunoprecipitation and immunoblot analyses, a glycoprotein of approximately 160 kD that has subsequently been identified as desmoglein 1 (dsg1). Pemphigus vulgaris antigen is a glycoprotein of approximately 130 kD with significant homologies to dsg1, and it has been designated as dsg3. The serum of paraneoplastic pemphigus patients recognizes by immunoprecipitation a complex of four polypeptides of 250, 230, 210, and 190 kD. The 250 and 210 kD antigens have been identified as desmoplakin I and II respectively, and the 230 kD corresponds to bullous pemphigoid antigen 1. The 190 kD antigen has not yet been identified.

Pathogenesis

Pemphigus autoantibodies are pathogenic. This was demonstrated by in vitro studies with pemphigus vulgaris IgG in which autoantibodies induced acantholysis of human skin in organ culture model systems. In vivo studies have been performed in pemphigus foliaceus, pemphigus vulgaris, and paraneoplastic pemphigus. The purified IgG from patients infused intraperitoneally into neonatal BALB/c mice has induced the production of acantholysis and intraepidermal vesiculation in the mice. Human IgG is detected by direct IF in the intercellular spaces of lesional skin of these mice. The disease process in mice is dependent on the titers of the infused pemphigus foliaceus or pemphigus vulgaris IgG. Other studies have demonstrated that acantholysis can be induced in the absence of complement or by the injection of $F(ab')_2$ fragments of pemphigus foliaceus IgG. However, the precise mechanism for acantholysis in pemphigus vulgaris and pemphigus foliaceus remains unknown. It has been reported that acantholysis induced by pemphigus autoantibodies may be caused by activation of proteinases such as plasminogen activator.

THERAPY

Based on the data outlined in the previous sections the initial goals of therapy are to clear the blistering disease and to allow the healing of previous lesions. Since pemphigus autoantibodies are known to be pathogenic, the aim of the therapy should be to eliminate pemphigus autoantibodies from the patient's serum and skin. Two clinical signs are employed to evaluate therapy in pemphigus patients—the estimated number of new lesions formed per week, and the rate of healing of these new lesions. In addition, pemphigus antibody titers should be performed every 4 to 6 weeks. Combining these clinical and serologic parameters provides the best means for judging the effectiveness of therapy. Therapy with steroids or immunosuppressants must be reduced to the lowest levels required to maintain a clinical remission and lessen side effects.

Currently mortality from pemphigus vulgaris has decreased to about 10 percent over a 5-year period, and approximately 30 to 40 percent of the patients remain in clinical remission off all therapy following successful treatment. Currently, the major cause of death in these patients is secondary to complications of high doses of corticosteroids and/or immunosuppressive therapy. Side effects from steroid therapy are a major, if not the most important, clinical problem in the management of pemphigus patients. Consequently, a history of duodenal ulcers, diabetes, hypertension, osteoporosis, cataracts, or exposure to tuberculosis must be obtained prior to starting therapy. A routine complete blood count (CBC) with differential and urinalysis must also be obtained. Baseline chest radiograph and purified protein derivative (PPD) are recommended prior to initiating steroids and, if positive, isoniazid therapy should be considered. Kidney and liver function should be monitored if immunosuppressive agents are used, since these agents are generally metabolized by these organs. Potential bone marrow toxicity from immunosuppressive agents should also be monitored with a weekly CBC during the first month and every 2 to 4 weeks thereafter.

Corticosteroids

Corticosteroids represent the first-line therapy in pemphigus vulgaris management, but they may need to be combined with an immunosuppressive agent in order to reduce side effects. Patients must initially be treated with enough steroids to suppress the blistering disease. Following the suppression of the disease, the serum is monitored for antibody levels. After they have disappeared the skin is examined by direct IF for the presence of antibody deposition at the cell surfaces of the epidermis. Once the autoantibodies can no longer be detected in the patient's serum or in the skin, steroids should be gradually tapered. Following the complete tapering of steroids patients are observed clinically and serologically, every 3 to 4 months for pemphigus disease activity.

Therapy is usually started at a dose equivalent to 1 to 2 mg per kilogram of prednisone daily in divided doses, depending on disease severity. If blister formation diminishes, prednisone can be consolidated into a single morning dose and rapidly reduced at first (approximately 5 to 10 mg per week) and then more slowly when nearing a dose of 40 mg per day. If the disease remains under control at 40 mg daily, then an attempt to change to an alternate-day therapy should be made by gradually tapering the dose given every other day to zero. The 40 mg every other day should then be tapered as tolerated. However, if after 6 to 8 weeks the patient continues to demonstrate new blister formation, the prednisone dose should be increased by 50 percent of the dose that the patient was receiving, and 50 percent increases of the dose should be done every week until the disease is controlled. Then, the usual tapering rate of prednisone is lower (5 to 2.5 mg per week). Once this dose has been tapered to a level of 80 mg per day, alternate-day tapering is recommended.

Immunosuppressive Agents

If high maintenance doses are required or if the patient is not tolerating prednisone, then addition of an immunosuppressive agent should be considered. The combination of immunosuppressive drugs with low doses of steroids not only controls the disease, but also has a pronounced steroid-sparing effect, resulting in the decreased occurrence of steroid side effects. Cytotoxic agents that have been used in various combinations to treat pemphigus include azathioprine, cyclophosphamide, and methotrexate. These agents take several weeks to take effect and are not drugs of first choice for treating the acute phase of pemphigus vulgaris. They are usually not started until the prednisone has been tapered to about 40 mg daily. When steroids have been discontinued, the immunosuppressive agent should be tapered over a 1- to 2-month period. Cyclophosphamide (Cytoxan) is usually the drug of choice. It is given in doses of 75 to 150 mg per day. Significant adverse effects include bone marrow suppression, hemorrhagic cystitis, bladder fibrosis, sterility, and increased risk of developing malignancies. The risk of cystitis can be reduced by encouraging patients to maintain a high fluid intake. Azathioprine (Imuran) is given in doses of 100 to 200 mg per day. Its major side effects are bone marrow suppression, an increased risk of developing malignancies, and hepatotoxicity. When methotrexate is used, 25 to 50 mg per week are given either intramuscularly (single dose) or orally (divided in three doses given 12 hours apart). Hepatotoxicity is the main side effect of methotrexate. Routine liver function tests as well as liver biopsies (both pretreatment and during therapy) are recommended if long-term treatment is anticipated.

Other Treatments

Intravenous pulse glucocorticosteroid therapy, using supraphysiologic doses of corticosteroids (1 g per day given for 3 days), offers an alternative approach to uncontrollable pemphigus patients. Although there are generally fewer side effects, serious complications also exist, including psychological disturbances, seizures, hypertension, sinus bradycardia, increased blood glucose, and severe arthralgia. After the pulse has been administered, oral glucocorticosteroids in tapering doses are usually required and sometimes, several pulses are necessary to control the disease.

Plasmapheresis, a technique in which antibody-containing plasma is removed from the circulation and replaced with a plasma substitute, has been a useful alternative in patients poorly controlled on high-dose prednisone and/or immunosuppressive agents. It is currently considered an experimental therapy, but it may be contemplated in patients with severe, refractory disease. It should be undertaken while the patient is receiving concomitant treatment with steroids and immunosuppressants. Complications include immunosuppression caused by removal of immunoglobulins and depletive coagulopathy.

Gold therapy has been shown to be effective in the treatment of patients with pemphigus vulgaris. Weekly doses of gold (25 to 50 mg) must be given to reach a cumulative dose of 1,500 mg or higher before any therapeutic effect can usually be detected. After the disease is controlled, the weekly doses of gold can be reduced to once a month and then discontinued. Patients treated with gold can achieve clinical and serologic remissions. Oral gold is now the preferred form of therapy. Complications of this therapy include thrombocytopenia, bone marrow suppression, glomerulonephritis, pneumonitis, and mucocutaneous eruptions.

Dapsone has been used in older individuals in which the concomitant use of steroids and immunosuppressants may be difficult. The standard dose is 50 to 100 mg per day.

Cyclosporine has also been used in the treatment of pemphigus vulgaris, and although there have been several favorable uncontrolled studies, it appears that cyclosporine is ineffective as a single therapy and is associated with a high rate of renal toxicity.

A few patients with drug-resistant pemphigus vulgaris have been successfully treated with extracorporeal photopheresis. However, this procedure is an experimental form of treatment, and therefore more experience is needed before it can be used on a routine basis.

Topical care for crusted lesions and erosions includes wet aluminum subacetate compresses and silver sulfadiazine three to four times daily, which removes crusts, decreases discomfort, and reduces the risk of infection. Patients with oral involvement may benefit from a soft diet and viscous lidocaine before meals; topical steroids in an adherent base may also be of some help.

Treatment of Other Pemphigus Variants

Pemphigus foliaceus is usually a relatively benign and self-limited disorder. The cutaneous eruption of the majority of patients will respond to treatment with systemic corticosteroids alone at 40 to 60 mg of prednisone per day. The disease can usually be controlled in a few weeks, and steroids may be rapidly tapered to every other day and maintained until autoantibodies are not detected. In some patients, however, the disease runs a chronic course and verrucous plaques develop on the trunk that are extremely resistant to therapy. Local fluorinated steroids may be used as an adjuvant to systemic therapy. Immunosuppressive drugs and gold compounds have also been used successfully. In drug-induced pemphigus it is extremely important to discontinue the suspected agent. Most cases will then resolve rapidly and need no further therapy. However, some patients may follow a chronic course similar to idiopathic pemphigus foliaceus or pemphigus vulgaris and will require analogous therapy. Most patients with paraneoplastic pemphigus follow a progressive course that is refractory to all treatments. Although a few patients may improve with therapies used to treat pemphigus vulgaris, most will only have improvement in their cutaneous disease if the malignancy is in remission or cured.

SUGGESTED READING

Becker BA, Gaspari AA. Pemphigus vulgaris and vegetans. Dermatol Clin 1993; 11(3):429–452.

Crosby DL, Diaz LA. Endemic pemphigus foliaceus. Dermatol Clin 1993; 11(3):453–462.

Pye RJ. Bullous eruptions. In: Champion RH, Burton JL, Ebling FGJ, eds. Rook/Wilkinson/Ebling textbook of dermatology. 5th ed. Oxford: Blackwell Scientific Publications, 1992: 1623–1673.

Stanley JR. Pemphigus. In: Fitzpatrick TB, Eisen AZ, Wolff K, et al, eds. Dermatology in general medicine. 4th ed. New York: McGraw-Hill, 1993: 606–615.

PEMPHIGOID: BULLOUS AND CICATRICIAL

LAWRENCE S. CHAN, M.D.
DAVID T. WOODLEY, M.D.

BULLOUS PEMPHIGOID

Bullous pemphigoid (BP) is an immune-mediated blistering disease of the skin, manifested as tense bullae (either generally or locally) on inflammed or urticarial skin. The mean age of onset of the disease is the late 60s. In the case of generalized involvement, the lesions preferentially occur in the intertriginous areas. In rare cases, the disease is manifested as pruritic urticarial plaques without clinically visible blisters or even as generalized pruritus without skin lesions. Classically, the histology of bullous pemphigoid is characterized by subepidermal blister formation accompanied by an eosinophilic dermal infiltrate. Direct immunofluorescence microscopy of a perilesional skin biopsy typically reveals the linear deposition of immunoglobulin G and complement at the dermal-epidermal junction. In the majority of cases, circulating anti–basement membrane antibodies of the immunoglobulin G class are detected by indirect immunofluorescence microscopy. These autoantibodies bind to hemidesmosomal components of the basal keratinocyte apposed to the cutaneous basement membrane zone. These autoantibodies are targeted to a 230,000 Daltons and/or a 180,000 Daltons glycoprotein associated with hemidesmosomes. If salt-split skin substrate is used, these autoantibodies bind to the epidermal roof. After proper therapy, the disease usually heals without scarring.

Therapy

The treatment plan for bullous pemphigoid should be tailored to suit the individual patient, depending on the severity of the disease and the patient's clinical response. For generalized bullous pemphigoid, systemic corticosteroids are the mainstay of treatment and should be started as soon as the clinical diagnosis is confirmed by lesional histology and perilesional direct immunofluorescence microscopy. Most patients with generalized bullous pemphigoid respond well to a single daily dose of oral prednisone in the range of 0.5 to 1.0 mg per kilogram body weight. Prednisone taken after breakfast is better tolerated than afternoon or evening administration. The mechanism of action of prednisone on bullous pemphigoid is most likely due to its anti-inflammatory effects.

Oral azathioprine (100 to 250 mg per day) often is used as an adjunct treatment. It was thought that the addition of azathioprine would allow lower total doses of prednisone. However, there is no documentation in the literature that this occurs, and this notion is being challenged. Since azathioprine is a slow-acting drug, it should be initiated early in the treatment regimen. The mechanism of action of azathioprine on bullous pemphigoid is unknown. It may act by decreasing the number of leukocytes through bone marrow suppression. Accordingly, the patient's leukocyte and platelet counts should be monitored monthly. The duration and magnitude of the azathioprine clinical effects correlate with tissue level, but not plasma level, of the metabolite thiopurine nucleotide. Therefore, blood levels of the drug have little predictive value for therapy. Unlike pemphigus vulgaris, the circulating anti–basement membrane antibody titers in patients with BP do not correlate with disease severity. Therefore, indirect immunofluorescence has little value in assessing disease activity or adjusting the dosages of medications. The adjustment of medication should be dependent primarily upon the clinical response of the patient. In general, one expects a decrease in new blisters approximately 1 week after the initiation of therapy of oral prednisone. Healing of the blisters occurs in the subsequent weeks.

Adjunctive topical corticosteroid (mid to high potency) may be added to selected areas in some BP patients. The application of a topical corticosteroid may reduce the need for high doses of oral prednisone. Since blistered skin may increase the chance of systemic absorption, the possible sparing of systemic steroids by the use of topical steroids may not be significant.

The timing for tapering oral prednisone is important, since tapering too early may result in flare of the disease and tapering too late may increase the chance of unnecessary corticosteroid side effects. Two weeks after the cessation of new blister formation and the initiation of healing, tapering of the oral prednisone may begin. In most cases, tapering the prednisone by 5 mg per day every 2 to 3 weeks can be achieved. Some physicians taper oral prednisone using an alternate-day schedule to further reduce potential complications. Our usual approach is to taper the daily prednisone to 20 to 40 mg and then initiate an alternate-day regimen. There are several schedules for converting daily prednisone to an alternate-day regimen. Our preference is to simply double the current daily dose of prednisone but to give it every other day. The patient is then on the same total weekly dose of prednisone. After a week or two on this regimen, we again begin to taper the alternate day prednisone by 5 mg each week.

If oral azathioprine is part of the therapeutic regimen, it should be kept constant while the prednisone is tapered. After the patient is completely off prednisone and remains disease free for several months, azathioprine can then be decreased, usually by 50 mg every week until it is completely discontinued.

When the patient has widespread blisters, erosions, and crusts, topical or systemic antibiotics should be administered to prevent secondary infection or sepsis resulting from denudation of the skin. Systemic antibiotics are usually dicloxacillin, erythromycin, or cephalexin at 1 g per day in divided doses. If the patient becomes febrile, blood cultures should be obtained to monitor for the possibility of sepsis.

Although most patients with generalized bullous pemphigoid respond well to low to medium doses of oral prednisone (with or without adjunctive agents such as azathioprine or topical corticosteroid), some patients respond poorly and may require higher doses of prednisone, longer duration of treatment, and/or more potent immunosuppressants. When dealing with poorly responsive cases, it is recommended that the diagnosis be throughly reevaluated. Indirect immunofluorescence on salt-split skin and immunoblotting should be performed to rule out other more difficult-to-treat diseases such as epidermolysis bullosa acquisita. Cyclophosphamide (daily dose of 1 to 2 mg per kilogram is a good alternative to azathioprine. We have had severe bullous pemphigoid patients who failed on azathioprine, but then rapidly responded to cyclophosphamide. Nevertheless, one must closely monitor the potential side effects of cyclophosphamide such as bone marrow suppression and hemorrhagic cystitis. A complete blood count and urinalysis should be performed on at least a semiweekly schedule.

For those patients who require long-term oral prednisone, one should consider using therapeutic measures to impede for steroid-induced bone loss. The use of a "triple therapy" (calcium 1 g per day, vitamin D 1,000 IU, diphosphonate EHDP 7.5 mg per kilogram) has been reported recently to impede bone loss in patients on systemic steroids.

Other medications have been used in generalized bullous pemphigoid with the hope of being able to use lower doses of systemic steroids to curtail the disease. Chlorambucil, an alkylating antineoplastic medication, has been used (0.1 mg per kilogram body weight) successfully to treat bullous pemphigoid in combination with low doses of systemic corticosteroid. The potentially serious side effects of chlorambucil include bone marrow suppression, especially thrombocytopenia, and leukemia.

Methotrexate, an antimetabolite, also has been reported to be a good adjunctive medication (weekly single dose of less than 20 mg) for bullous pemphigoid in combination with oral prednisone. The potential hepatotoxicity of methotrexate must be closely monitored by following liver enzymes on a biweekly basis.

A minority of patients respond well to sulfa-containing medications such as dapsone. These agents possess antineutrophil motility effects and may be anti-inflammatory in nature. Since potentially fatal hemolysis may occur in patients with a genetic G6PD deficiency, all patients should be checked for G6PD prior to dapsone treatment (100 to 400 mg per day).

Some patients with bullous pemphigoid respond to oral niacinamide (1.5 to 2.5 g per day in three divided doses) in combination with oral antibiotics such as tetracycline or erythromycin (both given at 2 g per day in four divided doses). Topical steroid creams or ointments may be added to this regimen. This therapy is particularly worth trying in elderly patients with milder disease who can be observed closely and are compliant. Like dapsone, tetracycline and erythromycin are anti-inflammatory in nature because of their inhibitory effects on inflammatory cells such as the neutrophils. Anti-inflammatory effects may be responsible for the clinical response. The treatment of bullous pemphigoid with cyclosporin, an antilymphocyte medication, has been tried but appears to give variable results.

For localized bullous pemphigoid, the potential morbidity and mortality are low. It can be treated with mid to high potency topical corticosteroids alone. In some cases, a low dose of oral prednisone may be added for a short duration to stop the development of new blister formation.

CICATRICIAL PEMPHIGOID

Cicatricial pemphigoid, as currently defined, is not a homogeneous, but rather a heterogeneous group of diseases. In general, cicatricial pemphigoid is characterized clinically by inflammation and blister formation on mucosal surfaces and histologically by a full subepithelial blister and linear immune deposits at basement membrane zone when mucosal biopsy specimens are examined by direct immunofluorescence microscopy. Circulating anti–basement membrane antibodies are detected in only a small percent of patients. Scarring may result from the inflammatory process, mostly involving ocular mucosae.

The heterogeneity of the currently defined cicatricial pemphigoid is illustrated by several recent findings. On one hand, a subset of patients who have predominantly mucosal disease and minor skin involvement has been found to have autoantibodies directed against a lower lamina lucida component laminin-5 (also known as kalinin/nicein/BM600/epiligrin). On the other hand, another subset of patients have pure ocular disease and are distinguished from bullous pemphigoid and other mucosal pemphigoid by the high frequency of fibrin deposition at the basement-membrane zone and a virtual absence of circulating antibodies against the basement-membrane zone. Yet another subgroup of patients has only oral mucosal disease without much cicatrization. This appears to be another unique disease entity. In addition, HLA-DQB1* 0301, a specific allele in the class II major histocompatibility complex gene region, was found to be significantly increased in patients with pure ocular cicatricial pemphigoid. Thus at least three distinct subsets of cicatricial pemphigoid can currently be defined—anti–laminin-5 mucosal pemphigoid, pure ocular cicatricial pemphigoid, and oral mucosal pemphigoid.

Therapy

As for bullous pemphigoid, the treatment for cicatricial pemphigoid as a group should be tailored to suit each patient, according to the particular organ involved. For patients who have ocular disease, the physician will face great difficulties in managing the disease. On one hand, untreated or insufficiently treated ocular disease will result in ocular mucosal scarring and potentially lead to blindness. On the other hand, proper treatment of ocular disease requires aggressive usage of potent immunosuppressives. Our initial treatment is oral prednisone (1 mg per kilogram body weight) plus azathioprine (100 to 300 mg per day). If no response occurs in 2 weeks, we add dapsone (100 to 300 mg per day). If no significant response is observed in 2 months with this combination therapy, we then use cyclophosphamide (1 to 2 mg per kilogram body weight) as a replacement for azathioprine. For those patients who cannot tolerate cyclophosphamide because of cystitis or other complications, the alternate therapy is chlorambucil. Patients who require long-term strong immunosuppressives should be properly informed about the potential side effects, such as bone marrow suppression, leukemia and other malignancies, and severe infection. Immunization for influenza and common bacterial infections are recommended. It should be noted that medical treatments do not reverse the formed scar, although they may stop further scar formation. Surgical correction of ocular scarring is not recommended because of the high rate of rescarring. Patients with ocular disease should be managed and monitored by both dermatologists and ophthalmologists.

For patients who do not have ocular disease, treatment should be less aggressive. Usually, a mid to high potency topical corticosteroid should be used as the initial treatment. Since secondary candidiasis may occur as a complication to steroid treatment, a compound medication containing both anticandida and corticosteroid such as Lotrisone cream may be used. In patients with severe oral disease, we give a short course (1 to 2 months) of low dose oral prednisone (20 to 40 mg per day) in conjunction with a topical steroid (Kenalog in orabase or Temovate gel) and/or topical cyclosporin A. Topical cyclosporin A used as a "swish-and-spit" agent is too expensive. We recommend that a small amount of full-strength cyclosporin A solution be poured into a small cup and the patient should then use a cotton applicator to soak the solution and press against the mucosal lesions for 5 minutes, repeated three times a day.

SUGGESTED READING

Foster CS, Wilson LA, Ekins MB. Immunosuppressive therapy for progressive ocular cicatricial pemphigoid. Ophthalmology 1982; 89:340–353.

Krain LS, Landau JW, Newcomer VD. Cyclophosphamide in the treatment of pemphigus vulgaris and bullous pemphigoid. Arch Dermatol 1972; 106:657–661.

Milligan A, Hutchinson PE. The use of chlorambucil in the treatment of bullous pemphigoid. J Am Acad Dermatol 1990; 22:796–801.

Paul MA, Jorizzo JL, Fleischer AB, White WL. Low-dose methotrexate treatment in elderly patients with bullous pemphigoid. J Am Acad Dermatol 1994; 31:620–625.

Rogers RS, Sheridan PJ, Nightingale SH. Desquamative gingivitis: Clinical, histopathologic, immunopathologic, and therapeutic observations. J Am Acad Dermatol 1982; 77:729–735.

Thivolet J, Barthelemy H, Rigot-Muller G, et al. Effects of cyclosporin on bullous pemphigoid and pemphigus. Lancet 1985; 1:334–335.

ERYTHEMA MULTIFORME

MARCIA G. TONNESEN, M.D.

Erythema multiforme (EM) is an acute, self-limited inflammatory disorder of the skin and mucous membranes, characterized by distinctive skin lesions and histopathologic changes. Currently the classification of EM is evolving as distinct subsets are identified and diagnostic criteria are established. Two clinical forms of EM have been designated EM minor and EM major.

Successful therapeutic intervention in any form of EM is hindered by the fact that specific pathogenic mechanisms of tissue injury have not yet been well defined, and few controlled studies have been performed to evaluate therapeutic effectiveness. A rational approach to therapy should be based on careful consideration of suspected etiologic factors; clinical characteristics, including extent and severity of mucocutaneous lesions and patient discomfort; and potential complications. Elimination of any identified or presumed precipitating factors is of prime importance. Optimal therapy should combine symptomatic and supportive measures with observation for and treatment of associated complications, depending on the severity of the episode (Tables 1 and 2).

ERYTHEMA MULTIFORME MINOR

EM minor is a relatively mild cutaneous illness that is frequently recurrent and usually occurs in young adults. The typical clinical picture is the sudden onset of a symmetric erythematous eruption with a predilection for the extensor aspects of the extremities (hands, elbows, knees). Mucosal involvement, when present, is usually limited to development of a few oral erosions. Skin lesions begin as fixed erythematous papules and may progress to become bullous. At least some of the lesions evolve with concentric zones of color change to form characteristic target lesions, the clinical hallmark of EM minor. Individual lesions, usually symptomless but occasionally associated with burning or itching, appear in successive crops which may coalesce, and then resolve within 2 to 4 weeks, leaving residual postinflammatory hyperpigmentation. Some patients suffer from recurrent episodes, often averaging one every 4 to 5 months. Most, if not all, cases of classic recurrent EM minor are associated with herpes simplex virus (HSV) infection and typically occur 7 to 14 days after the appearance of a recurrent HSV lesion (oral, genital, or other location). Current evidence supports the concepts that HSV is the major precipitating factor of EM minor, and that recurrent herpes-associated EM minor represents an HSV-specific host immune response in the skin.

Preferred Therapeutic Approach (Table 1)

Patient Education. Patients should be reassured regarding the usual benign, self-limited course and educated regarding the frequent association of EM minor with recurrent herpes simplex viral infection.

Symptomatic Measures. Since most episodes of EM minor are mild, symptomatic care is often sufficient. For pruritic or painful skin lesions, systemic antihistamines (hydroxyzine hydrochloride, 25 to 50 mg taken orally four times a day or diphenhydramine hydrochloride, 50 mg taken orally four times a day) or analgesics (acetaminophen, 650 mg taken orally four times a day) may provide relief.

Skin Care. For crusted erosive skin lesions, mild drying, debridement, and cleansing can be achieved with open, wet compresses of tepid water or aluminum acetate (Burow's solution diluted 1:20, or one Domeboro tablet dissolved in 1 pint of water) applied for 10 minutes twice a day. After cleansing, an antibacterial ointment (Polysporin or Bacitracin) followed by a bandaid or sterile dressing should be applied to eroded lesions.

Mouth Care. Liquid antacids or topical anesthetics such as dyclonine, viscous lidocaine, or a 1:1 mixture of Kaopectate and elixir of diphenhydramine used as a mouthwash will provide relief from painful erosions.

Table 1 Therapy for EM Minor

Patient Education
  Emphasize:
    Self-limited course
    Association with recurrent herpes simplex virus (HSV) infection

Symptomatic Measures
  Antipruritics:
    Hydroxyzine, 25-50 mg PO q.i.d. *or*
    Diphenhydramine HCl, 50 mg PO q.i.d.
  Analgesics:
    Acetaminophen, 650 mg PO q.i.d.

Skin Care for Erosions
  To dry, debride, and cleanse:
    Open, wet compresses of tepid water *or* aluminum acetate (Burow's solution) for 10 min b.i.d.
  To promote healing:
    Bacitracin or Polysporin antibacterial ointment
    Bandaid or sterile dressing

Mouth Care for Oral Erosions
  To relieve discomfort:
    Liquid antacid *or*
    Topical anesthetic such as:
      Dyclonine
      Viscous lidocaine
      Kaopectate/diphenhydramine 1:1
  To maintain hydration and nutrition:
    Liquid or soft diet

Preventive Measures for Frequent Recurrences of Herpes–Associated EM Minor
  To prevent or decrease recurrences of herpes simplex infection:
    Avoid sun
      Sunscreens (SPF 15 or greater)
      Sunstick (sunscreen in chapstick)
      Protective clothing
      No sun exposure 10 AM-3 PM
    Minimize stress
    Prophylactic oral antiviral therapy
      Acyclovir 400 mg PO b.i.d. for 6 months or longer; taper as tolerated
  For continuous or overlapping episodes:
    Stop treatment with systemic glucocorticosteroids or immunosuppressive drugs
    Institute oral acyclovir prophylaxis

A liquid or soft diet is usually better tolerated and therefore contributes to the maintenance of hydration and nutrition.

Preventive Measures. Because of the strong etiologic association between recurrent HSV infections and recurrent EM minor, measures that attempt to prevent recurrences of herpes simplex should lessen the frequency of subsequent episodes of EM. Avoidance of sun exposure through the use of sunscreens (SPF 15 or greater), sunsticks (sunscreen-containing chapstick), and protective clothing, and by minimizing sun exposure from 10 AM to 3 PM (the peak period for UVB solar irradiation) may reduce ultraviolet light-induced HSV recurrences on sun-exposed skin. Attempts should be made to minimize stress, a well-known precipitating factor in recurrent HSV.

Thus far, topical antiviral preparations have not been clearly shown to prevent or abort recurrent HSV infections. However, in several uncontrolled studies, prophylactic administration of oral acyclovir has resulted in abolition of recurrent HSV infections and of ensuing episodes of EM minor. Acyclovir does not shorten the duration of an episode of EM once begun, nor does it prevent an EM episode if therapy is started during the antecedent HSV infection. Therefore, in patients with frequently recurrent and debilitating herpes–associated EM minor, the treatment of choice is prophylactic daily oral acyclovir for a period of 6 months or longer. The recommended starting dose is 400 mg orally twice daily, with tapering of the dose after the disease is brought under control. Because of the self-limited nature of EM minor, the known occurrence of acyclovir resistance, and the unknown long-term side effects of chronic acyclovir therapy, the drug should be stopped periodically and the need for its continuance reassessed.

Because systemic glucocorticosteroid or immunosuppressive therapy has been linked to development of continuous or overlapping episodes of EM minor, such therapy is not recommended and should be stopped prior to initiation of a course of prophylactic oral

Table 2 Therapy for EM Major

Patient Education
- Emphasize:
  - Self-limited, potentially severe course
  - Association with drugs or infection (*Mycoplasma;* HSV)

Elimination of Etiologic Factors
- Drug:
  - Immediate withdrawal and future avoidance
- *Mycoplasma* infection:
  - Erythromycin, 250-500 mg PO q.i.d. *or*
  - Tetracycline, 250-500 mg PO q.i.d.

Supportive Care
- Hospitalization often necessary
- To maintain hydration and nutrition:
  - Parenteral nutrition, tube feedings, or liquid or soft diet, if tolerated

Symptomatic Measures
- Antipruritics:
  - Hydroxyzine, 25-50 mg PO q.i.d. *or*
  - Diphenhydramine HCl, 50 mg PO q.i.d.
- Analgesics/Antipyretics: Acetaminophen, 650 mg PO q.i.d.

Skin Care for Erosions
- To dry, debride, and cleanse:
  - Open, wet compresses of tepid water *or* aluminum acetate (Burow's solution) for 15 to 20 min b.i.d.
- To soothe and cleanse:
  - Baths in tepid water for 30 min b.i.d.
- To promote healing:
  - Bacitracin antibacterial ointment and sterile dressing or synthetic wound dressing

Mouth Care for Oral Erosions
- To relieve discomfort:
  - Liquid antacid
  - Topical anesthetic such as:
    - Dyclonine
    - Viscous lidocaine
    - Kaopectate/diphenhydramine 1:1
- To treat infection:
  - Erythromycin, 250 mg PO q.i.d. *or*
  - Tetracycline, 250 mg PO q.i.d. for 10 days

Eye Care
- Careful monitoring and early consultation with ophthalmologist

Reduction of Morbidity and Mortality
- For progressive disease:
  - Consider course of Prednisone 1 to 2 mg/kg/day; discontinue when no further disease progression
- For extensive involvement (>10% to 20% total body surface area):
  - Early referral to burn unit
  - Measures to guard against infection:
    - Withdrawal from systemic steroids
    - Limit antibiotic use to culture-proven infections
    - Minimize indwelling lines and catheters
    - Perform daily cultures of skin, blood, and urine
    - Aggressively treat sepsis if it occurs
  - Supportive care:
    - Air-fluidized bed
    - Respiratory and physical therapy
    - Parenteral nutrition or tube feedings
    - Adequate pain relief
    - Avoidance of all unnecessary medications
  - Skin care to facilitate rapid re-epithelialization:
    - Gentle debridement followed by synthetic or biologic dressing

acyclovir. Topical steroid therapy is of little benefit in the treatment of EM.

ERYTHEMA MULTIFORME MAJOR

EM major, also known as bullous EM or as Stevens-Johnson syndrome, is a severe, self-limited, variable mucocutaneous illness characterized by an extensive eruption with areas of epidermal detachment, often accompanied by significant involvement of mucosal surfaces, especially the mouth and conjunctivae. A prodrome with constitutional symptoms may herald the onset of the eruption. Skin lesions begin as papules and may evolve to form raised or flat atypical target lesions. Central blister formation may produce areas of epidermal necrosis and detachment. Painful mucosal erosions result in a foul-smelling mouth, typical hemorrhagic crusting of the lips, and decreased oral intake. Ocular involvement may produce red eyes, photophobia, and, if severe, an erosive, exudative conjunctivitis with residual scarring and lash and lacrimal abnormalities. Permanent visual loss may occur.

Certain drugs, particularly sulfonamides, nonsteroidal anti-inflammatory agents, anticonvulsants, penicillins, and allopurinol are important and well-documented etiologic factors in EM major. Infectious agents associated with EM major are *Mycoplasma pneumoniae* and HSV. The duration of erythema multiforme major, reflecting more severe mucocutaneous damage, is typically 4 to 6 weeks. Recurrences are infrequent. EM major is associated with significant morbidity and may be fatal.

Toxic epidermal necrolysis (TEN), characterized by the abrupt, rapid development of extensive mucocutaneous areas of confluent erythema and blistering with sheet-like, full-thickness epidermal necrosis and detachment resembling scalding, is considered by some to be a severe form of EM major, but is viewed by many as a distinct disease entity. Drugs are now believed to be the only documented cause of TEN. TEN can be considered a manifestation of "acute skin failure" with abnormal barrier function resulting in fluid, electrolyte, and protein loss; increased susceptibility to infection; impaired thermoregulation; altered immune status; and increased energy expenditure. Morbidity is significant and the mortality rate is at least 30 percent. The leading cause of death is sepsis.

A new classification for EM major, based on the morphology of skin lesions as well as on the extent of epidermal loss, has recently been formulated in an attempt to standardize diagnosis. Proposed division into five categories and extent of detachment are bullous erythema multiforme (<10 percent), Stevens-Johnson syndrome (<10 percent), overlap Stevens-Johnson–TEN (10 to 30 percent), TEN with discrete lesions (>30 percent), TEN without discrete lesions (>10 percent). Until specific subsets are further identified and defined, the erythema multiforme disease spectrum and its treatment will continue to be controversial.

Preferred Therapeutic Approach (Table 2)

Because of the extensive epidermal and mucosal necrosis that can occur in EM major, careful monitoring is critical, hospitalization is often required, and supportive care is usually necessary.

Patient Education. Patients should be advised that the course is self-limited but potentially severe and educated regarding the frequent association of EM major with drugs or, less commonly, with infection (*Mycoplasma,* HSV).

Elimination of Etiologic Factors. Any suspected or unnecessary drug should be withdrawn and avoided in the future. In particular, no drugs associated with EM major (especially sulfonamides and penicillins) should be used to treat any manifestation of the EM syndrome. If *Mycoplasma pneumoniae* infection is diagnosed or strongly suspected, systemic treatment should be initiated with erythromycin or tetracycline, 1 to 2 g per day. If HSV infection is diagnosed or strongly suspected, measures should be taken to prevent recurrence (see Table 1).

Supportive Care. Hospitalization is often advisable, and intravenous fluid therapy and nasogastric or parenteral feeding may be necessary to maintain hydration and nutrition.

Symptomatic Measures. For pruritic or painful skin lesions, systemic antihistamines (hydroxyzine hydrochloride, 25 to 50 mg taken orally four times a day or diphenhydramine hydrochloride, 50 mg taken orally four times a day) or analgesics (acetaminophen, 650 mg taken orally four times a day) may provide relief.

Skin Care. For bullous or crusted erosive skin lesions, mild drying, debridement, and cleansing can be achieved with open, wet compresses of tepid water or aluminum acetate (Burow's solution diluted 1:20, or a Domeboro tablet dissolved in 1 pint of water) applied for 15 to 20 minutes four times a day. Frequent bathing (30 minutes twice a day) in lukewarm to cool water has a soothing antipruritic effect as well as serving to cleanse the skin lesions and minimize secondary infection. Lesions should be observed for signs of secondary infection, cultured when indicated, and treatment should be initiated with the appropriate systemic antibiotic. Erythromycin, 250 mg taken orally four times a day, is a good first choice, pending culture results. If lesions progress to extensive tissue necrosis with as much as 20 to 30 percent total body surface area involved, surgical intervention and transfer to a burn unit are advisable (see following discussion).

Mouth Care. When extensive painful mouth lesions are present, good oral hygiene is critical to minimize infection and discomfort. Liquid antacids or topical anesthetics such as dyclonine, viscous lidocaine, or a 1:1 mixture of Kaopectate and elixir of diphenhydramine, used as a mouthwash, will provide pain relief.

A liquid or soft diet is usually better tolerated and therefore contributes to the maintenance of hydration and nutrition. EM major patients who have extensive oral involvement, however, may be unable to eat or drink despite the use of topical anesthetics, thus necessitating parenteral nutrition or tube feedings. When oral lesions are extensive, purulent, foul smelling, and associated with tender cervical lymphadenopathy, systemic therapy with erythromycin or tetracycline, 1 g per day for 10 days, is appropriate to combat secondary bacterial infection.

Eye Care. Because of the potential for long-term sequelae, resulting in visual loss, careful monitoring of eye involvement is mandatory and early consultation with and continuing care by an ophthalmologist are strongly recommended. Suggested therapeutic measures might include irrigation and compresses to cleanse the eye, lysis of adhesions, and instillation of topical antibiotics when indicated.

Reduction of Morbidity and Mortality. Indication for the use of systemic glucocorticosteroids in EM major is a highly controversial issue, since no controlled studies have been conducted to document efficacy. However, because EM major and TEN can progress to widespread epidermal necrosis with a mortality rate as high as 30 percent, early use of systemic steroids in the progressive phase of the disease process in an attempt to decrease the extent of tissue damage is advocated by some. High-dose therapy (prednisone, 1 to 2 mg per kilogram per day) is administered only during the stage of active extension of lesions. In contrast, systemic steroid use is condemned by others since some retrospective reports have suggested that patients treated with systemic steroids have an increased incidence of complications and death.

If extensive, advanced tissue necrosis occurs or is already evident (approaching 20 percent total body surface area involvement), immediate transfer of the patient to a burn unit under the care of a surgical burn specialist is strongly advocated. Therapeutic recommendations for care in the burn unit consist of:

1. Measures to guard against iatrogenic infection, including withdrawal from systemic steroids; limitation of antibiotic use to specific culture-proven infections; avoidance of indwelling lines and catheters whenever possible; daily cultures of skin, blood and urine; and aggressive treatment of sepsis if it occurs;
2. Supportive care consisting of use of an air-fluidized bed, respiratory and physical therapy, parenteral nutrition or tube feedings, adequate pain relief, and continuing care by an ophthalmologist;
3. Avoidance of all unnecessary medications, particularly those which are known etiologic factors of EM-TEN, such as sulfonamides (including sulfa-containing eye preparations, diuretics, and topical dressings); and
4. Skin care with emphasis on early gentle debridement followed by application of a dressing to protect the denuded dermis from desiccation and to facilitate rapid re-epithelialization. Reduced mortality has been reported with the use of allografts and porcine xenografts.

THERAPEUTIC OUTCOME

Both EM minor and EM major are self-limited disorders which can be expected to resolve within 4 to 6 weeks. If the disease persists longer than 8 weeks the diagnosis of EM should be questioned and alternative diagnoses investigated.

SUGGESTED READING

Esterly NB, ed. Special symposium: Corticosteroids for erythema multiforme? Pediatr Dermatol 1989; 6:229–250.

Halebian PH, Madden MR, Finklestein JL, et al. Improved burn center survival of patients with toxic epidermal necrolysis managed without corticosteroids. Ann Surg 1986; 204:503–512.

Huff JC. Therapy and prevention of erythema multiforme with acyclovir. Semin Dermatol 1988; 7:212–217.

Lemak MA, Duvic M, Bean SF. Oral acyclovir for the prevention of herpes-associated erythema multiforme. J Am Acad Dermatol 1986; 15:50–54.

Levy M, Shear NH. *Mycoplasma pneumoniae* infections and Stevens-Johnson syndrome: Report of eight cases and review of the literature. Clin Pediatr 1991; 30:42–49.

Rasmussen JE. Erythema multiforme in children: Response to treatment with systemic corticosteroids. Brit J Dermatol 1976; 95:181–186.

RENAL DISEASE

IMMUNE-MEDIATED NEPHROTIC RENAL DISEASE

RICHARD J. GLASSOCK, M.D.

Nephrotic syndrome (NS) is a common manifestation of underlying glomerular disease. It may be defined as an abnormal biochemical state arising from the continued excretion of large amounts of protein in the urine. Typically, over 3.5 g of protein are excreted daily in the adult. Characteristic abnormalities also include hypoproteinemia (hypoalbuminemia), hyperlipidemia, and a hypercoagulable state. Edema is variable and may be absent or very severe (anasarca).

The fundamental abnormality underlying the nephrotic syndrome is enhanced permeability of the glomerular capillary wall to plasma proteins. This abnormality can arise consequent to a variety of causes, some of which are presumably immunologic in nature. Metabolic disorders (e.g., diabetes mellitus), hereditary diseases (e.g., Alport's syndrome), hemodynamic abnormalities (e.g., hypertension, toxemia), and other disorders (e.g., obesity) may also give rise to the nephrotic syndrome.

Among the disorders causing nephrotic syndrome that are believed to be immunologically based, two general categories are described—disorders in which the kidney is the sole or predominant organ involved and in which clinical manifestations are the direct result of the abnormality in glomerular permeability (primary glomerular diseases) and disorders in which many organs, including the kidney, are involved and in which the clinical features are a combination of disease-related organ involvement and the underlying abnormality in glomerular permeability. Table 1 provides a brief classification of the causes of the nephrotic syndrome.

This chapter deals with the management of primary glomerular diseases that evoke nephrotic syndrome and are believed to have an immune basis. The secondary glomerular diseases such as lupus nephritis, Goodpasture's disease, amyloidosis, and systemic vasculitis, are addressed elsewhere.

MINIMAL CHANGE DISEASE

Minimal change disease is defined on the basis of the absence of structural glomerular lesions by light microscopy. Characteristically, immunofluorescence studies reveal only scanty immunoglobulin deposition, typically IgM, in the mesangial zones associated with diffuse foot process effacement by electron microscopy. Minimal change disease is believed to be caused by the secretion of a nonimmunoglobulin permeability factor from T lymphocytes. The nature of the stimulus, the precise origin, and the chemical nature of the putative permeability factor involved in the pathogenesis of this disease remain unknown. Most commonly, it affects children between the ages of 4 and 8, but it may also develop in young adults and older patients. It tends to present with the abrupt onset of nephrotic syndrome and has a marked tendency for spontaneous remission and relapse, particularly in children. The overall long-term prognosis is quite favorable with less than 5 percent of patients developing chronic renal failure.

Although 30 to 40 percent of patients will ultimately experience a spontaneous remission, treatment is usually initially indicated because of the adverse effects of nephrotic syndrome such as hyperlipidemia or increased tendency to thrombosis and edema. Glucocorticoid therapy (prednisone or prednisolone) will result in a complete remission of abnormal proteinuria in over 90 percent of patients, but relapses will occur in approximately 50 percent of the responding patients during or after withdrawal of glucocorticoid therapy. Pediatric patients appear to respond earlier and more completely than adults, with most children achieving complete remission within 8 weeks of an oral glucocorticoid regimen. On the other hand, 12 to 20 weeks of glucocorticoid therapy may be required to induce a complete remission in adults. The reasons for this difference in responsiveness to glucocorticoids remain unknown.

Initial treatment in children usually consists of oral prednisone or prednisolone 60 mg per square meter (80 mg per day maximum) for 4 to 6 weeks, followed by 35 to 40 mg per square meter taken every other day, for an additional 4 to 6 weeks. The entire daily dose is usually administered in a single dose in the morning. Initial treatment of adults usually consists of 1 mg per kilogram

Table 1 Classification of Nephrotic Syndrome (NS)

Immune-Mediated NS
Primary glomerular disease
Minimal change disease
Membranous glomerulonephritis
Focal sclerosis (?)
Membranoproliferative glomerulonephritis
IgA nephropathy
Secondary glomerular disease
Systemic lupus erythematosus (SLE)
Goodpasture's disease
Henoch-Schönlein purpura
Vasculitis
Amyloidosis
Neoplasia
Drugs (e.g., NSAIDs)
Infection (e.g., HIV)
Allograft rejection
Non–Immune Mediated NS
Metabolic
Hereditary
Hemodynamic
Miscellaneous (e.g., obesity)

per day (maximum 80 mg per day) of prednisone or prednisolone for 6 to 10 weeks, followed by 0.6 to 0.8 mg per kilogram taken every other day for an additional 6 to 10 weeks. Initiation of therapy with three intravenous "pulses" of 500 to 1,000 mg methylprednisolone may accelerate the occurrence of complete remissions. Patients failing to respond to this regimen after 8 to 12 weeks (children) or 12 to 20 weeks (adults) should be tentatively regarded as steroid resistant. However, it must be recognized that some patients will respond with a complete remission if therapy is continued for several weeks beyond these general treatment duration guidelines. This may be a part of the therapeutic response spectrum of minimal change disease, or it may indicate another underlying lesion missed at initial biopsy, most commonly focal and segmental glomerulosclerosis (focal sclerosis, see following discussion). If severe exogenous Cushing's syndrome has resulted from initial therapy, it would be best to consider adjunctive therapy rather than continuing to administer high-dose glucocorticoids (see following discussion). However, if therapy is well tolerated, it would be desirable to continue glucocorticoids in somewhat reduced dosage for another 4 to 6 weeks. Alternatively, the patient could be given three boluses of intravenous methylprednisolone, 500 to 1,000 mg each.

If a relapse of nephrotic syndrome occurs during the withdrawal of glucocorticoids, high-dose, daily glucocorticoid therapy should be reinstituted for about 4 weeks, followed by slow tapering to determine a threshold dose. If the threshold dose for relapse is less than 0.3 mg per kilogram taken every other day, then the patient may be maintained at this dose for 4 to 6 months followed by a subsequent slow taper. If the threshold dose is greater than 0.3 mg per kilogram taken every other day, then adjunctive therapy (see following discussion) should be considered. Infrequent relapses (less than two per year) can be treated with a repeat of the initial glucocorticoid course for two courses, unless complications (such as growth retardation) occur. Frequent relapses (three or more per year) should be considered an indication for adjunctive therapy (see following discussion).

Adjunctive therapy consists of the addition of an alkylating agent (either chlorambucil or cyclophosphamide) to the regimen. These agents will reduce or eliminate the tendency for relapse in about 50 to 60 percent of patients and will induce complete remissions in some glucocorticoid-resistant patients. Oral cyclophosphamide is preferred, 2 mg per kilogram per day, for 10 to 12 weeks, usually given after a glucocorticoid-induced remission and given concomitantly with 15 to 20 mg of prednisone or prednisolone every other day. There does not appear to be any advantage to initiating adjunctive therapy with intravenous cyclophosphamide. On the other hand, some prefer to give oral chlorambucil in doses of 0.1 to 0.2 mg per kilogram per day for 8 to 10 weeks with alternate-day prednisolone. Monitoring of white blood cell counts and platelets is required to avoid serious marrow toxicity. Gonadal damage is infrequent when the cumulative dose of cyclophosphamide is kept at less than 200 mg per kilogram and chlorambucil at less than 17 mg per kilogram. A relapse after an initially successful course of cyclophosphamide or chlorambucil can be retreated with the combination regimen on one occasion but repeated treatment may be associated with an increase in side effects. Patients with continued relapses after alkylating agent–based adjunctive therapy are uncommon but represent difficult clinical challenges. Continuation of high-dose glucocorticoid therapy will eventually produce disabling side effects and continued retreatment with alkylating agent-based regimens is too risky.

The use of oral cyclosporin A (CsA) appears to be the best approach in these patients. Oral CsA in doses of 5 mg per kilogram per day in adults and 100 to 150 mg per square meter in children combined with 10 to 20 mg of prednisolone taken every other day will result in a complete remission in a high percentage (>80 percent) of patients with frequently relapsing glucocorticoid-sensitive minimal change disease. If after 4 months of treatment with CsA the patient fails to achieve a complete remission, all therapy should be withdrawn. A remission following CsA therapy can be maintained by gradual reduction in dosage to 3 to 4 mg per kilogram per day and continued for one year. Following 1 year of continual therapy in remission, CsA can be gradually withdrawn. Many patients who previously relapsed with withdrawal of cyclosporin may enter long-term remissions. Renal function should be closely monitored during CsA therapy. A repeat renal biopsy may be required to evaluate possible CsA nephrotoxicity. Withdrawal of CsA too early is often associated with a relapse. Alternatively, frequently relapsing patients unresponsive to alkylating agent-adjunctive therapy can be treated with low-dose levamisole and alternate-day prednisone. Oral angiotensin converting enzyme inhibitors may reduce proteinuria in some patients but seldom result in complete remissions. In exceptional circumstances, long-term treatment (1 year or more) with oral azathioprine (2 mg per kilogram per day) may result in remission.

FOCAL AND SEGMENTAL SCLEROSIS

Focal and segmental sclerosis is characterized by sclerotic lesions affecting some glomeruli (focal) and in which the sclerotic lesions involve only a portion of the glomerular tuft (segmental). Heavy IgM and C3 deposits are found in the sclerotic lesions by immunofluorescence, but these probably have occurred on a nonspecific basis. Diffuse foot process effacement and markedly abnormal visceral epithelial cells are seen by electron microscopy. The etiology and pathogenesis of the lesion are uncertain but it has been suggested that circulating nonimmunoglobulin permeability factors may participate. Similar lesions may also occur in a variety of disease processes, such as human immunodeficiency viral infection, obesity, nonsteroidal antiinflammatory drug use, and vesicoureteral reflex.

The lesion of focal sclerosis is more commonly found in young and older adults with nephrotic syndrome and is a more steroid-resistant lesion than minimal change disease. Progressive renal failure is common among patients, particularly in association with continued heavy proteinuria and/or hypertension. Spontaneous remissions are uncommon. The idiopathic form of focal sclerosis accounts for 10 to 20 percent of all cases of idiopathic nephrotic syndrome. As stated previously, it may represent an evolutionary stage of minimal change disease or may appear de novo without a pre-existing diagnosis of minimal change disease. The onset is usually insidious and some patients may present with persistent non-nephrotic proteinuria. The majority of patients present with the nephrotic syndrome, which at times may be very severe.

Overall, 30 to 40 percent of patients with focal sclerosis can be induced into a complete remission with prolonged courses of oral glucocorticoids. Initial treatment, therefore, should consist of 1 mg per kilogram per day of prednisone or prednisolone (80 mg per day maximum) for at least 8 weeks, followed by approximately 0.8 mg per kilogram taken every other day for an additional 16 to 20 weeks. Patients who experience complete or partial remissions of proteinuria should have treatment slowly tapered. In all likelihood a reduction of proteinuria to non-nephrotic levels beneficially affects long-term prognosis. Patients who fail to respond after 6 months of treatment or who immediately relapse following a complete or partial remission upon withdrawal of glucocorticoids can be considered for adjunctive therapy.

Adjunctive therapy consists of 10 to 12 weeks of treatment with oral cyclophosphamide or chlorambucil given in a fashion similar to that described for minimal change disease. Alternatively, patients may be given CsA 5 mg per kilogram per day for 3 to 4 months, along with low-dose, alternate-day prednisone or prednisolone. Only about 20 to 30 percent of steroid-resistant patients will completely respond to these regimens, but a substantial reduction in proteinuria to non-nephrotic levels is likely to be associated with an improved prognosis. Patients who fail to respond to treatment with glucocorticoids, alkylating agents, and/or CsA should be placed on long-term angiotensin converting enzyme inhibitor therapy in the hope that a reduction in protein excretion will result in an improved prognosis.

Experimental approaches to focal sclerosis include plasma exchange, lipid apheresis, immunoabsorption, tacrolimus, and aggressive regimens involving high-dose intravenous methylprednisolone combined with oral or intravenous cyclophosphamide. These more aggressive regimens are incompletely evaluated at the present time and may be associated with substantial risks or side effects. Overall, long-term prognosis is guarded, especially in those patients with very heavy proteinuria (>10 g per day) who fail to respond to the regimens described above. Recurrences in renal allografts are common (30 to 50 percent). Post-transplant treatment with plasma exchange, sometimes combined with high-dose cyclosporin, may be beneficial in the treatment of recurrent disease.

MEMBRANOUS GLOMERULONEPHRITIS

This disorder is characterized by immunoglobulin containing electron-dense deposits on the subepithelial aspect of the glomerular capillary wall. This is presumably the consequence of autoantibody formation to an antigen present on the surface of glomerular visceral epithelial cells resulting in the in situ formation of immune complexes. It is a common cause of idiopathic nephrotic syndrome in adults but is quite rare in children. It may also be associated with a wide variety of diseases, such as systemic lupus erythematosus, chronic hepatitis B viral infection, cancer, and drugs.

The onset of the disease is usually insidious and overt nephrotic syndrome may be preceded by months or even years of asymptomatic proteinuria. The overall prognosis is reasonably favorable with 25 to 40 percent of patients entering spontaneous remissions. However, approximately 30 percent of patients will progress to end-stage renal disease within the first 10 to 15 years after diagnosis. Heavy proteinuria, male sex, increased serum creatinine at the time of discovery, and advanced glomerular and tubulointerstitial lesions on renal biopsy are predictive of an adverse outcome.

The treatment of this disorder is controversial, but general agreement exists that efforts to exclude potentially treatable diseases, such as drug ingestion, neoplasia, and certain infections (e.g., hepatitis B) should be carried out in patients suspected at being at risk for these conditions. Therefore, elderly patients should be investigated for the possibility of an occult carcinoma (lung, colon, stomach).

Assuming that secondary causes of membranous glomerulonephritis can be excluded, the decisions regarding treatment of the idiopathic disorder should be based on five aspects: (1) What is the risk of a complicating event relating to the nephrotic syndrome, such as a thromboembolic event or coronary arterial atherosclerosis? (2) What is the risk of progressive renal failure? (3) What is the likelihood of a spontaneous remission? (4) What is the likelihood of a complication related to treatment? (5) What is the likelihood of a treatment-related remission?

Obviously, estimation of these parameters for individual patients utilizing population-based data can be fraught with errors and uncertainties. Nevertheless, careful therapeutic decision making on an individual basis may avoid risky and unnecessary treatment in some patients or minimize the possibility of withholding treatment from other patients at high risk of progression. Some clinicians view idiopathic membranous glomerulonephritis as a disorder whose natural history is so benign as to indicate a very conservative approach in most patients, applying therapy only in those who demonstrate clear evidence of a progressive disease. On the other hand, others advocate a preemptive approach treating all patients with membranous glomerulonephritis and nephrotic-range proteinuria with a relatively standardized regimen. Both camps agree that specific therapy of patients with asymptomatic non-nephrotic proteinuria is unnecessary. Between the two polar therapeutic views lies an approach that selects patients for active treatment who demonstrate clinical and pathologic features indicative of a poor prognosis or a high complication rate related to nephrotic syndrome and in whom the risk of therapy is low.

Generally speaking, this group will be middle-aged males with persistent, heavy proteinuria (over 8 g per day for longer than 6 months) with hypoalbuminemia ($\leq$ 2.5 g per deciliter) whose renal biopsy shows moderately advanced glomerular lesions with or without chronic interstitial fibrosis and tubular atrophy. In this scenario, a young woman with 4 g of protein per day, mild hypoalbuminemia, a normal serum creatinine, and only mild glomerular capillary wall abnormalities would be managed conservatively. This more selective approach has one disadvantage—some patients destined to progress will be treated late in the course of disease when they may be less responsive to treatment. Whether this potential loss of efficacy by delayed therapy is too great a price to pay remains a matter of debate, but it must be counterbalanced by the fact that with a "treat all" approach, some patients will unnecessarily receive potentially hazardous treatment when a spontaneous remission was destined to occur.

Therapeutic regimens employed in membranous glomerulonephritis are quite varied, but strong evidence exists that oral glucocorticoids alone are relatively ineffective in inducing long-term remissions. Exceptional patients (<10 percent of the total population) may exhibit glucocorticoid treatment–related remissions and relapses. A regimen of intravenous "pulse" methylprednisolone (1.0 g intravenously for three successive daily doses) followed by oral glucocorticoids in doses of 0.5 mg on alternate days for several months will modestly increase remission rates and may offer some protection from chronic renal failure. The most effective regimen appears to be a combination of an alkylating agent with glucocorticoids. Two such regimens are popular, but the relative efficacy and safety have not been tested in a side-by-side comparison. One involves the cyclical administration of intravenous methylprednisolone, oral prednisolone, and oral chlorambucil (Milan regimen). Methylprednisolone is given in 1 g intravenous doses on three successive days, followed by 0.5 mg per kilogram per day of prednisolone for 27 days, then prednisolone is stopped and chlorambucil 0.2 mg per kilogram per day is given for 30 days. Then this cycle is repeated twice. The chlorambucil dosage is adjusted according to the peripheral white blood cell count. With this regimen, about 70 to 80 percent of patients will experience complete or partial remissions and the risk of progressive renal functional impairment is decreased to less than 10 percent. Another protocol involves combination of daily oral cyclophosphamide (2 mg per kilogram per day) with alternate-day prednisone (20 to 40 mg taken every other day) for 6 to 9 months. A 3-day course of intravenous methylprednisolone can be added to these regimens at the beginning of the regimen. The results are similar to those described for the cyclical methylprednisolone-prednisolone-chlorambucil regimen described above, but this therapeutic approach has been studied with much less intensity.

Side effects of cyclical methylprednisolone-prednisolone-chlorambucil are relatively uncommon (< 10 percent) except in elderly patients or those with renal insufficiency. These side effects usually consist of leukopenia, infections (especially herpes zoster), azoospermia, and gastrointestinal discomfort. Cyclophosphamide-based regimens may be associated with cystitis, alopecia, hepatitis, azoospermia, infection, and leukopenia. Both regimens theoretically can increase the later development of a myelodysplastic syndrome or leukemia, but this has seldom been observed when the courses of treatment are limited to less than 1 year.

Patients whose disease has already progressed to renal insufficiency (serum creatinine 1.5 to 3.5 mg per deciliter) can also be treated with similar regimens although the side effect profile will likely be increased. In addition, many fewer patients will experience complete remissions. Nevertheless, with this "rescue" approach to treatment, renal function may stabilize or improve and the need for maintenance dialysis may be forestalled. Additionally, combinations of prednisolone and oral azathioprine may slow the rate of progression. Patients with very advanced disease (serum creatinine > 3.5 mg per deciliter) in association with marked chronic tubulointerstitial fibrosis and atrophy on renal biopsies are unlikely to benefit from therapy and are probably best treated conservatively.

Additional therapy that should be given to most patients includes careful management of blood pressure, preferably with angiotensin converting enzyme inhibitors, which can also be given to nonhypertensive patients for their antiproteinuric effects. Hypercholesterolemia should probably be managed with HMG-coreductase inhibitors or probucol. The latter may also exhibit an antiproteinuric effect.

The role of prophylactic warfarin anticoagulation is debated. There is little doubt that patients with membranous glomerulonephritis are at increased risk for thromboembolic disease, including renal vein thrombosis and pulmonary embolism. Patients with serum albumin concentrations of 2.5 g per deciliter or less seem to be at highest risk. Because of a favorable benefit-risk ratio, prophylactic administration of warfarin (to an INR of about 1.5 to 2.0) is advocated for patients with serum albumin concentrations of 2.5 g per deciliter or less. All patients who have had a documented thromboembolic event, regardless of the serum albumin concentration, should also receive warfarin therapy. The duration of therapy required is unknown, but continuation of warfarin is recommended for as long as the patient has a protein excretion greater than 3.5 g per day and/or a serum albumin concentration of 2.5 g per day or less, unless serious bleeding complications ensue.

Experimental therapy, not yet at a stage where broad clinical recommendations are appropriate, include oral CsA and parenteral immunoglobulins. Cyclosporin may yet find a place in the management of patients with progressive disease who fail to respond to alkylating agent-prednisolone combinations. Intravenous immunoglobulin treatment may be an approach to induce remissions in early but not severe disease where an approach using alkylating agents is relatively contraindicated.

IgA NEPHROPATHY (BERGER'S DISEASE)

IgA nephropathy is a very common form of glomerulonephritis, but a rather infrequent cause of the nephrotic syndrome. It is characterized by mesangial deposition of IgA frequently accompanied by complement (C3) deposition. By light microscopy, a variety of structural lesions are observed, and those patients presenting with the nephrotic syndrome may have very mild or no observable changes by light microscopy, thus resembling minimal change disease. A more common presentation of IgA nephropathy is episodes of gross hematuria, often accompanied by non-nephrotic proteinuria. Ten to twenty-five percent of patients will slowly progress to end-stage renal failure over 10 to 20 years, and a minority will have more rapidly progressive disease. Persisting heavy proteinuria, hypertension, and advanced glomerular and/or tubulointerstitial lesions are indicative of an unfavorable prognosis.

For most patients, a conservative approach to treatment is indicated. Patients presenting with nephrotic syndrome accompanied by minimal glomerular abnormalities can be treated in a fashion similar to that described for minimal change disease. There is a high likelihood of a beneficial response and few patients will later progress to renal failure. The treatment of patients with heavy proteinuria with episodic hematuria accompanied by hypertension and obvious structural glomerular and tubulointerstitial lesions is more problematic. Glucocorticoids alone do not appear to be very effective. Angiotensin-converting enzyme inhibitors will often decrease the magnitude of proteinuria and may delay the onset of progressive renal insufficiency. Large doses of ω-fatty acids (combination of eicosopentanoic and doxosohexanoic acid) reduce the likelihood of progressive renal insufficiency but often do not have beneficial effects on proteinuria. Immunosuppressive agents, such as cyclophosphamide, or CsA, do not appear to be effective and are not indicated in the treatment of most patients with this disorder. Azathioprine may slow the rate of progression of the disease. However, patients with very rapidly progressive disease, associated with very extensive glomerular crescents, may be successfully managed by combinations of high-dose intravenous methylprednisolone, plasma exchange, and immunosuppression. Patients with exacerbations associated with acute renal failure and only modest glomerular involvement (< 30 percent crescents) may be treated conservatively because a spontaneous recovery is likely.

Patients with episodic macroscopic hematuria and slight proteinuria (< 500 mg per day) have a favorable prognosis, particularly if renal biopsies show only mild glomerular and/or tubulointerstitial lesions. Progression to nephrotic levels of proteinuria and the development of hypertension or renal insufficiency indicate an unfavorable prognosis and may be reasons for a more aggressive approach to treatment, including the use of angiotensin converting enzyme inhibitors. Experimental approaches to treatment, not yet fully evaluated, include combinations of dipyridamole and low-dose warfarin, antigen-elimination diets, and inhibitors of platelet aggregation.

MEMBRANOPROLIFERATIVE GLOMERULONEPHRITIS

Membranoproliferative glomerulonephritis is a rather uncommon form of glomerulonephritis observed in patients with nephrotic syndrome. It is characterized by the presence of subendothelial or intramembranous electron-dense deposits, frequently accompanied by complement (C3) and immunoglobulin. By light microscopy, it is characterized by diffuse increase in mesangial matrix and hypercellularity with extensions of cells, matrix, and new basement membrane synthesis into the peripheral capillaries. A similar lesion may be associated with a wide variety of underlying diseases, including chronic hepatitis C viral infection, cryoimmunoglobulinemia, monoclonal immunoglobulin disease, and systemic lupus erythematosus. The idiopathic (primary) disorder is most frequently seen in children and young adults. In addition to the nephrotic syndrome, common manifestations include hematuria, hypertension, and progressive renal insufficiency.

The treatment of this disorder is quite controversial. In children, long-term treatment with modest doses of prednisone or prednisolone on an every-other-day basis (e.g., 30 to 40 mg taken every other day) may reduce proteinuria, retard the rate of progression of renal insufficiency, and improve the glomerular abnormalities. However, the overall efficacy of this approach has not been unequivocally established in randomized prospective clinical trials. Initiation of treatment with daily prednisone or prednisolone may be associated with severe exacerbations of hypertension, and patients should be carefully monitored. Immunosuppressive drugs, such as cyclophosphamide, azathioprine, or CsA are not generally effective. Combinations of dipyridamole (150 to 300 mg) and aspirin (375 mg) taken daily have been shown to slow the rate of progression in patients with heavy proteinuria and impaired renal function. Hypertension, if present, should be treated aggressively, most likely with angiotensin converting enzyme inhibitors. Experimental treatments, not yet proven to be effective, include plasma exchange and intravenous immunoglobulins. Overall, the prognosis for membranoproliferative glomerulonephritis is guarded, with many patients developing progressive renal insufficiency, especially in association with persisting heavy proteinuria, hypertension, and advanced glomerular or tubulointerstitial lesions. The disease may recur in renal allografts.

SUGGESTED READING

Donadio JV, Bergtralh E, Offord KP, et al. A controlled trial of fish oil in IgA nephropathy. N Engl J Med 1994; 331:1194–1199.

Glassock RJ. Therapy of idiopathic nephrotic syndrome in adults. Am J Nephrol 1995; 15:422–428.

Imperiale TF, Goldfarb S, Berns J. Are cytotoxic agents beneficial in idiopathic membranous glomerulopathy? A meta-analysis of controlled trials. J Am Soc Nephrol 1995; 5:1553–1558.

Meyrier A, Nöel H, Auriche P, et al. Long-term renal tolerance of cyclosporin A treatment of adult idiopathic nephrotic syndrome. Kid Int 1994; 45:1446–1456.

Ponticelli C, Passerini P. Treatment of nephrotic syndrome associated with primary glomerulonephritis. Kid Int 1994; 46:595–604.

ACUTE HYPERSENSITIVITY INTERSTITIAL NEPHRITIS

PETER S. HEEGER, M.D.
ERIC G. NEILSON, M.D.

Acute tubulointerstitial nephritis, often referred to as simply "acute interstitial nephritis," accounts for nearly 15 percent of cases of acute renal failure. Individuals with acute interstitial nephritis (AIN) typically experience a sudden decrease in renal function, with the hallmarks of acute interstitial injury on renal biopsy manifested by mononuclear cell infiltrates (lymphocytes and plasma cells), occasional eosinophils, tubular destruction, and relatively normal glomeruli. It is also important that as many as 25 percent of patients with chronic renal failure have sustained injury from the concealed, long-term sequelae of what probably began as acute interstitial inflammation. In such patients, biopsy reveals progressive pathologic injury involving interstitial fibrosis, tubular atrophy, and tubular dropout with or without senescent glomerular tufts. Largely because of the work done in experimental systems, there is a growing knowledge of the pathophysiologic mechanisms involved in the production of interstitial injury. Applying this insight to human renal disease has resulted in a reasoned clinical method for evaluating patients suspected of having acute interstitial nephritis and in a firmer groundwork for the discussion of therapeutic options. The approach we use emphasizes the establishment of a diagnosis, the removal of potentially causative agents, and the attempt to treat the destructive lesion with chemotherapy when necessary.

CLINICAL FEATURES

The wide variety of etiologic factors that have been implicated in the development of AIN can be divided into three broad categories: pharmacologic agents, infectious diseases, and autoimmune phenomena (Table 1). Rarely, the presentation of interstitial nephritis is simply idiopathic. A thorough exploration of these potential causes is essential. The initial approach to the treatment of AIN is to remove any inciting agents and to treat any underlying disease.

The diagnosis of interstitial nephritis is relatively straightforward in the classic setting in which a rapidly rising serum creatinine level (0.3 to 0.5 mg per deciliter per day) accompanied by fever, rash, and eosinophilia occurs 10 to 15 days after beginning treatment with a pharmaceutical agent. Unfortunately, this presentation of a hypersensitivity reaction is the exception, not the rule. Skin rash occurs in less than 50 percent of patients, fever in approximately 75 percent, eosinophilia in about 80 percent, and the triad is found in less than 30 percent. Therefore when AIN is suspected, the physician must first systematically exclude prerenal and obstructive causes of acute renal failure from the differential diagnosis and then proceed to distinguish interstitial nephritis from acute tubular necrosis, glomerulonephritis, or vasculitis. A careful urinalysis is usually helpful in this regard. In interstitial nephritis, the urinalysis reveals mild-to-moderate proteinuria (although the nephrotic

Table 1 Etiology of Acute Interstitial Nephritis

Drugs
Antibiotics (e.g., penicillin derivatives, cephalosporins, rifampin, sulfonamides, fluoroquinolones)
Nonsteroidal anti-inflammatory drugs (NSAIDs)
H_2-blockers
Diuretics
Others (phenytoin, allopurinol, alpha-interferon)
Infectious Diseases
Diptheria
Scarlet fever
Subacute bacterial endocarditis
Leptospirosis
Human immunodeficiency virus
Epstein Barr virus
Legionella
Syphillis
Autoimmune Diseases
Systemic lupus erythematosis
Sjögren's syndrome
Sarcoidosis
Antitubular basement membrane disease
Tubulointerstitial nephritis-uveitis syndrome
Idiopathic

syndrome has been reported, especially with use of alpha-interferon and nonsteroidal anti-inflammatory drugs [NSAIDs]), and microscopic hematuria may be present. Sterile pyuria and/or white blood cell casts are usually encountered, but red blood cell casts are so rare that their presence should suggest the alternative diagnosis of glomerular injury. Additionally, the presence of eosinophiluria, as demonstrated by Hansel's stain, supports the diagnosis of interstitial nephritis. This finding is not entirely sensitive or specific, however, and must be considered in the context of the clinical setting.

Often, the available clinical data are insufficient to provide a definitive diagnosis without a renal biopsy. There are many reported cases of clinically unsuspected AIN diagnosed by renal biopsy, as well as multiple reports of biopsy-documented acute tubular necrosis in patients clinically suspected as suffering from AIN. Additionally, renal biopsy can provide important prognostic information based on the extent and character of the renal lesion. The presence of advanced renal insufficiency with significant fibrosis and an extensive mononuclear infiltrate on biopsy, for example, portend a poor renal outcome. In such a situation, it may be best to institute conservative treatment with preparation for renal replacement therapy, and to avoid the potential complications of immunosuppressive therapy. Establishment of a firm diagnosis must be made as quickly as possible because minimizing the time that elapses from the onset of renal injury to the institution of appropriate therapy allows the greatest possibility for return of normal renal function. In experimental interstitial nephritis, substantial irreversible interstitial fibrosis can develop in as little as 10 days. We recommend rapidly obtaining a tissue diagnosis in all cases of suspected interstitial nephritis, provided that the patient is medically stable enough to tolerate a biopsy, and there are no contraindications to immunosuppressive therapy.

MECHANISMS OF DISEASE

A general understanding of the underlying pathophysiologic processes leading to interstitial injury is helpful in the selection of appropriate therapy. We believe that virtually all forms of human interstitial nephritis have an immunologic basis, and several reports in the clinical literature are consistent with this view. Most of the detailed information, however, comes from studies in experimental animals. Rodent models of interstitial nephritis implicate humoral and/or cellular arms of the immune system in the expression of the disease. In some experimental models, animals with a genetic predisposition to interstitial nephritis lose their protective immunologic tolerance to self-antigens and subsequently develop an immune response against themselves. In other situations, molecular mimicry from infectious agents and drugs acting as a hapten-bridge with the tubulointerstitium can target an immune response towards previously unrecognized (or unexposed) self-antigens. Other drugs can damage interstitial structures through toxic mechanisms and thereby produce novel antigens that are immunogenic. Obviously, avoidance or removal of exogenous factors that mimic or lead to antigen expression is the first step in the treatment of interstitial nephritis.

Once the target nephritogenic antigen is recognized by the immune system, several immunoregulatory factors, including suppressor T-cell networks, anti-idiotypic networks, and the regulation of major histocompatibility complex (MHC) molecular expression, can modulate the severity of disease. Therapies that make use of these endogenous control mechanisms are at the forefront of immunologic research and are discussed at the end of this chapter.

Actual damage to the kidney can be mediated by several effector mechanisms, including complement activation, and the release of proteases, leukotrienes, superoxides, and peroxides by infiltrating eosinophils, basophils, and mast cells. The hallmark of AIN, however, is the presence of mononuclear cells, particularly T lymphocytes. These T cells cause injury through several discrete mechanisms including (1) delayed-type hypersensitivity with the release of inflammatory lymphokines, (2) cell-mediated cytotoxicity through protease release, and (3) the production of lymphokines that modulate the biosynthesis of extracellular matrix in epithelial cells and fibroblasts. The majority of therapeutic interventions probably modify some element of this effector response, although the exact mechanisms are not clear.

TREATMENT

Once the diagnosis of AIN has been firmly established, the first and most obvious intervention is to identify and discontinue the use of any potential offending drugs or to treat any underlying systemic infection. In some cases, this may constitute definitive therapy. Renal function, as assessed by daily blood urea nitrogen (BUN) and/or creatinine measurements, should improve within several days of removal of the potential inciting immunogenic stimuli.

For those patients whose condition does not improve or in whom the disease process appears to be secondary to an autoimmune disease or to be idiopathic treatment with corticosteroids should be considered as adjunctive therapy. The decision to treat with corticosteroids must be based on biopsy documentation of histologic AIN without evidence of significant renal fibrosis. We do not recommend steroid therapy without a biopsy, and we feel that immunosuppressive therapy in the presence of significant fibrosis would subject the patient to the risks of treatment without significant potential benefit. The decision to begin corticosteroid treatment should be additionally tempered by the marginal published clinical data to support its widespread use. One often quoted report of 14 patients with methicillin-induced interstitial nephritis suggests that treatment with corticosteroids leads to a faster (9 days versus 54 days) and fuller recovery of renal function (a lower final creatinine level) than with supportive therapy alone. This study is methodologically flawed, however, in that it is retrospective, nonrandomized, and nonblinded. Other similar reports and anecdotes pervade the clinical literature, some suggesting a marked efficacy of corticosteroid treatment, while others showing that the treatment has no effect on outcome. No properly designed study has yet been published. Nevertheless, many physicians have treated patients with AIN whose conditions have improved temporally (and probably causally) with the initiation of steroid therapy. We therefore recommend beginning steroid treatment in a patient with biopsy-proven interstitial nephritis of noninfectious etiology, which does not demonstrate significant fibrosis, and has not immediately responded to withdrawal of potential inciting factors. Since the likelihood of recovery of renal function decreases when azotemia persists for more than 1 to 2 weeks, therapy should be initiated early. We recommend a 4 to 6 week course of prednisone in a dose of 1 mg per kilogram per day (or in a patient incapable of oral intake, an equivalent dose of intravenous prednisolone), followed by a taper over an additional 2 to 3 weeks. Although shorter courses of therapy are endorsed by some authors, occasional patients with AIN will exhibit a clinical exacerbation following 10 days of treatment alone.

It should be noted that steroids themselves improve the glomerular filtration rate by 10 to 25 percent independent of any specific effect they may have on the destructive tubulointerstitial lesion. The mechanism for this is not fully known, but it seems to be related to volume expansion. As a result of this nonspecific effect, one may anticipate aggravated heart failure or preexisting hypertension. Also, because steroid treatment results in accelerated protein catabolism, the patient with renal failure is at higher risk for developing hyperkalemia, hyperphosphatemia, and hyperuricemia out of proportion to the degree of renal compromise. The diabetic patient will additionally develop a worsening of serum glucose that may require a change in insulin therapy. Despite these potential side effects, we believe that the risk-benefit ratio of a well-defined course of steroid therapy is favorable. Although the risks of long-term steroid treatment are more significant, we are unaware of any cases of AIN in which the maintenance of improved renal function has been dependent on steroids, except in the setting of AIN from sarcoidosis.

The mechanism whereby corticosteroids exert a beneficial influence in the treatment of AIN can only be inferred from their known effects on other immunologic processes. A specific assessment of their action has not been made in either human or experimental interstitial nephritis. Corticosteroids are known to impair cell-mediated immunity and have been shown to abrogate delayed-type hypersensitivity responses in humans. Numerous investigators have noted that pharmacologic doses of steroids inhibit production of interleukin 1, interleukin 2, and gamma interferon by macrophages and T cells and may impair T-cell responsiveness to these and other lymphokines. There is some evidence that steroids suppress antibody production. In addition, steroids stabilize lysosomal membranes, and thereby suppress the release of proteolytic enzymes. It is therefore reasonable to speculate that the beneficial effects of corticosteroids in interstitial nephritis interrupt the effector phase of the immune response through one or more of the above mechanisms.

In a small number of patients with AIN who do not respond to steroid therapy alone, a more aggressive intervention may be required to produce a remission. In the occasional patient who has little to no fibrosis on renal biopsy and who has not responded to the removal of inciting factors and to 1 to 2 weeks of daily prednisone treatment, cytotoxic treatment may be offered. Under these conditions, it would be reasonable to begin cyclophosphamide at a dosage of 2 mg per kilogram per day in addition to the steroids. If no response is noted within 5 to 6 weeks, the cyclophosphamide should be discontinued and the steroids tapered over several weeks. On the other hand, if an improvement in renal function coincides with the initiation of cyclophosphamide therapy, then, based on anecdotal experience, treatment should be continued for 1 year. As always, with cyclophosphamide, the white blood cell count must be monitored closely and the drug discontinued or decreased in dosage if the total white blood cell count decreases to less than 3,500 per cubic millimeter (2,000 neutrophils). We do not believe that cyclophosphamide poses a serious oncogenic threat within this time frame, and there is only a small chance of its limiting fertility. Given that fertility is likely to be decreased with chronic renal failure, we tend to accept these risks with consultation and guidance from the patient. Although there is no controlled clinical data to support the use of cyclophosphamide, there are anecdotal reports in which a response was noted in several patients. In addition, cyclophosphamide is extremely effective in preventing irreversible damage in experimental interstitial nephritis, provided that it is given early at an appropriate

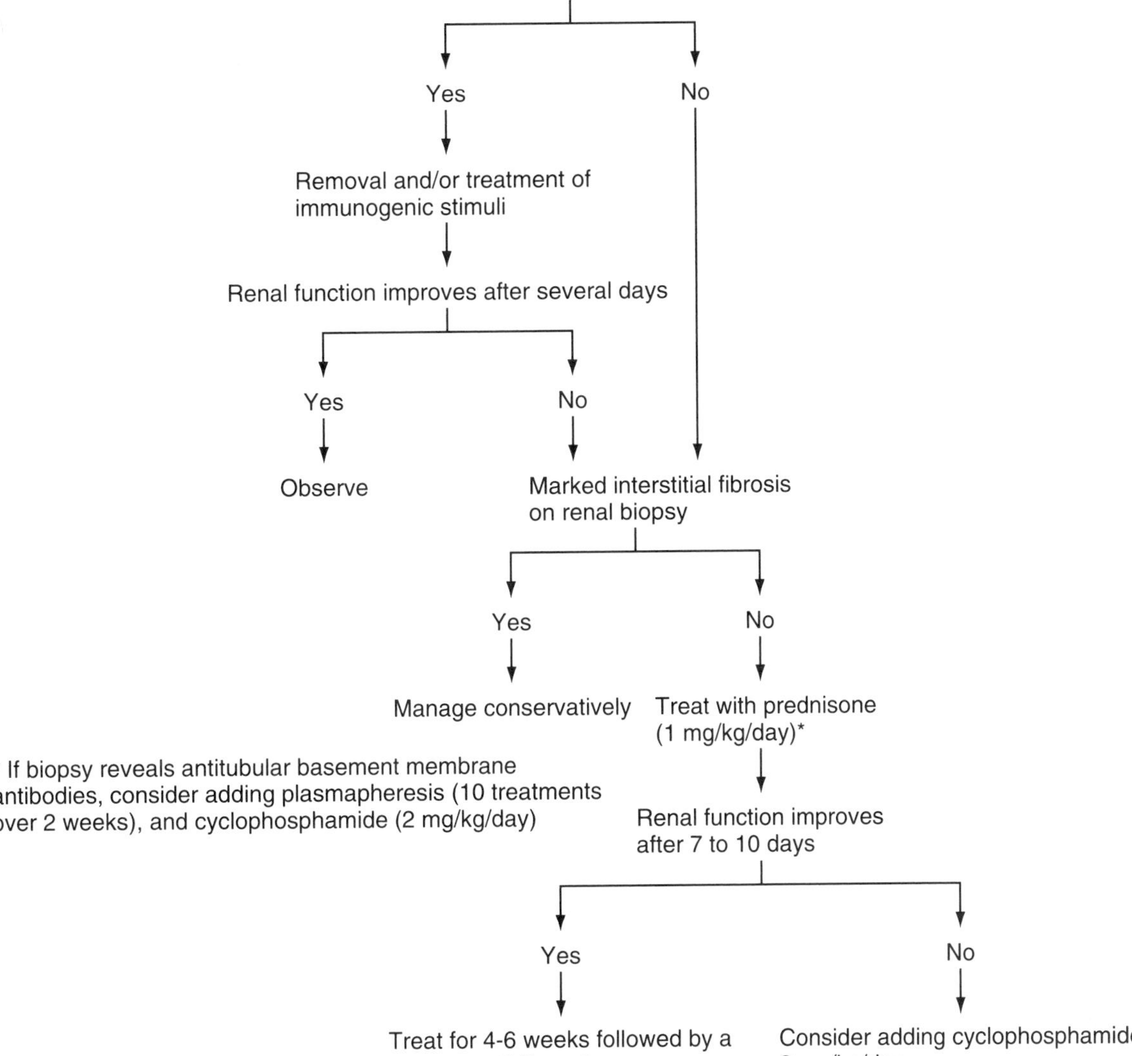

Figure 1 Treatment of acute interstitial nephritis.

dosage. Unfortunately, because of the limited numbers of patients, it is not likely that cytotoxic therapy will be systematically evaluated in controlled trials.

The possible beneficial effect of cyclophosphamide seems to be mediated through the functional inhibition of T cells, in that cyclophosphamide has been demonstrated to abrogate the delayed-type hypersensitivity response in experimental animals, without an effect on the humoral immune response.

Finally, one of the most important features of immunosuppressive management is knowing when to stop treatment. With all of the interventions mentioned above, it takes time for the maximum effect to be achieved. Within several weeks, however, one should be able to make a rational decision to provide no further treatment. Protracted treatment in patients with renal failure can lead to metabolic and infectious complications that occasionally prove fatal. The positive renal transplant experience and the consistent improvement in dialytic techniques have demonstrated that patient survival and well-being must always take precedence over attempts to treat hopeless renal failure. It is clearly preferable, at some point, to accept the irreversibility of progressive renal insufficiency and plan for chronic dialysis and/or renal transplantation rather than prolong treatment with powerful immunosuppressive agents. Our overall approach to the treatment of AIN is summarized in Figure 1.

EXPERIMENTAL THERAPY

Data from experimental animal studies support the use of cyclosporin A in the therapy of acute interstitial nephritis. This drug has been shown to be an effective prophylactic and therapeutic agent probably by direct inhibition of T-cell activation. With a small but growing experience with this therapy in the treatment of autoimmune diseases in humans, we can anticipate the occasional use of cyclosporin A in the treatment of interstitial nephritis. Nevertheless, since its long-term administration in some transplant settings has raised questions about cyclosporin A's ability to induce fibrogenesis and since the number of steroid-unresponsive cases of AIN are relatively small, it remains unlikely cyclosporin A will be extensively studied as a treatment modality for this disease entity. We believe, however, that further evaluation of the beneficial effects of cyclosporin A is warranted, since it is likely that the drug will be used for only a limited time in any given patient.

The use of plasmapheresis may also be considered in those rare patients who, in addition to meeting the criteria for cyclophosphamide therapy, have antitubular basement membrane antibodies demonstrable by renal immunofluorescence. The rationale for this is parallel to the rationale for treating antiglomerular basement membrane disease with plasmapheresis, cyclophosphamide, and steroids—antitubular basement membrane antibodies are playing a critical role in the disease process and their removal disturbs an immune effector mechanism that contributes to renal injury. Normally we would use 3- to 4-liter exchanges every day for 5 days, and every other day for a second week. Anecdotal reports on its limited use have been mixed.

On the forefront of immunologic research is the use of antigen-specific therapy in the treatment of immune-mediated diseases. The ultimate goal of these approaches is to eliminate or inhibit autoreactive, disease-producing T lymphocytes, while leaving the rest of the immune system intact, thus avoiding the complications of global immunosuppression. Towards this goal, studies in experimental interstitial nephritis have shown that the induction of a specific suppressor T-cell response, or the induction of specific anti-idiotypic antibodies (antibodies directed towards unique gene products of the T-cell receptor region that are in or near the antigen-binding site) can prevent or decrease the severity of interstitial injury, even after the disease is well established. The use of T-cell receptor vaccines and the induction of specific T-cell tolerance through antigenic peptide antagonists are additional modalities under evaluation. Although there are many practical obstacles to overcome before such therapy can be used in humans, these novel approaches hold considerable promise for the future.

SUPPORTIVE THERAPY

While a variety of specific renal tubular disorders, electrolyte abnormalities, and acid-base disturbances accompany the development of chronic interstitial nephritis, the complications of AIN are, in essence, the general complications of acute renal failure. Thus, the supportive therapy of AIN may involve the treatment of volume overload, hyponatremia, hyperkalemia, hypocalcemia, hyperphosphatemia, and acidosis. (These aspects of patient care are discussed in standard textbooks of nephrology and therefore will not receive further attention here.) Some recent evidence also suggests the potential efficacy of dietary protein restriction in slowing the progression of some forms of chronic renal insufficiency. Interestingly, the cellular lesions of experimental interstitial nephritis can be largely attenuated by dietary protein restriction, probably through a nonspecific inhibition of T-cell function. Bearing in mind that this finding has not been formally investigated in humans, one may consider decreasing protein intake to approximately 0.5 to 0.6 g per kilogram per day in those patients left with chronic renal insufficiency after an episode of acute tubulointerstitial nephropathy. However, considering the overall catabolic and relatively malnourished state of most hospitalized patients with acute renal failure, protein restriction during the acute phase is probably best delayed until ambulatory health is fully established and the patient may be treated on an outpatient basis.

SUGGESTED READING

Buysen JGM, Houthoff HJ, Krediet RT, Arisz L. Acute interstitial nephritis: A clinical and morphological study in 27 patients. Nephrol Dial Transplant 1990; 5:94–99.

Galpin JE, Shinberger JH, Stanley TM, et al. Acute interstitial nephritis due to methicillin. Am J Med 1978; 65:756–765.

Hannedouche T, Grateau G, Noel LH, et al. Renal granulomatous sarcoidosis: Report of six cases. Nephrol Dial Transplant 1990; 5:18–24.

Koselj M, Kveder R, Bren AF, Rott T. Acute renal failure in patients with drug-induced acute interstitial nephritis. Renal Failure 1993; 15:69–72.

Laberke HG, Bohle A. Acute interstitial nephritis: Correlations between clinical and morphological findings. Clin Nephrol 1980; 14:263–273.

Neilson EG. Pathogenesis and therapy of interstitial nephritis. Kidney Int 1989; 35:1257–1270.

ORGAN TRANSPLANT RECIPIENTS

TERRY B. STROM, M.D.
MANIKKAM SUTHANTHIRAN, M.D.

IMMUNOLOGIC CONSIDERATIONS

Organ transplantation is the preferred treatment for many patients suffering from cardiac, pulmonary, liver, or end-stage renal disease, and for some patients with insulin-dependent diabetes mellitus. Many individual centers, each employing somewhat different protocols, report excellent graft and patient survival. No absolute consensus has developed on how to achieve optimal immunosuppression. Immunologic considerations, including maintenance immunosuppression and antirejection therapy, are organized around a few general principles:

1. Careful patient selection and preparation, and, in the circumstance of renal transplantation, selection of the best available ABO-compatible, human-leukocyte-antigen (HLA) match, in the event that several potential living-related donors are available for organ donation.
2. Use of a multidrug approach to immunosuppressive therapy, similar in principle to that used in chemotherapy, in which several agents are used simultaneously, each of which is directed at a different and pertinent molecular target (Fig. 1, Table 1). Additive-synergistic effects are achieved through the low-dose administration of each therapeutic, thereby limiting the toxicity of each individual agent while increasing the total immunosuppressive effect.
3. High doses of immunosuppressive drugs and/or a greater number of individual immunosuppressive drugs are required to gain early engraftment; evermore intensive therapy is required to treat established rejection, whereas far less intensive immunosuppression is needed in the long-term for maintenance. Hence, intensive induction and lower dose maintenance drug protocols are used.
4. Careful investigation of each episode of post-transplant graft dysfunction, realizing that most of the common causes of graft dysfunction, including rejection, can (and frequently do) coexist. Successful therapy therefore often involves several simultaneous therapeutic maneuvers.
5. The appropriate reduction or withdrawal of an immunosuppressive drug when that drug's toxicity exceeds its therapeutic benefit.

TRANSPLANT THERAPY

Pretransplant Transfusions

Although pretransplant random whole blood transfusion was a powerful adjunct to transplant therapy when cyclosporine (CsA) was not available, the short-term benefits of random transfusion have recently been more difficult to demonstrate in the CsA era. There is no agreement concerning the role of donor-specific transfusions (DST) for recipients of HLA-mismatched living-related donor renal transplants (LDR). Occasionally DST produces adverse presensitization to the donor. Because these sensitized patients cannot be transplanted with tissues procured from the transfusion donor, many units do not employ routine DST. Owing to the powerful tolerogenic effects of DST in experimental models, several active and very interesting clinical trials are evaluating various forms of preoperative-perioperative donor blood element infusions into graft recipients as a therapeutic modality.

Therapy Designed to Prevent Rejection

Antirejection protocols are aimed at interrupting several discrete stages in the immune activation pathway leading to allograft rejection. When possible, selection is undertaken using HLA matching to minimize histoincompatibility between donor and recipient. All post-transplant immunosuppressive protocols use at least two agents, each directed at a discrete site in the T-cell activation cascade (see Fig. 1, Table 1).

Immunopharmacology of allograft rejection

Cyclosporine and Tacrolimus Cyclosporin

CsA, a small neutral hydrophobic cyclic peptide of fungal origin, and tacrolimus (FK506), a water-soluble macrolide lactone produced by *Streptomyces tsukubaenis,* block the Ca^{2+} dependent T-cell activation pathway that is triggered through activation of the T–cell receptor-CD3 complex. Oral doses of both agents are erratically absorbed. Because the absorption of CsA requires bile, and FK506 does not, the absorption of FK506 is not influenced by clamping a T-tube. In this limited respect, the treatment of liver transplant recipients with FK506 provides superior bioavailability.

The immunosuppressive effects of CsA and FK506 are dependent upon the formation of heterodimeric complexes that consist of the native compound, CsA or FK506, and its respective cytoplasmic "immunophilin" receptor protein, cyclophilin or FK-binding protein (FKBP). Both CsA-cyclophilin and FK506-FKBP complexes bind calcineurin, a calcium and calmodulin sensitive phosphatase, and inhibit its catalytic activity (see Fig. 1; Table 1). CsA/FK506-mediated inhibition of calcineurin phosphatase activity prevents the dephosphorylation of cytoplasmic NF-AT, and thereby impedes subsequent import of this critical DNA-binding protein

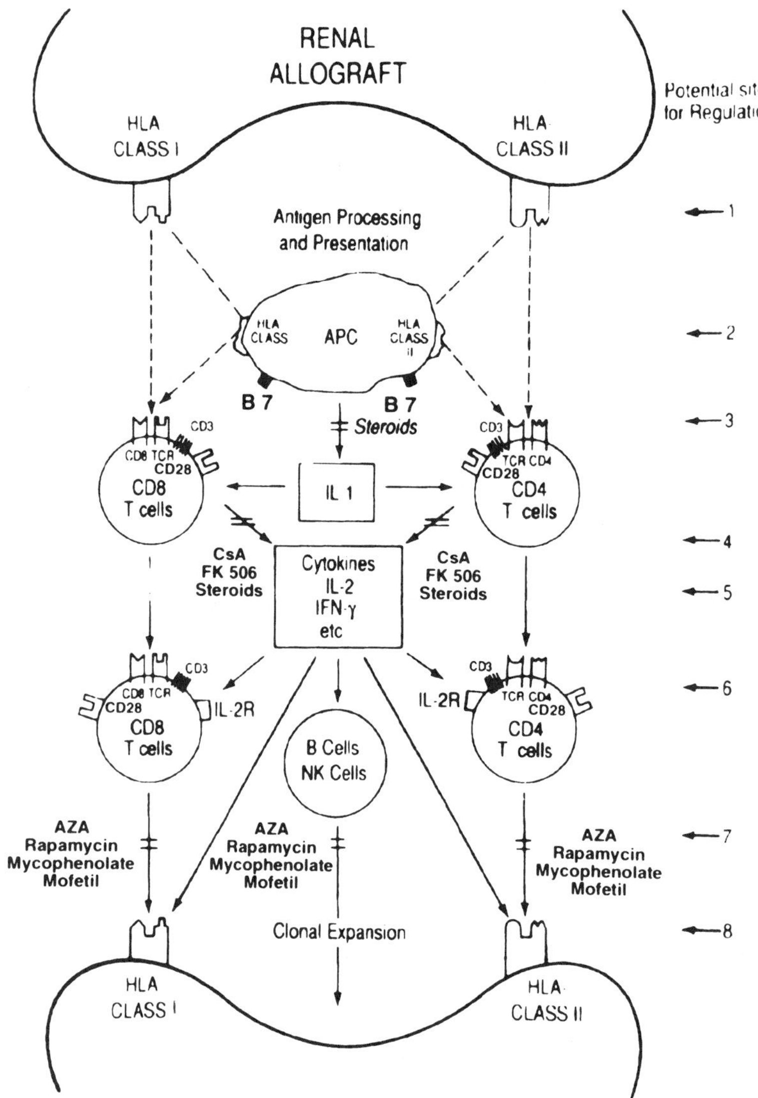

Figure 1 The antiallograft response. Schematic representation of HLA, the primary stimulus for the initiation of the anti-allograft response, cell surface proteins participating in antigenic recognition and signal transduction, contribution of the cytokines and multiple cell types to the immune response, and the potential sites for the regulation of the antiallograft response. *Site 1:* Minimizing histoincompatibility between the recipients and the donor (e.g., HLA matching); *Site 2:* Prevention of monokine production by APCs (e.g., corticosteroids); *Site 3:* Blockade of antigen recognition (e.g., OKT3 mAbs); *Site 4:* Inhibition of T-cell cytokine production (e.g., CsA); *Site 5:* Inhibition of cytokine activity (e.g., anti–IL-2 antibody); *Site 6:* Inhibition of cell cycle progression (e.g., anti–IL-2 receptor antibody); *Site 7:* inhibition of clonal expansion (e.g., azathioprine); *Site 8:* prevention of allograft damage by masking target antigen molecules (e.g., antibodies directed at adhesion molecules). (HLA-class 1: HLA-A, HLA-B, and HLA-C antigens; HLA-class 2: HLA-DR and HLA-DQ antigens; APC: antigen presenting cell; CsA: cyclosporine; AZA: azathioprine; IL-2: interleukin-2; IFN-γ: interferon-γ; NK cells: natural killer cells).

Table 1 Mechanism of Action of Immunosuppressants

Agent	*Mechanism of Action*
CsA/FK506	Blocks Ca^{2+}-dependent T-cell activation pathway via binding to calcineurin
Corticosteroids	Blocks cytokine gene expression
Azathioprine	Inhibits purine synthesis
Mycophenolate mofetil	Inhibits a lymphocyte-selective guanosine synthesis pathway
Rapamycin	Inhibits the response of antigen activated lymphocytes to growth factor

into the nucleus. CsA/FK506 not only inhibits the expression of NF-AT but also the activities of other DNA-binding proteins such as NF-kB and AP-1 factors. The phosphorylation status of transcription factors not only affects their ability to migrate into the nucleus but also their DNA-binding ability and interaction with the cellular transcriptional machinery (e.g., c-Jun).

CsA/FK506 inhibits activation of several T-cell cytokine genes, including interleukin-2 (IL-2), interleukin-4 (IL-4), and gamma interferon (IFN-γ); however, this activity does not totally account for the antiproliferative effect of CsA/FK506 upon activated T cells. Inhibition of expression of protooncogenes (e.g., H-ras, c-myc) as well as prevention of expression of receptors for cytokines (e.g., the IL-2 alpha chain receptor) are likely to be critical in this regard.

It is clearly significant that CsA, in striking contrast to its inhibitory activity on the induced expression of IL-2, enhances the expression of transforming growth factor-beta (TGF-β), which is known to exert antiproliferative properties in several systems. Because TGF-β is a potent inhibitor of IL-2– and IL-4–stimulated T-cell proliferation and the generation of antigen specific CTL, enhanced expression of TGF-β is likely to contribute to the immunosuppressive activity of CsA. This novel effect of CsA also suggests a mechanism for some of the complications (e.g., renal fibrosis) of CsA therapy since TGF-β is a fibroblast growth factor.

Corticosteroids

Corticosteroids were first used in clinical transplantation to reverse acute rejection reactions in patients receiving maintenance doses of azathioprine. It is now customary to use modest doses of a corticosteroid in maintenance protocols that also utilize CsA or tacrolimus with or without azathioprine. A short course of a very high dose of corticosteroids is often used to treat acute rejection episodes. Corticosteroids inhibit T-cell proliferation, T-cell–dependent immunity, and cytokine gene transcription (including IL-1, IL-2, IL-6, IFN-γ, and tumor necrosis factor-alpha (TNF-α) genes (see Fig. 1, Table 1). Although no individual cytokine can totally reverse the inhibitory effects of corticosteroids upon mitogen–stimulated T-cell proliferation, a combination of cytokines is effective.

Some cytokine genes possess a glucocorticosteroid response element in the 5′ regulatory region that serves as a target for the heterodimeric complex formed by the association of corticosteroids with the intracellular glucocorticosteroid receptor protein. Binding of this complex to the glucocorticosteroid response element can, in theory, block gene expression. Blockade of IL-2 gene transcription, however, involves impairment of the cooperative effect of several DNA-binding proteins, although the IL-2 gene does not possess a glucocorticosteroid response element.

How do glucocorticoids block T-cell activation? Glucocorticoids block expression of numerous genes through the noncovalent association of the interaction of the activated hormone-receptor complex with the c-Jun–c-fos heterodimer (activation protein-1, AP-1). c-Jun and c-fos heterodimers bind to the AP-1 site of the promoter of many cytokine genes (e.g., IL-2). Indeed, glucocorticoids interfere with IL-2 gene expression through prevention of nuclear transcription factors binding to the AP-1 and NF-AT sites. Moreover, glucocorticoids inhibit the pretranscriptional calcineurin-dependent pathways for T-cell activation. Inhibition of cytokine production by corticosteroids represents an important rationale for their use in controlling the antiallograft response (see Fig. 1, Table 1).

Azathioprine

Azathioprine is the 1-methyl-4-nitro-5-imidazolyl derivative of 6-mercaptopurine, and this purine analogue functions as a purine antagonist and inhibits cellular proliferation (See Fig. 1, Table 1). Allopurinol blocks the catabolism of azathioprine, causing a dramatic increase in bone marrow suppression, which is occasionally lethal. Azathioprine is often used in conjunction with CsA or tacrolimus and corticosteroids in maintenance protocols. Although application of azathioprine diminishes the incidence and intensity of rejection episodes, it is not valuable in the therapy of ongoing rejection.

Mycophenolate Mofetil

An agent now available, mycophenolate mofetil, blocks purine metabolism through its inhibitory effect upon inosine monophosphate dehydrogenase, an enzyme in the de novo purine biosynthetic pathway. The effects of mycophenolate mofetil upon purine metabolism are semiselective for activated lymphocytes. As a consequence, mycophenolate mofetil competes with azathioprine for use in some drug regimens.

OKT3 Monoclonal Antibody (mAb)

The multimeric CD3 complex proteins are noncovalently associated to the alpha- and beta-chains of the T-cell receptor for antigen. The CD3 complex is expressed on the surface of all mature T lymphocytes. OKT3 binds to the sigma-chain of the CD3 complex; OKT3 binding to T cells leads to modulation of all components of the TCR-CD3 complex from the T-cell surface, either by shedding or internalization. Moreover, T cells virtually disappear from the peripheral blood following the administration of OKT3 mAb.

Maintenance Immunosuppressive Regimens

The basic immunosuppressive protocol used in most transplant centers involves the use of multiple drugs, (usually CsA or FK506 and corticosteroids with or without azathioprine or mycophenolate mofetil) each directed at a discrete site in the T-cell activation cascade (see Fig. 1, Table 1) and each with distinct side effects. CsA, FK506, azathioprine, and corticosteroids are already approved by the FDA, whereas the clinical efficacy of rapamycin (an agent that inhibits the proliferative signal imparted by IL-2, IL-4, or IL-7 to antigen-activated T cells) is being explored in clinical trials.

Alternative Approaches: Sequential Immunotherapy

Following the lead of Soulillou and associates, a number of other centers have adopted an alternative approach to antirejection prophylaxis. OKT3 mAb or polyclonal antilymphocyte antibodies are used in many transplant centers as induction therapy in the immediate post-transplant period. Administration of antilymphocyte globulin (ALG) or OKT3 in conjunction with corticosteroids, azathioprine, and greatly reduced doses of CsA/FK506 are applied in the immediate post-transplant period. This protocol establishes a potent immunosuppressive umbrella that enables initial engraftment without immediate use of high dose CsA/FK506 during the early post-transplant period, and it enables engraftment without use of high dose CsA/FK506 in the critical early post-transplant days during which time renal grafts are highly sensitive to the nephrotoxic effects of CsA/FK506. The incidence of early rejection episodes is reduced by the prophylactic usage of antilymphocyte antibodies. Any incipient rejection is treated by the use of what we view as essentially antirejection strategies to induce immunosuppression. This protocol is particularly beneficial in the long term for patients at high risk for immunologic graft failure (e.g., broadly presensitized or retransplant patients).

Therapy Designed to Treat Established Rejection

Low-dose prednisone, CsA/FK506, and azathioprine maintenance drug therapy is effective in the prevention of acute cellular rejection; each drug blocks a different facet of T-cell activation. However, these drugs are ineffective in blocking the activity of already activated T cells or late-acting elements of the allograft response that no longer require helper T-cell input. Thus, these agents do not readily abrogate established acute rejection episodes or prevent chronic rejection. Treatment of acute rejection requires the use of agents that act against already fully activated T cells. High-dose corticosteroids, polyclonal antilymphocyte antibodies, or OKT3 are often successfully used as therapies for the treatment of acute cellular rejection.

Approximately, two-thirds of acute cellular rejections will respond to high-dose corticosteroid boluses. Steroid-sensitive rejection episodes are typically characterized by a dense infiltration of T cells in the medullary regions of the graft. We often treat the first rejection episode with 1 g of IV methylprednisolone daily for 3 consecutive days. The mechanism by which corticosteroids act to reduce the intensity of leukocytic infiltration in a rejecting allograft has not been fully elucidated; however, release of numerous cytokines is blocked by high-dose steroids, and T-cell trafficking patterns are altered.

OKT3-treated T cells lose their antigen receptor proteins and become literally blinded to the presence of the allograft; thus, rejection abates. OKT3 is superior to standard high-dose corticosteroid therapy for reversing allograft rejection (90 versus 70 percent success). More than 90 percent of first rejections and a high percentage of second-rejection episodes respond to OKT3 therapy. Nonetheless, OKT3 is often reserved as treatment for corticosteroid-resistant rejection episodes. As antirejection treatment, OKT3 is given as a daily 5 mg IV bolus for 5 to 10 consecutive days.

While prophylactic administration of OKT3 to patients in the immediate post-transplant period is well tolerated, administration of the first and occasionally second dose of OKT3 to patients treated for ongoing rejection often causes a "capillary leak" syndrome that can lead to severe ARDS-type pulmonary edema, hypotension, and/or aseptic meningitis. This syndrome is caused by the release of lymphokines from the OKT3 targeted activated T cells. Because of these troublesome symptoms as well as additional expense, we reserve OKT3 therapy for steroid-insensitive rejection episodes. Subsequent doses are well tolerated. Approximately 75 percent of patients develop IgG or IgM anti-idiotype or anti-isotype antibodies against OKT3. Azathioprine at doses of 1 to 2 mg per kilogram per day and prednisone at 30 mg per day are employed to limit the frequency and delay the onset of occurrence of host anti-OKT3 antibodies. OKT3 is not efficacious in patients who have developed high titer anti-idiotypic antibodies against OKT3. Anti-isotypic antibodies do not neutralize the immunosuppressive properties of OKT3.

Polyclonal or antilymphocyte antibody preparations are derived from animals immunized with human lymphocytes. The antibodies are directed against both lymphocyte-specific and more broadly expressed antigens. More than 80 percent of steroid-resistant first-rejection episodes will respond to these polyclonal antibodies. Patients are skin tested with 0.1 mg of a 1:1,000 dilution of polyclonal antilymphocyte antibodies prior to administration of the first dose and pretreated before each dose with diphenhydramine and steroids. Antilymphocyte antibodies, often at a dosage of 10 to 15 mg per kilogram, are administered daily by slow IV infusion over 4 to 8 hours for 10 to 14 days. Adverse reactions include anaphylaxis; hemolysis; thrombocytopenia; neutropenia; dyspnea; chills; fever; hypotension; chemical phlebitis; pruritus; serum sickness; and chest, flank, and back pain. Unlike the first-dose complications noted with OKT3, the severity of anaphylactoid side effects to these polyclonal antilymphocyte preparations can increase with subsequent doses. Frank anaphylaxis can occur anytime during treatment. The use of polyclonal antilymphocyte antibodies has decreased because OKT3 is less toxic and comparably effective in reversing rejection.

We rarely treat a kidney transplant recipient for more than three rejection episodes in the early post-transplant period because third and fourth rejections tend to be vasculitic forms that are therapeutically resistant, and the risks to the patient from zealous immunosuppression are unacceptably high by that point. In contrast, patients with cardiac allografts who will die with the cessation of cardiac function are treated more vigorously because complete rejection, in the absence of retransplantation, is fatal.

Although current drug protocols are far superior to those employed a decade ago, the situation is far from ideal. Most allografts eventually succumb to chronic rejection. Long-term therapy is mandatory. We anticipate clinical application, in the near future, of more refined immunosuppressive regimens—new drugs, humanized mAbs, and fusion proteins that target discrete steps in antigen recognition, signal transduction, and effector immunity. We are also optimistic regarding the inducibility of antigen-specific tolerance in the clinical setting, but a delivery date cannot yet be guaranteed.

SUGGESTED READING

Almawi WY, Hadro ET, Strom TB, et al. Abrogation of glucocorticosteroid-mediated inhibition of T cell proliferation by the synergistic action of IL-1, IL-6, and IFN. J Immunol 1991; 146:3523–3527.

Eugui EM, Almquist SJ, Muller CD, Allison AC. Lymphocyte-selective cytostatic and immunosuppressive effects of mycophenolic acid in vitro: Role of deoxyguanosine nucleotide depletion. Scand J Immunol 1991; 33:161–173.

Flanagan WM, Corthesy B, Brown RJ, Crabtree GR. Nuclear association of a T-cell transcription factor blocked by FK506 and cyclosporine. Nature 1991; 352:802–807.

Franklin TJ, Cook JM. The inhibition of nucleic acid synthesis by mycophenolic acid. Biochem J 1969; 113:515.

Fruman DA, Klee CB, Bierer BE, Burakoff SJ. Calcineurin phosphatase activity in T lymphocytes is inhibited by FK506 and cyclosporin A. Proc Natl Acad Sci USA 1992; 89:3686–3690.

Li B, Sehajpal PK, Khanna A, et al. Differential regulation of transforming growth factor beta and interleukin-2 genes in human T-cells: Demonstration by usage of novel competitor DNA constructs in the quantitative polymerase chain reaction. J Exp Med 1991; 174:1259–1262.

Li B, Sehajpal PK, Subramaniam A, et al. Suthanthiran M. Inhibition of interleukin-2 receptor expression in normal human T cells by cyclosporine. Transplantation 1992; 53:146–151.

Opelz G. Correlation of HLA matching with kidney graft survival in patients with or without cyclosporine treatment. Transplantation 1985; 40:240–243.

Paliogianni F, Raptis A, Ahuja SS, et al. Negative transcriptional regulation of human interleukin-2 (IL-2) gene by glucocorticoids through interference with nuclear transcription factors AP-1 and NF-AT. J Clin Invest 1993; 91:1481–1487.

Schreiber SC. Immunophilin-sensitive protein phosphatase activation in cell signalling pathways. Cell 1992; 70:365–368.

Sollinger HW, Eugui EM, Allison AC. RS-61443: Mechanisms of action, experimental and early clinical results. Clin Transplant 1991; 5:523–526.

Takemoto S, Terasaki PI, Cecka JM, et al. Survival of nationally shared, HLA-matched kidney transplants from cadaveric donors. The UNOS Scientific Renal Transplant Registry. N Engl J Med 1992; 327:834–839.

Thistlethwaite JR Jr, Cosimi AB, Delmonico FL, et al. Evolving use of OKT3 monoclonal antibody for treatment of renal allograft rejection. Transplantation 1984; 38:695–670.

Zanker B, Walz G, Wieder KJ, Strom TB. Evidence that glucocorticosteroids block expression of the human IL-6 gene by accessory cell. Transplantation 1990; 49:198–201.

LUPUS NEPHRITIS

CLAUDIO PONTICELLI, M.D., F.R.C.P. (Edin.)
GABRIELLA MORONI, M.D.

Renal disease is very common in patients with systemic lupus erythematosus (SLE). At presentation, about half of the patients have some clinical signs of kidney involvement, but renal disease may eventually develop in about three-fourths of the patients. Most cases of renal involvement in SLE are caused by glomerulonephritis, which can eventually result in arterial hypertension, nephrotic syndrome, and renal failure with related complications.

PRESENTATION AND COURSE OF LUPUS NEPHRITIS

Lupus nephritis, or lupus glomerulonephritis, may present with a nephrotic syndrome (proteinuria more than 3.5 g per day, hypoalbuminemia, hypercholesterolemia, various degrees of edema), a nephritic syndrome (macroscopic or microscopic hematuria, erythrocyte or hemoglobin casts, proteinuria, hypertension, impairment of renal function), or an already established renal insufficiency. In rare but dramatic instances, postpartum or postabortum acute anuric renal failure with or without microangiopathic hemolytic anemia is the first manifestation of kidney involvement or even of SLE. However, many patients may have lupus nephritis without any particular symptoms, and it is diagnosed only by routine analysis. It is possible that underlying, sometimes progressive renal disease may be present in these asymptomatic patients. From a practical point of view it is recommended that blood pressure, serum creatinine, and urinalysis be regularly checked, even in patients with minimal or no signs or symptoms of disease-related renal activity. It is also important to study the urinary sediment. The amounts of erythrocytes and leukocytes and the presence of erythrocyte and leukocyte casts are often related to the renal activity of SLE.

The clinical outcome of lupus nephritis is highly variable and may be strongly influenced by therapy. Some patients continue to have minimal urinary abnormalities during follow-up, but others with mild renal disease at presentation may later develop nephrotic proteinuria, hypertension, and renal insufficiency. About half of the patients with nephrotic syndrome at presentation may slowly progress towards uremia, but others maintain stable renal function, with fluctuation of proteinuria and sometimes complete remission.

In patients with nephritic syndrome the extrarenal activity of SLE is often severe. The clinical course of these patients is punctuated by renal flare-ups alternated with periods of clinical quiescence often induced by therapy. If untreated, most nephritic patients will develop end-stage renal disease within a short time. Despite aggressive treatment, a few patients have tumultuous progressive courses with severe hypertension, heart failure, and rapidly progressive renal insufficiency. Black race, severe anemia, and renal insufficiency at presentation are associated with poor prognoses.

Renal failure and infections are the most frequent causes of death in the first few years after diagnosis of lupus nephritis. In the long-term, many deaths are related to atherosclerotic disease. Prolonged glucocorticoid therapy, persistent immunologic activity of SLE, hypertension, and nephrotic syndrome may all contribute to the development of cardiovascular disease. Renal failure, infection, and malignancy account for most of the other deaths during long-term follow-up.

RENAL PATHOLOGY AND CLINICOPATHOLOGIC CORRELATIONS

Although some clinicians think that the therapeutic decisions for lupus nephritis can be made even without the help of renal histology, there are few doubts that a kidney biopsy may provide reliable information about the type and the severity of renal involvement. Any form of glomerulonephritis (GN), from the mildest to the most severe, can be seen in SLE patients. Several classifications of renal lesions in SLE have been proposed. Although not universally accepted, the World Health Organization's (WHO) classification remains the most commonly adopted. According to that classification, there are five main patterns of glomerular disease: class I: Normal glomeruli; class II: Mesangial glomerulonephritis; class III: Focal proliferative glomerulonephritis; class IV: Diffuse proliferative glomerulonephritis; class V: Membranous glomerulonephritis. The different types of glomerulonephritis usually have different clinical presentations, natural outcomes, and responses to therapy (Table 1). It must be remembered, however, that the correlation between the findings of the initial biopsy and ultimate survival is weakened by the variable courses of each subtype of glomerulonephritis by transformation from one class to another and by possible overlap of two classes.

The sum of the semiquantitative scores of certain glomerular vascular and tubulo interstitial features provides activity and chronicity indexes (Table 2). An elevated activity index means that there are many lesions that can progress to irreversible damage, and it is a good indication for aggressive treatment. A high chronicity index shows that there are irreversible lesions that are hard to modify by therapy. Unfortunately, there are important differences among pathologists' interpretations that may limit the clinical impact of these important indices.

THERAPY

Treatment of lupus nephritis remains controversial. Therapy can reduce the disease activity, improve proteinuria, and prevent renal insufficiency. On the other hand, therapy can expose patients to disabling and even life-threatening complications. Therefore, the indica-

Table 2 Renal Pathology Score System in Lupus Nephritis

*Activity Index 0-3**	*Chronicity Index 0-3**
Glomerular Changes	
1. Fibrinoid necrosis ×2† Karyorrhexis	1. Glomerular sclerosis
2. Cellular proliferative	2. Fibrous crescents ×2†
3. Cellular crescents	
4. Hyaline thrombi	
5. Leukocyte infiltration	
Tubulointerstitial Changes	
1. Mononuclear cell infiltration	1. Interstitial fibrosis
	2. Tubular atrophy

From Austin HA III, Muenz LR, Joyce KM, et al. Prognostic factors in lupus nephritis. Am J Med 1983; 75(3):382-391; with permission.
*Each factor is scored from 0 to 3.
†Fibrinoid necrosis and cellular crescents are weighted by a factor of 2 because such lesions are disproportionately more ominous than the other active lesions.

Table 1 Clinical Characteristics of the Different Histologic Classes of Lupus Nephritis According to WHO Classification

Class	*I*	*II*	*III*	*IV*	*V*
Histology	Normal glomeruli	Mesangial GN	Focal proliferative GN (50%)	Diffuse proliferative GN	Membranous GN
Frequency	Quite rare	10%-30%	10%-25%	40%-60%	10%-20%
Renal signs and symptoms	No urine abnormalities	Mild proteinuria and urine sediment abnormalities	Proteinuria; hematuria	Heavy proteinuria; telescoped sediment; hypertension; renal failure	Proteinuria; often nephrotic syndrome
Renal prognosis	Excellent	Excellent if no transformation	Good	Severe if untreated	Renal failure 30%-50%; remission 30%
Transformation	To class II or IV 15%-20% To class V, 2%-5%	To class IV 20%-40%	To class V, 2%-5%	To class III or V 5%-10%	Rare

tions to treatment, the choice of drugs, and their dosage are of utmost prognostic importance.

Indications for Therapy

The therapeutic decisions for patients with lupus nephritis present peculiar difficulties that are related not only to the low therapeutic indexes of the available drugs but also to the heterogeneous nature of the disease and to the possible discrepancies between clinical features and histologic patterns. In principle, however, the type of therapy should be dictated by the severity of the clinical and histologic features rather than by the diagnosis of lupus nephritis or by immunologic parameters.

Patients with minor renal abnormalities (proteinuria less than 1 g per day, inactive urine sediment, normal renal function and blood pressure) and with minimal or pure mesangial lesions in a renal biopsy do not require "specific" treatment. However, because of the possibility of clinico-histologic worsening, periodic clinical surveillance of these patients is mandatory. Therapeutic measures should be aimed at checking the extrarenal activity of SLE when present. Arthralgias, arthritis, myalgias, and fever can often be controlled with salicylates and nonsteroidal anti-inflammatory drugs. Hydroxychloroquine and quinacrine are effective against most dermatologic manifestations. Hemolytic anemia, leukopenia, and thrombocytopenia usually respond to moderate doses of glucocorticoids. Lupus-related inflammations of the lung or heart may be controlled by prednisone, at an initial dose of 1 mg per kilogram per day. Cerebral thromboembolism, often related to the presence of antiphospholipid antibodies, requires anticoagulation. The diffuse central nervous system manifestations caused by primary angiopathy do not always respond to high-dose glucocorticoids, administered either orally or intravenously. Better results have been obtained with a combination of glucocorticoids with intravenous high-dose cyclophosphamide, 1 g per 1.73 square meters.

Whether or not to treat patients with focal proliferative lesions affecting only a minority of glomeruli is optional. If there are neither clinical nor histologic features of lupus activity, we prefer to use symptomatic treatment alone. Others suggest the use of small doses of glucocorticoids (prednisone, 10 to 20 mg per day) and/or immunosuppressive agents (cyclophosphamide, 1 mg per kilogram per day or azathioprine, 1.5 to 2 mg per kilogram per day) to inhibit the immunologic activity of SLE and to prevent potential transformation into more severe forms of lupus nephritis. There is no evidence, however, that such an approach is of any benefit. Patients with focal lesions affecting more than 50 percent of glomeruli and associated with proteinuria more than 2 g per day, elevated serum creatinine, and/or active nephritic sediment should be treated as patients with class IV lupus nephritis.

Patients with membranous glomerulonephritis, nonnephrotic proteinuria, and stable renal function usually have an excellent natural outcome. These patients do not require any specific treatment. Symptomatic therapy may also be useless, since extrarenal activity is usually mild. The indications for glucocorticoid and/or immunosuppressive therapy of patients with membranous nephritis and nephrotic syndrome are still under discussion. Since the natural course of class V nephritis is relatively good, with many patients maintaining normal renal function over time, a number of clinicians use symptomatic therapy alone. However, some patients do progress to renal failure and others are exposed to the potential complications of the nephrotic syndrome, such as intravascular thrombosis, cardiovascular disease, malnutrition, and so on. There are no prognostic clues at presentation to indicate which patients will have a favorable evolution and which will not. Since a 6-month treatment of alternating glucocorticoids and cytotoxic agents may obtain remission of the nephrotic syndrome in about two-thirds of cases and may prevent progression to renal failure in responders, we are in favor of such a treatment. Good results with cyclosporine have also been reported.

Diffuse proliferative nephritis (class IV) is the most severe form of renal disease in SLE, although there are considerable variations in clinical presentation and outcome between one patient and another. Whether or not to treat patients with class IV nephritis as evidenced by a renal biopsy but without clinical signs of renal activity (clinical silent form) is still a matter of controversy. Low-dose prednisone (10 to 20 mg per day) has been advocated to prevent possible evolution to chronic histologic lesions and deterioration of renal function, but there is no proof that such an approach is really useful. These patients should be checked regularly over time and aggressive treatment should be started when there is an increase in serum creatinine or in proteinuria to more than 2 g per day (see following discussion). Most patients with class IV nephritis have a nephritic syndrome, a nephrotic syndrome, or renal insufficiency at presentation or in their early follow-up. These patients need vigorous therapy with high-dose glucocorticoids and/or immunosuppressive agents in order to cure the potentially reversible inflammatory lesions. Careful surveillance is necessary even for cases showing improvement or normalization of renal signs in order to recognize SLE flare-ups early. Ideally, serum complement levels should be normal and anti-DNA antibodies should be negative. However, we prefer to assess the activity of lupus nephritis and to modulate therapy based on the levels of serum creatinine, the amount of daily proteinuria, and the urine sediment, since a relationship between clinical and biologic parameters is often lacking.

Glucocorticoids

There is general agreement that glucocorticoids have improved the survival of patients with lupus nephritis. Although these agents are universally considered for the first-line therapeutic approach, there is no absolute guide in lupus nephritis for the dosage and type of administration. The early experiences clearly showed that low-dose prednisone is unable to interfere with the unfavorable course of severe class IV lupus nephritis. Thus, for patients with severe diffuse proliferative lupus nephritis, many clinicians today start prednisone at doses of 1 to 2 mg per kilogram per day. The doses are tapered off only when renal disease and serologic parameters improve. However, in some patients this may happen only after several months, while progressive renal disease unresponsive to increased dosage of prednisone can develop in another 30 to 40 percent of patients. Moreover, independently of the clinical response, many patients given high-dose prednisone for a long time are prone to the devastating side effects of glucocorticoids, which include hypertension, infection, accelerated atherosclerosis, cushingoid features, obesity, diabetes, aseptic bone necrosis, cataracts, myopathy, and growth retardation in children.

Since low-dose prednisone is ineffective and high-dose prednisone is toxic, an intermediate approach is advisable. For patients with moderate disease, prednisone should be started at dosages not exceeding 1 mg per kilogram per day. It should be taken in a single dose, between 7 and 9 AM to mimic the circadian rhythm of endogenous cortisol, which is maximal in the morning. If lupus nephritis improves, prednisone may be tapered off to a low-dose maintenance (0.2 to 0.4 mg per kilogram per day). The dose should be reduced gradually and slowly over several months to prevent possible flare-ups. For those patients who tolerate low-dose prednisone without signs of renal and extrarenal activity, a switch to an alternate day regimen may be tried after some months. Such a therapeutic schedule may control lupus nephritis in many patients, but it is insufficient for more severe cases.

A number of patients may have frequent flare-ups that require repeated administration of high-dose prednisone. Alternative approaches for controlling SLE activity while reducing glucocorticoid toxicity are recommended in these instances. Several reports have shown that a short course of intravenous high-dose methylprednisolone pulses (generally one pulse of 1 g given every 24 hours for 3 consecutive days) can dramatically reverse extrarenal symptoms and can rapidly improve renal function, particularly in patients who have had a recent rise in serum creatinine.

Proteinuria is usually improved more slowly and it may take as long as 6 months. The clinical remission is often maintained with moderate doses of prednisone, thus reducing the iatrogenic risks related to intensive and prolonged glucocorticoid therapy. In some patients rapid injection of high-dose methylprednisolone may induce flushing, tremor, nausea, and altered taste, which spontaneously disappear within a few hours. More severe but very rare complications include seizures, anaphylaxis, and arrhythmia. The risk of these adverse effects can be minimized if methylprednisolone is infused over at least 30 minutes instead of being injected rapidly. Some investigators suggest the regular administration of a single pulse of IV steroid every month for 6 to 12 months or until immunologic improvement occurs.

In view of the large interpatient variability in the severity of the disease and in the responses to therapy, we suggest a more flexible strategy. We start with one methylprednisolone pulse (0.5 to 1 g each according to the size of the patient) for 3 consecutive days and then the patient is given oral prednisone in a single morning dose (0.5 to 1 mg per kilogram per day according to the severity of the disease). The dose is gradually tapered to the minimum amount possible, with conversion to the alternate-day regimen when possible. Whenever a flare-up of SLE occurs (increase in plasma creatinine of at least 30 percent over the basal value and/or increase in proteinuria of at least 2 g per day) a new course of IV methylprednisolone pulses is given and the oral prednisone dose is increased. For patients with persistent activity or with frequent flare-ups, an immunosuppressive agent is added (Fig. 1). With this therapeutic strategy, we have obtained satisfactory long-term clinical results in 58 patients with diffuse proliferative lupus nephritis (Fig. 2).

Immunosuppressive Agents

Immunosuppressive agents can interfere with both the immune and the inflammatory responses and are therefore of potential benefit in treating lupus nephritis. On the other hand, these agents may also have disquieting side effects in either the short-term or the long-term and should therefore be used with caution. Several drugs have been tried, including methotrexate, chlorambucil, and vincristine, but the two immunosuppressive agents most widely employed in SLE are cyclophosphamide and azathioprine. Whether or not they have any advantages over glucocorticoids is still disputed. Clinical experience shows, however, that immunosuppressive agents can be useful in the following instances: (1) for treatment of severe phases, (2) when glucocorticoids alone are unable to control the activity of the disease, and (3) for maintenance treatment if one needs to reduce the doses of glucocorticoids because of iatrogenic toxicity.

Since alkylating agents may be oncogenic and since the risk of neoplasia seems to relate to their cumulative doses, it is advisable to limit cyclophosphamide treatment to short periods, reserving longer courses for the more difficult cases. The risk of neoplasia seems to be lower (but not absent!) for azathioprine, which may be preferred for long-term treatment. Although not currently supported by pertinent studies, there is the clinical impression that cyclophosphamide is more effective in obtaining a clinical response, whereas azathioprine is better tolerated, having less bladder, gonadal, and bone marrow toxicity. One possible therapeutic strategy might be to add cyclophosphamide (1.5 to 2 mg per kilogram day) for those patients who show persistent proteinuria, renal insufficiency, and extrarenal activity in spite of adequate glucocorticoid treatment. If a good response is obtained with cyclophosphamide, the drug may be stopped after 2 to 3 months and then may be replaced by azathioprine (2 to 2.5 mg per kilogram per day for 12 to 24 months) for those cases that cannot be controlled with low-dose prednisone alone.

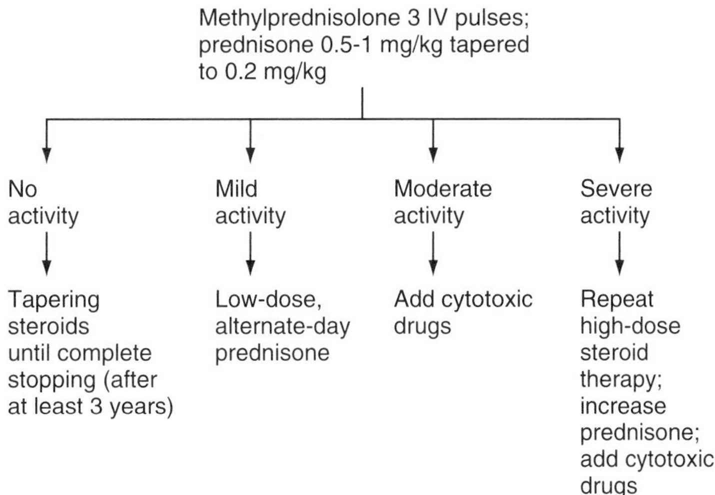

Figure 1 A possible flexible therapeutic strategy for patients with class III and class IV lupus nephritis.

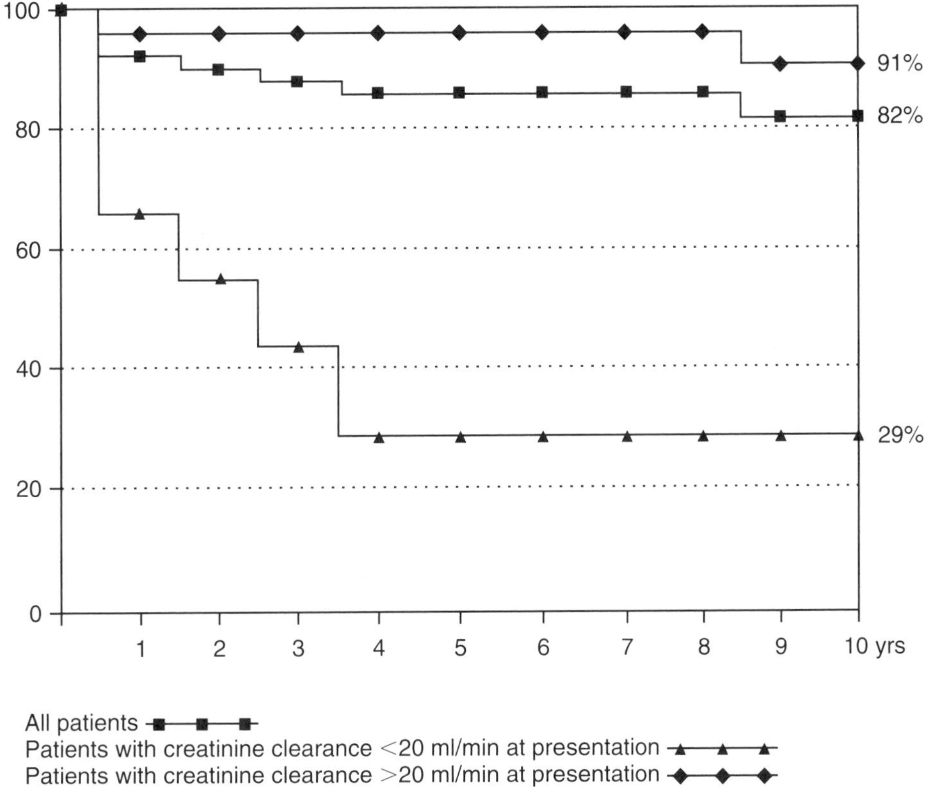

Figure 2 Survival with kidney functioning in 58 patients with diffuse proliferative lupus nephritis.

For several years, the National Institutes of Health (NIH) group has been administering cyclophosphamide as intermittent intravenous pulses. A controlled study showed that the 10-year kidney survival of patients with lupus nephritis was significantly better for patients given intravenous cyclophosphamide plus moderate doses of prednisone than for those given prednisone alone. Although there was a trend to a better outcome for patients assigned to intravenous cyclophospamide than for patients given various types and combinations of oral immunosuppressive drugs, this difference was not significant. Neither malignancy nor bladder toxicity developed in patients given intermittent pulses of cyclophosphamide.

In the first experience of the NIH group, pulses of 0.75 g per square meter were given indefinitely every 3 months. Then the administration was limited to 5 years or until remission was sustained for 2 years. More recent protocols are based on the administration of intravenous cyclophosphamide (0.75 g per square meter) every month for 6 months, followed by one pulse of cyclophosphamide every 3 months for maintenance. Treatment is continued for at least 1 year after remission, as defined by inactive urinary sediment, reduction of proteinuria to a non-nephrotic range, and inactivity of extrarenal lupus.

Several groups from all over the world have confirmed the efficacy of intravenous cyclophosphamide. Forced diuresis and intravenous hydration are recommended to protect from bladder toxicity. Nausea and vomiting are relatively frequent. Alopecia is common. In a few patients the white blood cell count may fall below 1,000 per cubic millimeter, with increased risk of infection. A major problem is represented by ovarian failure. The risk of sterilization may be reduced but not eliminated by administering the cyclophosphamide pulse at the time of menstruation.

Other Treatments

Alternative approaches to glucocorticoids and immunosuppressive agents have been tried for patients with lupus nephritis. Several uncontrolled studies of intensive plasma-exchange therapy in patients with severe disease reported good results. However, an American multicenter controlled study did not show any benefit from plasmapheresis.

The experience with cyclosporine is still preliminary and lacks controlled studies. In view of antiproteinuric properties, this drug might be indicated for patients with nephrotic syndrome refractory to treatment. Cyclosporine might also replace glucocorticoids for maintenance therapy in patients with severe hypercorticism. However, because of its nephrotoxicity, cyclosporine should be used with caution. Patients with renal insufficiency, hypertension, or severe tubulointerstitial lesions in a kidney biopsy are at increased risk for renal toxicity and should not be treated with cyclosporine. The initial doses should not exceed 5 mg per kilogram per day and should be gradually tapered to a maintenance dose of 3 to 4 mg per kilogram per day, if possible. Serum creatinine, blood trough levels of cyclosporine, and blood pressure should be carefully monitored in patients receiving cyclosporine treatment.

Impressive results have been reported for the defibrinogenating agent ancrod. Unfortunately, the studies were not controlled, and the drug has been tested by only one group.

Thromboxane antagonists might potentially have some role, but no clinical experience with these agents in lupus nephritis has been reported.

Fish oil may improve lipid parameters, but it neither improves renal function nor reduces the activity of the disease.

SUGGESTED READING

Austin HA III, Muenz LR, Joyce KM, et al. Prognostic factors in lupus nephritis. Am J Med 1983; 75:382–391.

Boumpas DT, Austin HA III, Vaughn EM, et al. Controlled trial of pulse methylprednisolone versus two regimens of pulse cyclophoshamide in severe lupus nephritis. Lancet 1992; 340:741–745.

Cameron JS. Lupus nephritis in childhood and adolescence. Pediatr Nephrol 1994; 8:230–249.

Ponticelli C. Current treatment recommendations for lupus nephritis. Drugs 1990; 40(1):19–30.

GOODPASTURE'S SYNDROME

ANDREW J. REES, M.B., Ch.B., M.Sc., F.R.C.P.

The term *Goodpasture's syndrome* was originally applied to all patients with necrotizing glomerulonephritis and pulmonary hemorrhage. Today it is used most frequently to describe only those patients in whom the syndrome is caused by autoantibodies to the glomerular basement membrane (anti-GBM). Nevertheless, it is important to remember that anti-GBM antibodies are responsible for the pulmonary hemorrhage and nephritis in less than half the patients who present with these conditions. Other causes include various types of systemic vasculitis associated with antineutrophil cytoplasmic antibodies (ANCA), systemic lupus erythematosus, and occasionally cryoglobulinemia. This chapter deals exclusively with the management of the anti-GBM antibody-mediated disease except where differences in clinical presentation are contrasted.

Two aspects of antibody-mediated Goodpasture's syndrome have ensured that its importance far exceeds its prevalence, and both have obvious consequences for therapy. First, anti-GBM disease is almost always severe and is frequently life-threatening. It may evolve with great rapidity, sometimes with complete loss of renal function within 24 hours, or the loss of several liters of blood into the lungs within a similar time frame. Thus, treatment is urgent and the disease should be regarded as a medical emergency. Second, anti-GBM disease is the first type of glomerulonephritis in which the pathogenesis (autoimmunity to the GBM) is known and can be quantified by measurement of circulating anti-GBM antibodies. This means that is possible to diagnose the disease noninvasively, to design rational therapies to remove anti-GBM antibodies, and to monitor disease activity. It has also been possible to study the relationship between circulating anti-GBM antibodies and the damage they cause. Such studies have demonstrated the influence of secondary factors such as intercurrent infection and cigarette smoke on the natural history of the disease. Thus, a better understanding of pathogenesis has improved management.

CLINICAL ASPECTS

Anti-GBM disease affects people of both sexes and of all ages. It presents most commonly during the third decade of life but there is a second peak in incidence in patients older than 60 years of age. Originally it was suggested that most patients were men, but this greatly exaggerates the sex difference, and most current series record male to female ratios of less than 2:1. Some authors have found elderly female patients to be less severely affected than other groups, but this has not been my experience.

The anti-GBM antibodies react with the same antigen in all patients and have highly restricted specificity. The target has been identified as the carboxy-terminal NCI domain of the α_3 chain of type (IV) collagen (α_3[IV]NCI), with very little cross-reactivity with NCI domains from other collagen chains. The gene encoding α_3(IV)NCI has been cloned and expressed in *Escherichia coli* and insect cells, but only the latter has the correct conformation to bind anti-GBM antibodies with similar affinity to the natural antigen. The antibodies are usually IgG with subclasses IgG_1 or IgG_4 predominating. Some patients also have IgA or IgM antibodies and in very rare instances isolated IgA anti-GBM antibodies have been described.

It is not known why tolerance to α_3(IV)NCI is lost, but there is strong evidence of an inherited predisposition. The frequency of the class II major histocompatibility molecules HLA-DR15 (present in 70 percent to 80 percent of patients compared to 25 percent of controls) and HLA-DR4 are increased in patients, and those of DR1 and DR7 are decreased. There is also an association with immunoglobulin allotypes; inheritance also appears to influence the severity of anti-GBM nephritis. Even so, it is unclear what initiates anti-GBM antibody synthesis. Despite repeated claims and a few convincing anecdotes, there is no real evidence to link anti-GBM disease with exposure to hydrocarbon fumes. The evidence that specific viral infections cause anti-GBM disease is equally unconvincing. An association with Hodgkin's disease (or its treatment) has been reported. Perhaps the simplest explanation for these findings is that anti-GBM disease can occur in a genetically susceptible individual when there is local inflammation or injury to the kidney. Recent reports of the development of anti-GBM disease after lithotripsy is perhaps the clearest example of this.

Patients with anti-GBM antibodies usually present with glomerulonephritis, which is associated with hemoptysis or a past history of hemoptysis in one-half to three-quarters of patients. It is uncommon for patients to have signs or symptoms suggestive of generalized disease such as rashes, arthralgia, myalgia, or fever; these are much more characteristic of other types or rapidly progressive nephritis. Typically, the glomerulonephritis is severe and progresses to renal failure in weeks or months if left untreated, but exceptional patients have more indolent disease. However, progression can be much more rapid in the presence of intercurrent infection and renal function can be destroyed within hours or days. At present it is impossible to tell whether an individual who presents with comparatively little renal injury is at risk of sudden deterioration or whether they have truly indolent disease. Evidence from renal biopsies, including those from patients who have already developed renal failure, suggests an explosive final event, in that necrosis and extracapillary proliferation (crescents) in glomeruli all appear to be at a similar stage of evolution. This contrasts with the appearances in biopsies from patients with other forms of rapidly progressive nephritis in whom crescents are found in all phases of evolution from cellular to fibrous, which implies repeated episodes of disease activity.

The severity of pulmonary hemorrhage is highly variable. It is found in 50 to 70 percent of patients and usually precedes evidence of nephritis, sometimes by many years. It is episodic, and varies in severity from mild hemoptysis to severe respiratory failure. It is the most common aspect of the disease in exceptional patients. These differences are not due to the specificity of anti-GBM antibodies, which bind α_3(IV)NCI regardless of clinical presentation. Thus, environmental factors must determine whether the lungs are affected, and exposure to cigarette smoke is the best characterized of these. This is evidenced by the observation that almost all current cigarette smokers who develop Goodpasture's syndrome have pulmonary hemorrhage, but its occurrence is rare in nonsmokers. Cigarette smoke also appears to precipitate acute pulmonary hemorrhage, as can intercurrent infection, fluid overload, and high concentrations of inspired oxygen (at least experimentally in rodents). Cocaine inhalation can also provoke lung hemorrhage. Avoidance of circumstances known to aggravate damage caused by anti-GBM antibodies is as crucial to effective management of antibody-mediated nephritis as are attempts to control antibody levels and to suppress inflammation.

The effectiveness of therapy is greatly influenced by the speed of diagnosis because of the rapidity with which anti-GBM disease can destroy the kidneys. Anti-GBM disease can often be suspected clinically, even in the absence of pulmonary hemorrhage, for example, in patients with deteriorating renal function and a diagnosis of nephritis (evidenced by the urinalysis and microscopy) not accompanied by vasculitis or the signs of generalized illness. Glomerulonephritis should be confirmed by renal biopsy and pulmonary hemorrhage by the presence of hemoptysis, alveolar shadows on chest radiographs, or an increased diffusing capacity for carbon monoxide after correction for lung volumes and for the patient's hemoglobin concentration (κCO). The specific diagnosis is confirmed by demonstrating the presence of anti-GBM antibodies either in the serum by solid phase immunoassays (older tests using indirect immunofluorescence are too insensitive) or in kidney tissue by immunohistochemical demonstration of linear deposition of immunoglobulin along the GBM. The antibodies are most frequently IgG with or without IgM. Occasional patients have been reported with isolated IgA anti-GBM antibodies. Linear staining of the alveolar basement membrane is variable, and its absence on biopsy specimens cannot be used to exclude the diagnosis. This is probably because of variable accessibility of α_3(IV)NCI to circulating anti-GBM antibodies.

Serum and tissue diagnoses are equally effective, but the radioimmunoassay has the advantage of serial measurements that can be used to follow the patient's response to treatment to ensure that anti-GBM antibodies are undetectable before renal transplantation is undertaken. The main conditions that need to be distinguished from anti-GBM disease are other types of rapidly progressive glomerulonephritis (principally those associated with vasculitis), pneumonia complicated by acute tubular necrosis, toxins such as paraquat that damage lungs and kidneys, and finally, any cause of renal failure complicated by pulmonary edema. The principal difficulties usually come either from confusing rapidly progressive glomerular nephritis (RPGN) accompanied by anemia with chronic renal failure, or failing to distinguish anti-GBM disease from systemic vasculitis. The recent demonstration that active systemic vasculitis and idiopathic RPGN are both very strongly associated with antibodies to neutrophil cytoplasmic antigen (ANCA) has greatly facilitated the distinction, even though up to 5 percent of patients may have ANCA as well as anti-GBM antibodies.

APPROACHES TO TREATMENT

The immediate aim of treatment in anti-GBM disease is to control pulmonary hemorrhage and glomerular inflammation as swiftly as possible, thereby providing the best chance of healing and repair. Simultaneously, it may be necessary to treat infection and to support renal and pulmonary function. The longer term objective is to suppress anti-GBM antibody synthesis permanently. Before discussing our preferred regimen, it is important to recognize the grim prognosis for untreated patients. In their 1973 survey, Wilson and Dixon reported that 25 of their 53 patients died and only seven retained useful renal function. Although the general availability of dialysis and better diagnosis of less severely affected cases have improved prognosis, less than 15 percent of untreated patients in reported series of more than five patients who presented with raised plasma creatinine have retained useful renal function.

Immunosuppressive drugs by themselves appear to have little influence on the course of anti-GBM antibody-mediated nephritis, regardless of whether they are prescribed singly or in combination; this observation is in contrast with their effectiveness in treating other types of rapidly progressive nephritis. It is possible that pulmonary hemorrhage can be controlled by drugs more easily than nephritis, since intravenous boluses of methylprenisolone have been reported to be effective. However, this has not been my experience, and pulmonary hemorrhage tends to be episodic. In the past, bilateral nephrectomy was advocated for treating severe pulmonary hemorrhage in patients with anti-GBM disease. The original rationale for bilateral nephrectomy was that removal of the GBM would minimize the stimulus to further anti-GBM synthesis. However, nephrectomy has no effect on anti-GBM antibody titres. This is not surprising since the autoantigen is found in the lungs as well as the kidneys, and with hindsight, the case reports that originally suggested benefit are unconvincing. This approach is strongly contraindicated and should be abandoned as ineffective and potentially dangerous.

Against this background, it was argued that effective treatment should combine measures to rapidly reduce the concentration of anti-GBM antibodies with those to limit their synthesis and to suppress inflammation. Thus, a treatment regimen was developed that combined repeated large volume plasma exchange with cytotoxic drugs and steroids. Ideally, this regimen should have been assessed by a prospective controlled trial, but unfortunately this has proved impossible because of the rarity of anti-GBM disease and the rapidity with which it progresses. Consequently, the usefulness of the therapy has to be judged by its ability to control anti-GBM antibody titers and to suppress disease activity, and also by the frequency and severity of the complications.

MANAGEMENT

Specific Therapy

Our standard regimen for treating Goodpasture's syndrome is outlined in Table 1. It consists of daily whole volume (4 L for adults) plasma exchanges for albumin, combined with 60 mg of prednisolone daily, and cyclophosphamide, 100 to 150 mg per day administered orally, depending on weight. Originally we used azathioprine as well, but this proved unnecessary and its use has been abandoned. The regimen is modified in patients older than 55 years of age who are rarely given more than 100 mg cyclophosphamide. Plasma exchanges are performed for 14 days or until clinical evidence of continuing injury has subsided. They are restarted if disease activity recurs or if the anti-GBM antibody titre increases rapidly after the first course has been completed; both circumstances are relatively uncommon. Five plasma exchanges are the routine when a second course is required. Other groups have reported on the use of less intensive plasma exchange, and so their results are not directly comparable. It should be emphasized that daily whole volume exchanges combined with immunosuppressive drugs are needed to ensure rapid lowering of anti-GBM antibody

Table 1 Plasma-Exchange Regimen

Plasma exchange:	Daily 4 L exchanges for albumin for 14 days
Corticosteroids:	Prednisolone 60 mg daily for 7 days; thereafter 45, 30, 25, 20, 15, 10, 5 mg for 1 week each
Cytotoxic drugs:	Cyclophosphamide 100-150 mg/day given for 8-12 weeks
	Cyclophosphamide 100 mg/day in patients over 55 years of age

concentrations in all patients. Cyclophosphamide is discontinued after 8 to 12 weeks, provided that anti-GBM antibody titers are no longer detectable. The prednisolone dose is also reduced rapidly. Patients receive 60 mg of prednisolone daily for 1 week, and then the dose is reduced at weekly intervals to 45 mg daily, 30 mg daily, 25 mg daily, and 20 mg daily. Thereafter, the dose of prednisolone is reduced by decrements of 5 mg weekly until it is stopped after 8 to 12 weeks. The prolonged use of immunosuppressive drugs is unnecessary in this condition provided that anti-GBM antibodies remain undetectable.

Plasma Exchange

The development of automatic techniques for plasma separation by centrifugation or filtration opened the way for therapeutic plasma exchange. This is a technique in which whole blood is removed from a patient and separated into its plasma and cellular constituents before the cells are reinfused with fresh albumin instead of the patient's plasma, which is discarded. A single 4 L plasma exchange removes approximately 90 percent of an intravascular marker injected at the start of plasma exchange, and results in a 45 percent decrease in the serum concentration of IgG, and thus is a highly effective way to remove circulating autoantibodies. Unfortunately, anti-GBM antibodies are rapidly resynthesized, and repeated exchanges, as well as the concurrent administration of immunosuppressive drugs, are needed to reliably reduce their concentration in most patients.

Veno-venous circuits are inadequate for plasma exchange of this intensity and central vein catheters are most suitable. All types of cell separators are effective at removing IgG, and so the choice between centrifugation and filtration or the recently developed immunoabsorption columns, which remove IgG specifically, is a personal one and depends on the facilities available. Albumin solutions should be used as the plasma substitute and should have potassium and calcium added in sufficient amounts to bring their concentrations into the physiologic range. Plasma exchange removes coagulation factors as well as immunoglobulins. These are returned as 2 U of fresh frozen plasma at the end of exchange in all patients who are at risk from bleeding. Clearly this should include those with fresh pulmonary hemorrhage or who have had recent renal biopsies. The anticoagulation needed to prevent clotting in the extracorporeal circuit also poses a potential danger for these patients, but only a slight one because most of the anticoagulant is discarded with the patient's plasma rather than being returned to the patient.

Table 2 Practical Considerations to Minimize the Dangers of Plasma Exchange

Proper extracorporeal techniques to prevent air embolism
Accurate volume replacement to maintain blood volume
Sterile techniques to minimize the risk of infection
Use of albumin solutions not contaminated with vasoactive substances
Addition of potassium chloride and calcium glucose to each 400 ml unit of albumin to prevent acute electrolyte disturbances
Diluting replacement albumin solutions given to hypoalbuminemic patients because of the risk of acute hypervolemia
Prevention of chronic fluid overload caused by sodium loading imposed by exchanges

Plasma exchange shares the complications of all extracorporeal circuits, such as infection of vascular access sites and embolism. In addition, there is a tendency to overload patients with renal failure with sodium because the sodium concentration of most plasma substitutes is greater than that of plasma. Thus, each whole volume exchange is often associated with a sodium load of 100 to 150 mmol. Fluid overload should be anticipated by daily measurement of body weight, and excess fluid should be removed by appropriate use of diuretics or dialysis. Acute hypervolemia associated with severe hypertension can be a problem, especially in children, because of rapid redistribution of fluid, which is caused by the sudden increase of plasma albumin concentration to normal levels in previously hypoalbuminemic patients. Finally, repeated plasma exchange can cause thrombocytopenia because of platelet destruction in the extracorporeal circuit. Table 2 outlines practical steps to minimize the complications.

Cytotoxic Drugs

Anti-GBM antibody titers rapidly return to pre-exchange values without the concomitant use of cytotoxic drugs. The main drug used is the alkylating agent cyclophosphamide. It is rapidly converted by hepatic microsomes to a series of active metabolites, which are incorporated into host DNA at all stages of the cell cycle; cells are killed only during division. In humans, cyclophosphamide suppresses primary antibody responses when given in daily doses of more than 2 mg per kilogram. It has been found to shorten significantly the duration of anti-GBM antibody synthesis in Goodpasture's syndrome when given to patients being treated by plasma exchange. The principal early complication of cyclophosphamide is myelotoxcity. It can occur at any stage of treatment and should be anticipated by daily measurement of the leuckocyte count and prevented by appropriate reduction of the dosage. Later complications include hemorrhage cystitis caused by excretion of toxic metabolites, infertility (especially in men), and a small but perceptible risk of malignancy. Eight- to 12-week courses in the doses advocated here have minimal short-term and long-term risks.

Prednisolone

Corticosteroids are the most powerful anti-inflammatory drugs available, and they also have some immunosuppressive properties. The pharmacologic aspects of these drugs are discussed extensively in other chapters. In anti-GBM antibody-mediated disease, corticosteroids are used predominantly for their anti-inflammatory properties and are prescribed in short, intensive courses to control the inflammatory response until anti-GBM antibody synthesis has been suppressed. There is no rationale for continuing their use beyond this point.

Supportive Treatment

Renal Failure

Patients with Goodpasture's syndrome may progress to end-stage renal failure within 24 hours and so need to have their renal function assessed daily in the early stages of their disease. Dialysis may be needed either because of azotemia or fluid retention (exacerbated by plasma exchange or blood transfusion), which can cause new life-threatening pulmonary hemorrhage.

Respiratory Failure

The treatment of respiratory failure in patients with anti-GBM disease is also controversial. Although hypoxemia may need to be corrected by increasing the inspired concentration of oxygen, there are sound experimental reasons for being anxious about such therapy. Oxygen toxicity exacerbates anti-GBM antibody-mediated pulmonary injury in rats and rabbits, probably increasing alveolar-capillary-endothelial cell permeability and thus the accessibility of the GBM to circulating antibody. It is impossible to test whether high concentrations of inspired oxygen have similar effects in patients with Goodpasture's syndrome; however, it seems prudent to limit the inspired oxygen concentration to the absolute minimum necessary to maintain safe levels of arterial oxygen concentration. Continuous positive airway pressure should be used as required.

Anemia

Some patients with Goodpasture's syndrome are severely anemic and may present with a hemoglobin concentration of less than 5 g per deciliter. Care must be taken to avoid hypervolemia, which exacerbates pulmonary hemorrhage, when blood transfusions are given.

Infection

Intercurrent infection is the most powerful cause of relapse with anti-GBM disease and appears to produce the effect by enhancing the potency of inflammatory mediators rather than by changing anti-GBM antibody synthesis. Recent experimental evidence has implicated the release of cytokines such as tumour necrosis factor and interleukin-1 in this phenomenon. Meticulous care must be taken to prevent infection during the course of treatment, especially because the risks substantially increase by the presence of indwelling catheters (intravenous, peritoneal, or urinary) and by the use of high doses of steroids.

Other Nonspecific Measures

Cigarette smoking has been identified as an important cause of pulmonary hemorrhage in patients with Goodpasture's syndrome, and resumption of smoking can precipitate relapse. These data provide exceptionally powerful reasons for patients with this disease to stop smoking. Goodpasture's syndrome has frequently been associated with exposure to hydrocarbon fumes. Whether or not the nature of this association and its effects are analogous to those of cigarette smoke is impossible to tell; it seems prudent to limit such exposure as much as possible.

RESULTS OF THERAPY

At the Hammersmith Hospital, we have used plasma exchange to treat antibody-mediated Goodpasture's syndrome for the past 15 years and during this time have treated 63 patients. Since 1980, we have also performed serial assays of anti-GBM antibodies and advised on the management of many more patients treated in other units throughout the United Kingdom.

Control of Anti-GBM Antibody Titer

Anti-GBM antibody titers fell immediately after the start of therapy in all patients treated with the combination of plasma exchange and immunosuppressive drugs, and there has been little tendency for anti-GBM antibody titers to increase once the concentrations have been reduced to background values. Long-term, possibly permanent, disappearance of anti-GBM antibodies was achieved within 8 weeks in 29 to 30 patients who received a full course of a plasma exchange regimen. A full course was defined as at least 12 plasma exchanges and at least 8 weeks of treatment with cyclophosphamide. By contrast, anti-GBM antibodies persisted for much longer in patients who did not receive complete treatment, and only three of 33 patients were cleared of antibodies by 8 weeks; the autoantibodies persisted for more than 1 year in 12 of these patients. Thus, it appears that cyclophosphamide and plasma exchange act synergistically to promote long-term control of anti-GBM antibody synthesis.

Renal Function

Nephrons that have been destroyed cannot regenerate, and so it comes as no surprise that the degree of

Table 3 Outcome at Two Months of Patients with Anti-GBM Disease Treated with Plasma Exchange

Presenting Creatinine	*Independent Renal Function*	*Dialysis*	*Deaths*
Dialysis (30)	4 (13%)	19	7
>600 μmols/L (8)	4 (50%)	3	1
<600 μmols/L (2)	18 (86%)	2	1
Total (59)	26 (44%)	24	9

improvement of renal function depends on the severity of injury at the time that treatment is initiated (Table 3). The plasma exchange regimen has been used on 30 dialysis-dependent patients with anti-GBM disease under our direct supervision, and only four regained useful renal function despite control of autoantibody titers. Similarly, the results in patients whose serum creatinine exceeds 600 μmols per liter (6.8 mg per deciliter) at the start of treatment were only moderately encouraging, with improvement in only four to eight such patients. By contrast, renal function improved in 18 of 21 patients with plasma creatinines that were rapidly increasing, but were less than 600 μmols per liter (6.8 mg per deciliter). Improvement in these patients was evident as soon as the plasma-exchange regimen was started, which argues strongly that it was a direct result of treatment. Seven patients with biopsy-proven nephritis and whose serum creatinine levels were within the normal range were also treated. They all improved as assessed by changes in serum creatinine levels within normal range or by improvement of the urine sediment. Thus, the plasma-exchange regimen is effective treatment for nephritis in Goodpasture's syndrome provided that it is introduced before the kidneys have been severely damaged. Late deterioration of renal function because of progressive fibrosis has occurred in a few patients without recurrence of detectable anti-GBM antibody synthesis. These patients have not been treated by reintroduction of plasma exchange or drug therapy, but have received nonspecific treatment until dialysis or transplantation.

Pulmonary Hemorrhage

Pulmonary hemorrhage in anti-GBM antibody-mediated disease has a much greater tendency to be episodic than does nephritis, and the lungs have a much greater capacity to recover. The patients who died of respiratory failure had pulmonary hemorrhage that was aggravated by intercurrent infection, hypervolemia, or the resumption of cigarette smoking in various patients. None of the surviving patients has developed clinically detectable pulmonary fibrosis, possibly because the lung injury is highly focal even when pulmonary hemorrhage is widespread.

Mortality

The overall mortality rate at 8 weeks in patients treated at Hammersmith Hospital was 15 percent (nine of 59 patients). In three patients, death was unrelated to the treatment regimen, but rather to unsuitability for long-term dialysis in two and an acute myocardial infarct in the third; pulmonary hemorrhage was the cause of death in the remaining five patients.

MONITORING THE EFFECTS OF THERAPY

The effects of treatment should be monitored meticulously by repeated assessments of disease activity and fluid balance, and for the possibility of complications. Routine investigations include daily measures of body weight, urine microscopy, serum creatinine, and complete blood count. Chest radiographs and κCO are assessed three times weekly when clinically indicated. Cultures of urine, sputum, and vascular access sites are taken three times weekly, but antibiotics are given only when clinically indicated. Whenever possible, it is helpful to frequently monitor anti-GBM antibody titers. Anti-GBM antibody concentrations are measured daily for the first 2 weeks and three times weekly thereafter. Many clinicians do not repeat assays as frequently as we do; however, it is important to measure antibody titers at presentation to confirm the diagnosis, and also at the end of therapy to assess the need for continued immunosuppression. Titres should also be measured in all patients with deteriorating renal function to distinguish active disease from progressive scarring and before transplantation in patients who develop end-stage renal failure.

PATIENT SELECTION

The plasma-exchange regimen described here is arduous and exposes the patient to discomfort as well as some risk. It should not be used indiscriminately, but should be reserved for those patients who are likely to benefit. Presently, we use plasma exchange in all patients with active pulmonary hemorrhage and all those with nephritis and declining renal function. We also treat the majority of patients with nephritis and creatinine levels within the normal range if they have clinical or morphologic evidence of active nephritis. Patients who are anuric but do not have pulmonary hemorrhage are not usually treated unless the renal biopsy contains a surprising number of glomeruli with patent capillary loops; similarly, dialysis-dependent patients who are still passing 500 to 1,000 ml of urine per 24 hours are also sometimes treated. Occasionally, treatment is given to limit the duration of anti-GBM antibody synthesis and to allow earlier renal transplantation.

Although this plasma-exchange regimen appears to be the first consistently effective treatment for anti-GBM disease, it is clearly unsatisfactory because it is cumbersome and lacks specificity. Presently, understanding of autoimmunity and the control of autoantibody responses are advancing rapidly, and it is hoped that the development of more specific ways to suppress anti-GBM antibody synthesis will result. It is also a depressing fact that many patients present after their kidneys have been destroyed, and this clearly indicates the need for earlier diagnosis.

ANTI-GBM DISEASE IN ALPORT'S SYNDROME

The development of anti-GBM antibodies after renal transplantation provides a special case. Alport's Syndrome is an X-linked disease that results in progressive renal failure usually caused by mutations of the α_5- or α_6-chains of type IV collagen. These chains are present in the same specialized basement membranes that express the α_3- and α_4-chains, and probably form a distinct collagen network with them. Thus, patients with Alport's Syndrome do not express α_3(IV)NCI in glomeruli. Transplantation of a normal kidney into patients with Alport's Syndrome is sometimes followed by the development of anti-GBM antibodies; in this instance, of course, they are alloantibodies rather than autoantibodies. It was originally thought that anti-GBM antibodies were directed against the α_3(IV)NCI as is the case in the autoimmune form of the disease. However, we have recently developed more specific assays using conformationally correct recombinant α_3(IV)NCI and α_5(IV)NCI and have shown that this is not the case. Anti-GBM antibodies after renal transplantation in patients with Alport's are usually specific for α_5(IV)NCI and have minimal cross-reactivity with α_3-chains. This has serious implications for the diagnosis and the monitoring of anti-GBM antibody responses in this setting. Apparently low antibody titres in conventional anti-GBM assays may conceal very high anti–α_5-activity. It follows that patients with Alport's Syndrome need to be very carefully monitored after renal transplantation preferably with an anti-α_5 (NCI) specific assay. Treatment is with plasma exchange and cyclophosphamide in addition to or as partial substitution for conventional anti-rejection therapy.

SUGGESTED READING

Herody M, Bobrie G, Gonarin C, et al. Anti-GBM disease: Predictive value of clinical, histological and serological data. Clin Nephrol 1993; 40:249–255.

Turner AN, Lockwood CM Rees AJ. In:Shrier RW, Gottschalk CW, eds. Diseases of the kidney. 5th ed. Boston: Little Brown, 1993: 1865.

IMMUNOLOGICALLY MEDIATED NEPHRITIC RENAL DISEASE

GERALD B. APPEL, M.D.
STEVEN SMITH, M.D.

Glomerulonephritis may be caused by a number of immunologically mediated mechanisms. The clinical presentations and the potential therapeutic options are variable. Some of the diseases present with mild clinical manifestations such as asymptomatic microhematuria or proteinuria. Others commonly present with an explosive onset of the classic nephritic picture of dark urine attributable to hematuria, oliguria, hypertension, edema, and azotemia. Still others have an indolent course and present only in late stages with severe chronic renal insufficiency. Some immunologically mediated glomerular diseases may present with a spectrum of the above clinical findings.

Although all of these forms of glomerulonephritis have an immune pathogenesis, the nature of the immunologic insult varies greatly. Some are caused by immune complex deposition in the mesangium or subendothelial location along the glomerular capillary loops. Others are caused by the deposition of antiglomerular basement membrane antibodies directed against intrinsic components of the glomerular capillary wall. In others, endothelial damage may be produced or initiated by antineutrophil cytoplasmic antibodies, antiphospholipid antibodies, or other less defined mechanisms of immune damage. Treatment of these disorders likewise varies from supportive care to intensive therapy with intravenous glucocorticoids and cytotoxic medications, depending on the severity of the histologic and clinical manifestations. The common etiologies of immunologically mediated glomerulonephritis are listed in Table 1.

IgA NEPHROPATHY

IgA nephropathy is one of the most common causes of glomerulonephritis worldwide and may account for up to 20 percent of all primary glomerulopathies. IgA nephropathy is most often idiopathic, but it can occur in association with cirrhosis of the liver, celiac disease, psoriasis, and ankylosing spondylitis. Although the light microscopy typically shows proliferation of mesangial cells and less commonly endothelial or extracapillary proliferation (crescents), the diagnosis is established by immune deposits containing IgA on immunofluorescence. Young patients usually present with macroscopic hematuria in association with infections and exercise, whereas older individuals often develop asymptomatic microscopic hematuria and mild proteinuria. The progression of the renal disease is variable. Some have spontaneous remission of their signs and symptoms, others continue to manifest mild signs and symptoms, and about 20 percent progress to end-stage renal disease

Table 1 Immunologically Mediated Glomerulonephritic Diseases

IgA nephropathy
Henoch-Schönlein purpura
Poststreptococcal glomerulonephritis
Other postinfectious glomerulonephritides
Membranoproliferative glomerulonephritis
Wegener's granulomatosis
Polyarteritis nodosa
Idiopathic rapidly progressive glomerulonephritis
Systemic lupus erythematosus*
Antiglomerular basement membrane disease†
Light chain deposition disease
Antiphospholipid antibody syndrome
Fibrillary glomerulonephritis

*See the chapter "Lupus Nephritis."
†See the chapter "Goodpasture's Syndrome."

(ESRD) over a 20-year period after diagnosis. Features suggestive of a worse prognosis include older age at onset, absence of gross hematuria, hypertension, greater degrees of proteinuria and severe proliferation, sclerosis, and crescents on renal biopsy.

There is no proven effective treatment for IgA nephropathy, and controlled therapeutic trials are difficult given the varied presentation and rate of progression. Aspirin, dipyridamole, phenytoin (which can decrease serum IgA levels), tonsillectomy, and/or antibiotic therapy to prevent recurrent infections have all proven unsuccessful. Rarely, a patient with celiac disease–associated IgA nephropathy will respond to gluten removal from the diet. For the majority of patients with mesangial disease and asymptomatic or mild clinical manifestations no specific treatment is indicated. Supportive care should include blood pressure control and reassurance for patients with frightening but usually harmless episodes of gross hematuria. Use of angiotensin converting enzyme (ACE) inhibitors in several studies has consistently been documented not only to control blood pressure but also to slow the progression to renal failure.

Therapy with oral fish oils may modify the production of inflammatory mediators of glomerular injury such as thromboxanes and leukotrienes. Although several small prospective studies failed to detect a benefit of fish oil therapy in IgA nephropathy, a recent large controlled trial of 106 patients found a slower decline in renal function when proteinuric patients were treated with 12 g per day of fish oils. Neither the use of glucocorticoids nor the use of cytotoxics has given consistent beneficial results in patients with IgA nephropathy. Many nephrologists would treat only those patients with clinical and histologic features suggestive of a poor prognosis. For those with nephrotic range proteinuria a course of high dose oral glucocorticoids given daily (prednisone 60 mg per day) or every other day (prednisone 120 mg every other day) for a trial period of 4 to 12 months has been effective in some patients. For those with a rapidly progressive course to renal insufficiency and a crescentic pattern on biopsy both intravenous pulse glucocorticoids in high doses (1 g methylprednisone daily for 3 days) repeated monthly with low-dose glucocorticoid treatment in between pulses may be effective in reversing the renal failure and delaying the need for dialysis. Likewise, 6 monthly doses of intravenous cyclophosphamide (up to 1 g per square meter) in conjunction with high doses of oral glucocorticoids tapered to low doses (less than 30 mg per day) over 3 months has been successful in some patients. A few patients have been treated with immunosuppressive regimens in conjunction with plasma exchange with conflicting results. Although the short-term prognosis for patients with crescentic IgA nephropathy can dramatically improve, many are eventually left with so much glomerular damage by the crescentic process that they ultimately progress nonimmunologically to renal failure.

Although cyclosporin (4 to 6 mg per kilogram per day) taken orally has been used to treat patients with IgA nephropathy with reduction of proteinuria, resolution of hypoalbuminemia, and signs and symptoms of the nephrotic syndrome, relapse on cessation of therapy is common. Cyclosporin levels must be monitored carefully to prevent nephrotoxicity. Recent uncontrolled studies have shown success with high-dose polyvalent IgG (2 g per kilogram per month) for 3 months followed by IM IgG for 6 months, but this has yet to be proven in controlled trials.

HENOCH-SCHÖNLEIN PURPURA

Henoch-Schönlein purpura, most commonly a childhood disease, is associated with a small vessel vasculitis of the skin, intestinal tract, kidneys, and joints. Clinically, patients present with lower extremity purpura, arthralgias-arthritis, abdominal pain and gastrointestinal bleeding, and nephritis. Microscopic hematuria and mild proteinuria are the most common manifestations of renal involvement. Gross hematuria and nephrotic-range proteinuria are infrequent, and a nephritic picture with oliguria and acute renal failure is rarely observed. The renal histologic picture is indistinguishable from the more severe forms of IgA nephropathy with IgA immune deposits and a proliferative glomerulonephritis.

In general, the prognosis for recovery in Henoch-Schönlein purpura is excellent, and there is no proven treatment. Only a small percentage of patients have adverse outcomes whether from gastrointestinal catastrophes or progressive renal failure. Supportive care with attention to electrolyte balance and blood pressure control is usually adequate treatment. If infection intervenes, appropriate antibiotics should be given. Patients with severe abdominal symptoms are often treated with a short course of high-dose corticosteroids, but there is no evidence that glucocorticoids or cytotoxic agents affect the course of the renal disease. However, patients with the nephrotic syndrome, oliguric acute renal failure, or progressive renal failure should be treated in a fashion similar to those with serious forms of IgA nephropathy with corticosteroids and cytotoxics. IV gammaglobulin (2 g per kilogram per month for 3 months) has also been used in a few patients with anecdotal success.

POSTSTREPTOCOCCAL GLOMERULONEPHRITIS

Poststreptococcal glomerulonephritis occurs 1 to 3 weeks following pharyngitis or dermal infections caused by nephritogenic strains of group A beta-hemolytic streptococci and is due to an acute immune complex deposition in the kidney. Patients with clinical symptoms usually manifest hematuria and proteinuria with only some nephritic findings. Most recover within 6 weeks, and the prognosis for full recovery of renal function is excellent in children. Some adults may be left with residual proteinuria, hypertension, or renal insufficiency. Only rarely will a patient develop a rapidly progressive course to renal failure with this form of glomerulonephritis.

The treatment of poststreptococcal disease is primarily supportive. A low-salt diet to prevent fluid accumulation and judicious use of potent loop diuretics (but not potassium-sparing diuretics) are all helpful. Dialysis is indicated for either fluid accumulation unresponsive to diuretics or the rare cases that progress to uremia. Hypertension may be treated with calcium channel blocking drugs, ACE inhibitors, and vasodilators. Antibiotics may be used to treat the original streptococcal disease and prevent the spread of nephritogenic strains, but they have no effect on the course of the renal disease. For the vast majority of patients, the use of glucocorticoids and other immunosuppressives is unnecessary and potentially hazardous. For patients with a rapidly progressive course and a renal biopsy showing severe extracapillary proliferative features (crescentic glomerulonephritis) a short course of intravenous or oral glucocorticoids (methylprednisolone 500 to 1,000 mg intravenously daily for 3 to 5 days or prednisone 120 mg every other day for 1 to 2 weeks) has been effective. There are no controlled trials, however, to document the efficacy of this regimen in the very small population with such a severe clinical presentation.

OTHER POSTINFECTIOUS GLOMERULONEPHRITIDES

Immune complex–mediated postinfectious glomerulonephritis can occur with bacterial endocarditis, deep visceral bacterial infections, bacterial pneumonias and empyemas, osteomyelitis, and infected cerebroventricular shunts. *Staphylococcus aureus* and *Streptococcus viridans* remain common organisms associated with endocarditis-induced glomerulonephritis. Gram-negative organisms and fungal organisms are reported in drug addicts with endocarditis and glomerulonephritis. *Staphylococcus epidermidis* is the most frequent offender in shunt nephritis and with endocarditis in patients with prosthetic valves. Most patients present with signs and symptoms related to their underlying infectious illness. The renal manifestations vary from microscopic hematuria and mild proteinuria to acute renal failure with irreversible renal damage. Patients with endocarditis are more likely to present with renal insufficiency and a nephritic picture, whereas almost 30 percent of patients with shunt nephritis have the nephrotic syndrome. The severity of the renal disease is usually related to the nature of the infection, the presence of embolic phenomena as well as the immune complex glomerulonephritis, and the duration of the disease before appropriate antibiotic therapy has been instituted. Primary therapy should be directed at identifying the nature and source of the infection and its eradication with antibiotic therapy and/or surgical removal of infected material. The use of glucocorticoids, which has been used only anecdotally and in uncontrolled trials, is potentially hazardous in patients with an ongoing infection.

MEMBRANOPROLIFERATIVE GLOMERULONEPHRITIS

Membranoproliferative glomerulonephritis (MPGN) is a histologic pattern of glomerular injury that may be associated with viral hepatitis and other chronic infections, systemic lupus erythematosus (SLE), paraprotein deposition disease, and certain thrombotic microangiopathies. Idiopathic MPGN most commonly causes a nephrotic picture, but patients may also present with asymptomatic urinary abnormalities or an acute nephritic picture. The pathogenesis is incompletely understood but involves immune complex deposition and activation of the complement cascade with inflammation, cellular proliferation, and repair expanding the mesangial matrix and reduplicating the glomerular basement membrane. Idiopathic MPGN has been divided into types I, II, and III on the basis of the electron micrographic localization of the immune deposits, but the prognosis and course of each appear similar. Poor prognostic factors on presentation include hypertension, decreased glomerular filtration rate (GFR), the nephrotic syndrome, and crescents (extracapillary glomerular proliferation) or severe tubulointerstitial changes on the renal biopsy.

Treatment of MPGN is controversial. Corticosteroids and other immunosuppressive medications have been used to decrease proteinuria and preserve renal function. Cyclophosphamide, at a dose of 1 to 2 mg per kilogram per day, with or without anticoagulation, given for many months, may decrease proteinuria, preserve GFR, and prevent progressive renal failure in some patients. Some studies have found improved renal function in patients treated with daily antiplatelet agents and anticoagulants (dipyridamole, aspirin, and warfarin). In children, a large, randomized, well-controlled trial of long-term, alternate-day corticosteroids (2 mg per kg every 48 hours) led to greater remissions of the nephrotic syndrome and preservation of renal function. Although no such study exists in adults, many would treat adult patients with idiopathic MPGN and the nephrotic syndrome in a similar fashion.

ESSENTIAL MIXED CRYOGLOBULINEMIA AND HEPATITIS C–RELATED CRYOGLOBULINEMIC GLOMERULONEPHRITIS

Cryoglobulins are immunoglobulins that reversibly precipitate at decreased temperature. The cryoprecipitate may be made up of monoclonal immunoglobulin (type I), polyclonal IgG and monoclonal IgM (type II-mixed), or polyclonal IgG and polyclonal IgM (type III-mixed). Collagen vascular diseases, chronic infections, and lymphoproliferative disorders have been implicated in the pathogenesis of the mixed cryoglobulins. Recently, many cases of essential mixed cryoglobulinemia have been documented to have hepatitis C virus (HCV) antibodies and HCV RNA identified in their cryoprecipitate.

Mixed cryoglobulins act like immune complexes and cause complement-mediated vasculitis and inflammation. Patients present with fever, weakness, arthralgias, hepatosplenomegaly, Raynaud's, purpuric necrotizing skin lesions, and nephritis. Laboratory test findings include decreased complement (especially C1q-C4), positive rheumatoid factor, and detectable circulating cryoglobulins. Those with renal disease often have cryoglobulins consisting of polyclonal IgG and monoclonal IgM with rheumatoid factor activity (type II).

Up to 50 percent of patients with essential mixed cryoglobulinemia develop renal involvement at some time during the course of their disease. Most have an indolent protracted course with some proteinuria, hematuria, and decreased GFR. Twenty-five percent may present with acute nephritis with hematuria, proteinuria, hypertension, and acute renal dysfunction, and a small percentage may have severe acute oliguric renal failure. Renal biopsies often show an MPGN-type pattern.

Essential mixed cryoglobulinemia is a disease with acute episodes of nephritis and then remission with about 10 percent progression to ESRD. There has been no consistently effective treatment in controlled trials. However, given the recently identified role of HCV in this disease, some trials of alpha-interferon therapy (3 million units SC three times per week for 6 months) have demonstrated decreased proteinuria, increased GFR, and decreased circulating cryoglobulins, as well as clearance of HCV RNA from the circulation. Others have not been able to show an improvement in GFR, and relapse is common when therapy is stopped. Patients with severe progressive disease often respond to immunosuppressive therapy with pulse methylprednisone (1 gram administered IV per day for 1 to 3 days) followed by high-dose prednisone (60 mg daily) and/or oral cyclophosphamide (1 to 2 mg per kilogram per day). Similar therapy has even been used in patients with HCV-related cryoglobulinemia and glomerulonephritis. Once their glomerular disease has stabilized some of these patients have been treated with interferon. Plasma exchange has also been used to remove the circulating cryoglobulins in severe disease in both idiopathic and HCV-related disease, but the efficacy of this procedure remains unproven.

RAPIDLY PROGRESSIVE GLOMERULONEPHRITIS

Rapidly progressive glomerulonephritis (RPGN) refers to a form of glomerular damage in which there is a rapid decline in renal function over weeks to months. Histologically there is prominent extracapillary epithelial cell proliferation with crescent formation attributable to a number of inflammatory processes that cause rupture of glomerular capillaries into Bowman's space. Timely diagnosis and aggressive therapy are important in order to halt or reverse the renal injury. RPGN may be divided into three groups based on the immune pathogenesis of the disease. Type I is due to antiglomerular basement membrane antibodies and has linear immunofluorescent staining for immunoglobulin along the glomerular basement membrane (see the chapter on Goodpasture's Disease). Type II rapidly progressive glomerulonephritis is due to immune complex deposition as seen in some patients with collagen vascular disease and with infections such as poststreptococcal disease and endocarditis. The treatment is as defined for each entity causing the glomerular lesion. In Type III RPGN, there are no immune deposits (pauci-immune RPGN) and anti-GBM antibodies are not found. Of these patients, 90 percent have antineutrophil cytoplasmic antibodies (ANCA) in their circulation.

The pauci-immune ANCA positive vasculitides represent a spectrum of diseases including idiopathic crescentic glomerulonephritis, Wegener's granulomatosis, and polyarteritis nodosa, each involving different size vessels and presenting with and without systemic manifestations. ANCA have more than one specificity. P-ANCA is directed against myeloperoxidase and often is associated with isolated renal disease with RPGN or with a clinical picture of microscopic PAN, often with systemic signs. C-ANCA is directed against proteinase 3 and is most frequently found in patients with glomerular disease, often fulfilling the clinical criteria for Wegener's granulomatosis. Among patients with ANCA-positive glomerulonephritis there is no difference in renal or patient survival in either the presence or absence of systemic vasculitis. ANCA itself may be directly involved in the pathogenesis of the glomerular injury by activating neutrophils and monocytes that produce vascular injury within the glomeruli and elsewhere.

Idiopathic pauci-immune RPGN generally refers to cases with renal limited disease and no evidence of systemic vasculitis, although some have argued that a limited form of renal vasculitis is responsible. Patients with rapidly progressive glomerulonephritis usually present with acute nephritis with active urinary sediment and hematuria, hypertension, a decreasing glomerular filtration rate, and often oliguria. Many patients will be uremic at presentation or shortly thereafter and require dialysis. Poor prognostic signs include severe oliguric renal failure, extensive glomerular crescent formation, and extensive tubulointerstitial damage on renal biopsy.

Some investigators have successfully used aggressive therapy including pulse methylprednisone 30 mg per kilogram per day given daily or every other day for three doses followed by oral prednisone 1 mg per kilogram per day or 2 mg per kilogram per every other day for 3 to 6 months. Most patients respond in 4 to 6 weeks. However, most nephrologists would treat this disease with either oral or IV cyclophosphamide. Cyclophosphamide IV (up to 1 g per square meter, given at intervals of 2 to 4 weeks) or oral cyclophosphamide (1 to 2.5 mg per kilogram per day), in addition to corticosteroids, has been highly successful in reversing acute renal failure and restoring renal function even in dialysis-dependent patients. Because those glomeruli with extensive necrosis and crescents usually become obsolete, rapid institution of aggressive therapy is probably more important than the precise formula by which it is administered. In addition to cytotoxic therapy and corticosteroids, plasma exchange has been used in several trials. It has not been proven to have an added beneficial effect except perhaps in the subgroup of patients with severe renal failure. Blood pressure control and methods to prevent nonimmunologic progression of the renal disease should also be instituted to prevent later loss of glomerular function.

WEGENER'S GRANULOMATOSIS

Pathologically, the classic triad of Wegener's granulomatosis involves (1) upper and/or lower respiratory tract granulomatous inflammation, (2) systemic necrotizing vasculitis, and (3) focal, segmental necrotizing and crescentic glomerulonephritis without immune deposits. Clinically, patients can present with inflammatory rhinitis, sinusitis, cough, hemoptysis, and cavitary lung lesions on chest radiograph. As many as 75 percent of patients will have renal involvement at some point in their disease manifested by proteinuria, hematuria, and often rapid progression to renal failure. C-ANCA against proteinase 3 is thought to be present in the majority of cases with renal involvement. These antibodies may be involved in the pathogenesis of the disease by activating neutrophils under certain conditions to cause vessel wall injury. ANCA titers may correlate loosely with disease activity in some cases, but clinical judgment seems to be more important as a guide to therapy in following these patients.

The prognosis for patients with Wegener's granulomatosis depends on the aggressiveness of the disease process, the degree of renal and extrarenal involvement, and the speed at which appropriate therapy is instituted. The use of cyclophosphamide has dramatically improved both overall prognosis and the renal survival of these patients. Thus, while untreated patients in the pre-steroid era had a mean survival of about 5 months, currently 90 percent have improvement and 75 percent get complete remission of their disease often for years and even decades. Therapy is effective even in dialysis-dependent patients.

Standard therapy includes cyclophosphamide at a dose of 1 to 2 mg per kilogram per day orally combined with oral glucocorticoids. This immunosuppressive regimen should be maintained (with tapering of the glucocorticoid dose) for 6 months to 1 year after all signs of disease activity have resolved since relapses can occur with earlier discontinuation of therapy. An alternate regimen, especially for severely ill patients, consists of administering the dose of cyclophosphamide intravenously (at doses of up to 1 g per square meter) in conjunction with oral or intravenous glucocorticoids. These intravenous doses should be given initially at two to three weekly intervals as the leukocyte count allows; when the disease has been brought under control the doses may be spread out to a monthly maintenance schedule for at least 1 year. The literature and experts in this area have conflicting opinions as to the comparative efficacy and safety of intravenous versus oral cyclophosphamide. Although some patients have been successfully treated with other immunosuppressive regimens (including azathioprine, methotrexate, chlorambucil, and cyclosporin), cyclophosphamide is at present still the first-line drug of choice for this disease.

Trimethoprim-sulfamethoxazole has been used with anecdotal benefit for local regional disease of the respiratory tract, but its utility in renal disease is unclear.

There is no supportive evidence for the use of plasmapheresis in several trials for the treatment of renal disease; however, it may be useful as adjunctive therapy in cases of massive pulmonary hemorrhage with a severe progressive renal course despite the use of cyclophosphamide and steroids.

POLYARTERITIS NODOSA

Classic macroscopic polyarteritis nodosa refers to a systemic necrotizing vasculitis that primarily affects the medium-sized muscular arteries and leads to aneurysms and localized infarcts distal to the lesions. The kidney, heart, and gastrointestinal tract are often involved with relative sparing of the lungs and skin. Microscopic polyarteritis is a necrotizing inflammation of smaller arteries, arterioles, capillaries, and venules that typically involves the lungs and skin and in which aneurysm formation is rare. Hypertension and ischemic glomerular lesions leading to proteinuria and decreased glomerular filtration rate are common with macroscopic polyarteritis. With the microscopic form of the disease, hypertension is less common, and glomeruli are involved by a proliferative, necrotizing, and crescentric pauci-immune glomerulonephritis (RPGN-Type III). A nephritic presentation with hematuria and oliguric renal failure is common in microscopic polyarteritis. Although the etiology of these diseases remains unknown, a number of systemic diseases such as bacterial endocarditis, collagen vascular diseases, and hepatitis B infection can present with similar clinical findings and should be excluded before a diagnosis of idiopathic polyarteritis is made and treatment is instituted. Although there is no laboratory test that is specific for polyarteritis, many patients (especially those with microscopic polyarteritis) will have a positive test result for ANCA (predominantly P-ANCA).

The natural history of untreated polyarteritis is poor with a median survival of 3 months, and less than 15 percent survive 5 years. The major cause of early death is active vasculitis leading to renal failure, gastrointestinal hemorrhage, myocardial infarction, and cerebrovascular accidents. The use of glucocorticoids improved mean survival from 3 to 63 months with 50 percent of patients surviving 5 years. The addition of cytotoxic therapy has improved these statistics further, with remissions in greater than 80 percent and 5-year survival in over 80 percent.

Cyclophosphamide (1 to 2 mg per kilogram per day taken orally) is the most widely used therapy and appears to be the drug of choice. Cyclophosphamide therapy is usually initiated in combination with glucocorticoids (prednisone 1 to 2 mg per kilogram per day) with a taper of the glucocorticoid dose over time. The glucocorticoids may also eventually be administered as alternate-day therapy to minimize side effects. Regimens using pulse intravenous glucocorticoids and cyclophosphamide have also been used successfully. Therapy adjunctive to the use of immunosuppression should include blood pressure control and methods to minimize the nonimmunologic progression of the renal disease (reduction of intraglomerular and systemic hypertension and low-protein diets).

LIGHT CHAIN DEPOSITION DISEASE

Light chain deposition disease is caused by the overproduction and extracellular deposition of a monoclonal immunoglobin light chain. It is a systemic process and similar to AL amyloidosis except the deposits do not form beta-pleated sheets and thus do not stain congo red positive. Older males are predominantly affected and most have a lymphoplasmacytic B cell disease compatible with multiple myeloma.

Glomeruli on light microscopy have eosinophilic mesangial glomerular nodules. A single class of immunoglobin light chain (kappa in 80 percent of cases) stains in a diffuse linear pattern along the glomerular basement membranes (GBMs), in the nodules, and along the tubular basement membranes.

Moderate albuminuria is common and the nephrotic syndrome is found in one-half of patients at presentation often accompanied by hypertension and renal insufficiency. Therapy is directed at the abnormal clone of B cells with melphalan or cyclophosphamide and prednisone as for multiple myeloma and can lead to significant renal and patient survival.

FIBRILLARY GLOMERULOPATHY AND IMMUNOTACTOID GLOMERULOPATHY

Fibrillary glomerulopathy and immunotactoid glomerulopathy are likely a result of deposition of immunoglobins of the IgG class or other proteins in the glomeruli that polymerize to form nonamyloid, congo–red negative, fibrillar structures ranging in size from 12 to 49 nm. In fibrillary GN the fibrils are 20 nm in diameter and deposited in the GBM. They are 30 to 50 nm in diameter in immunotactoid GN and may be associated with a plasma cell dyscrasia.

Proteinuria is found in almost all patients, and hematuria, the nephrotic syndrome and renal insufficiency, is eventually found in the majority of cases. Patients progress to ESRD in a mean of 2 to 4 years. Corticosteroid therapy has not proven successful, but some patients with a crescentic pattern on light microscopy have been treated successfully with cyclophosphamide and corticosteroids.

ANTIPHOSPHOLIPID SYNDROME

Some patients with circulating antibodies directed against phospholipids will have the antiphospholipid syndrome with venous and arterial thromboses, cerebrovascular events, repeated spontaneous abortions, thrombocytopenia, and livedo reticularis. Recently, patients with these antiphospholipid antibodies have been documented to have glomerular damage from microthromboses of the glomerular capillary loops. Patients with anticardiolipin antibodies and a thrombotic event or glomerular thromboses should be anticoagulated, as long as the circulating antiphospholipid antibody persists. There is no consensus on therapy for patients with high titer antiphospholipid antibodies without evidence of a thrombotic event. Some experts favor anticoagulation, some favor low-dose aspirin, and others would merely monitor the patients. In general, in patients with SLE and the antiphospholipid syndrome, the titer of the antiphospholipid antibody does not correlate with clinical SLE disease activity or the titer of the anti-DNA antibodies.

SUGGESTED READING

Appel GB. Immune complex glomerulonephritis, deposits with interest. N Engl J Med 1993; 328:505–506.

Couser WG. Rapidly progressive glomerulonephritis classification, pathogenetic mechanisms, and therapy. Am J Kidney Dis 1988; 11:449.

D'Agati VD, Appel GB. Polyarteritis, Wegener's granulomatosis, Charg-Strauss syndrome. . . ." In: Brenner B, Tischer C, eds. Renal pathology. 2nd ed. Philadelphia: JB Lippincott, 1994:1087.

D'Amico G, Ferrario F. Mesangiocapillary glomerulonephritis. J Am Soc Nephrol 1992; 2:S159-S166.

Donadio J, Bergstralh E, et al. A controlled trial of fish oil in IgA nephropathy. N Engl J Med 1994; 331(18):1194–1199.

Falk RJ, Hogan S, Carey FS, et al. Clinical course of antineutrophil

cytoplasmic autoantibody associated glomerulonephritis and systemic vasculitis. Ann Intern Med 1990; 113:656–663.
Glassock R. Treatment of immunologically mediated glomerular disease. Kidney Int 1992; 42(suppl 38):S121-S126.
Johnson RJ, Gretch DR, Yamabe H, et al. Membranoproliferative glomerulonephritis associated with hepatitis C viral infection. N Engl J Med 1992; 117:573–577.
Kunis CL, Kiss B, Williams G, et al. Treatment of rapidly progressive glomerulonephritis with IV pulse cyclophosphamide. Clin Nephrol 1992; 37:1–8.
Misiani R, Bellavita P, Fenili D, et al. Interferon alpha therapy in cryoglobulinemia associated with HCV. N Engl J Med 1994; 330:751–756.
Ponticelli C, Passerini P. Treatment of nephrotic syndrome associated with primary glomerulonephritis. Kidney Int 1994; 46:595.
Tarshish P, Bernstein J, Tobin J, Edelmann C. Treatment of mesangiocapillary glomerulonephritis with alternate day prednisone: A report of the international study of kidney disease in children. Pediatr Nephrol 1992; 6:123–130.

THERAPEUTIC APPROACHES TO RENAL TRANSPLANTATION

DILIP S. KITTUR, M.D., Sc.D.
JAMES F. BURDICK, M.D.

Over the past 10 years renal transplantation has become the preferred modality of treatment for patients with end-stage renal disease (ESRD) who have no precluding risks. Patients prefer transplant over dialysis because of improved quality of life. Moreover, from an economic point of view transplantation is more cost-effective than long-term dialysis. The current immunosuppression, which includes cyclosporine or 7k506, is more specific and effective and at the same time is associated with less harmful side effects. Consequently, the criteria for selecting patients for transplantation have been liberalized to include those with more risk factors such as advanced age. However, the supply of organs has not improved and the shortage of kidneys is acute. Because of this discrepancy between supply and demand, living-unrelated donors and cadaveric donors with some risk factors (e.g., hypertension and advanced age) are being used with increasing frequency. The overall success of transplantation is good despite a diminished emphasis on HLA matching. Graft survival after cadaveric transplantation is very good and is even better with living donors as shown in Table 1. A number of new immunosuppressive drugs are nearing clinical use. The most outstanding problem in renal transplantation for which there is no effective treatment is chronic rejection.

PATIENT SELECTION

The main considerations in selecting patients for transplantation is their ability to withstand the surgical procedure, the subsequent fluid shifts caused by diuresis, and the issues that would compound the risks of immunosuppression. Selecting recipients for renal transplantation is a careful but expeditious process. In general, patients are on dialysis before they undergo transplantation. However, uremic patients that are close to dialysis are also considered. Hypertension and diabetes are etiologic factors in a significant number of potential recipients. In these patients, especially, the cardiovascular status is evaluated more carefully, commonly by an echocardiogram and a stress test.

All patients are also carefully screened for past infections, including hepatitis B and C, HIV, and other common opportunistic viruses such as cytomegalovirus (CMV) and Epstein Barr virus (EBV). Seropositivity with the latter common viruses does not constitute a contraindication to transplantation but rather provides prognostic parameters. For example, patients that are CMV seronegative are highly prone to developing serious CMV infection with a seropositive donor kidney unless they are treated with prophylactic immunoglobulins. Regarding the former viruses, HIV is the only absolute contraindication for renal transplantation. Disseminated malignancy is another absolute contraindication; localized malignancy, if resected with a disease-free in-

Table 1 UNOS Registry Kidney Transplant Results

	n	*3-Month Survival (%)*	*1-Year Survival (%)*	*2-Year Survival (%)*	*3-Year Survival (%)*
Cadaveric–Donor Graft Survival	38,599	86.4	80.3	74.5	68.7
Cadaveric–Donor Patient Survival	38,629	96.4	93.2	90.4	87.5
Living–Donor Graft Survival	10,926	94.0	91.2	87.7	83.7
Living–Donor Patient Survival	10,931	98.7	97.3	95.9	94.3

Modified from 1994 Annual Report of The U.S. Scientific Registry of Transplant Recipients and The Organ Procurement and Transplantation Network (Transplant Data: 1988-1993). United Network for Organ Sharing. U.S. Department of Health and Human Services, Public Health Services, Health Resources and Services Administration, Division of Organ Transplantation.

terval of 1 to 2 years, is generally not a contraindication for transplantation. Other factors considered in selection of patients are psychosocial factors such as compliance to medications, since these factors are important for the long-term success of renal transplantation. The algorithm for evaluating recipients is shown in Table 2.

DONOR SELECTION

In response to the increased number of recipients awaiting renal transplantation, donor criteria have been relaxed in recent years. We and other centers have continued to emphasize living donation. Living-unrelated donors are also being used with increased frequency. The psychosocial evaluation of the unrelated donors tends to be more comprehensive than that of a related donor. Both types of living donors are critically evaluated regarding their ability to maintain normal physiology with a single kidney. Low creatinine clearance or proteinuria raise a warning flag. History of renal disease in the family is of concern but does not necessarily rule out living donation. To keep the morbidity and mortality of living donation very low, the potential donors are screened for cardiorespiratory problems.

Brain-dead but heart-beating cadaveric donors constitute almost two-thirds of the total donor pool. In addition, some centers have used non–heart beating cadavers with satisfactory results. Brain death is documented by the attending physician with the help of neurologists or neurosurgeons. Subsequent to brain death, the physiology of the donor is supported by the intensive care unit team with help from organ procurement agencies. Adequate hydration of the donor to prevent hypotension and electrolyte imbalance is crucial to subsequent functioning of the organs. The families of cadaveric donors find donation to be a positive outcome in the midst of their tragedy.

Table 2 Patient Evaluation Algorithm for Kidney Transplantation

Screening
- Patient is on dialysis or has severe uremia near requiring dialysis
- Kidney disease not high risk for recurrence (e.g., cystinosis, active lupus)
- Patient desires transplantation
- No absolute contraindication (e.g., HIV-positive, extremes of age, unable to be rehabilitated)

Workup
- General systems work-up reveals no uncontrollable diseases (heart, lungs, liver, neurologic)
- Surgical anatomy appropriate (iliac artery atherosclerosis, postphlebitic iliac vein obliteration) or reconstructible (bladder augmentation or ileal loop)

Donor
- If living donor is available proceed with this; if not, register patient as candidate for cadaver transplant on the UNOS waiting list

Donors with risk factors ("expanded-criteria" donors) are being used with greater frequency because of a drop in donation resulting from safer driving practices and from an increasing incidence of donors that must be ruled out because of concern about HIV. As part of the expanded-criteria donors, kidneys from donors with adequately controlled hypertension or diabetes, as well as those from older donors (<60 years of age) are accepted by many centers, including ours, for transplantation. Because there is some (as yet undefined) risk of early failure in organs from these donors, the kidneys from expanded-criteria donors are generally used in patients that would otherwise have difficulties in obtaining a kidney such as patients that are highly sensitized to HLA antigens because of multiple transfusions or pregnancies and older patients. Although the long-term outcome from these kidneys is unknown, the expanded-criteria donors have prevented a decline in organ acquisition and in transplantation.

PERIOPERATIVE MANAGEMENT OF THE TRANSPLANT RECIPIENT

The kidney transplant operation has remained standard for the last several years. The urgency of performing the operation is different when the organ is from a cadaveric source than when it is from a living-related donor; renal transplants from cadaveric donors are done on an emergent basis, whereas those from living donors have the advantage of being scheduled selectively. The immediate preoperative evaluation in both instances involves laboratory work that is necessary to determine the electrolyte balance, rule out active infections, and assess cardiorespiratory adequacy. Regardless of donor source, a crossmatch is performed between the donor's leukocytes and the recipient's serum to determine if the recipient has preformed antibodies against the donor HLA antigen. In the absence of significant contraindications and if the crossmatch test is negative, the recipient operation proceeds expeditiously.

The kidney is transplanted heterotopically in the retroperitoneum in the iliac fossa. The arterial supply comes from the external iliac arteries and the venous drainage is into the external iliac vein. The donor ureter is anastomosed to the recipient's bladder either by an extra-vesicle or an intravesicle approach. The recipient is kept well hydrated during the operative procedure since studies have indicated that the function of transplanted kidneys is recovered more promptly if the central venous pressure is kept in the high normal ranges. Prior to reperfusion of the transplanted kidney, Lasix and mannitol are generally administered to expedite renal function and prevent ischemia reperfusion injury. Prompt renal function occurs in 60 to 70 percent of patients; in the remainder there is a period of nonfunction, which is commonly referred to as acute tubular necrosis (ATN). The majority of patients with ATN recover within a period of a few days to a few

Table 3 Common Complications After a Kidney Transplant

Technical
- Wound hematoma
- Urine leak
- Peritoneal fluid leak
- Transient postbiopsy bleeding

Rejection
- Acute
- Chronic

Infection
- Atypical viral, bacterial, fungal

Late Complications
- Ureteral stenosis
- Lymphocele
- Arterial stenosis
- Chronic rejection

Table 4 Kidney Transplant Immunosuppression

Preoperative or on call: Azathioprine 2 mg/kg IV
Intraoperative: Methylprednisolone 500 mg IV

Presuming No Rejection
First week
- After meththylprednisolone 125 q6 X 6 then prednisone 30 mg/d (20 mg if >55 y.o.)
- Azathioprine 1.5 mg/kg
- Cyclosporine 4 mg/kg PO or nasogastric tube b.i.d., adjust to level above 200, or tacrolimus 0.05 mg/kg PO b.i.d., adjust to blood level about 10 ng/dl

Fourth week
- Prednisone: 20 mg/day
- Azathioprine: 1.5 mg/kg
- Cyclosporine or tacrolimus: same dosage as first week

Maintenance
- Prednisone: 15 mg/d by 6 mo, 10 mg/d by 9 mo

For Rejection
- Initial treatment: methylprednisolone pulse; if no response, go to OKT3

weeks. The incidence of permanent primary nonfunction is currently less than 5 percent in cadaveric renal transplant.

When the renal allograft comes from a living donor, the recipient and donor operation proceed simultaneously. The donor kidney is excised carefully through a flank incision. The recipient operation is identical to that described above. The main difference between the two operations is in the outcome after living donation. The renal graft from a living donor suffers a significantly shorter period of cold ischemia since the preservation time is usually less than an hour. Therefore, in a vast majority of these cases renal function starts promptly. Additional complications following renal transplantation are outlined in Table 3.

RENAL ALLOGRAFT REJECTION

Of the three types of rejection—hyperacute, acute, and chronic—the latter two are commonly encountered after renal transplantation. Hyperacute rejection is mediated by preformed antibodies and has been successfully prevented by emphasis on pretransplant crossmatch (described earlier). On the other hand, approximately 40 percent of patients develop acute rejection after renal transplantation. The underlying mechanism in acute rejection is alloantigen presentation by antigen presenting cells (APCs) and endothelial cells followed by clonal T-cell proliferation. Clinically, acute rejection commonly manifests as elevated serum creatinine and decreased urine output. In severe cases, graft rejection is associated with tenderness over the graft, fever, and leukocytosis. Renal scan and ultrasound are routinely performed in suspected cases of rejection. Reduced renal flow is a common finding in both of these tests. Confirmation is usually obtained by a biopsy. Moderate to dense lymphatic filtration and endothelitis are pathognomonic features of acute rejection.

The clinical course of chronic rejection is more indolent than that of acute rejection. A gradual rise in serum creatinine occurs over a period of months. Differentiating nephrotoxicity caused by therapy with cyclosporine or tacrolimus (Prograf) from rejection is more difficult in chronic rejection than it is in acute rejection. Renal biopsy is the most reliable diagnostic test. Thickening of the subintima of moderate size arterioles and glomerulosclerosis are common features that distinguish chronic rejection from other diagnoses. The treatment of both types of rejection is outlined in the following discussion and in Table 4.

IMMUNOSUPPRESSION IN RENAL TRANSPLANTATION

Since the goal of current immunosuppressive therapy is to prevent rejection, recipients of renal transplants are placed on maintenance immunosuppression immediately following transplantation. Cyclosporine used in conjunction with steroids and azathioprine (Imuran) has been the mainstay of immunosuppression in the last decade. Maintenance immunosuppression starts intraoperatively and is usually more intense in the early postoperative period. Intraoperatively intravenous steroids are administered and are part of induction immunosuppressive therapy. The induction therapy also consists of both azathioprine and cyclosporine if the renal function is adequate. When renal function is not adequate, an antilymphocyte agent such as OKT3 or antithymocyte globulin (ATG) may be administered initially, and cyclosporine is deferred for a week or so. Steroids are usually tapered rapidly to a maintenance dose of prednisone 30 mg administered orally after the third post-transplant day. Once renal function is stabilized, cyclosporine is administered in doses required to maintain a blood level of 150 to 250 ng per milliliter.

Subsequently, most patients are maintained indefinitely on triple drug therapy, including steroids, azathioprine, and cyclosporine, until the renal allograft remains functional.

Newer immunosuppressive drugs are rapidly going through clinical trials and will probably be used in immunosuppressive regimens in the next few years. Tacrolimus (FK506), a newer immunosuppressive drug, has actions similar to cyclosporine A on IL-2 production by T lymphocytes. Both agents inhibit IL-2 gene transcription, thus leading to decreased T-cell proliferation. Tacrolimus has side effects similar to cyclosporine, namely nephrotoxicity, neurotoxicity, and an increased tendency to hypertension. In preliminary studies, the nephrotoxicity of cyclosporine and tacrolimus appears to be equivalent. Tacrolimus appears to produce more gastrointestinal disturbances than cyclosporine. Preliminary studies in renal transplant patients have not revealed superiority of either agent over the other. Thus, it is conceivable that cyclosporine will be the immunosuppressive agent in common use. Tacrolimus has been useful in instances where cyclosporine therapy fails and patients continue to have rejections. The latest immunosuppressive to be licensed in the United States is a purine metabolite inhibitor specific for T and B lymphocytes called mycophenolate mofitil (Cellcept).

Despite being on maintenance immunosuppressive therapy, several recipients have acute episodes of rejection. These patients receive additional immunosuppressive agents, which are slowly tapered after the rejection episode is reversed. In acute episodes the first line of therapy is usually large doses of steroids administered intravenously. Approximately 75 percent of rejection episodes are reversed by these steroid boluses. If the rejection episode is resistant to steroids or if the episode is severe as indicated by a fast-rising creatinine, antilymphocyte antibodies are commonly used preparations. The two preparations in general use are ATG and OKT3. The former is a polyclonal serum while the latter is a monoclonal antibody directed against a portion of the CD3 structure on T cells. The efficacy of OKT3 is considerably better than that of ATG; OKT3 reverses more than 90 percent of rejection episodes. After reversing the rejection episode, the patients are generally maintained on higher doses of steroids, which are eventually tapered to maintenance levels.

Untoward Effects of Immunosuppression

The most common effects of immunosuppression are increased incidence of infection and malignancies. The infections that are common in these patients are usually of an atypical opportunistic nature (Table 5). Viral infections are more common in the early phases of immunosuppression, whereas atypical bacteria and fungi are more common in the later phases. In regard to viruses, CMV is perhaps the most frequently encountered viral infection in immunosuppressed recipients. Since approximately 40 percent of normal population is CMV positive, a CMV-negative recipient has a significant probability of receiving a CMV-positive organ. The severity of CMV illness in these instances is quite high unless prophylactic measures are undertaken. Prophylaxis with intravenous immunoglobulin preparations has reduced the incidence and severity of CMV disease considerably in transplant recipients. These preparations also reduce the intensity of reactivation of CMV disease in recipients that are CMV positive prior to transplantation. Gancyclovir is employed if CMV infection becomes clinically manifested by hyperpyrexia and/or CMV pneumonia. The two other common viruses encountered in immunosuppressed patients are herpes simplex and herpes zoster. In our center all recipients receive prophylaxis with acyclovir to decrease of the incidence of herpes infection.

Table 5 Infections After a Kidney Transplant

Bacterial wound or bladder infection
Yeast (*Candida*) wound or bladder infection
Cytomegalovirus (CMV)
Herpes simplex or zoster
Pneumocystis carinii
Cryptococcal meningitis
Aspergillosis

Two commonly encountered atypical bacteria in immunosuppressed patients are *Pneumocystis carinii* and legionella. Patients generally receive Bactrim prophylaxis to reduce the chance of pneumocystis infections. It is also noteworthy that staphylococcal pneumonias are more common in these patients than is generally observed in normal populations. In some regions of the United States tuberculosis has become an important pathogen in the immunocompromised individual. All prospective recipients are tested for active tuberculosis infection by ATP and chest radiograph before transplantation. Patients with active tuberculosis are not transplanted, but those with a positive PPD can be transplanted under INH coverage.

The incidence of lymphoid malignancies is significantly higher in immunocompromised recipients than that seen in normal populations. A related disorder that is being recognized with increasing frequency is lymphoproliferative disorder (LPD), which is associated with EBV. Patients under heavy immunosuppression appear to be more susceptible to polyclonal lymphoproliferation. Although the disorder is not as malignant as monoclonal lymphoproliferation, it is nonetheless a considerable concern in the transplant recipient. LPD can be life-threatening, and at the very minimum requires a drastic reduction in immunosuppression and can require complete cessation of immunosuppression. In all other lymphoid malignancies, the recommended course of action is cessation of immunosuppression, in addition to definitive treatment of the malignancy.

Other untoward effects of immunosuppression are related to the cardiovascular system. Prednisone predisposes these patients to hypercholesterolemia and hyperlipidemia. Cyclosporine and tacrolimus are also vasoactive agents in the sense that they increase patient susceptibility to hypertension. Consequently, the cardiovascular morbidity in transplant recipients is higher than that in the normal population.

RESULTS OF RENAL TRANSPLANTATION

Excellent graft and patient survival with minimal morbidity is currently possible with modern immunosuppression. Current graft survival averages between 80 and 85 percent 1-year survival, depending on the type and HLA matching of the donor (see Table 1). The best results are obtained in a six antigen match or a zero antigen mismatched donor recipient situation. For a variety of reasons living donors, even if poorly matched, also lead to a good outcome. Patient survival with modern immunosuppression is usually greater than 95 percent over 1 year. This compares quite favorably with patient survival on dialysis.

SUGGESTED READING

Braun WE, Marwick TH. Coronary artery disease in renal transplant recipients. Clev Clin J Med 1994; 61(5):370–385.

Browne BJ, Kahan BD. Renal transplantation. Surg Clin North Am 1994; 74(5):1097–1116.

Flechner SM. Current status of renal transplantation. Patient selection, results, and immunosuppression. Urol Clin North Am 1994; 21(2):265–282.

Hibberd PL, Rubin RH. Renal transplantation and related infections. Semin Respir Infect 1993; 8(3):216–224.

Morris PJ. Rejection—unanswered questions. Hum Immunol 1990; 28:104–111.

Suthanthiran M, Strom TB. Renal transplantation. N Engl J Med 1994; 331(6):365–376.

ANAPHYLACTIC SYNDROMES

CHEMICAL SENSITIVITY

ABBA I. TERR, M.D.

The term chemical sensitivity does not define a specific disease or group of diseases because sensitivity (i.e., immunologic hypersensitivity or allergy) is caused by one or more environmental allergens, which are always "chemical," whether natural or man-made. Furthermore, there are several distinct types of immunologic hypersensitivities with corresponding clinical expressions in allergic disease. In recent years, however, a concept has appeared that chemical sensitivity is a new and unique disease caused by synthetic chemicals in the environment. The proposed disease, called multiple chemical sensitivity, has created great controversy and confusion among clinicians. Proper management of a patient with suspected chemical sensitivity requires an accurate diagnosis, which in turn demands a thorough evaluation of both the patient and his environment.

For effective treatment, an adequate history of the illness with particular attention to specific symptoms and their timing with respect to the patient's location is essential and should include information about the home environment, workplace, and leisure time activity. A thorough physical examination is required to verify objectively the presence and extent of anatomical and functional abnormalities, since allergic, irritant, and toxic diseases all induce some form of inflammation. On the other hand, nonspecific tests of organ function, such as pulmonary function tests, imaging studies, and specific tests that indicate the existence of a particular type of immune response such as wheal-erythema skin tests must be interpreted with reference to the clinical findings.

Cases of suspected chemical sensitivity may require an equally rigorous and expert examination of the patient's environment, usually the workplace, sometimes the home, and occasionally a neighborhood site such as a nearby landfill, watertable, or even the ambient air quality. This type of examination requires the services of an industrial hygienist with appropriate expertise and equipment. Such a process is usually very costly, but recommendations for certain treatment strategies and their potential impact on the patient's current and future health may justify the need for such information.

In the case of suspected chemical sensitivity the patient may present with a list of chemicals of concern, or the history may uncover the possibility of certain chemicals to be considered as the cause of the patient's illness. Manufacturers of chemicals or commercial products maintain and supply documents known as material safety data sheets (MSDS) for each product. These documents (Table 1), as well as toxicology texts, are useful as initial sources of information for identifying the known irritant and toxic properties of the chemical in question, but they may not be helpful when some form of immunologic sensitivity is suspected. The MSDS also gives limited advice about protective measures and antidotes for treatment.

ALLERGY

Although all allergens are chemicals, a number of occupational allergies have been documented in which the patient is allergic to a defined low or high molecular weight synthetic chemical, in contrast to high molecular-weight naturally occurring substances, usually proteins, that account for the usual nonoccupational allergic diseases. Occupational allergic contact dermatitis is by far the most prevalent condition in this category. Some of the more common occupational contact allergens are listed in Table 2. Occupational asthma can be caused by specific allergic sensitivity to either low molecular-weight compounds that are believed to act as haptens in the induction of the sensitized state or to high molecular-weight chemicals that may be capable of allergenicity per se. Examples of such allergens are listed in Table 3. Hypersensitivity pneumonitis is almost always caused by natural allergens rather than by synthetic chemicals.

Diagnosis

A thorough history and physical examination and relevant laboratory or imaging tests, along with an appropriate examination and analysis of workplace or other environmental exposures, will generally reveal the diagnosis of the illness, but specific allergy testing is then necessary to identify the causative allergen. Patch testing is the accepted standard method for allergen identifica-

Table 1 Material Safety Data Sheet

Identification
Physical data
Hazardous ingredients
Fire and explosion hazard data
Health hazard data
Toxicity data
Classification (poison, irritant, etc.)
Effects of overexposure
Emergency and first-aid procedures
Reactivity data
Spill or leak procedures
Special protection information
Special precautions

Table 2 Common Chemical Allergens in Allergic Contact Dermatitis

Balsam of Peru
Benzocaine
Chromium
Cinnamic aldehyde
Colophony
Epoxy resins
Ethylene diamine
Formaldehyde
Imidazolidinyl urea
Lanolin alcohol
Mercapto compounds
Neomycin
Nickel
p-phenylenediamine
Quaternium compounds
Thiuram

Table 3 Chemical Allergens in Occupational Asthma

Low Molecular-Weight Allergens	*High Molecular-Weight Allergens*
Inorganic chemicals	Animal products
Ammonium persulfate	Antimicrobials
Metal salts:	Crustaceans
Aluminum	Foods
Chromium	Fungi
Cobalt	Enzymes
Nickel	Gums
Platinum	Insects
Organic chemicals	Mites
Acrylates	Pollens
Amines	
Acid anhydrides	
Azo compounds	
Isocyanates	
Plicatic acid	
Polyvinyl compounds	
Styrene compounds	

tion in allergic contact dermatitis and immediate wheal-erythema prick and intradermal skin testing for occupational asthma. Availability of the allergen, irritant, or toxic effects of the chemical, and dosage for testing are limiting factors. Bronchial inhalation challenge testing with the suspect chemical is considered the standard for diagnosis in occupational asthma, but the same limitations for skin testing apply here as well, in addition to the technical difficulties and danger inherent in the bronchial provocation procedure. The presence of precipitating antibodies to the allergen has traditionally been used for diagnostic allergen testing in hypersensitivity pneumonitis, but experience has shown that the presence of these antibodies in the serum is evidence of exposure to the chemical, but not necessarily proof of disease.

Treatment

The therapy of specific allergic diseases, whether caused by natural allergens or synthetic chemicals, is discussed in other chapters of this book. Avoidance of occupational allergens may require special control measures in the workplace, job alterations, or vocational rehabilitation.

IRRITATION SYNDROMES

Almost any chemical compound encountered in the environment has the potential to cause irritation to the skin, mucous membranes, conjunctivae, or the respiratory tract from contact or from inhalation. The mechanisms for irritation are many, and they are specific to the chemical and physical properties of the chemical. Absorption of an environmental chemical can cause reversible, transient effects on internal organs. For example, transient neurologic symptoms of spaciness, incoordination, and sedation commonly occur from inhalation of many organic solvents. These tissue and organ effects are considered irritative if they are reversible and leave no residual organ dysfunction.

Diagnosis

The diagnosis of chemical irritation is usually obvious upon history and examination of the patient, but the nature of the chemical exposure must be known. There is a dose-response relationship, and there may be a range of dosage for the threshold of irritation for each chemical. The fact that some individuals experience irritative phenomena at unusually low doses of certain compounds does not imply an immunologic mechanism, but rather an idiosyncratic tissue or organ susceptibility.

Treatment

Treatment of chemical irritation is symptomatic only, so specific measures depend on the affected organ and the nature of the response. Correct diagnosis permits the patient to take proper precautions to avoid irritant quantities of the chemical in the future.

TOXICITY

Chemical toxicity, like irritation, is specific to the chemical and physical properties of the chemical and is dose related. Unlike allergy, toxicity can occur in any exposed individual, but the threshold and severity may vary over a range of dosage. The adage "the dose makes the toxin" means that every chemical is both toxic and nontoxic, depending upon dose. Toxicity may be acute or chronic, and, in some cases, notably carcinogenesis, the onset may be delayed, even as long as years.

Diagnosis

Toxicity to environmental chemicals may arise from exposure through inhalation, ingestion, injection, or direct skin contact. Absorption from any of these routes of exposure can result in toxic effects on remote organs. Therefore, a high degree of suspicion may be required to make the diagnosis. In contrast to allergy in which evidence of both exposure and the presence of the relevant immune response mediating an allergic reaction can be obtained by the appropriate testing, chemical toxicity must usually be diagnosed by history and examination alone to seek the objective clinical findings known to be associated with the particular chemical suspected in each case. In exceptional cases, such as lead or arsenic poisoning, quantitation of the element in certain body tissues may establish the diagnosis.

Treatment

As in the case of chemical irritation, therapy is specific to the chemical, the target site, and severity of the tissue damage. Removal of residual toxin (e.g., chelation therapy for lead poisoning) may be indicated. In every case, knowledge of the environmental source of the chemical is essential to avoid future recurrences.

BUILDING-RELATED ILLNESS

Increasingly, illnesses caused by chemicals or allergens present in building construction materials or contents are being recognized. In these cases small epidemics of disease occur among the building occupants. It is necessary in each case to identify the type of illness and the building-related cause, which can be an infectious microorganism, allergen, irritant, toxin, or other agent. One well-known example is Legionnaire's disease. "Sick building syndrome" is a term for illness related to the building air quality, which might be caused by offgassing of chemicals from the building or its contents, inadequate air exchanges, or improper humidity.

Diagnosis

The diagnosis of suspected building-related illness is based on an epidemiologic investigation of the incident, which may include the medical history and physical examination of cases and controls, questionnaire surveys, and relevant examination of the building itself.

Treatment

Therapy of affected building occupants depends upon the nature of the specific illness, which may include infection, toxicity, irritation, or allergy.

MULTIPLE CHEMICAL SENSITIVITY

The term multiple chemical sensitivity refers to a controversial condition of numerous subjective symptoms without significant abnormal physical signs or laboratory abnormalities in persons who attribute their symptoms to multiple environmental chemicals. The condition typically causes significant disability. There is ongoing debate about the etiology, because there are a number of theories that encompass allergic, immunotoxic, neurotoxic, and psychologic mechanisms to explain symptoms, and therefore many different treatment strategies have been advocated.

Diagnosis

Attempts to establish a case definition have not been productive, so a clinical diagnosis rests entirely on the patient's own perception of an environmental cause for symptoms. However, it is necessary to rule out the presence of any recognized physical disease that might explain some or all of the symptoms by appropriate examination, testing, and referral. It is equally important to avoid unnecessary laboratory tests based on unproven theories of multiple chemical sensitivity such as extensive testing of blood lymphocyte counts, autoantibodies, antibodies to a variety of environmental chemicals, and levels of chemicals in various body fluids, unless there is compelling clinical evidence that the results of such tests would confirm an a priori suspicion of an immune dysfunction or autoimmune disease. The same admonition holds for imaging studies of the brain. In many cases psychiatric evaluation may be indicated because of the pattern of symptomatology.

Treatment

To date no form of medical "treatment" based on any of the various theories of pathogenesis of multiple chemical sensitivity has been shown to be effective and none has been subjected to a rigorous clinical trial. These include excessive avoidance of environmental chemicals often leading to major lifestyle changes, sublingual or subcutaneous "neutralization" therapy, IV gamma globulin, and sauna "detoxification." In fact, chemical avoidance treatment based on the immunotoxic theory enhances unfounded environmental fears, thereby increasing the number and severity of symptoms that these patients experience.

Pending definitive studies, physician management of multiple chemical sensitivity must be an individualized cooperative doctor-patient effort to reduce symptoms and enhance coping with everyday environmental exposures. This requires frequent visits with short-term practical goals for the patient to gain progressive control over existing fears and prohibitions. Regular physical exercise and relaxation techniques may help. Clinical depression and anxiety can be relieved with appropriate medication. Psychotherapy is indicated for many patients with this condition, although they typically reject this suggestion. Behavioral modification and biofeedback may be useful tools if the expertise is available

Regularly scheduled visits to discuss progress and to permit the patient to verbalize his or her concerns will help to avoid crisis intervention.

SUGGESTED READING

Bernstein DI, ed. Guidelines for the diagnosis and evaluation of occupational lung disease. J Allergy Clin Immunol 1989;84:791–844.

Sparks PJ, Daniell W, Black DW, et al. Multiple chemical sensitivity syndrome: A clinical perspective. I. Case definition, theories of pathogenesis, and research needs. J Occup Med 1994;36:718–730.

Sparks PJ, Daniell W, Black DW, et al. Multiple chemical sensitivity syndrome: A clinical perspective. II. Evaluation, diagnostic testing, treatment, and social considerations. J Occup Med 1994;36:731–737.

Terr AI. Environmental illness. A clinical review of 50 cases. Arch Intern Med 1986; 146:145–149.

DIAGNOSING FOOD INTOLERANCES IN CHILDREN

HUGH A. SAMPSON, M.D.

Adverse food reactions, or any untoward event resulting from the ingestion of a food, are common in children. They may be the result of *food hypersensitivities* (allergy), adverse immunologic reactions, or *food intolerances,* adverse physiologic reactions. Food intolerances are secondary to toxic or pharmacologic substances found in some foods such as chemical or microbial contaminants, or metabolic disorders of the patient such as lactose intolerance. Food aversions may mimic an adverse food reaction, but cannot be reproduced when the patient ingests the food unknowingly or in a blinded challenge. True food allergies are most frequent in young children, occurring in up to 6 percent of children less than 3 years of age and then declining to about 1.5 percent to 2 percent in older children.

When evaluating a child for suspected adverse food reactions, the initial effort should be directed at distinguishing whether the reaction is most likely due to an intolerance or a hypersensitivity response. Table 1 lists a number of disorders associated with food intolerances, but a full discussion of the evaluation of these disorders is beyond the scope of this chapter. Table 2 lists a number of food hypersensitivity (allergic) disorders, which can be diagnosed with methods outlined in this chapter.

DIAGNOSING FOOD HYPERSENSITIVITIES

As outlined in Figure 1, the evaluation of a patient for suspected adverse food reactions involves a thorough history, physical examination, and laboratory tests. With the history, an attempt is made to establish whether the patient is suffering from an intolerance or hypersensitivity reaction, and if the latter, whether a non–IgE or IgE-mediated mechanism is involved. The presence of atopic features on physical exam, especially atopic

Table 1 Differential Diagnosis of Adverse Food Reactions

- Gastrointestinal disorders (vomiting and/or diarrhea)
  - Structural abnormalities
    - Hiatal hernia
    - Pyloric stenosis
    - Hirschsprung's disease
    - Tracheoesophageal fistula
  - Enzyme deficiencies (primary versus secondary)
    - Disaccharidase deficiency (lactase, sucrase-isomaltase, glucose-galactose)
    - Galactosemia
    - Phenylketonuria
  - Malignancy
  - Other
    - Pancreatic insufficiency (cystic fibrosis, Schwachman-Diamond syndrome)
    - Gallbladder disease
    - Peptic ulcer disease
- Contaminants and additives
  - Flavorings and preservatives
    - Sodium metabisulfite, monosodium glutamate
  - Dyes
    - Tartrazine, other azo dyes (?)
  - Toxins
    - Bacterial (*Clostridium botulinum, Staphylococcus aureus*)
    - Fungal (aflatoxins, trichothecenes, ergot)
    - Seafood associated
      - Scrombroid poisoning (tuna, mackerel)
      - Ciguatera poisoning (grouper, snapper, barracuda)
      - Saxitoxin (shellfish)
    - Infectious organisms
      - Bacteria (*Salmonella, Shigella, Escherichia coli, Yersinia, Campylobacter*)
      - Parasites (*Giardia, Trichinella*)
      - Virus (hepatitis, rotavirus, enterovirus)
- Mold antigens (?)
- Accidental contaminants
  - Heavy metals (mercury, copper)
  - Pesticides
  - Antibiotics (penicillin)
- Pharmacologic agents
  - Caffeine (coffee, soft drinks)
  - Histamine (fish, sauerkraut)
  - Serotonin (banana, tomato)
  - Tyramine (cheeses, pickled herring)
  - Glycosidal alkaloid solanine (potatoes)
  - Alcohol
  - Theobromine (chocolate, tea)
  - Typtamine (tomato, plum)
  - Phenylethylamine (chocolate)
- Psychologic reactions

Modified from Sampson HA. Differential diagnosis in adverse reactions to foods. J Allergy Clin Immunol 1986; 78:212-219.

eczema, increases the likelihood of an IgE-mediated mechanism. In IgE-mediated syndromes, the clinical impression may be re-enforced by skin tests or in vitro diagnostic tests (e.g., RAST). Diets *completely* eliminating suspected food allergens are utilized both in the initial evaluation and subsequent therapy of food allergy.

History

Although critical to the evaluation of food hypersensitivity, the parental history may be misleading and in most series involving double-blind placebo-controlled food challenges [DBPCFC's], historical reports of adverse food reactions are verified about 30 to 40 percent of the time. However, a thorough history is essential for delineating further evaluation. Several points should be established: (1) the identity and quantity of the food allergen suspected of provoking the reaction, (2) the time elapsed between the ingestion of the suspected food and the onset of symptoms, (3) a complete description of the symptoms elicited and the duration of the reaction, (4) whether similar symptoms have occurred in the past when the food was eaten and the therapeutic measures taken, and (5) whether other factors (e.g., exercise) appear necessary for the development of symptoms. Reactions that occur within minutes to hours of ingesting a specific food and conform to a pattern of signs and symptoms outlined previously are more likely to represent a food hypersensitivity. In general, the history is used in an effort to exclude a number of disorders that may mimic food allergic reactions (Table 1) and to determine which laboratory studies would be worthwhile (e.g., skin tests, IgA antigliadin antibody).

Table 2 Food Hypersensitivity Disorders

Gastrointestinal
IgE-mediated
Oral allergey syndrome (oral and perioral pruritus and angioedema, throat tightness)
Gastrointestinal anaphylaxis (nausea, cramping, emesis, diarrhea)
Allergic eosinophilic gastroenteritis (subset)
Infantile colic (~15% of infants with colic)
Non-IgE-mediated
Food-induced enterocolitis (1-3 hr postingestion: emesis, diarrhea, failure to thrive, and rarely, hypotension)
Food-induced colitis (2-12 hr postingestion; blood in stools)
Allergic eosinophilic gastroenteritis (postprandial nausea, emesis, weight loss)
Food-induced malabsorption syndrome ("celiac-like"; nausea, steatorrhea, weight loss)
Celiac disease
Cutaneous
IgE-mediated
Acute (common) and chronic (rare) urticaria
Atopic dermatitis (pruritic morbilliform rash leading to eczematous lesion)
Non–IgE-mediated
Dermatitis herpetiformis
Contact hypersensitivity
Contact irritation (especially with acidic fruits and vegetables)
Respiratory
IgE-mediated
Rhinoconjunctivitis
Laryngeal edema
Asthma (both acute wheezing and increased bronchial hyperreactivity)
Non–IgE-mediated
Heiner's syndrome (rare form of pulmonary hemosiderosis)
Other: Mechanism Unknown
Migraine (rare)
Irritability with other symptoms of hypersensitivity
(?) Arthritis (rare subset)
(?) Nephritis (rare subset of recurrent glomerulonephritis)

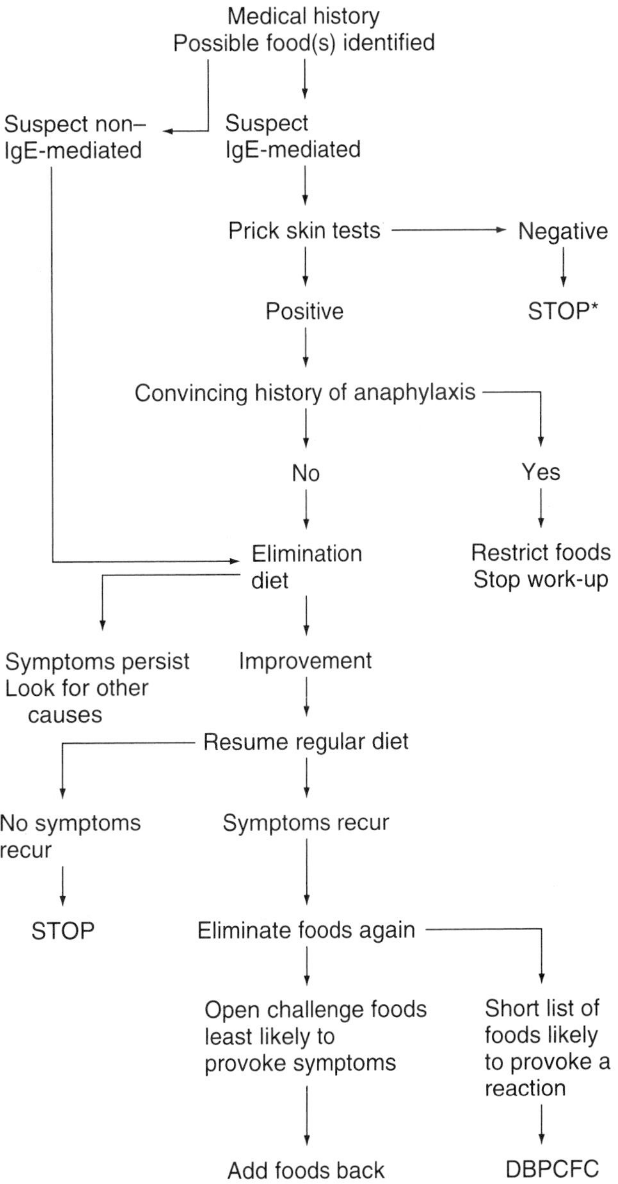

Figure 1 Evaluation of possible food hypersensitivity reactions.

Diet diaries are sometimes used as an adjunct to the history. Parents keep a chronological record of all items ingested by the child over a set period of time, generally no longer than a week, and any symptoms occurring during this time. The diary is reviewed in an effort to correlate ingestion of specific foods with the development of symptoms, but in these times of processed foods and prepackaged meals, this is helpful only occasionally.

Skin Testing

If an IgE-mediated food sensitivity is suspected, skin testing with food extracts by the prick or puncture method may be helpful. Routine intradermal skin tests with food extracts are not indicated because of the number of excessive false-positive results and increased risk. *A positive skin test indicates the presence of allergen-specific IgE antibodies on cutaneous mast cells; it does not mean the patient will develop symptoms when ingesting the specific food.* The positive predictive values of most prick skin tests are less than 50 percent. However, negative predictive accuracies are excellent and IgE-mediated allergic reactions are extremely rare in the face of negative skin tests.

Food extracts for skin testing may be purchased from a number of companies (weight:volume = 1:20), although extract quality varies somewhat from one company to another. The use of the "prick + prick" method (inserting the needle into the food and then pricking the skin) with fresh foods is frequently necessary for testing most fruits and vegetables and when a skin test is negative in the face of a strongly suggestive history. Wheals 3 mm or more greater than the negative control wheal are considered positive and are seen in virtually all patients having IgE-mediated allergic reactions to foods.

In Vitro Tests of Food-Specific IgE Antibodies

Skin testing is not feasible or recommended in the following clinical situations: patients with extensive skin disease, significant and prolonged dermatographism, a history of exquisite sensitivity (i.e., exposure to minute quantities of a specific food resulting in a life-threatening reaction), or patients using long-acting antihistamines (e.g., astemizole). In such cases, in vitro diagnostic tests are used to demonstrate the presence of food allergen–specific IgE antibodies, not clinical reactivity.

Radioallergosorbent Test (RAST)

The RAST has been the standard in vitro test for demonstrating allergen-specific IgE antibodies. A number of similar tests utilizing enzyme-linked or fluorescein-linked antibodies are also available. These tests are slightly less sensitive than skin testing in the evaluation of allergic reactions to foods. The Pharmacia CAP System appears to provide improved sensitivity and an increased dynamic range compared to the standard RAST.

Basophil Degranulation Tests

Commercial assays have become available to measure the amount of histamine released by basophils in response to a food allergen. To date, the diagnostic value of basophil degranulation tests for distinguishing *symptomatic* food allergy has not been demonstrated.

Elimination Diets

If the history and/or preliminary laboratory studies indicate that certain foods may be provoking symptoms in a child, those foods and all "hidden" sources of that food should be totally eliminated from the child's diet for a period of 1 to 2 weeks. If symptoms clear *completely,* further characterization of the sensitivity should be pursued (e.g., endoscopy and biopsy, blinded challenge). Prick skin testing should be performed if not done before initiating the elimination diet. The presence or absence of food allergen–specific IgE antibodies is useful for counseling the patient about the potential danger of accidental food ingestion, and, in young infants, the likelihood of both "outgrowing" the sensitivity and developing other food sensitivities. In chronic disorders such as atopic dermatitis, asthma, or chronic diarrhea, factors in addition to the food sensitivity may be triggering symptoms, so failure to see resolution of symptoms does *not* necessarily rule out a food hypersensitivity.

In cases where food hypersensitivity or intolerance are suspected but no specific foods can be incriminated, a brief trial (i.e., 2 to 4 weeks) of an oligoantigenic diet may be helpful. In young infants (< 4 months of age), an extensively hydrolyzed casein formula (Alimentum, Nutramigen, or Pregestimil) or an amino acid–derived formula (Neocate) should be utilized. In older children the following diets may be utilized: *4 to 8 months of age:* infant diet + rice cereal + pears; *9 to 24 months of age:* 4 to 8-month diet + rice + squash + lamb; *older than 24 months of age:* 9- to 24-month diet + fresh lettuce + potato + safflower oil + tea + sugar; or elemental formulas may be tried (e.g., Vivonex TEN or Tolerex with flavor packs, or Neocate 1^+).

Double-Blind Placebo-Controlled Food Challenge [DBPCFC]

The DBPCFC is the "gold standard" for diagnosing food allergies and has been used successfully in children for diagnosing virtually all food-related complaints. The choice of foods utilized in DBPCFCs is based upon history, skin test (or RAST) results, and/or foods suspected on the basis of a preliminary elimination diet. In practice, open or single-blind oral food challenges may be used to "screen" for food allergic reactions. However, if a child appears to have multiple food allergies, positive responses should be confirmed by DBPCFC. Even in very young infants it is often necessary to blind challenges because an infant and young child forced to drink or ingest something he or she does not want frequently becomes irritable and upset, which may provoke cutaneous erythema and or scratching, and occasionally wheezing and emesis. Failure to use appropriate blinding and placebo controls may lead to misinterpretation of such challenges.

In order to maximize the positive predictive value of DBPCFCs, it is best to eliminate suspect foods for 10 to 14 days, and up to 1 month in some gastrointestinal disorders. Ideally all medication should be discontinued. Antihistamines should be stopped long enough to allow the return of a normal histamine skin test, for example, diphenhydramine, 3 to 6 days; hydroxyzine, 7 to 14 days; astemizole, 4 to 8 weeks. Systemic corticosteroids should be discontinued for 4 to 8 weeks prior to admission, inhaled corticosteroids and cromolyn for at least 12 hours, oral theophylline for 8 hours, and inhaled beta-adrenergic medications for at least 6 to 8 hours before beginning all DBPCFCs. In children with unstable asthma or chronic urticaria, it is not always possible to discontinue all medications, but every effort should be made to minimize drugs to levels sufficient to prevent breakthrough of acute symptoms. In a study where challenges were performed in patients continuing antihistamines, skin symptoms were partially masked, but there appeared to be little effect on gastrointestinal or respiratory symptoms. In children with asthma and food hypersensitivity, inhaled beclomethasone or sodium cromoglycate did not prevent wheezing or changes in airway hyper-reactivity in many patients.

In order to optimize the probability of the food challenge providing a definitive diagnosis, the child's symptoms must be stabilized before initiating the challenge. For example, patients with atopic dermatitis or unstable asthma may require aggressive topical therapy in the hospital to obtain a stable baseline with minimal symptoms. Performing challenges on patients with active symptoms is an exercise in frustration, and may place the child at increased risk of a severe reaction since early mild symptoms may be overlooked.

The food challenge should be administered in the fasting state, starting with a dose unlikely to provoke symptoms (25 to 500 mg powdered food in liquid or capsules). As indicated in Table 3, foods for use in challenges are readily accessible and can be hidden in a number of vehicles. The dose is generally doubled every 15 to 60 minutes, depending upon the type of reaction suspected. During the challenge, activities (e.g., games, videos, television) should be available so that the patient does not focus on symptoms. In young children, it is generally very useful to observe their activity level; they will often become quiet and withdrawn when symptoms start to develop. Early symptoms may include pruritus or tingling of the tongue or palate, itching or tightness in the throat (sometimes inducing a sensation of itching in the inner ear), nausea, and abdominal cramps.

Challenges must be randomized and an equal number of placebo and food antigen challenges must be administered to adequately control for potential confounding factors such as variability in symptoms of chronic diseases, temporal effects, psychogenic factors, patient or observer bias, and so on. When evaluating suspected immediate food hypersensitivity, administration of test foods should be separated by an observation period of 24 hours; longer periods are required for "delayed" or "late" reactions.

If a patient suspected of IgE-mediated hypersensitivity tolerates 10 g of powdered food, clinical reactivity is generally ruled out. *However, all negative blinded challenges must be followed by an open feeding of the food in usual quantities under observation to rule out the rare false-negative challenge.* Although loss of reactivity to peanuts, tree nuts, fish, and shellfish is extremely unlikely, many children and adults will lose their symptomatic hypersensitivity to other foods after maintaining a strict allergen elimination diet for several years.

The diagnosis of many non–IgE-mediated food

Table 3 Sources of Food for Double-Blind Placebo-Controlled Food Challenges

*Food**	*Challenge Substances*	*Food**	*Challenge Substance*
Egg	Dehydrated whole egg†	Rye	Rye flour
Milk	Dry skim milk powder‡	Corn	Corn meal or corn flour
Soy	Soy flour	Oat	Oat flour
Wheat	Wheat flour§	Rice	Brown rice flour
Peanut	Peanut flour, peanut butter, or ground peanut (food processor or coffee grinder)	Potato	Potato flour, instant potato flour
		Nuts	"Piston-packed" nut butter, crushed or ground nut
Fish	16 gm lightly broiled fish‖	Meats	16 gm baby food chicken, turkey, ham, lamb, beef‡
Barley	Barley flour		

Vehicles for Use in Food Challenges

Fruit juices are rapidly absorbed and disguise mild flavors. Apple, fruit punch, orange, cranberry, and grape juices are commonly selected by patients

Tolerex, Vivonex TEN, or Neocate 1^{+} mask the taste of most challenge substances; flavor packets (vanilla, cherry-vanilla, raspberry, orange-pineapple, lemon-lime) may further mask the taste of strong flavors

Baby fruits such as applesauce, bananas, pears, peaches, or plums can be used as a vehicle for administering challenges

Hot cereals (instant grits, oatmeal, and cream of wheat cereals) can be used to administer peanut or nut challenges; flavor with other nut butters or with artificial nut flavors

*Except where specified, use 10 g of the substance, unless the history suggests a larger quantity may be necessary.

†Bakery suppliers sell dehydrated whole eggs. It must be 100% egg with nothing added.

‡The dry skim milk powder and baby food meats may be purchased from grocery stores.

§Some cake flours are 100% wheat, whereas others contain barley or malt. Flours should be purchased prepackaged.

‖Fish can be masked in canned tuna fish, to which children rarely, if ever, react. Fresh fish may be purchased from a grocery store or market.

hypersensitivities (e.g., food-induced enterocolitis or colitis syndromes) generally is established with an open oral food challenge, which consists of administering 0.4 to 0.6 g per kilogram of the suspected protein allergen. In the enterocolitis syndrome, a positive challenge results in vomiting and diarrhea within 1 to 6 hours, and occasionally (in about 15 percent of challenges) may be accompanied by hypotension. A positive challenge is accompanied by a rise in the absolute neutrophil count (greater than 3,500 cells per cubic millimeter) 4 to 6 hrs after symptoms develop, and neutrophils, eosinophils, and occasionally red blood cells are generally seen in the stools. In the colitis syndrome, gross or occult blood should appear in the stools within 24 to 48 hours. In addition, characteristic mucosal findings on sigmoidoscopy and biopsy are seen in this syndrome.

Quantitation of IgA antigliadin and IgA antiendomysial antibodies appear promising as screening tests for celiac disease. However, the diagnosis is dependent on demonstrating biopsy evidence of villous atrophy and inflammatory infiltrate while the patient is ingesting gluten, resolution of biopsy findings after 6 to 12 weeks of gluten elimination, and recurrence of biopsy changes following reinstitution of gluten.

Patients should be observed for at least 2 hours following the challenge when evaluating IgE-mediated responses and up to 4 to 6 hours in cases of milk-induced enterocolitis. In general DBPCFCs should be conducted in a clinic or hospital setting, especially if an IgE-mediated reaction is suspected, and trained personnel and equipment should be available for treating systemic anaphylaxis. Emergency medications should be at hand and the appropriate doses calculated to treat anaphylaxis. Normally, challenges should not be performed to a food suspected of causing a life-threatening anaphylactic reaction, especially if the presence of IgE-specific antibodies is confirmed. However, in cases where the causative antigen cannot be conclusively determined by history, a challenge should be conducted in the intensive care unit of a center that frequently deals with food allergic reactions.

Evaluation of largely subjective complaints, such as chronic abdominal pain, recurrent headaches, or behavioral problems, may be carried out safely on an outpatient basis. Often such symptoms are said to require several ingestions of the responsible food to reproduce the complaint. With such subjective symptoms, it is generally necessary to perform three placebo-controlled challenges to rule out random chance (i.e., $p < 0.05$). Patients are given weekly supplies of capsules or liquid challenges, which have been randomized to provide three sets of test food and placebo, and they are required to record all symptoms in a daily diary. At the end of the 6-week period, the diary is reviewed to determine whether symptoms occurred during the active or placebo arms of the challenge series. A cause-and-effect relationship can be inferred only if there are no responses to placebo and repeated responses to the food allergen.

THERAPY OF FOOD ALLERGIC DISORDERS

Strict *elimination* of the offending allergen is the only proven therapy for food hypersensitivities. Fortunately clinical reactivity to food allergens is generally very specific, and patients rarely react to more than one member of a botanical family or animal species. An elimination diet must be prescribed only to foods to which the child is reactive; there is no reason to prescribe broad elimination diets. Elimination of large numbers of foods have been reported to lead to malnutrition, eating disorders, adverse family psychosocial interactions, and other psychological problems.

One of the most common failures in the treatment of food allergic disorders is to properly educate patients (parents) so that all "hidden" sources of a food can be avoided. Patients must learn to recognize label ingredients that indicate the presence of a particular food (e.g., caseinate, whey, or lactalbumin for milk), to identify hidden sources of food antigens (e.g., casein or soy in canned tuna fish, egg in wheat noodles), and to substitute "safe" foods for allergenic foods. A dietitian knowledgeable in food allergy diets can ensure a nutritionally balanced diet, provide appropriate substitutes for specific food allergens, and anticipate any potential dietary deficiencies (e.g., calcium on a milk-free diet). The Food Allergy Network (10400 Eaton Pl., Suite 107, Fairfax, VA 22030) provides invaluable material to assist patients in complying with allergen elimination diets.

H_1-and H_2-antihistamines, ketotifin, and corticosteroids have been used to modify symptoms to food allergens, but overall they have minimal efficacy or their side effects are unacceptable. Results of trials with oral sodium cromolyn are conflicting, but most well-controlled studies have failed to demonstrate efficacy. To date, appropriately designed trials have never demonstrated efficacy for the use of *oral* desensitization, injection immunotherapy, or *subcutaneous* provocation and neutralization.

Despite concerted efforts to avoid food allergens, accidental ingestions are not uncommon and children (or their caregivers) must be prepared for inadvertent ingestion of a food allergen. The treatment of food allergic symptoms is similar to that for allergic symptoms provoked by other factors. Laryngeal or pulmonary symptoms following an inadvertent food exposure should be treated immediately with epinephrine and inhaled bronchodilators. The treatment of food-induced anaphylaxis requires subcutaneous or intravenous epinephrine, H_1- and H_2-antihistamines, aggressive volume expansion, bronchodilators, oxygen, and possibly other vasopressors. Early administration of epinephrine may abort an anaphylactic reaction; therefore, children with IgE-mediated food allergies, especially those with asthma; a history of a previous severe allergic reaction; or sensitivity to peanut, nuts, or seafood, must have injectable epinephrine available (Epi-Pen or Ana-Guard). Daycare centers and schools should have a list of emergency telephone numbers with backups to be called. Following an epinephrine injection for systemic reactions, the child should be taken to a medical facility immediately. All patients with IgE-mediated food allergy, especially those children with asthma, should be warned about the possibility of developing a severe anaphylactic reaction and should be educated in the appropriate treatment measures to be taken in case of an accidental ingestion.

SUGGESTED READING

Barnes-Koerner C, Sampson HA. Diets and nutrition. In: Metcalfe DD, Sampson HA, Simon R, eds. *Food allergy; Adverse reactions to foods and food additives.* Boston: Blackwell Scientific Publications, 1991; 332.

Bock SA, Atkins FM. Patterns of food hypersensitivity during sixteen years of double-blind placebo-controlled food challenges. J Pediatr 1990; 117:561–567.

Bock SA, Sampson HA, Atkins FM, et al. Double-blind placebo-controlled food challenge as an office procedure: A manual. J Allergy Clin Immunol 1988; 82:986–997.

James JM, Sampson HA. An overview of food hypersensitivity. Pediatr Allergy Immunol 1992; 3:67–78.

Sampson HA. Differential diagnosis in adverse reactions to foods. J Allergy Clin Immunol 1986; 78:212–219.

Sampson HA, Mendelson L, Rosen JP. Fatal and near-fatal food-induced anaphylaxis in children. New Engl J Med 1992; 327: 380–384.

FOOD ALLERGY IN ADULTS

JOHN CONDEMI, M.D.
DEAN D. METCALFE, M.D.

Food allergy is the result of immunologically mediated reactions to ingested food antigens. In adults, food allergy is infrequent and may present with a wide variety of symptoms. Although gastrointestinal symptoms (nausea, vomiting, and diarrhea) and cutaneous symptoms (urticaria, eczema, and angioedema) predominate, respiratory symptoms (bronchospasm and rhinoconjunctivitis) and anaphylaxis may be observed in allergic individuals. When considering the diagnosis of food allergy, nonimmunologically mediated adverse reactions to food must be excluded (Table 1). Corroboration of the patient's history may be obtained by positive prick skin test reactions to food extracts demonstrating mast cell–bound IgE to a food antigen, the elimination of symptoms on exclusion of the suspected food(s) from the diet, and in selected patients, the reproduction of the symptoms on double-blinded placebo-controlled oral food challenge. Because skin testing and diagnostic oral food challenges pose a potential risk to the patient, only physicians skilled in these procedures, with support facilities to manage severe allergic reactions, and following informed consent, should perform these diagnostic tests. In general, it is rarely necessary to challenge a patient with a positive history and skin test to the suspected food. Challenges are usually reserved for skin test negative patients to prove that the food is not responsible for the reaction.

Table 1 Examples of Adverse Food Reactions Caused by Nonimmunologic Mechanisms

Enzyme Deficiencies	*Toxins*
Lactase deficiency	Bacterial toxins
Sucrase deficiency	Botulism
Phenylketonuria	Staphylococcal toxin
	Endogenous toxins
Gastrointestinal Disease	Certain mushrooms—α-amannitine
Hiatal hernia	Seafood-associated
Peptic ulcer	Saxitoxin (Shellfish)
Gallbladder disease	Scombroid poisoning (tuna, skipjack, mackeral)
Postsurgical dumping syndrome	Ciguatera poisoning (snapper, grouper)
Neoplasia	
Inflammatory bowel disease	
Pancreatic insufficiency	
Additives and Contaminants	*Fungi*
Dyes	Aflatoxins
Tartrazine	Ergot
Exogenous chemicals	
Nitrates and nitrites	*Other Disorders*
Monosodium glutamate	Collagen vascular disease
Sulfiting agents	Endocrine disorders
Antibiotics	
Pesticides	*Psychologic Reactions*
Endogenous chemicals	Bulimia
Caffeine	Anorexia nervosa
Tyramine	
Phenylethylamine	
Alcohol	
Theobromine	
Tryptamine	
Histamine	
Serotonin	

THERAPY

Once a food allergy has been identified and confirmed, the management consists of dietary avoidance to prevent the allergic reaction and pharmacologic therapy of symptoms resulting from inadvertent ingestion. A treatment plan must be individualized to account for the number and types of food involved, the degree of sensitivity, and the nature and severity of the symptoms.

Diet

The treatment of choice in food allergy is elimination of the offending food(s) from the patient's diet.

Table 2 Classification of Foods from Plant Sources

Grain family	**Poppy family**	**Spurge family**	**Heath family**	**Composite family**	**Grape family**
Wheat	Poppy seed	Tapioca	Cranberry	Leaf lettuce	Grape
Graham flour	**Plum family**	**Arrowroot family**	Blueberry	Head lettuce	Raisin
Gluten flour	Plum	Arrowroot	**Gooseberry family**	Endive	**Myrtle family**
Bran	Prune	**Arrum family**	Gooseberry	Escarole	Allspice
Wheat germ	Cherry	Taro	Currant	Artichoke	Cloves
Rye	Peach	**Buckwheat family**	**Honeysuckle family**	Dandelion	Pimento
Barley	Apricot	Buckwheat	Elderberry	Oyster plant	Paprika
Malt	Nectarine	Rhubarb	**Citrus family**	Chicory	Guava
Corn	Almond	**Potato family**	Orange	**Legume family**	**Mint family**
Oats	**Laurel family**	Potato	Grapefruit	Navy bean	Mint
Rice	Avocado	Tomato	Lemon	Kidney bean	Peppermint
Wild rice	Cinnamon	Eggplant	Lime	Lima bean	Spearmint
Sorghum	Bay leaf	Red pepper	Tangerine	String bean	Thyme
Cane	**Olive family**	Green pepper	Kumquat	Soybean	Sage
Mustard family	Green olive	Bell pepper	**Pineapple family**	Lentil	Marjoram
Mustard	Ripe olive	Chili	Pineapple	Black-eyed pea	Savory
Cabbage	**Ginger family**	Tabasco	**Papaw family**	Pea	**Pepper family**
Cauliflower	Ginger	Pimento	Papaya	Peanut	Black pepper
Broccoli	Turmeric	**Lily family**	**Birch family**	Licorice	**Nutmeg family**
Brussel sprouts	Cardamon	Asparagus	Filbert	Acacia	Nutmeg
Turnip	**Pine family**	Onion	Hazelnut	Senna	**Walnut family**
Rutabaga	Juniper	Garlic	**Mulberry family**	**Morning glory family**	English walnut
Kale	**Orchid family**	Leek	Mulberry	Sweet potato	Black walnut
Collard	Vanilla	Chive	Fig	Yam	Butternut
Celery cabbage	**Madder family**	Aloes	Hop	**Sunflower family**	Hickory nut
Kohlrabi	Coffee	**Goosefoot family**	Breadfruit	Jerusalem artichoke	Pecan
Radish	**Tea family**	Beet	**Maple family**	Sunflower seed	**Cashew family**
Horseradish	Tea	Spinach	Maple syrup	**Pomegranate family**	Cashew
Watercress	**Pedalium family**	Swiss chard	**Palm family**	Pomegranate	Pistachio
Gourd family	Sesame seed	**Parsley family**	Coconut	**Ebony family**	Mango
Pumpkin	**Mallow family**	Parsley	Date	Persimmon	**Beech family**
Squash	Okra	Parsnip	Sago	**Rose family**	Beechnut
Cucumber	Cottonseed	Carrot	**Legythis family**	Raspberry	Chestnut
Cantaloupe	**Banana family**	Celery	Brazil nut	Blackberry	**Fungi family**
Muskmelon	Banana	Celeriac	**Sterculia family**	Loganberry	Mushroom
Honeydew melon	Plantain	Caraway	Cocoa	Boysenberry	Yeast
Persian melon		Anise	Chocolate	Dewberry	
Casaba		Dill		Strawberry	
Watermelon		Coriander			
Apple family		Fennel			
Apple					
Pear					
Quince					

Care must be taken to provide optimal nutrition while completely eliminating the food(s) provoking adverse reactions. Palatability is an important consideration, because the success of the diet depends on patient compliance. Diets that eliminate one or two foods are generally easy to design, but may become difficult to employ when common foodstuffs are to be avoided. For example, the dietary sources of milk and egg are numerous because of their widespread use in common foodstuffs. Elimination of these two foods alone results in a major loss of common commercially prepared foods from the diet. Hidden sources of these food and others must be identified by the patient to reduce unexpected exposure to an offending food. The patient should be instructed to be wary of meals prepared by others, who may include foods to which the patient may be sensitive.

There have been reports of cases in which patients with extreme sensitivities have experienced anaphylaxis, with subsequent death after such inadvertent exposures. Knowledge of the botanical families, as well as the classification of foods from animal sources, is necessary because cross-reacting antigens sometimes may be found among foods in the same group. For example, patients sensitive to shrimp often exhibit symptoms after ingestion of other crustaceans, such as crab, lobster, and crayfish. Cross-reactivity in other food groups is not uniform, and diets should be planned in accordance with the patient's history of tolerance to these foods. Examples of these classifications of food groups are listed in Tables 2 and 3.

The approach to a patient with multiple food sensitivities should involve the skills of a dietician. Patients with multiple food sensitivities have subjective symptoms only and negative skin tests but believe that they are sensitive to a large number of foods. In these patients one must perform a complete history and a physical examination with appropriate laboratory tests to determine if an underlying disease is responsible for

Table 3 Classification of Foods from Animal Sources

Mollusks	Crustaceans	Fish
Abalone	Crab	Sturgeon
Mussel	Crayfish	Hake
Oyster	Lobster	Anchovy
Scallop	Shrimp	Sardine
Clam	**Reptiles**	Herring
Squid	Turtle	Haddock
Amphibians	**Birds**	Bass
Frog	Chicken	Trout
Mammals	Duck	Salmon
Beef	Goose	Whitefish
Pork	Turkey	Scrod
Goat	Guinea hen	Shad
Mutton	Squab	Eel
Venison	Pheasant	Carp
Horsemeat	Partridge	Codfish
Rabbit	Grouse	Halibut
Squirrel		Catfish
		Sole
		Pike
		Flounder
		Drum
		Mullet
		Weakfish
		Mackerel
		Tuna
		Pompano
		Bluefish
		Snapper
		Sunfish
		Swordfish

Table 4 Lamb and Rice Diet

Foods Allowed

Brown rice: natural long grain, short grain; parboiled
White rice: enriched, converted; cook without added fat
Brown or white rice, rice flour
Brown rice cakes, containing only brown rice and salt (if desired)
Puffed rice cereal, containing only brown rice
Lamb
Water
Salt

All food must be prepared without added fat. Rice, lamb, salt, and water are the only allowable foods. No food containing any other ingredients is to be eaten. Check labels. Salt or baking soda should be used to brush the teeth

Eliminate

All foods not listed above, especially coffee, tea, soft drinks, and juices. Vitamins, aspirin, and any medication not ordered by a doctor must be eliminated

Possible Menu

Breakfast	*Lunch*	*Dinner*	*Snack*
Rice mush	Rice patties Pan-fried lamb chops	Rice and lamb sauté	Rice cakes

Instructions

Stay on basic diet for ______ days.

Then, on ___ add ______ all by itself, first thing in the AM
Then, on ___ add ______ all by itself, first thing in the AM
Then, on ___ add ______ all by itself, first thing in the AM
Next, on ___ add ______ all by itself, first thing in the AM
Next, on ___ add ______ all by itself, first thing in the AM

Continue food additions one at a time at ___ day intervals until most or all other foods in the diet have been tested. Keep a diet diary as indicated. Add foods in large amounts, and eat them several times a day during addition period

their symptoms. Once a systemic disease is ruled out, the patient should be referred to a dietician to determine if the patient's diet may result in malnutrition or a vitamin deficiency. If that potential exists, then appropriate supplements such as calcium and vitamins may be prescribed. For foods that are essential to prevent malnutrition, a plan for introduction of the food is discussed with the patient.

The open challenge is utilized in patients who have continued to have symptoms in spite of severe food restrictions and desire advice on what type of foods to eat. These patients cook and prepare the food in their usual fashion and eat it in the presence of a nurse or physician. If the patient has no adverse events then the food remains in the diet. After the introduction of several foods in the office without an unusual event, the patient can often be advised to introduce foods on their own at home. These patients will continue to have symptoms but will no longer lose weight or become malnourished. Once the patient has achieved enough variety in their diet the physician can then attempt to treat symptoms.

In patients who have modified their diet and are convinced that foods are continuing to cause symptoms, a well-defined, limited diet (Table 4) with supplemental nutrition (e.g., Vivonex and Ensure) can be prescribed. If there is no improvement in symptoms, the patient should by this time be convinced that foods are not responsible for their symptoms and be willing to increase their diet by adding one food every two days (Table 4). Foods that the patient does not suspect are introduced in an open fashion. Foods that the patient does suspect, and are essential for proper nutrition, are introduced in a single-blind fashion. It is possible to perform these challenges in the office setting with night shades over the eyes and a nose plug so that the patient cannot see or smell the food. Foods can also be masked in tuna fish.

When treatment is first instituted, strict avoidance of all sources of the offending food should be observed. If the initial diagnosis is correct and compliance is maintained, improvement in the patient's condition should result. Eventually, in the absence of anaphylactic sensitivity, small amounts of the offending food may be tolerated on cautious reintroduction into the diet. For example, small amounts of egg may be tolerated when used as an ingredient in the preparation of other foods. In addition, certain foods not tolerated raw or partially cooked may be ingested without difficulty when completely cooked. Usually by practical experience, most patients learn the method of preparation and the volume of a particular food that may be ingested without inducting symptoms, thereby making the diet more manageable.

Medications

Even the most careful patient may inadvertently ingest a food to which he or she is sensitive. When the resulting symptoms of this exposure involve sites distant from the gastrointestinal tract, the treatment for each specific symptom is the same as that for similar allergic reactions. For example, the treatment of food-induced urticaria is the same as the treatment of idiopathic urticaria. Asthma resulting from food ingestion is managed in the same way as asthma provoked by other allergens, including the administration of an aerosolized beta-agonist by inhaler or nebulizer. The treatment for anaphylaxis caused by a food allergy differs only slightly from the treatment of other anaphylactic reactions. In addition to the standard therapy of anaphylaxis, gastric lavage may be necessary to reduce further antigen absorption and exposure.

The patient with anaphylactic sensitivity should be taught how to self-administer epinephrine and should have an epinephrine-containing syringe (e.g., Epi-Pen or ANA kit) and antihistamine available at all times. An identification tag stating the patient's sensitivity is also mandatory. If a patient has epinephrine (two doses), does not have a history of previous life-threatening anaphylaxis, and is within 15 to 20 minutes of medical help, the patient may wait to see if symptoms develop following accidental ingestion of a small amount of food to which he or she is sensitive. If symptoms of an allergic reaction occur such as hoarseness or difficulty in breathing, the patient should administer one dose of subcutaneous epinephrine and seek medical attention. As in bee sting hypersensitivity, the early administration of epinephrine appears to greatly reduce the likelihood of a fatal outcome. Patients with a history of life-threatening anaphylaxis or hypersensitivity to foods who do not have injectable epinephrine should seek medical attention immediately. Patients with a known history of anaphylaxis to foods should avoid the use of beta-blockers and angiotensin converting enzymes (ACE) inhibitors, which will increase the severity of anaphylaxis. These patients may require IV glucagon for adequate treatment of the cardiovascular effects of anaphylaxis.

Gastrointestinal symptoms following inadvertent food ingestion are usually treated with antihistamines. An H_1-antihistamine, such as diphenhydramine hydrochloride in 25 to 50 mg doses three to four times daily, may be administered. As with other members of the ethanolamine series, diphenhydramine has marked sedative properties that may be undesirable in certain patients. Chlorpheniramine, an alkylamine, has a less sedative effect in most patients and may be given initially in doses of 4 mg three to four times daily. Alternatively, newer nonsedative antihistamines may be prescribed.

Antihistamines, in addition to sedative effects, occasionally cause other CNS side effects, such as ataxia, dizziness, and difficulty in concentration. The anticholinergic properties of these drugs may lead to manifestations of atropine poisoning in susceptible patients or when given in large doses. The role of H_2-antihistamines such as cimetidine or renitidine in the treatment of gastrointestinal food reactions has not been determined.

Glucocorticoids are rarely used in the treatment of food allergy. Eosinophilic gastroenteritis and protein-losing gastroenteropathy associated with food allergy are two conditions in which glucocorticoid use may be instituted and the dosage tapered as symptoms resolve. Prednisone in oral dosages up to 60 mg a day may be required initially to ameliorate symptoms. When prolonged glucocorticoid therapy is required, alternate-day therapy with the minimal dosage required to control symptoms should be used. In these instances 10 to 15 mg of prednisone every other day is usually sufficient. Prolonged glucocorticoid therapy should be reserved for severe cases owing to the numerous side effects of this drug.

CONTROVERSIES IN FOOD ALLERGY

Controversy exists over the possible association of food allergy with poorly defined neurologic and behavioral complaints. It has been hypothesized for many years that symptoms such as depression, tension, and fatigue are associated with immunologically mediated reactions to foods. In spite of the longstanding nature of such claims, as yet no firm evidence has been presented to establish such an association. Thus, these problems should not be considered to be secondary to immunologically mediated food reactions.

Other areas of controversy center around two additional modes of treatment of food allergy. The first is whether parenteral or oral administration of dilute concentrations of food extract provides superior efficacy. Controlled studies of sublingual treatment have demonstrated that it is no more effective than placebo. The second area of controversy concerns the prophylactic oral administration of cromolyn sodium or other drugs with mast cell–stabilizing properties. Insufficient clinical evidence exists to support use of such drugs in food allergy, and they are not approved by the Food and Drug Administration for use in this disorder.

SUGGESTED READING

Atkins FM, Steinberg SS, et al. Evaluation of immediate adverse reactions to foods in adults. I. Correlation of demographic, laboratory, and prick skin test data with response to controlled oral challenge. J Allergy Clin Immunol 1985; 75:348–363.

Condemi JJ. Unproved diagnostic and therapeutic techniques. In: Metcalfe DD, Sampson HA, and Simon RA, eds. Food allergy: Adverse reactions to foods and food additives. Boston: Blackwell Scientific Publications, 1991:392–404.

Metcalfe DD. Allergic reactions to foods. In: Frank MM, et al, eds.

Samter's immunologic diseases. 5th ed. Boston: Little, Brown, 1995:1357–1366.
Pearson DJ, Rix KJB. Allergy mimetic reactions to food and pseudofood allergy. In: Dokor P, et al, eds. Pseudoallergic reactions. Vol 4. Basel: Karger, 1985:59.
Terrill EE, Hill SR, et al. A checklist of names for 3,000 vascular plants of economic importance. Agriculture handbook 505. Washington, DC: United States Department of Agriculture. Agricultural Research Service, October 1986.
Yunginger JW, Sweeney KG, et al. Fatal food-induced anaphylaxis. JAMA 1988; 260:1450–1452.

PENICILLIN ALLERGY

MICHAEL S. KAPLAN, M.D.

IMMUNOLOGIC REACTIONS TO PENICILLIN

Penicillins are capable of producing a broad spectrum of immunologic reactions. The scope of these reactions is depicted in Table 1 in approximate order of decreasing frequency. The true incidence of immunologic reactions is unknown but may be as high as 8 percent of all treatment courses in adults and children. The majority of reactions are cutaneous in nature and not serious. A maculopapular or morbilliform nonpruritic eruption occurs in 9 percent of treatment courses with ampicillin. The incidence approaches 100 percent in patients with infectious mononucleosis and is also increased in patients who are receiving allopurinol. This rash and the maculopapular nonpruritic rash associated with penicillin therapy are not IgE mediated, tend to occur late in the course of therapy, are not associated with a risk of anaphylaxis, and can dissipate with continued therapy. The rash can begin even after the penicillin or ampicillin has been discontinued. Reactions encompassing four Gell and Coombs classes of immunopathic responses have been described with the penicillins and are depicted in Table 2. This chapter is devoted to a discussion of type I hypersensitivity.

Table 1 Hypersensitivity Reactions to Penicillins (in Approximate Decreasing Frequency)

Maculopapular rash
Urticarial rash
Fever
Bronchospasm
Vasculitis
Serum sickness
Exfoliative dermatitis
Stevens-Johnson syndrome
Anaphylaxis
Interstitial nephritis

IgE-MEDIATED REACTIONS

Type I hypersensitivity reactions can occur at any dose and with oral, topical, or parenteral preparations. Reactions may occur without previous known exposure. Hidden exposures are thought to occur in foods of animal origin when animals are treated with penicillin injections; from airborne penicillin particles inhaled by health care or pharmaceutical workers; or from small amounts of penicillin in penicillium mold–contaminated foods.

IgE-mediated reactions to penicillin have been classified according to onset of reaction. *Immediate reactions* occur within minutes to 1 hour after a dose of penicillin and present as urticaria, angioedema, laryngeal edema, bronchospasm, or anaphylaxis. *Accelerated reactions* occur within 1 to 72 hours after starting penicillin, manifesting with urticaria, angioedema, laryngeal edema, or bronchospasm. *Late reactions* occur more than 72 hours after penicillin exposure. Late reaction symptoms include morbilliform rash, interstitial nephritis, hemolytic anemia, neutropenia, thrombocytopenia, serum sickness, drug fever, Stevens-Johnson syndrome, and exfoliative dermatitis. These reactions are not IgE mediated, but represent a heterogeny of immune mechanisms. IgE-mediated reactions to penicillin occur in about 2 percent of adult treatment courses.

Anaphylaxis to penicillin is rare, occurring in 0.04 percent to 0.2 percent of treated individuals. Fatal anaphylaxis occurs in one of every 100,000 treated patients; only one-third of patients who had previously received penicillin had a history of a prior reaction. Anaphylaxis may occur after oral penicillin administration or even during skin testing with penicillin determinants. Atopic predisposition is not a factor contributing to overall risk of a hypersensitivity reaction to penicillin, nor is sensitivity to penicillium mold. However, fatal anaphylactic penicillin reactions tend to occur in atopic individuals, and serum sickness reactions to desensitization may occur more frequently in patients with an IgE-mediated penicillin hypersensitivity.

PENICILLIN SKIN TESTING

Who Should Be Tested?

Skin testing all individuals who are to receive penicillin is neither practical nor cost effective. Three

Table 2 Classification of Immunopathic Responses to Penicillins

Gell and Coombs Class	*Mechanism*	*Reaction*	*Comments*
Type I	IgE immediate hypersensitivity	Urticaria; flushing; laryngeal edema; bronchospasm; abdominal pain; diarrhea; hypovolemic shock	Skin testing with PPL, MDM, Pen G; avoid Pcn or desensitize
Type II	IgG, IgM, C′ cytoxic	Hemolytic anemia; thrombocytopenia; nephritis	Pcn determinants bound to cell surface; Coombs-positive anemia; skin test and desensitization not applicable
Type III	Soluble immune complexes, C′, and in some patients IgE	Serum sickness	Circulating immune complexes may be positive; ICs plus C′ on biopsy of involved tissue; some patients have intense IgE response; avoid Pcn, desensitization *not* applicable
Type IV	Delayed hypersensitivity	Contact dermatitis	DH skin test or patch test; avoid Pcn contact

MDM, Minor determinants; *Pcn,* penicillin; *Pen G,* penicillin G; *PPL,* penicilloyl polylysine.

to 10 percent of the adult population will have positive skin tests to penicillin irrespective of a positive history. Patients with a history of only skin reactions to penicillin will have less than a 30 percent skin test reaction rate using accurate test reagents. If the history is one of a morbilliform eruption, the skin test reactivity rate is less than 10 percent.

One school of thought recommends that penicillin skin testing be done only in those patients who have a positive history and in whom therapeutic intervention is imminent. The penicillin testing is valid only for the immediate therapeutic course. If skin testing is negative, the subsequent course of penicillin rarely resensitizes the patient. Testing is recommended before each future treatment course, depending on the severity of prior reactions, skin test responses, and subsequent rechallenges. There is a refractory period of skin test unresponsiveness immediately following a treatment course of penicillin, particularly high-dose therapy. Skin reactivity to penicillin determinants returns within 1 to 3 months.

The incidence of positive skin tests in children with a history of penicillin reactions is low (10 percent), yet many children carry a lifelong label of penicillin allergy. One approach to "clear the air" regarding penicillin sensitivity is to skin test history positive children when penicillin therapy is desirable. If the skin test is negative, then an oral challenge with penicillin is given under observation for 1 hour. The oral challenge is likely to be negative in the face of negative skin tests. Skin test–negative, oral challenge–negative patients can then be given a full therapeutic course of penicillin. Only a few patients will develop a rash under those circumstances, but not a serious systemic reaction. Retesting 4 to 6 weeks after completion of the treatment course will detect patients who have become resensitized or initially sensitized. The incidence of a subsequent positive skin test is low (10 percent). If the skin test is positive, the risk of subsequent reaction is 40 to 73 percent. Approximately one-half of these reactions will be systemic, and one of ten systemic reactions is fatal or near fatal.

Unfortunately, there are no clear-cut risk factors for fatal anaphylaxis. Two-thirds of fatal anaphylactic reactions occur in individuals who have had penicillin before, but without a reaction. However, patients with penicillin hypersensitivity have a higher incidence of other drug reactions, and fatal anaphylaxis tends to occur more frequently in atopic individuals and asthmatics with active disease. Using the above information, the best risk profile for fatal anaphylaxis may be those *atopic individuals,* especially *asthmatics* with *other drug sensitivities* who have received penicillins before, regardless of a history for a prior reaction. The use of beta-blockers is an additional risk when combined with the above factors.

Skin test reactivity to penicillin declines with time. Seventy to 100 percent of history-positive patients will have a positive skin test for at least one of the reagents when tested 2 weeks to 3 months after a penicillin reaction. By 5 years after a reaction, 50 percent of history-positive patients are skin-test negative. Skin-test positivity declines to 20 to 30 percent by 10 years. At any given time, the skin tests are 96 percent reliable. Four percent of history-positive, skin-test negative patients will react to penicillin treatment with approximately 1 percent as accelerated reactions and 3 percent as mild, cutaneous reactions. In one large study, anaphylaxis did not occur in skin-test negative patients.

In vitro assays for specific penicilloyl IgE antibodies are less sensitive than skin tests. Radioallergosorbent test (RAST) or enzyme linked immunosorbent assay (ELISA) for penicilloyl specific IgE antibodies detects only 60 to 95 percent of patients who have a positive skin test to penicilloyl polylysine (PPL).

An in vitro enzyme-linked immune assay for the detection of histamine release from peripheral blood leukocytes (basophils) holds some promise in early trials for detecting penicillin-induced histamine release. Its use as a diagnostic tool is still investigational.

SKIN-TEST REAGENTS

Ninety-five percent of benzylpenicillin is metabolized to the penicilloyl moiety (the major determinant). The remainder is metabolized to a variety of minor determinants which include benzylpenicilloate and penilloate. These metabolic products of penicillin combine easily with serum proteins, creating immunogenic complexes. Thus the penicillins are one of the most common drugs to cause adverse immunologic reactions.

The penicilloyl moiety has been combined with polylysine and is commercially available as PrePen. A positive skin test to PPL is thought to reflect a risk for non–life-threatening reactions such as urticaria, whereas a positive skin test to minor determinants indicates a risk for anaphylaxis.

The minor determinants are not commercially available. Alternatively, fresh benzylpenicillin G has been used along with PPL as a skin-test reagent. Skin testing to penicillin G (Pen G) alone would miss approximately 60 percent of allergic individuals. Aging Pen G to generate minor determinants has no advantage over fresh Pen G when minor determinants are unavailable. If there is a history of serious reaction, then epicutaneous testing (scratch or prick) with a 5 unit per milliliter concentration is used. If the history of a reaction is vague or mild in nature or if the initial skin test with 5 units per milliliter is negative, epicutaneous testing is then performed with a 10,000 unit per milliliter solution. Patients with negative or equivocal responses to the above testing are tested intradermally with 0.02 to 0.04 ml of a 10,000 unit per milliliter mix. A net wheal of 2 mm diameter or greater after 15 to 20 minutes compared to a diluent or saline control is considered positive. A positive histamine control is also used: one drop of 1 mg per milliliter histamine phosphate for epicutaneous tests and 0.02 to 0.04 ml of 0.1 mg per milliter for intradermal tests.

The semisynthetic penicillins contain the same 6 aminopenicillic acid nucleus as benzylpenicillin G. Thus there is a great deal of cross-reactivity with Pen G. Extensive studies indicate that a negative skin test with penicillin G determinants excludes patients at risk for a reaction to semisynthetic penicillins. There may be a small risk for patients to react to antigenic determinants unique to the semisynthetic penicillins. The reagents for these determinants are not commercially available. Serial testing can be done with the specific agent by epicutaneous techniques using concentrations of 0.25 mg per milliliter, 2.5 mg per milliliter, and 25 mg per milliliter. If the epicutaneous tests are negative or equivocal, then intradermal testing can be done serially with concentrations of 2.5 mg per milliliter and 25 mg per milliliter. The testing is interpreted by the same criteria as penicillin G. Skin test reactivity may predict the safe starting level for desensitization. Patients with prick test or low-dose intracutaneous test sensitivity may have to start at one-one thousandth of step 1 doses as listed in the desensitization protocols in Tables 5 and 6. An algorithm for skin testing and treatment is presented in Figure 1.

DESENSITIZATION

If any of the skin tests are positive and an alternative antibiotic (non–beta-lactam) cannot be used, then a protocol to desensitize to penicillin must be employed. It is unclear whether benzylpenicillin G desensitization will provide protection from a reaction to the semisynthetic penicillins or the cephalosporins. It is probably best to desensitize with the specific agent to be used in therapy, employing a modified protocol based on benzylpenicillin desensitization. The mechanism for desensitization is unknown. The overall incidence of immunologic reactions to penicillin during desensitization and subsequent therapy is 27 percent. Most of these reactions are consistent with an IgE-mediated mechanism, but one must also watch for other immunologic reactions such as serum sickness, hemolytic anemia, and interstitial nephritis. The later reactions occur in 5 percent of desensitized patients. Complications encountered during and after desensitization are listed in Table 3. Most reactions encountered during desensitization are fleeting, mild, cutaneous reactions, rhinitis, or wheeze. These reactions can be treated while desensitization proceeds. Skin tests can revert to negative during desensitization.

A checklist as depicted in Table 4 for patients undergoing desensitization is a useful safeguard. Oral desensitization (Table 5) is associated with fewer anaphylactic reactions than parenteral desensitization. This may be a dose-dependent factor. Parenteral desensitization (Table 6) allows visualization for local reactions to allow adjustments in the protocol. If a reaction begins to occur during parenteral desensitization, a tourniquet can be placed proximal to the injection site and ice applied.

Doses are given 15 to 20 minutes apart. Any dose that provokes a mild systemic reaction should be repeated until the patient tolerates that dose, then resume the protocol. Serious systemic reactions should be treated appropriately. If desensitization is continued, then the dose is withheld until the patient has been stabilized. The dose is then reduced by two, ten-fold dilutions and advanced per protocol as tolerated. In general, it is not advisable to pretreat with antihistamines or corticosteroids. This may mask milder reactions that signal a need to alter the desensitization protocol. There is also no firm evidence that such pretreatment is effective for IgE-mediated anaphylaxis. Once therapeutic doses are achieved, the course of therapy should not be interrupted. A lapse of 10 to 12 hours between doses may breach tolerance.

Chronic desensitization is applicable for individuals who are at risk for serious reactions and who frequently encounter beta-lactam antibiotics; examples include nurses or pharmacists who mix penicillin powders and

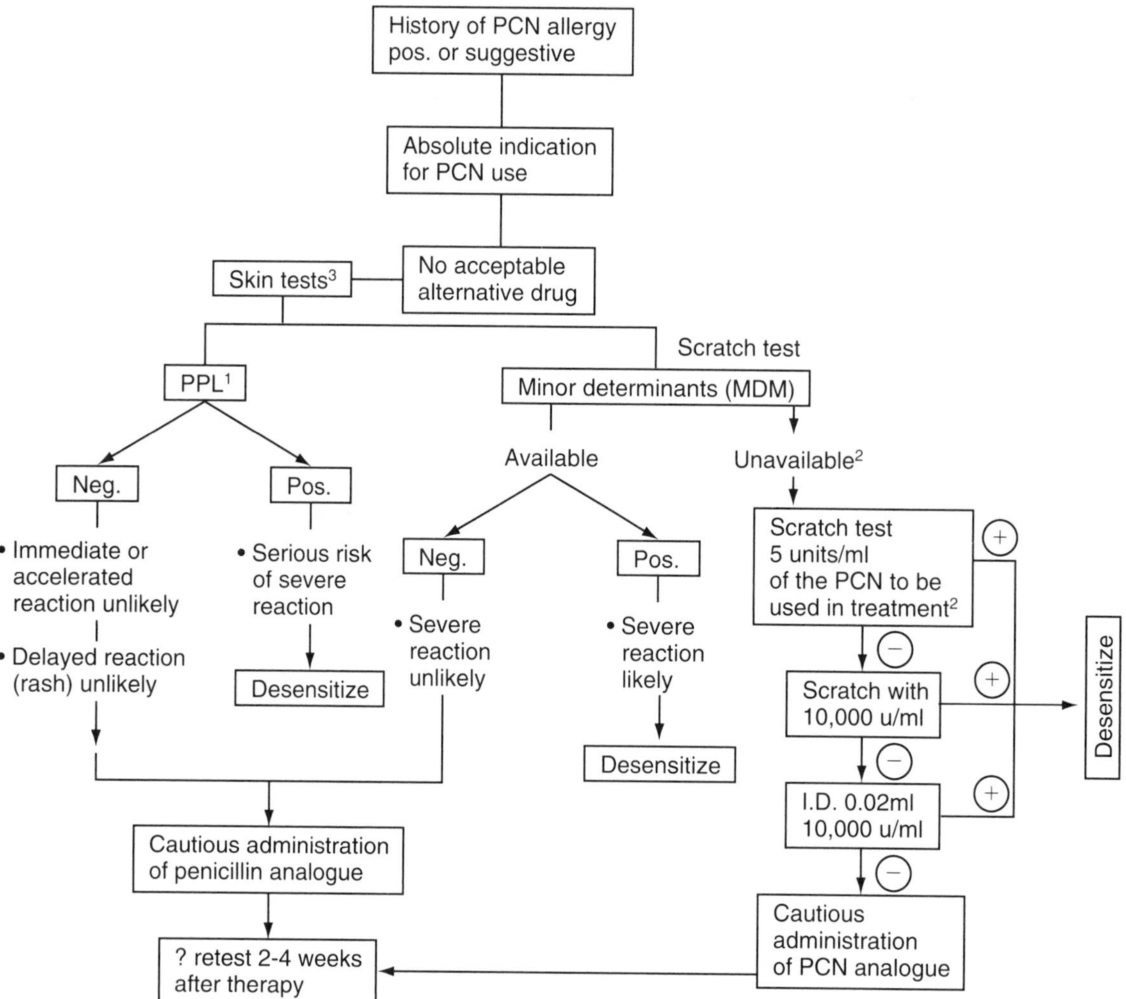

[1] Kremers-Urban Co., Milwaukee, WI.
[2] Fresh Benzyl potassium penicillin 1 million unit vial reconstituted to 100,000 units/ml (stock vial: good for one week). Make 10,000 unit/ml and 5 unit/ml fresh daily; MDM made fresh daily.
[3] Epicutaneous tests are done first; if negative after 20 minutes intradermal tests are done with the same, diluted, reagent as indicated.

Figure 1 Skin testing and treatment.

certain patients with frequent bacterial infections. This may be achieved by daily administration of 250 mg tablets of Pen G. As in acute desensitization, treatment must not lapse more than 8 to 12 hours in order to maintain tolerance.

When a rapid desensitization is needed, such as in a pregnant woman with syphilis, a protocol such as in Table 7 can be used. For exquisitely sensitive patients, a lower starting dose may be used.

Carbipenems

The carbipenems have a bicyclic nucleus analogous to penicillin. It is not surprising that studies have demonstrated a high degree of cross-reactivity between penicillin and imipenem skin-test reagents. Penicillin allergic individuals should also be considered sensitive to carbipenems.

Monobactams

There is no evidence that aztreonam cross-reacts with penicillin. Penicillin-sensitive patients have been treated with aztreonam without adverse sensitivity reactions.

Cephacarbams

Cross-reactivity to penicillin has not been determined.

Table 3 Complications During Desensitization (or as a Consequence of Continued Drug Exposure)

Complication	*Comments*
Cutaneous (not uncommon) Morbilliform Urticarial Maculopapular Angioedema	Do not give higher doses of Pcn when reaction begins to develop Treat with oral antihistamine (AH) For reactions resistant to AH, use Prednisone 20-40 mg per day for 4-7 days (0.5-1 mg/kg/day for children <60 lbs) Continue protocol by resuming at 50% of last tolerated dose (2 steps back from the dose that caused the reaction) Can resume while rash is still present
Respiratory (rare) Asthma Angioedema	Stop protocol. Stabilize respiratory function Restart protocol at 1/100 of original step 1
Anaphylaxis (rare)	Stop protocol. Treat anaphylaxis Re-examine risks vs. benefits of continuing desensitization May resume "low and slow." Restart protocol at 1/100 or less of original step 1. Proceed in half-steps of the original protocol
Serum Sickness (late response)	Patients with IgE-mediated Pcn reactions may be at more risk Prolonged treatment with Prednisone
Nonallergic Serious Reactions Toxic epidermal necrolysis Exfoliative dermatitis Stevens-Johnson syndrome Hepatitis Nephritis Hemolysis Systemic Vasculitis	Contraindicated to continue Pcn

Table 4 Penicillin Desensitization Check List

1. **Document** the absolute need for penicillin
   Life-threatening infection
   No acceptable alternative drug
2. **Informed consent.** Document that risks and benefits were explained to patient or patient's proxy
3. If patient has asthma, **stabilize asthma** first
   Peak flow rate ≥85% of personal best, *or*
   ≥80% of predicted value
4. Perform desensitization **in hospital,** preferably on intensive care unit
   Adequate **personnel** for close observation and monitoring
   Appropriate **equipment and medications** in the immediate area to treat anaphylaxis
   Discontinue beta-blocking agents
5. Start at **lower dose** for patients with stronger skin test responses (i.e., prick vs. intracutaneous response)
6. Ultimately, the **route of administration** by which the drug is to be given should be part of the desensitization protocol
7. Successful desensitization should **proceed immediately into the therapeutic regimen.** Breaks in dosing can result in hypersensitivity reactions
8. **Monitor vital signs frequently** during desensitization and for the first 12 hours on full therapy
9. Ordinarily do not use antihistamines or corticosteroids to premedicate. These agents may mask signs of impending anaphylaxis that allow proper adjustments of the protocol

Cephalosporins

General Considerations

The beta-lactam nucleus of penicillin is attached to a five-member thiazolidine ring. Cephalosporins have a six-member dihydrothiazine ring attached to the beta-lactam nucleus. Cephalosporins are metabolized to the major determinant cephaloyl moiety, which cross-reacts with the penicillin major determinant. Cross-reactivity of penicillin and cephalosporin minor determinants is limited. In a large survey of adverse drug reactions, penicillin accounts for 10.4 percent of all adverse reactions whereas cephalosporins account for 1.3 percent.

The risk of an adverse reaction to cephalosporin in a penicillin-sensitive patient is somewhat controversial. Sullivan reported an overall 51 percent skin test reactivity rate to cephalosporin in 123 penicillin skin test–positive patients. Cephalosporin challenge was not performed in the study; but in another study, 27 history-positive, skin-test positive penicillin-allergic patients were challenged with cephalosporin and none reacted. Cephalosporin skin test was not done. The expected cephalosporin reaction rate in penicillin allergic patients would be 6 or 7 patients (27 patients × 0.51 cross-reaction rate × 0.5 expected reaction rate to challenge in history positive–skin test positive patients). Petz reported an overall reaction rate of 8 percent to

Table 5 Oral Desensitization Protocol

*Step**	*Phenoxymethyl† Penicillin (U/ml)*	*Amount (ml)*	*Dose (U)*	*Cumulative Dosage (U)*	*Cumulative Time Course*
1	1,000	0.1	100	100	
2	1,000	0.2	200	300	
3	1,000	0.4	400	700	
4	1,000	0.8	800	1,500	
5	1,000	1.6	1,600	3,100	
6	1,000	3.2	3,200	6,300	
7	1,000	6.4	6,400	12,700	
8	10,000	1.2	12,000	24,700	
9	10,000	2.4	24,000	48,700	
10	10,000	4.8	48,000	96,700	
11	80,000	1.0	80,000	176,700	
12	80,000	2.0	160,000	336,700	
13	80,000	4.0	320,000	656,700	
14	80,000	8.0	640,000	1,296,700	260 min
		Observe patient for 30 minutes			
	Change to benzylpenicillin G administered IV				
15	500,000	0.25	125,000		
16	500,000	0.50	250,000		
17	500,000	1.0	500,000		
18	500,000	2.25	1,125,000		350 min
19	**Continue with regular therapeutic doses. NOTE: A break in dosing risks a systemic reaction.**				

From Sullivan TJ. Penicillin allergy. In: Lichtenstein LM, Fauci AS, eds. Current therapy in allergy, immunology and rheumatology. Toronto: BC Decker, 1985:60.
*Interval between steps: 20 minutes.
†Solution 1: Stock solution prepared fresh 400,000 U/5 ml (80,000 U/ml).
Solution 2: Take 2 cc of solution 1 and add 14 cc sterile water (= 10,000 U/ml).
Solution 3: Take 2 cc of solution 2 and add 18 cc sterile water (= 1,000 U/ml).

Table 6 Parenteral Desensitization Protocol

*Step**	*Concentration of β-Lactam Drug (mg/ml)*	*Benzyl-penicillin (Units/ml)*	*Amount (ml subcutaneously)*	*Cumulative Time Course*
1	0.1	100	0.10	
2	0.1	100	0.20	
3	0.1	100	0.40	
4	0.1	100	0.80	
5	1	1,000	0.15	
6	1	1,000	0.30	
7	1	1,000	0.60	
8	10	10,000	0.10	
9	10	10,000	0.20	
10	10	10,000	0.40	
11	10	10,000	0.80	
12	100	100,000	0.15	
13	100	100,000	0.30	
14	100	100,000	0.60	
15	1,000	1,000,000	0.10	
16	1,000	1,000,000	0.20	
17	1,000	1,000,000	0.40	
18	1,000	1,000,000	0.50	340 min
		Observe patient for 30 minutes		
19	1,000	1,000,000 U/hr continuous	IV (0.5g)	370 min
20	1,000	Continuous IV	IV (1.5 g)	400 min
		NOTE: A break in dosing risks a systemic reaction.		

From Sullivan TJ. Penicillin allergy. In: Lichtenstein LM, Fauci AS, eds. Current therapy in allergy, immunology and rheumatology. Toronto: BC Decker, 1985:61.
*Interval between steps, 20 minutes.

Table 7 An Example of Rapid Desensitization to Benzathine Penicillin

Concentration (units/cc)	*Dose (units/0.1 cc)*	*Cumulative Dose (units)*	*Elapsed Time*
1	0.1 SC	0.1	
10	1.0 SC	1.1	
100	10 SC	11.1	
1,000	100 SC	111.1	
10,000	1,000 SC	1,111.1	
100,000	10,000 SC	11,111.1	
1,000,000	100,000 SC	111,111.1	
	200,000 IM	311,111.1	
	2.1 million IM	2,411,111.1	170 min

cephalosporins in 450 penicillin-sensitive patients. The risk of cross-reaction with penicillin differs among the various cephalosporins; in general, it is more common with the first- and second-generation cephalosporins (Cephaloridin 16.5 percent, Cephalothin 5 percent, Cephalexin 5.4 percent). In Petz's survey only one patient of 9,385 without a history of penicillin sensitivity had an anaphylactic reaction to a cephalosporin (0.1 percent). The risk for anaphylaxis to cephalosporins in penicillin-sensitive patients was 0.4 percent. The rate of urticarial reactions to cephalosporins was 1.3 percent in penicillin-sensitive patients and 0.4 percent in patients without a history of penicillin sensitivity. However, the reaction rate to immunologically unrelated drugs is also of this magnitude in penicillin-allergic patients. Since cephalosporin skin testing was not done in this survey, the precise relationship between cephalosporin and penicillin cross-reactivity is unclear.

The extent of cross-reactivity among the cephalosporins is unknown. It is likely to be low if the clinically relevant antibodies are side-chain specific. Antibodies to the monobactam, aztreonam are side-chain specific and therefore do not cross-react with either penicillin or cephalothin. Ceftazidine, which has an identical aminothiazolyl side-chain, can inhibit aztreonam antibodies in vitro.

Cephalosporin Skin Tests

The predictive value of using native cephalosporins as skin-test reagents is unknown. The nature of the haptenic determinants is also unknown. Native cephalosporins in concentrations of 1 mg per milliliter or greater cause nonspecific skin reactivity. The skin test reagent for cephalosporin is prepared by making a 10^{-3} mol per liter solution in phosphate-buffered saline. This stock solution is made fresh. Sequential epicutaneous tests are then done with 1:10,000, 1:1,000, and 1:100 dilutions. Negative or equivocal reactions are followed by intradermal testing in the same sequence. The use of penicillin skin-test reagents to predict cephalosporin sensitivity is not completely clear since the studies that suggest cross-reactivity did not challenge patients with cephalosporins, and challenge studies in penicillin-sensitive patients did not look at cephalosporin skin reactivity. On the other hand, the rate of reactions to cephalosporins in penicillin-sensitive patients is low and usually limited to cutaneous reactions and the occurrence of anaphylaxis is very low. At this time a positive skin test to dilute native cephalosporin should be interpreted as reflecting a risk for a hypersensitivity reaction. However, a negative skin test does not rule out this risk and should be taken as "no information."

Before treating with a cephalosporin, patients with a history of penicillin sensitivity should be skin tested with penicillin reagents. Those patients with a negative skin test may be treated with penicillin or cephalosporin. The reaction rate is likely to be very low and limited to cutaneous reactions. Patients who are history-positive and skin-test positive to penicillin should be skin tested with the cephalosporin of choice. Individuals who are also cephalosporin skin-test positive should avoid both drugs. Alternatively, cautious administration of cephalosporin as dictated by the clinical situation should follow the desensitization model used for penicillin.

REMARKS

The risk of a reaction to penicillin is dependent on such factors as a history of prior reaction, a history of multiple drug sensitivities, time interval since the prior penicillin reaction, and persistence of specific IgE antibodies. From a procedural point of view, the most useful parameter in assessing a patient's risk is skin-test response to major and minor determinants or penicillin G if the minor determinant mix is unavailable. A positive reaction identifies a patient at risk for a serious reaction to penicillin or a cross-reacting beta-lactam drug. Such medications should then be avoided or a desensitization protocol should be used if alternative medication is undesirable.

SUGGESTED READING

Anderson JA. Cross-sensitivity to cephalosporins in patients allergic to penicillin. Pediatr Infect Dis J 1986; 5:557–561.

Cameron W, Windt M, Borish L, et al. A complicated case of penicillin allergy. Ann Allergy 1984; 53:455.
Green G, Rosenblum A, Sweet L. Evaluation of penicillin hypersensitivity: Value of clinical history and skin testing with penicilloyl-polylysine and penicillin G. J Allergy Clin Immunol 1977; 60:339–345.
Levine BB. Immunologic mechanisms of penicillin allergy. A haptenic model system for the study of allergic disease of man. N Engl J Med 1966; 275:1115–1125.
Lin RY. A perspective on penicillin allergy. Arch Intern Med 1992; 152:930–937.
Petz LD. Immunologic reactions of humans to cephalosporins. Postgrad Med J 1971; 47(suppl):64–69.
Saxon A, Beall GN, Rohr AS, Adelman DC. Immediate hypersensitivity reactions to beta-lactam antibiotics. Ann Int Med 1987; 107:204–215.
Sogn DD, Evans R III, Shepherd GM, et al. Results of the NIAID collaborative clinical trial to test the predictive value of skin testing with major and minor penicillin derivatives in hospitalized adults. Arch Intern Med 1992; 152:1025–1032.
Sullivan TJ, Wedner H, Shatz G, et al. Skin testing to detect penicillin allergy. J Allergy Clin Immunol 1981; 68:171–180.
Weiss ME, Adkinson NF. Immediate hypersensitivity reactions to penicillin and related antibiotics. Clin Allergy 1988; 18:515–540.

DRUG REACTIONS

RICHARD D. DESHAZO, M.D.
DAVID L. SMITH, M.D.

EPIDEMIOLOGY

Adverse reactions to drugs (ADRs) occur in 15 to 30 percent of hospitalized patients. Most of these reactions are not severe, although deaths occur in up to 0.1 percent. No more than 10 percent of ADRs are due to drug allergy. The worst of these, anaphylaxis, has been most often reported with beta-lactam antibiotics. For instance, anaphylaxis to penicillin occurs in 0.002 percent of drug courses. Adverse drug reactions are a special problem in the elderly.

CLASSIFICATION OF DRUG REACTIONS AND SOME GENERAL PRINCIPLES

ADRs are classified as predictable or unpredictable (Table 1). A *predictable drug reaction* is related to the pharmacologic actions of the drug, is seen in otherwise normal patients, and although uncommon, is known to occur. *Unpredictable reactions* are related to immunologic responses (hypersensitivity reactions) or to genetic differences in susceptible patients (idiosyncrasy or intolerance). A subtype, the *pseudoallergic* reaction, mimics an allergic reaction, but has nonimmunologic mechanisms (Table 2).

Table 1 Classification of Adverse Drug Reactions with Some Representative Examples

Predictable Adverse Reactions

I. Toxicity due to overdosage; seizures secondary to theophylline
II. Side effects: immediate or delayed; sedation with antihistamines
III. Secondary or indirect effects
  A. Related to drug alone; disturbance of bacterial flora
  B. Related to both disease and drugs; maculopapular rash to ampicillin with viral infections
IV. Interactions between or among drugs: bleeding with warfarin and cimetidine

Unpredictable Reactions

I. Intolerance: A known effect occurring with an unusually small dose; tinnitus due to small doses of aspirin
II. Idiosyncratic reactions in patients with abnormal metabolism (see Table 3)
III. Allergic (immunologic) or pseudoallergic reactions (see Table 2)

Modified from DeSwarte RD. Drug Allergy. In: Patterson R, ed. Allergic diseases: Diagnosis and management. 4th ed. Philadelphia: JB Lippincott, 1993:395.

Table 2 Pseudoallergic Reactions with Some Representative Examples

A. Anaphylactoid reactions (mast cell mediator release without IgE involvement): opiates, radiocontrast media, desferoxamine, vancomycin
B. Probably involving accumulation of bradykinin: cough, angioedema due to ACE inhibitors
C. Probably due to excess leukotriene production: aspirin-induced asthma or urticaria
D. Bronchospasm: inhaled or ingested sulfites, beta-blockade

RISK FACTORS FOR DRUG REACTIONS

A variety of *abnormalities of drug metabolism* occur and predispose to idiosyncratic and immunologic reactions (Table 3). In patients with the slow acetylator phenotype, drug metabolism may proceed by alternative pathways predisposing to the production of toxic metabolites. These metabolites can form haptens with tissue proteins and produce neoantigens. This occurs in the metabolism of sulfonamides to reactive hydroxylamines. Drug-induced lupus is also more common in slow acetylators. Serum sickness-like reactions to cefaclor may be due to variant metabolism because patients with this response usually tolerate other beta-lactam antibiotics.

Age-related abnormalities in drug pharmacology contribute to the fact that ADRs increase with age. Psychotropic and cardiovascular agents are the more common causes of serious ADRs in the elderly, perhaps because of the narrow therapeutic-toxic window with these drugs. Although drug absorption is probably normal in most elderly patients, abnormalities of drug distribution, metabolism, excretion, and cellular response to drugs are present. For instance, age-related decreases in serum albumin increase serum levels of highly protein-bound drugs. Changes in total body weight and lean body mass effect the volume of distribution and drug half-life. First-pass drug metabolism (oxidation, reduction, and hydroxylation) decreases with age while second-pass metabolism (biotransformation, acetylation, glucuronidation) is less affected. Age-related changes in creatinine clearance also have profound changes on serum drug concentrations.

Table 3 Examples of Genetic Variants in Drug Metabolism Predisposing to Drug Reactions

G6PD deficiency
- Hemolytic anemia: sulfonamides, nitrofurans, vitamin K analogues, sulfones, 8-aminoquinolones, aminosalicylic acid, probenecid, quinidine, aminopyrine, chloramphenicol, aspirin

Slow acetylation
- Drug-induced lupus: isoniazid, hydralazine, ? procainamide
- Drug toxicity: isoniazid

Slow acetylation or oxygenated amine detoxification phenotype
- Increased toxic oxidative metabolites: sulfonamides

Fast acetylation
- Hepatotoxicity: isoniazid (increased likelihood with rifampin, decreased with para-aminosalicylic acid)

Abnormal plasma cholinesterase
- Prolonged paralysis: succinylcholine

Epoxide hydrolase deficiency
- Toxicity: phenytoin

Hemoglobin Zurich
- Methemoglobinemia, hemolysis: sulfonamides

Hemoglobin H
- Hemolytic anemia: sulfonamides, nitrites, methylene blue

Subclinical myopathy with elevated CPK
- Malignant hyperthermia: succinylcholine, halothane

Coumarin resistance
- Decreased sensitivity: coumarin

Protein C deficiency
- Skin necrosis: coumarin

Selective IgA deficiency
- Anaphylaxis: blood products containing IgA

Specific HLA types
- Toxic epidermal necrolysis: sulfonamides (HLA B12)
- Agranulocytosis: levamisole (HLA B27)
- Drug-induced lupus: hydralazine (HLA DR4)
- Nephrotoxicity: gold, penicillamine (HLA DR3)
- Thrombocytopenia: gold (HLA DR3)

Developed partly from data of Van Arsdel PP Jr. Classification and risk factors for drug allergy. Immunol Allergy Clin North Am 1991; 11:475.

Specific HLA haplotypes are linked to an increased risk of developing immunologic reactions to certain medications (Table 3). Although atopy per se is not strongly linked to a risk for drug reactions, there may be a familial tendency to drug allergy independent of specific HLA associations. A multiple-drug allergy syndrome has been described in a group of patients who have had IgE-mediated reactions to many drugs. Drug allergy also appears to be more common in females than males.

Other risk factors include *bronchial hyper-reactivity and HIV infection.* Patients with bronchial hyper-reactivity may be sensitive to beta-blockers, including those in eye drops. Beta-blockers may also increase the severity of anaphylactic reactions and decrease the response to epinephrine used to treat them. Patients with HIV infections, especially those with AIDS, have frequent immunologic drug reactions, perhaps related to a deficiency of glutathione, which detoxifies hydroxylamines.

PATTERNS OF ADVERSE DRUG REACTIONS

Certain drugs predictably produce patterns of adverse drug reactions often involving specific organ systems. At least seven of these patterns exist (Table 4) and are briefly reviewed below:

Multisystem Patterns

Anaphylactic (IgE-mediated) or *anaphylactoid* (mast cell degranulation by mechanisms other than IgE) reactions frequently involve multiple organ systems. Common manifestations include urticaria and/or angioedema, itching, bronchospasm, laryngeal obstruction, and hypotension. Anaphylactic reactions may occur in response to any foreign protein to which the patient has been previously exposed. Most drugs have been reported to cause anaphylaxis and cross-allergenicity among chemically similar drugs appears common. For instance, patients with hypersensitivity reactions to sulfonamide antimicrobial agents may react to oral hypoglycemic drugs, or thiazide diuretics. Administration of opiates may activate dermal opiate receptors, which may lead to anaphylactoid reactions, primarily urticaria and hypotension. Iodinated radiocontrast media may cause anaphylactoid reactions, perhaps by activation of the complement system with subsequent mast cell degranulation via mast cell complement receptors. Other agents causing anaphylactoid reactions include vancomycin, dextran, and polymyxin B.

Table 4 Some Organ-Specific Patterns of Adverse Drug Reactions

I. Multisystem Patterns
Anaphylactic-anaphylactoid: antimicrobials, proteins, iodinated contrast media, NSAIDs, ethylene oxide, taxol
Stevens-Johnson syndrome or toxic epidermal necrolysis: sulfonamides, beta-lactam antibiotics, hydantoins, carbamazepine
Hypersensitivity syndrome: anticonvulsants, sulfonamides, allopurinol
Serum sickness or vasculitis: proteins, antimicrobials, allopurinol, thiazides, pyrazolones, hydantoins, propylthiouracil
Drug fever: bleomycin, amphotericin B, sulfonamides, beta-lactam antibiotics, methyldopa, quinidine, procainamide
Drug-induced lupus: hydralazine, procainamide, isoniazid, methyldopa, chloropromazine, quinidine, anticonvulsants

II. Dermatologic Patterns
Urticaria-angioedema: same as for anaphylactic reactions, plus opiates. Isolated angioedema: ACE inhibitors
Pruritus without urticaria: gold, sulfonamides
Morbilliform rashes: penicillins, sulfonamides, barbiturates, antituberculosis drugs, anticonvulsants, quinidine
Fixed eruption: phenolphthalein, analgesic-antipyretics, barbiturates, beta-lactam antibiotics, sulfonamides, tetracycline
Photoallergic photosensitivity: phenothiazines, sulfonamides, griseofulvin
Phototoxic photosensitivity: tetracyclines, sulfanilamide, chlorpromazine, psoralens
Contact dermatitis: local anesthetics, neomycin, paraben esters, ethylenediamine, antihistamines, mercurials

III. Hepatic Patterns
Cholestasis: macrolides, phenothiazines, hypoglycemics, imipramine, nitrofurantoin
Hepatocellular: valproic acid, halothane, isoniazid, methyldopa, quinidine, nitrofurantoin, phenytoin, sulfonylureas
Granulomatous: quinidine, allopurinol, methyldopa, sulfonamides

IV. Renal Patterns
Nephrosis (membranous glomerulonephritis): gold, captopril, NSAIDs, penicillamine, probenecid, anticonvulsants
Acute interstitial nephritis: beta-lactams (especially methicillin), rifampin, NSAIDs, sulfonamides, captopril, allopurinol

V. Respiratory Patterns
Rhinitis: reserpine, hydralazine, alpha–receptor blockers, anticholinesterases, iodides, levodopa, triethanolamine
Asthma: inhaled proteins (pancreatic extract, psyllium), beta-lactam antibiotics, sulfites, NSAIDs, β-receptor blockers
Cough: ACE inhibitors
Pulmonary infiltrates with eosinophilia: nitrofurantoin, methotrexate, NSAIDs, sulfonamides, tetracycline, isoniazid
Chronic fibrotic reactions: nitrofurantoin, cytotoxic chemotherapeutics

VI. Hematologic Patterns
Eosinophilia: gold, allopurinol, 5-ASA, ampicillin, tricyclics, capreomycin, carbamazepine, digitalis, phenytoin
Thrombocytopenia: quinidine, sulfonamides, gold, heparin
Hemolytic anemia (Coombs' positive)
  Hapten-carrier mechanism: penicillin, cisplatin
  "Innocent bystander," sulfonamides, quinines, chloropromazine, para-aminosalicylicacid
  Drug-induced autoimmune antibodies: methyldopa, penicillin
Granulocytopenia: sulfasalazine, procainamide, penicillins, phenothiazines

VII. Reticuloendothelial Patterns
Phenytoin, penicillin, aminosalicylic acid, dapsone

Modified from DeSwarte RD. Drug Allergy. In: Patterson R, ed. Allergic diseases: Diagnosis and management. 4th ed. Philadelphia: JB Lippincott, 1993:395.

Adverse reactions to local anesthetics, neuromuscular blockers, and nonsteroidal anti-inflammatory compounds (NSAIDs) require specific comments. Although frequently discussed, true anaphylaxis or anaphylactoid reactions to local anesthetics is rare or nonexistent. The usual causes of ADRs to these agents include vasovagal syncope and inadvertent systemic administration. Serious reactions to neuromuscular blockers may occur via specific IgE. However some neuromuscular blockers such as tubocurarine have intrinsic histamine-releasing activity.

The *Stevens-Johnson syndrome* (SJS), which may occur after the administration of penicillin, sulfa-based antimicrobials, and other drugs, is characterized by a macular rash (sometimes with necrotic centers), fever, stomatitis, and conjunctivitis. It overlaps with and may evolve into the syndrome of *toxic epidermal necrolysis* (TEN) associated with extensive epidermal loss and a scalded skin appearance. SJS and TEN are absolute contraindications to readministration of suspect drugs. The *hypersensitivity syndrome* is an ADR to aromatic antiepileptic agents and sulfonamides and is associated with an exanthematous to purpuric rash with one or more systemic manifestations. These include fever, lymphadenopathy, hepatitis, nephritis, carditis, eosinophilia, and atypical lymphocytes in the peripheral blood. It most frequently appears after 2 to 6 weeks of drug administration. *Serum sickness* is an immune complex reaction characterized by fever, lymphadenopathy, and cutaneous vasculitis beginning 10 to 14 days after administration of xenogenic proteins. Similar vasculitic reactions occur to beta-lactam antibiotics and may last up to several months. Cutaneous vasculitis is characterized by palpable purpura and may be accompanied by vasculitis in other organs. *Drug fever* may be associated with maculopapular or urticarial rashes and leukocytosis, or may occur alone. The latter is the case with bleomycin and amphotericin B.

Dermatologic Patterns

Cutaneous reactions to drugs occur in 2 to 3 percent of hospitalized patients. Certain patterns occur predictably to certain drugs. However, *urticaria and/or angioedema* has been reported with almost all drugs. Angiotensin converting enzyme (ACE) inhibitors may cause isolated angioedema, which begins as late as several months after beginning therapy, probably by increasing tissue levels of bradykinin. The pathophysiology of the *drug-related morbilliform dermatitis* associated with beta-lactam antibiotics is poorly understood. Most patients with this response remain otherwise asymptomatic, but in a small number, the rash may proceed to more serious reactions. The *fixed eruption,* a nummular eczema reoccurring in the same area on reexposure to a drug, is thought to be lymphocyte mediated. Eczematous *photoallergic reactions* are thought to be due to ultraviolet-induced immunogenic alterations of drugs in the skin, whereas blistering *phototoxic reactions* appear to be due to absorption and transmission of light energy by drugs. Numerous drugs, even diphenhydramine, applied topically may produce *contact dermatitis.* In a given medicinal, the culprit may be a preservative or other excipient rather than the active drug. After contact sensitivity occurs, administration of the drug by another route may lead to a generalized eczematoid reaction as is the case with contact dermatitis to ethylenediamine followed by a generalized dermatitis to aminophylline.

Hepatic Patterns

Hepatic reactions may mimic any acute or chronic hepatobiliary disease. *Cholestatic reactions* are characterized by jaundice without elevation of enzymes other than alkaline phosphatase; however, fever, rash, and eosinophilia may be present. Recovery is not always rapid after withdrawal of the drug and chronic cholestasis has been described. Erythromycin estolate has been implicated in such reactions more often than other erythromycin salts, probably because it is better absorbed. *Hepatocellular reactions* to drugs are characterized by hepatic enzyme elevations and may cause fulminant hepatic failure. Both hepatotoxic metabolites and immunologic mechanisms have been suggested, and antinuclear and smooth muscle antibodies are sometimes seen. Mixed patterns of cholestatic and hepatocellular disease occur, and variable hepatic necrosis may be seen with *granulomatous reactions.* Methotrexate may produce *cirrhosis* without prodromal enzyme elevations.

Renal Patterns

Drug-induced *nephrotic syndrome* appears related to drug-induced immune complexes. Resolution is usually rapid on drug withdrawal, but proteinuria may persist for several years. Drug-induced *interstitial nephritis* is a common cause of renal failure and hypersensitivity manifestations such as fever, rash, arthralgia, and eosinophilia, and eosinophiluria may coexist.

Respiratory Patterns

With the exception of reactions to triethanolamine, *drug-associated rhinitis* is felt to occur on a nonimmunologic basis. *Asthmatic reactions* to inhaled proteins are almost always IgE-mediated, but asthmatic reactions to inhaled or ingested sulfite generally occur by nonimmunologic mechanisms. *Cough* is the predominant symptom in the syndrome of drug-induced pulmonary infiltrates with eosinophilia (PIE). Cough also occurs as a response to ACE inhibitors. Reactions to nitrofurantoin are associated with cough and pleural effusions; pulmonary fibrosis occurs in as many as 1 of 750 long-term users. *Pulmonary edema* may occur in opiate overdoses, with toxic doses of salicylates, and with hydrochlorothiazide (but not other thiazide diuretics). Aspirin and other NSAIDs are prostaglandin synthetase inhibitors and may induce overproduction of leukotrienes, causing urticaria, anaphylaxis, or *exacerbations of rhinosinusitis and asthma* in some individuals (see the chapter *Aspirin Sensitivity in Rhinosinusitis and Asthma*). NSAIDs also cause a syndrome of *aseptic meningitis.*

Hematologic Patterns

Eosinophilia occurs with or without other manifestations of drug allergy. Eosinophilia without other manifestations requires observation but not necessarily drug withdrawal. Drug-induced *thrombocytopenia* and Coomb's positive *hemolytic anemia* include the "hapten-carrier" (chemical combination of a drug metabolite with cell surface) and the "innocent bystander" (antigen-antibody complexes associated with cell surface, with subsequent complement activation) types. In addition some drugs induce anti–red cell antibodies. Modification of the RBC membrane by cephalosporins results in nonspecific uptake of immunoglobulins and a positive Coombs' test without hemolysis.

Reticuloendothelial Patterns

Phenytoin may produce *depression of serum IgA* and cell-mediated immunity, leukopenia and lymphadenopathy. Rarely patients develop lymphoma even when the drug is stopped. *Angioimmunoblastic* (hyperglobulinemic) *lymphadenopathy* has been described with penicillin and phenytoin.

APPROACH TO THE PATIENT WITH A HISTORY OF A DRUG REACTION WHO REQUIRES DRUG TREATMENT FOR THE SAME INDICATION

For most patients with a history of drug reaction who require drug treatment for the same indication a systematic approach resolves the problem. This ap-

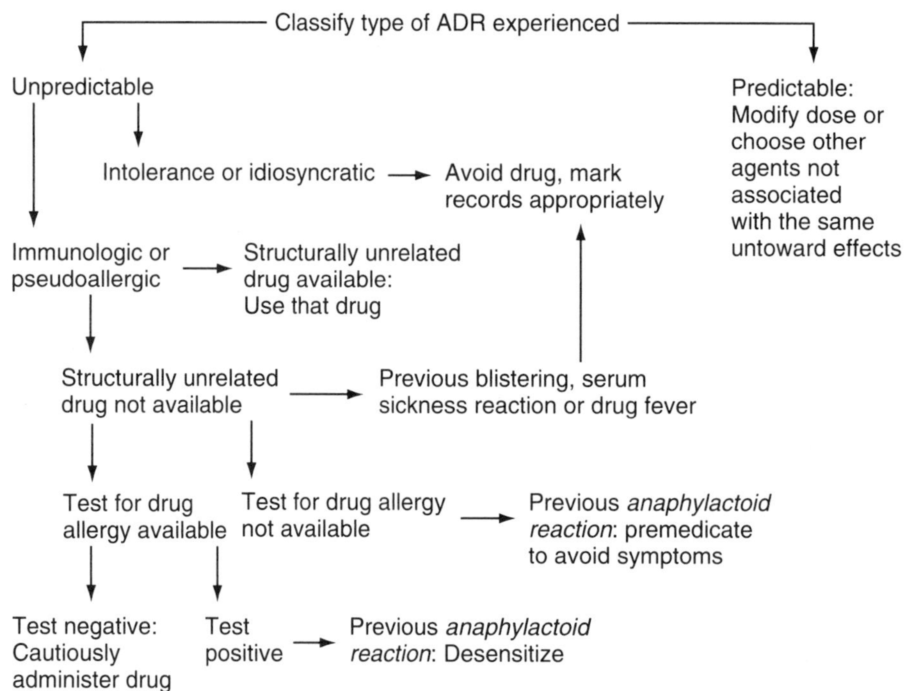

Figure 1 Approach to the patient with a previous ADR who requires treatment for the same indication.

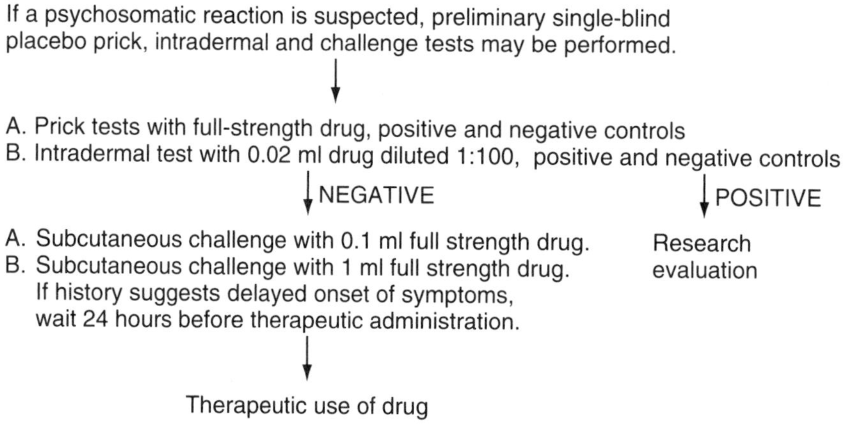

If a psychosomatic reaction is suspected, preliminary single-blind placebo prick, intradermal and challenge tests may be performed.

↓

A. Prick tests with full-strength drug, positive and negative controls
B. Intradermal test with 0.02 ml drug diluted 1:100, positive and negative controls

↓ NEGATIVE → A. Subcutaneous challenge with 0.1 ml full strength drug.
B. Subcutaneous challenge with 1 ml full strength drug.
If history suggests delayed onset of symptoms, wait 24 hours before therapeutic administration.

↓

Therapeutic use of drug

↓ POSITIVE → Research evaluation

Figure 2 Method of skin testing and provocative dose challenge for local anesthetics. (Modified from deShazo RD, Nelson HS. An approach to the patient with a history of local anesthetic hypersensitivity: Experience with 90 patients. J Allergy Clin Immunol 1979; 63:387.)

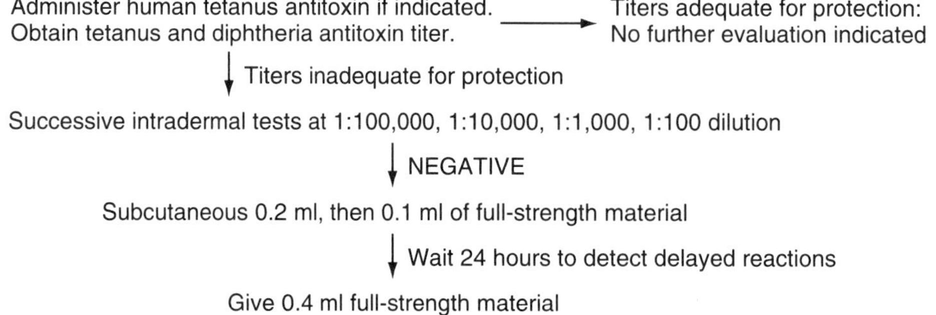

Figure 3 Suggested skin testing/challenge procedure for patients with possible hypersensitivity to tetanus/Diphtheria toxoid. (Modified from Jacobs RL, Lowe RS, Lanier BQ. Adverse reactions to tetanus toxoid. JAMA 1982; 247:40.)

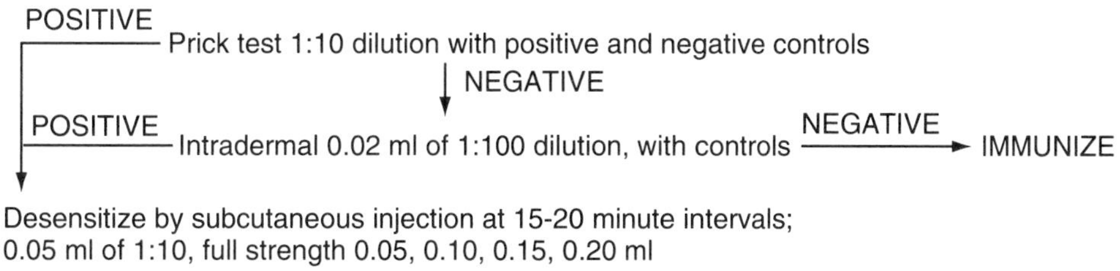

POSITIVE — Prick test 1:10 dilution with positive and negative controls
↓ NEGATIVE
POSITIVE — Intradermal 0.02 ml of 1:100 dilution, with controls — NEGATIVE → IMMUNIZE
↓
Desensitize by subcutaneous injection at 15-20 minute intervals;
0.05 ml of 1:10, full strength 0.05, 0.10, 0.15, 0.20 ml

Figure 4 Suggested skin testing/desensitization procedure for patients with possible sensitivity to MMR, influenza yellow fever vaccines. (Modified from Peter G, ed. Report of the Committee on Infectious Diseases. 22nd ed. Elk Grove Village, Ill: American Academy of Pediatrics, 1991:29.)

Table 5 A Protocol for Intravenous Desensitization to an Aminoglycoside Using Tobramycin

*Dose No.**	*Tobramycin Dose (mg)*	*Dose No.*	*Tobramycin Dose (mg)*
1	0.001	10	0.512
2	0.002	11	1
3	0.004	12	2
4	0.008	13	4
5	0.016	14	8
6	0.032	15	16
7	0.064	16	32
8	0.128	17	16
9	0.256	(Total dose of 80 mg)	

Modified from Earl HS, Sullivan TJ. Acute desensitization of a patient with cystic fibrosis allergic to both betalactam and aminoglycoside antibiotics. J Allergy Clin Immunol 1987; 79:477.

*Doses are given 30 minutes apart.

Table 6 A Protocol for Desensitization to Trimethoprim Sulfamethoxazole (T/S)

Day	*Dose*	*T/S*
1	1 ml of 1:20 pediatric suspension	0.4/2 mg
2	2 ml of 1:20 pediatric suspension	0.8/4 mg
3	4 ml of 1:20 pediatric suspension	1.6/8 mg
4	8 ml of 1:20 pediatric suspension	3.2/16 mg
5	1 ml of undiluted pediatric suspension	8/40 mg
6	2 ml of pediatric suspension	16/80 mg
7	4 ml of pediatric suspension	32/160 mg
8	8 ml of pediatric suspension	64/320 mg
9	1 tablet	80/400 mg
10	1 double-strength (DS) tablet	160/800 mg

Modified from Absar N, Daneshvar H, Beall G. Desensitization to trimethoprim/sulfamethoxazole in HIV-infected patients. J Allergy Clin Immunol 1994; 93:1001.

proach requires a knowledge of the material previously discussed and is outlined in Figure 1.

First, *determine what type of ADR the patient had experienced.* More often than not, the patient seen for evaluation of drug allergy has had a *predictable* drug reaction such as a side effect. In such a case the problem may resolve with a modification in dose or change in agent. Taking a more detailed history may reveal only a poorly characterized rash that occurred in early childhood, which is unlikely to recur. The physician should correct erroneous chart entries and stickers and educate the patient. If, after review of the history, a serious reaction on readministration is considered highly unlikely but further security is desired, the consenting patient may be given an initial small dose in a setting where anaphylaxis can be adequately treated. *Intolerance or idiosyncratic* reactions are not amenable to immunologic manipulation and require avoidance of the responsible drug and others of the same chemical class.

Evaluation and therapy for an *immunologic* drug reaction, such as with skin testing and/or desensitization, may result in anaphylaxis. Personnel familiar with and equipped to treat anaphylaxis must be available throughout the procedure, which should not be undertaken unless the drug is absolutely necessary. For instance, penicillin skin testing is not required if the patient does not require the drug. The patient should be assured that the physician is available if further consultation is required. If an alternative structurally unrelated drug is available, that drug may be used without further evaluation. If the reaction consisted of SJS, TEN, serum sickness, or a drug fever, avoid further administration of the drug. In the absence of a suitable alternate drug, evaluation usually consists of skin testing for IgE-mediated hypersensitivity where available; in vitro tests may be substituted in some cases but are generally regarded as being less reliable. For instance, skin testing has been successfully used to find a nonreacting neuromuscular blocker for patients with IgE-mediated sensitivity to one or more of these agents while in vitro testing frequently gives false-positive results (see Suggested Reading). Skin testing is often immediately followed by a challenge procedure if negative or desensitization if positive. Drugs for which skin testing may be followed by graduated challenge include local anesthetics (Figure 2) and tetanus toxoid (Figure 3). A skin test-challenge protocol for streptokinase consists of 0.1 ml of 1,000 IU per milliliter, with positive and negative controls. Testing and challenge-desensitization to MMR, yellow fever, and influenza vaccines (Figure 4) may be undertaken in the patient with clinical sensitivity (unable to eat) to eggs but is not required merely because of a positive skin test to egg. Drugs for which a positive skin test is often followed by desensitization include beta-lactam antibiotics (see the chapter *Penicillin Allergy*) and proteins, such as insulin (see the chapter *Insulin Allergy and Insulin Resistance*). Package inserts for heterologous serums give appropriate procedures for skin testing and desensitization.

Desensitization to a limited number of drugs has been successful even when skin testing is not available or is unreliable. Most regimens for prevention of anaphylactic reactions to such drugs, such as aminoglycosides (Table 5), give a doubling dose every 15 to 20 minutes such that a full therapeutic dose has been given after 3 to 8 hours. The patient will usually remain desensitized as long as the drug is administered at least every 12 hours, but if therapy is interrupted, desensitization may have to be repeated. Oral desensitization appears to be safer than parenteral desensitization. Desensitization for less acute immunologic reactions such as to trimethoprim-sulfamethoxazole has been most successfully performed over a period of several days to weeks (Table 6). Desensitization to NSAIDs (see the chapter *Aspirin Sensitivity in Rhinosinusitis and Asthma*) has been successful for asthmatic but not urticarial drug reactions. If the reaction was anaphylactoid in nature, premedication may serve to minimize or prevent symptoms on readministration. Premedication with corticosteroid and antihistamines has been shown to reduce the reaction rate to radiocontrast media to less than 5 percent (Table 7), and may be similarly effective for other anaphylactoid reactions such as those to taxol. Although premedication has not been shown to be similarly effective for anaphylaxis, it may be used when there is no choice but to give the drug.

Table 7 A Combination Regimen to Prevent Reactions to Radiocontrast Agents in Patients with Previous Reactions

Prednisone 50 mg PO or hydrocortisone 200 mg IV 13, 7, and 1 hour before radiocontrast procedure
PLUS
Diphenhydramine 50 mg PO or IV, 1 hour before procedure
PLUS
Ephedrine 25 mg PO, 1 hour before procedure (may be withheld in patient with contraindications such as angina)
PLUS
Use lower osmolarity radiocontrast media (e.g., iopamidol or iohexol)

Modified from Greenberger PA, Patterson R. The prevention of immediate generalized reactions to radiocontrast media in high-risk patients. J Allergy Clin Immunology 1991; 87:867.

APPROACH TO THE PATIENT EXPERIENCING A DRUG REACTION WHILE ON MULTIPLE DRUGS

Management of the patient who experiences a drug reaction while receiving multiple drugs may be difficult. The most recently administered drug is more often the culprit, but delayed-onset reactions such as serum sickness may occur to a drug previously administered. The clinical approach should be organized in such a way as to facilitate a resolution of the reaction, while at the same time providing useful information as to the culprit drug responsible for the reaction, if possible. One such approach is as outlined in Figure 5. The information provided in the preceding paragraphs and tables pro-

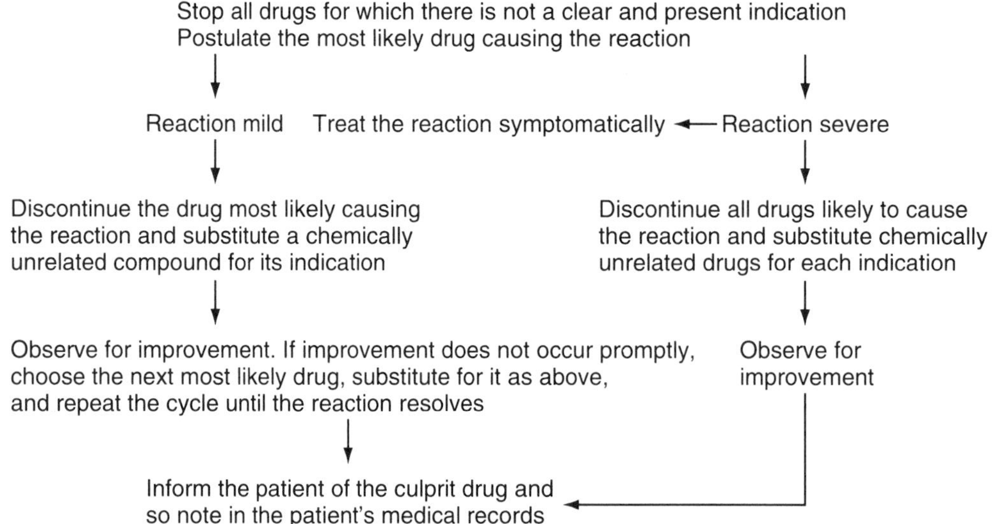

Figure 5 Approach to the patient with a drug reaction while on multiple drugs.

vides the basis for postulating the most likely drug causing the reaction. For instance, the most likely drugs causing multisystem reactions are antibiotics, including antituberculosis and antifungal drugs, diuretics, anticonvulsants, allopurinol, coumarin, heparin, oral hypoglycemics, and antiarrhythmic agents. The ADR provides an opportunity to review the patient's therapy and eliminate nonessential drugs.

SUGGESTED READING

Absar N, Daneshvar H, Beall G. Desensitization to trimethoprim/sulfamethoxazole in HIV-infected patients. J Allergy Clin Immunol 1994; 93:1001.

Anderson JA. Allergic reactions to drugs and biological agents. JAMA 1992; 268:2845.

DeSwarte RD. Drug Allergy. In: Patterson R, ed. Allergic diseases: diagnosis and management. 4th ed. Philadelphia: JB Lippincott, 1993:395.

Smith DL, deShazo RD. Systemic reactions to local anesthetics and neuromuscular blocking agents. Immunol Allergy Clin North Am 1995; 15:613–634.

Sullivan TJ. Drug allergy. In: Middleton E Jr, Reed CE, Ellis EF, Adkinson NF Jr, et al, eds. Allergy: principles and practice. 4th ed. St Louis: Mosby, 1993:1726.

INSECT STING ALLERGY IN ADULTS

DAVID F. GRAFT, M.D.

Allergic reactions to insect stings are a more serious problem in adults than in children since the reactions tend to be more severe and death occurs much more frequently. Stinging insects (honeybees, yellow jackets, hornets, wasps, and imported fire ants) are members of the order Hymenoptera. Honeybees are small fuzzy insects with alternating tan and black stripes. They are often seen pollinating clover and flowering plants, are relatively nonaggressive, and generally sting only when caught underfoot or if their hive is disturbed. The barbed stinger usually remains at the site of the sting, a feature that can be an important diagnostic clue. Another strain of honeybee ("African" bee or "killer bee") has been steadily migrating northward from Central and South America and has now reached Texas. They will probably continue to move gradually to the north until their progression is limited by climatic factors. These bees, as compared with the established "European" honeybees, exhibit strong defensive behavior, consider a much wider area to be part of their domain, and sting in large numbers when provoked. Bumblebees are large, slow-moving, noisy bees with hairy bodies of alternating yellow and black stripes. They are nonaggressive and account for only a small fraction of stings.

The vespids include yellow jackets, hornets, and wasps. Yellow jackets have alternating yellow and black body stripes and a characteristic hovering-darting flight pattern. They nest in the ground or in decaying logs and scavenge for food, frequenting garbage cans and picnics where they fly sorties at soda cans and other food stuffs. They are short tempered and sting upon minor provocation. Closely related are the yellow and white-faced hornets, which build teardrop-shaped nests in trees or shrubs. Not quite as aggressive as the other vespids, the thin-bodied paper wasps build nests in the eaves of buildings in which the hexagonal development cells are not covered by a paper envelope. Imported fire ants are primarily found in the Gulf Coast states. Their dirt mounds of one to two feet in height contain thousands of ants.

SPECTRUM OF REACTIONS

A normal reaction to a Hymenopteran sting is transient redness and itching at the sting site. About 10 percent of the population develop large local reactions. These vary in severity from just a few inches of swelling to involvement of an entire extremity and may last for several days. Fire ants usually cause a semicircle of vesicles at the sting sites that results from repetitive stinging as they pivot around, anchored by their mandibles to the victim.

Systemic IgE-mediated reactions occur in 0.4 to 0.8 percent of individuals and by definition involve body sites distant from the sting location. They usually commence within minutes after the sting but occasionally several hours may transpire before symptoms start. Milder reactions may be limited to generalized pruritus or urticaria; more severe manifestations include respiratory or cardiovascular symptoms. Systemic reactions tend to be more severe in adults than children. Furthermore, adults suffer almost all of the 40 to 50 deaths per year in the United States that are attributed to insect sting anaphylaxis.

A toxic reaction may result if a person receives a large number of stings in rapid fashion. These reactions are rare and tend to occur when a nest is disturbed. Over the past 20 years, incidents of 500 or more stings by Africanized honeybees have been reported. Some of these have been fatal, but a healthy adult may tolerate over 5,000 stings without sequelae. Several types of delayed adverse responses have been reported including serum-sickness-like reactions, transverse myelitis, and myocarditis. The pathophysiology of delayed reactions remains in doubt; immunologic mechanisms may not be involved.

ACUTE MANAGEMENT

Individuals presenting with anaphylaxis require careful observation. A subcutaneous injection of epinephrine (1:1,000) at a dose of 0.3 to 0.5 ml is the cornerstone of management and often is sufficient to terminate a reaction. This may be repeated in 10 to 15 minutes if necessary. An oral antihistamine such as diphenhydramine hydrochloride (Benadryl), 12.5 to 50 mg is also usually given. It may lessen urticaria or other cutaneous symptoms, but in more serious or progressive reactions, its use should not delay the administration of epinephrine. Diphenhydramine (Benadryl) may also be administered parentally (50 mg; 5 mg per kilogram per 24 hours) for more serious reactions.

Inhaled sympathomimetic agents such as isoproterenol or albuterol may decrease bronchoconstriction but do not address other systemic manifestations such as shock. Aminophylline may be helpful if bronchoconstriction persists following epinephrine. Severe reactions often require treatment with oxygen, H_2-antihistamines such as cimetidine (Tagamet), volume expanders, and pressor agents. Corticosteroids such as prednisone (0.5 to 2 mg per kilogram per 24 hours) are commonly used, but their delayed onset of action (4 to 6 hours) limits their effectiveness in the early stages of treatment. Intubation or tracheostomy is indicated for severe upper airway edema not responding to therapy. Allergic reactions are generally more severe in patients who take beta-blocker drugs. Furthermore, reactions in these patients may be more difficult to treat because beta-blockers impede the response to epinephrine and other sympathomimetic medications. Glucagon, 50 mg per kilogram given over 2 minutes intravenously, may be helpful in this clinical situation.

Systemic reactions commencing more than several hours after a sting usually manifest only mild symptoms. Most are easily managed with oral antihistamines and observation. Occasionally, anaphylaxis may be prolonged or biphasic in nature. Close observation and continued treatment are essential in this situation. The administration of corticosteroids as early in treatment as feasible may help to diminish later symptoms. Overnight hospitalization is indicated for patients who have experienced severe reactions or who have complicated medical problems.

Treatment recommendations for large local reactions include ice, elevation, and antihistamines. A short course of prednisone (0.5 to 2 mg per kilogram per day for 5 days), especially if initiated immediately after the sting, may be the best treatment to prevent symptoms in patients who usually develop massive, large local reactions.

DECREASING FUTURE REACTIONS

Preventing Stings

Future stings can be avoided by taking common sense precautions to significantly reduce exposure. Shoes should always be worn outside. Hives and nests around the home should be exterminated. Good sanitation should be practiced since garbage and outdoor food, especially canned drinks, attract yellow jackets. Perfumes and dark and floral-patterned clothing should be avoided.

Emergency Epinephrine

To encourage prompt treatment, epinephrine is available in emergency kits for self-administration. These are used by insect-sting–allergic individuals immediately after the sting to "buy time" to get to a medical facility. The Ana-Kit contains a preloaded syringe that can deliver two 0.3 ml doses of 1:1,000 epinephrine. Incremental doses may also be given. The physician who prescribes this kit must provide thorough instruction and must be confident that the patient can perform the injection procedure. These kits may be confusing to nonmedical personnel and some patients have a petrifying fear of needles. A practice self-injection with saline will help to allay such fears. The Epipen (0.3 mg epinephrine) and EpiPen Jr. (0.15 mg epinephrine) offer a concealed needle and a pressure-sensitive spring-loaded injection device that make them suited for patients and families who are uncomfortable with the injection process. Epinephrine, 1.3 to 3.9 mg by inhalation (6 to 18 puffs of Primatene Mist) may also be used to achieve a therapeutic plasma level and may be especially helpful for laryngeal edema and bronchospasm. Patients who are receiving maintenance injections of venom immunotherapy are advised that emergency self-treatment will probably not be required; however, they should have the kit available if they are distant from medical facilities. A Medic-Alert bracelet is also advised.

Venom Immunotherapy

The clinical history is the key to determining the need for venom immunotherapy (VIT). A careful history discloses the type, degree, and time course of symptoms, and often identifies the culprit insect. An individual who has experienced a sting-induced systemic reaction should be referred to an allergist who will perform skin tests with dilute solutions of honeybee, yellow jacket, yellow hornet, white-faced hornet, and *Polistes* wasp venoms and, if indicated, imported fire ant whole body extract. Radioallergosorbent testing (RAST) cannot replace venom skin testing but may provide additional information. Whole body extract materials were used before 1979 to diagnose and treat flying Hymenopteron allergy, but they were shown to be ineffective and venoms supplanted their use. To date, fire ant venom has only been available in small research quantities; fortunately, the fire ant whole body extract material seems more potent than those previously available for the other Hymenopteron and has been successfully used for skin testing and treatment. Table 1 lists the indications for VIT in adults. Some clinicians would recommend VIT for an adult who experienced any degree of systemic reaction. However, most individuals have a stereotypic response to a sting with the symptoms on subsequent stings closely resembling the first episode. Therefore, when only a mild reaction has occurred, the physician and patient may jointly decide whether to embark on a course of VIT.

Individuals with large local reactions or negative skin tests are not candidates for venom therapy. Finally, a positive venom skin test or RAST in the absence of a sting-induced systemic reaction is not an indication for therapy. Approximately 25 percent of the general population may have such evidence of sensitization to venom antigens, apparently resulting from past stings. This is usually transient, disappearing in 1 to 3 years.

Other factors may influence the decision concerning the need for VIT. Those with an increased risk of being stung such as landscapers or other individuals who engage in outdoor activities, especially those that take them far away from available medical care, will dispose the physician towards initiating venom treatment. Part of the morbidity associated with stinging insect allergy includes psychological effects of anxiety in the victim and family because of the threat of a sudden "unpreventable" systemic reaction. This high level of anxiety has frequently been exacerbated by a physician warning that "the next sting may be your last." Actually, most victims exhibit an individual pattern of anaphylaxis that varies only slightly in severity from one sting to another. Some investigators have proposed that a diagnostic sting challenge be used to select patients for VIT. Patients who did not react would not be placed on VIT. However,

Table 1 Indications for Venom Immunotherapy in Adults

Classification of Sting Reaction by History	*Venom Skin Test*	*Venom Immunotherapy*
Large local	Positive or negative	No
Systemic (mild)	Positive	Patient-MD decision
	Negative	No
Systemic (mod-severe)	Positive	Yes
	Negative	No
Toxic	Not indicated	No

Table 2 Typical Dose Schedule for Venom Immunotherapy*

1 μg/ml	*10 μg/ml*	*100 μg/ml*
1. 0.05 ml	5. 0.05 ml	9. 0.05 ml
2. 0.10 ml	6. 0.10 ml	10. 0.10 ml
3. 0.20 ml	7. 0.20 ml	11. 0.20 ml
4. 0.40 ml	8. 0.40 ml	12. 0.40 ml
		13. 0.60 ml
		14. 0.80 ml
		15. 1.00 ml

*Mixed vespid venom contains three times the venom per ml shown in this table.

a recent report described individuals who tolerated one sting challenge, but reacted later to a second challenge. Therefore, further study is needed before definitive recommendations can be made.

The venoms used for immunotherapy are the same as those used for skin testing (honeybee, yellow jacket, yellow hornet, white-faced hornet, and wasp). The regimen begins with an injection of 0.01 μg and advances weekly to 100 μg (Table 2). The maintenance dose of 100 μg (chosen empirically because it is about twice the venom content of a sting) is given every 4 weeks for a year, after which the interval is lengthened to 6 to 8 weeks. A trial of very rapid 1-day rush regimen had some success but caused many systemic reactions and had to be performed in a hospital. More recently, a 2- to 5-hour regimen of VIT in which 10 gradually increasing doses were administered every 10 to 15 minutes to achieve a total dose on day 1 of about 55 μg per venom was described. However, local reactions occurred in over half the patients, and 12 percent experienced mild systemic reactions. A recent report described individuals who had the maintenance interval lengthened to 3 months and then tolerated intentional challenge stings without problem. If these results are verified by further studies, the cost of VIT can be reduced.

Venom immunotherapy is extremely effective. Studies employing intentional stings have demonstrated a 97 to 100 percent protection rate in adults and children after 3 months of treatment. The small percentage of patients who were not protected experienced very mild reactions and perhaps more properly should be considered partial successes instead of failures. In most of the early studies regarding venom efficacy, the majority of the patients demonstrated sensitivity to vespid (usually yellow jacket) venom. The success rate in preventing future systemic reactions may be somewhat less with honeybee venom. Although one group advocates the use of a smaller maintenance venom dose (50 μg), data have been published that demonstrate a superior protective effect with 100 μg doses.

Patients usually receive all the venoms to which they show significant positive skin test results. The venoms are given in separate injections except in cases of multiple vespid sensitivity. In this common clinical situation, a single injection of a mixed-vespid preparation containing full doses of yellow jacket, yellow hornet, and white-faced hornet venom may be employed. Because of the cross-allergenicity of vespid venoms, patients usually have positive skin test results to more than one venom following a single vespid sting. Sometimes the wasp venom skin test is positive, but requires a higher concentration of venom to achieve this then for the other vespid venoms; in this particular situation, RAST inhibition studies can disclose whether patients are sensitive to a cross-reacting allergen or multiple unique allergens.

Venom injections, like other forms of allergen immunotherapy, are administered subcutaneously in the middle-third of the outer aspect of the upper arm. The usual care in matching patient and correct allergen extracts and doses, aspirating to be sure no blood is obtained (which, if present, would indicate intravascular placement of the needle and the need to select a different site), and observing the patient in the office for 30 minutes after the injection needs to be followed.

Most patients have short-lived erythema, itching, or swelling at the injection site. Large local reactions, which measure larger than 5 cm in diameter and last longer than 24 hours, occur in about 20 percent of patients. Interestingly, they tend to commence at venom doses between 10 and 30 mg. Generally, unless the local reactions are very large, the schedule of increasing doses is continued since these local reactions usually cease when the venom dose reaches 60 mg. Systemic reactions, including generalized pruritus, urticaria, angioedema, brochospasm, laryngeal edema, or hypotension, occur in a minority of patients. Treatment with epinephrine is the cornerstone of therapy, which may also include antihistamines, $beta_2$-agonists, glucocorticoids, and fluids. The next dose needs to be decreased before the schedule can be resumed. Sometimes large local reactions may continue to occur. Although some clinicians have recommended using a lower concentration of venom (by increasing the diluent and thus the total volume injected), others have employed the use of a higher concentration (using less diluent) with success.

Venom skin tests are generally repeated every 2 to 5 years. Most patients maintain positive venom skin tests, although many will demonstrate a tenfold or greater decline in venom sensitivity after 5 years. If a patient develops negative skin tests, venom immunotherapy is generally discontinued. A 5-year duration of therapy is sufficient for many venom-sensitive patients since studies have shown that 90 percent of such patients tolerate subsequent stings with impunity. However, patients with initial sting reactions that were graded as severe are more likely to react to post-VIT stings. Patients whose initial sting-induced reactions were of mild to moderate severity usually stop injections after 5 years. However, at this time, we recommend that those patients who have suffered severe reactions continue their injections indefinitely.

SUGGESTED READING

Golden DBK, Addison BI, Gadde J, et al. Prospective observations on stopping prolonged venom immunotherapy. J Allergy Clin Immunol 1989; 84:162.

Graft DF, Schoenwetter WF. Insect sting allergy: analysis of a cohort of patients who initiated venom immunotherapy from 1978 to 1986. Ann Allergy 1994; 73:481–485.

Keating MU, Kagey-Sobotka A, Hamilton RG, Yunginger JW. Clinical and immunologic follow-up of patients who stop venom immunotherapy. J Allergy Clin Immunol 1991; 88:339–348.

Reisman RE. Natural history of insect sting allergy: Relationship of severity of symptoms of initial sting anaphylaxis to re-sting reactions. J Allergy Clin Immunol 1992; 90:335–339.

Valentine MD. Allergy to stinging insects. Ann Allergy 1994;70: 427–432.

Van der Linden PWG, Struyvenberg A, Kraaijenhagen RJ, et al. Anaphylactic shock after insect-sting challenge in 138 persons with a previous insect-sting reaction. Ann Intern Med 1993; 118:161–168.

INSECT STING ALLERGY IN CHILDREN

RADVAN URBANEK, M.D.
PIA J. HAUK, M.D.

Systemic hypersensitivity reactions attributable to insect stings, mostly from Hymenoptera, have been reported to occur in 3 percent of the population. The morbidity rate is considerable for individuals with a higher exposure rate such as the family members of beekeepers. Patients of all ages who have experienced anaphylactic reactions are at risk of developing symptoms of unpredictable severity following subsequent stings. Some episodes can be fatal.

In the United States, yellow jackets are the principal cause of allergic reactions. In Europe, most hypersensitivity reactions occur because of stings from honeybees or from the Vespula species. Stings from hornets or bumblebees can also occasionally elicit hypersensitivity symptoms. In children, the overwhelming majority of allergic reactions to insect stings is caused by an IgE-mediated immediate-type allergy. Toxic reactions to venoms may occur after numerous simultaneous stings (50 to 100) and have clinical characteristics similar to anaphylaxis.

Approximately one-third of children who experience allergic reactions to stings have a history of atopic disease. However, children who suffer from other atopic diseases are not at higher risk of developing allergic reactions to insect stings than children who do not. Nevertheless, frequent exposure to large amounts of insect venom, as may occur in family members of beekeepers, stimulates the production of specific antibodies.

CLINICAL SYMPTOMATOLOGY

The usual reactions to insect stings are localized pain, erythema, and subsequent swelling at the site of the sting. More extensive local reactions are common in young children of preschool age. In addition, insect stings on the face and neck are associated with enlarged edemas, which deform the patient's appearance.

The clinical symptomatology of allergic reactions to insect stings covers a wide spectrum, ranging from large local reactions to life-threatening systemic reactions. In children, the severity of allergic reactions can be classified into four grades (Table 1). The more detailed differentiation provided by H. L. Mueller defines four grades of systemic reactions in adults. However, this has no advantage since there are no clinical criteria or in vitro predictors that can reliably identify children who are potentially at risk of anaphylaxis from insect stings. Furthermore, in comparison to the more precise reporting in adult patients, less accurate differentiation of symptoms is to be expected in children.

Table 1 Classification of Sting Reactions

0 =	Normal reaction (i.e., pain, erythema, local swelling)
I =	Large local reaction (i.e., swelling extending over two neighboring joints and lasting longer than 24 hours)
II =	Mild systemic reaction (e.g., urticaria, angioedema, generalized pruritus, nausea)
III =	Life-threatening reaction (e.g., dyspnea, unconsciousness, collapse, shock)

Clinically, an immediate-type reaction is characterised by the short time interval between the sting and the onset of the first clinical symptoms, which take between a few minutes and an hour to appear. Skin symptoms such as urticaria, flushing, itching, and angioedema occur most frequently. They are often followed by respiratory (20 to 25 percent) and gastrointestinal complaints (20 to 25 percent) and occasionally by cardiovascular symptoms (5 to 10 percent). The latter may appear alone but usually occur in combination with CNS symptoms such as dizziness, collapse, and unconsciousness. The most common gastrointestinal symptoms are nausea, vomiting, abdominal cramps, and diarrhea. Patients with respiratory symptoms experience difficulties in breathing and swallowing, itching in the throat, hoarseness of voice, rhinorrhoea, coughing, and wheezing. Besides the usual, immediate-type reactions, "unusual diseases" may also occur, appearing hours or several days after a sting. Vasculitis, nephrotic syndrome, encephalitis, and serum sickness have been reported in some adults, more than half of whom had previously experienced anaphylaxis. In children, these delayed unusual reactions are rare.

DIAGNOSTIC TESTS

Purified and freeze-dried venom from different types of insects (honeybee, yellow jacket, white-faced hornets, yellow hornets, and wasps) and mixed-vespid venoms (venom from yellow jackets, white-faced hornets, and yellow hornets in equal parts) are available for diagnosis and treatment. The diagnosis of IgE-mediated insect-venom allergy is routinely based on history, skin testing, and determination of venom-specific IgE antibodies.

Venom used for prick and intradermal skin tests should be diluted in human serum albumin to avoid loss of potency from adsorption on the tube surface. Venom dilutions should not be stored since they can lose their allergenic potency. A cutaneous reaction occurring 20 minutes after a skin-prick test with a venom concentration of 1 to 100 μg per milliliter or after an intradermal test with 0.1 to 1 μg per milliliter of venom indicates an IgE-mediated type allergy. The occurrence of a positive skin reaction to more than one venom concentration increases diagnostic specificity. We have never elicited a systemic allergic reaction by skin testing. When skin-test

Table 2 Score Scale Assessment of Potential Risk of Life-Threatening Reactions

		*Score**		*Score*
Systemic reaction	Mild	1	Life-threatening	2
Skin-prick test	Wheal <3 mm	1	Wheal ≥3 mm	2
Specific IgE level (RAST class)	Low (class 1)	1	High (class 2-4)	2

*A cumulative score >5 indicates patient at risk, immunotherapy advisable.

Table 3 Pharmacologic Treatment of Allergic Reactions to Insect Stings in Children

Indication	*Agent*	*Dosage*	*Side Effects*
Large local reaction	Corticosteroids	2 mg/kg prednisone equivalent	Hyperglycemia, fluid retention
Urticaria, itching	Antihistamine	1-2 mg clemastine or 25 mg diphenhydramine	Drowsiness, dry mouth
Angioedema	Epinephrine	0.01 mg/kg SC (epinephrine 1:1,000 dilution)	Palpitation, nervousness, tremor, hypertension
Bronchospasm	Epinephrine	Inhalation 5-10 puffs (1 puff = 0.35 mg) Epinephrine Medihaler or 0.01 mg/kg SC (epinephrine 1:1,000)	Palpitation, nervousness, tremor, hypertension
Hypotension, shock	Epinephrine	Epinephrine 0.01 mg/kg (1-5 ml of 1:10,000 dilution) intravenously,	Arrhythmias, hypertension
		Colloids 5-10 ml/kg,	Congestive heart failure
		Oxygen (SO_2 <80%)	None

reactivity is studied in relation to the interval between the last sting resulting in an allergic reaction and the time of testing, it shows a decline in skin sensitivity over a period of time. The highest cutaneous sensitivity appears 1 to 3 months after the index sting.

Laboratory tests such as the determination of venom-specific IgE antibodies are less sensitive than skin testing. On the other hand, the evidence of specific IgE is a better single predictor of clinical reactivity. In addition, the measurement of specific IgE can be used in children who are not available for skin testing or in individuals with extensive skin disease. Because of the fact that only some children and their parents can reliably identify the responsible insect, further investigation is necessary to confirm the culprit. Although skin tests and the determination of venom-specific IgE are the most important methods used in allergy practice, there is no correlation between the severity of a clinical reaction and the result of a skin test or the IgE level. It is therefore useful to make an assessment using a score scale system comprising clinical history, skin-test result, and specific IgE (Table 2). The score thus obtained helps in assessing the risk of a potential life-threatening reaction, but it also overestimates the number of patients who require immunotherapy. Patients who have experienced large local reactions are not considered in this score system because their risk of developing a systemic reaction to a subsequent sting is only about 5 percent.

Determination of venom-specific IgG antibodies and allergen-induced histamine release are additional in vitro tests used to prove sensitization to insect venoms. Measurements of plasma histamine and mast-cell tryptase following systemic allergic sting reactions permit the pathophysiology of the disease to be studied, but as prognostic parameters, they are only of little value.

From the natural history of insect-sting allergy we know that subsequent stings may induce life-threatening responses. However, such severe reactions are quite rare in children. Furthermore, sting challenges in allergic patients who have not undergone immunotherapy induce systemic symptoms again in only a low percentage of patients (i.e., 9 to 38 percent). Thus the challenge procedure may be offered in order to estimate a patient's individual risk. Sting challenges reassure those who are subsequently found to be protected and helps to identify those who need immunotherapy. In particular, children who are not sensitized to any insect venom according to standard diagnostic tests but who are believed to have experienced a systemic allergic reaction to an insect sting should be challenged in order to reveal their risk of experiencing life-threatening reactions to the insect in question.

THERAPY

The emergency treatment for systemic reactions caused by insect stings is the same as that for anaphylaxis of any other cause (Table 3). Depending on the clinical symptoms, antihistamines given orally or intravenously may alleviate urticaria and itching. Epinephrine hydrochloride in 1:1,000 dilution (0.1 ml per 10 kg of body weight = equivalent to 0.01 mg per kilogram) administered subcutaneously is indicated for cardiovascular and respiratory as well as for gastrointestinal and severe cutaneous symptoms. This dose can be repeated every 30

Table 4 Guidelines for Diagnostic and Therapeutic Procedures in Insect Venom–Allergic Children

Index Sting	*Sensitization (Skin Test, IgE)*	*Challenge*	*Emergency Kit*	*Venom Immunotherapy*
Large local reaction	No	No	No	No
	Yes	No	Yes	No
Mild systemic reaction (cutaneous symptoms)	No	On request	Yes	No
	Yes	On request	Yes*	On request
Life-threatening reaction	No	Recommended	Yes	No
	Yes	No	Yes*	Yes

*Patients who do not undergo venom immunotherapy.

minutes if required. Although aerosolized epinephrine helps to treat upper-airway edema, its insufficient absorption limits its use for other systemic symptoms. In shock, the intravenous application of volume using crystalloid or colloid solutions is required. The intravenous administration of epinephrine in 1:10,000 dilution is only required in cases of profound shock. Oxygen and bronchodilators are administered if necessary. The acute symptoms of anaphylaxis usually subside within 10 to 30 minutes.

Large local reactions are treated with 1 to 2 mg of prednisone equivalent (orally or parenterally) or by the immediate application of a topical steroid preparation (betamethasone dipropionate in propylene glycol as a vehicle) allowing rapid penetration.

To prevent insect stings, patients should be advised to refrain from using hair sprays and perfumes and not to eat out of doors so as not to attract insects. Patients at risk should carry an emergency kit containing an antihistamine preparation, corticosteroids, and an adrenaline medihaler. Epinephrine is available in prefilled syringes for self-administration (Epi Pen/Fastject junior 1 × 0.15 mg IM, SC application for SC application). However, it is important that precise instructions to give repeatedly to children at risk and to their parents.

VENOM IMMUNOTHERAPY

Specific hyposensitisation with Hymenoptera venoms has been proved effective in preventing anaphylaxis in more than 95 percent of children. Since in infancy and early childhood severe allergic reactions are rare and fatalities are almost unknown, venom immunotherapy (VIT) is recommended only in heavily exposed patients such as the children of beekeepers who exhibit severe systemic reactions. Individuals who have experienced only large local reactions or cutaneous symptoms should be instructed to use the emergency treatment kit previously mentioned. Immunotherapy has never been recommended in "unusual" reactions such as serum sickness.

In about 50 percent of cases, identification of the offending insect relies on diagnostic tests, which are frequently positive with more than one venom. In view of the extensive cross-reactivity between Vespula and Dolichovespula venoms, treatment with Vespula venom alone appears sufficient. The cross-reaction between honeybee and vespid venoms is less pronounced. Cutaneous sensitization and/or specific IgE antibodies do not always help to identify the insect that gave the index sting. In such cases, further diagnostic tests such as RAST inhibition and an in-hospital sting challenge are recommended before commencing immunotherapy based on clinical indications. In children, only one type of insect venom should be used for immunotherapy.

Selection guidelines for venom immunotherapy are given in Table 4. The generally recommended maintenance dose, corresponding to approximately 2 stings, is 100 μg of single venom, regardless of the patient's age. The initial dose in children is 1 μg, administered subcutaneously.

Many treatment schedules recommending various injection intervals have been developed. Rush protocols with dosing intervals of 1 hour provide rapid protection within a few days. However, they are associated with more side effects than slow schedules or cluster protocols. The maintenance dose is given at monthly intervals, which can be shortened or extended to up to 2 months if therapy continues successfully. No long-term adverse reactions to VIT have been reported.

Venom immunotherapy results in elevated concentrations of venom-specific IgG antibodies. The most significant increase is noted during the first 3 months of treatment, the period during which the largest amounts of allergen are administered. It can be assumed that the measurement of specific IgG antibody levels at regular intervals allows the effect of hyposensitization treatment to be assessed. However, there is a considerable overlap in the individual IgG levels of patients treated successfully and those of immunotherapy failures. Thus the venom-specific IgG level is more a parameter for evaluating the individual immune response rather than an absolute criterion for protection against insect stings.

In contrast, the concentration of specific IgE increases during the first few months of treatment and declines later on. The disappearance of venom-specific IgE antibodies is a reason for discontinuing immunotherapy. Although the majority of hyposensitized children never completely lose their specific IgE antibodies and/or skin-test sensitization, venom immunotherapy may be discontinued after 3 to 5 years. Subsequent field stings or challenge stings reveal a recurrence of anaphylactic reactions in 5 to 10 percent of such patients. However, the reactions are generally less severe than those induced by the index sting before treatment.

SUGGESTED READING

Day JH, Buckeridge DL, Welsh AC. Risk assessment in determining systemic reactivity to honeybee stings in sting-threatened individuals. J Allergy Clin Immunol 1994; 93:691–705.

Mueller U, Mosbech H, Blaauw P, et al. Emergency treatment of allergic reactions to Hymenoptera stings. Clin Exp Allergy 1991; 21:281–288.

Reisman RE. Insect stings. N Engl J Med 1993; 331:523–27.

Urbanek R, Forster J, Kuhn W, Ziupa J. Discontinuation of bee immunotherapy in children and adolescents. J Pediatr 1985; 107:367–371.

Valentine MD, Schuberth KC, Kagey-Sobotka A, et al. The value of immunotherapy with venom in children with allergy to insect stings. N Engl J Med 1990; 323:1601–1603.

SYSTEMIC ANAPHYLAXIS

ALEXANDRA S. WOROBEC, M.D.
DEAN D. METCALFE, M.D.

Systemic anaphylaxis is an acute allergic reaction involving the release of mediators from mast cells, basophils, and secondarily recruited inflammatory cells, which may occur within a few minutes to a few hours following exposure to a triggering agent. Literally meaning "anti-protection" from the Greek "ana" = no and "phylaxis" = protection, anaphylaxis is potentially life threatening and therefore constitutes a medical emergency that requires prompt recognition and therapy.

Anaphylactic reactions have been classically divided into two categories based on mechanism: (1) anaphylaxis that is traditionally considered to involve IgE, mast cells, and basophils; and (2) anaphylactoid reactions that may be due to other immunologic as well as nonimmunologic mechanisms. Recent murine work using an IgE knockout model is consistent with the hypothesis that non–IgE-mediated signal pathways may also initiate a systemic reaction resembling anaphylaxis. A representative list of etiologic agents involved in anaphylactic syndromes classified according to possible mechanism is included in Table 1. Nonetheless, these distinctions remain a matter of semantics since clinical symptomatology and treatment of all categories is essentially the same.

The signs and symptoms of anaphylaxis may be isolated to one or involve several organ systems. Cutaneous manifestations include erythema, flushing, pruritus, urticaria, and angioedema. Gastrointestinal symptoms include crampy abdominal pain, nausea, vomiting, and diarrhea. Uterine cramping may occur. Life-threatening manifestations most commonly involve respiratory distress secondary to upper airway obstruction from angioedema of the tongue, oropharynx, or larynx, or secondary to lower airway obstruction from bronchospasm. Cardiovascular symptoms are often severe and refractory and include hypotension, arrythmias, and hypovolemic shock. Involvement of the cardiovascular system constitutes the second most common cause of death in anaphylactic syndromes. In general, the magnitude of the anaphylactic response parallels the magnitude of the stimulus, with more severe reactions occurring closer temporally to the time of exposure to the inciting agent.

RECOGNITION AND TREATMENT OF ANAPHYLAXIS

Treatment of anaphylaxis requires early recognition of clinical symptoms associated with the syndrome and a history of possible antigen exposure. Several disorders may present with clinical manifestations not unlike anaphylaxis and hence, comprise the differential diagnostic list for this syndrome (Table 2). The vasovagal reaction is perhaps the most common diagnosis which is confused with anaphylaxis. It presents with symptoms of pallor, profuse sweating, weakness, bradycardia, hypotension, and occassionally syncope. Because bradycardia is an early manifestation of hypovolemic shock, heart rate cannot be used reliably to differentiate a vasovagal reaction from anaphylaxis. Indeed, the heart rate has been reported to be low, normal, or elevated during anaphylaxis. Elevated plasma histamine or tryptase levels, particularly the latter, are retrospective supportive findings in favor of a mast cell–mediated disorder such as anaphylaxis.

The immediate treatment of anaphylaxis begins with a rapid assessment of the patient's level of consciousness, along with the patient's airway, breathing, and circulation (ABCs). A broad outline of measures to be instituted in a patient with probable anaphylaxis is presented in Table 3. The management of anaphylaxis must take into consideration the severity of the reaction.

The first-line drug of choice for treating anaphylaxis is subcutaneous epinephrine. The dose of epinephrine injected subcutaneously is usually 0.3 ml of 1:1,000

Table 1 Classification of Anaphylactic Syndromes

Mechanism	*Etiologic Agents**
I. IgE Mediated	
Haptens	Most antibiotics: penicillins, cephalosporins, sulfonamides, tetracycline, bacitracin, nitrofurantoin, amphotericin
	Industrial chemicals: ethylene oxide, glue, formaldehyde
Complete Antigens	Allergen extracts: pollens, molds, danders
	Venoms: hymenoptera (including fire ant), snake, deer fly (Chrysops species), kissing bug (Triatoma species)
	Foreign proteins: chymopapain, horse serum
	Foods: peanut, milk, egg, seafood, grains, tree nuts
	Vaccines contaminated with egg protein: influenza
	Human proteins: insulin, vasopressin, serum, and seminal proteins
	Enzymes: streptokinase, trypsin, L-asparaginase
	Protamine
	Latex
	Immunomodulators: cyclosporine
	Ruptured hydatid cyst
II. Direct Mast-Cell Activation	Hypertonic solutions: radiocontrast media, mannitol
	Opiates
	Polysaccharides: Acacia, dextran, iron-dextran
	Muscle depolarizing agents: curare, d-tubocurarine
	Polymyxin B, vancomycin
	Some chemotherapeutic agents
III. Complement Mediated: C3a, C5a	Human proteins: immunoglobulins, plasma
	Dialysis membranes
IV. Arachidonic Cascade Mediated	Nonsteroidal anti-inflammatory agents, aspirin
V. Mechanism Unknown	
Exercise-induced anaphylaxis	
Idiopathic recurrent anaphylaxis	
Cholinergic urticaria with anaphylaxis	
Cold-induced urticaria with anaphylaxis	
Steroid preparations	Progesterone, hydrocortisone
Mastocytosis	
Sulfites	

*Examples only, list is not complete.

Table 2 Differential Diagnosis of Anaphylaxis

Pulmonary	*Endocrine*
Laryngeal edema	Hypoglycemia
Epiglottitis	Pheochromocytoma
Foreign body aspiration	Carcinoid syndrome
Pulmonary embolus	Catamenial (progesterone-induced) anaphylaxis
Asphyxiation	
Hyperventilation	
Cardiovascular	*Psychiatric*
Myocardial infarction	Vocal cord dysfunction syndrome
Arrhythmia	Munchausen's disease
Hypovolemic shock	Panic attack/Globus hystericus
Cardiac arrest	
CNS	*Other*
Vasovagal reaction	Hereditary angioedema
Cerebrovascular accident	Cold urticaria
Seizure disorder	Idiopathic urticaria
Drug overdose	Mastocytosis
	Serum sickness
	Idiopathic capillary leak syndrome
	Sulfite exposure
	Scombroid poisoning (tuna, bluefish, mackeral)

aqueous epinephrine in the adult, although the dosage may need to be decreased in the elderly (to say, 0.2 ml) or increased in patients receiving beta-adrenergic blockers (to 0.5 ml). Dosing of epinephrine in children is based on weight, or 0.01 ml per kilogram of a 1:1,000 dilution up to a maximum of 0.3 ml of epinephrine injected subcutaneously. A second epinephrine injection (0.1 to 0.2 ml of 1:1,000 epinephrine) may be given into the site of an insect sting, or drug or allergen injection site to delay systemic absorption of the agent if the antigen source is not a digit or other terminal region of the anatomy.

The 1993 report of the Working Group on Asthma in Pregnancy with the National Heart, Lung and Blood Institute (NIH publication #93–3279) considering the treatment of pregnant women with epinephrine (and likewise diphenhydramine) listed epinephrine as the initial pharmacologic agent of choice in the management of anaphylaxis. A second-line agent of choice for some obstetricians for the treatment of hypotension secondary to anaphylaxis in the pregnant patient is ephedrine, 10 to 15 mg, administered IV push. Although less effective than epinephrine, it is believed that its predominant beta-adrenergic activity may cause less reduction in uterine blood flow than epinephrine.

Along with the administration of epinephrine to increase systemic vascular resistance and elevate diastolic pressure, produce bronchodilation, and increase inotropic and chronotropic cardiac activity, additional measures may be required to stabilize and maintain

Table 3 Step-Wise Treatment of Systemic Anaphylaxis: General Measures*

NOTE: To be performed at the time of administration of the first dose(s) of epinephrine SC

1. Removal or discontinuation of inciting agent
   - Special case for insect sting or allergen injection:
     - Application of a loose tourniquet proximally if an allergen, injection, or sting is on an extremity with further loosening of the tourniquet q15min. The insect stinger should be gently flicked off. 0.1-0.3 ml of aqueous epinephrine may be administered SC at the site of antigen injection to delay its absorption
2. Examination of skin color, upper and lower airway patency. Secure and maintain adequate airway
3. Monitoring of vital signs: BP, pulse, respiratory rate
4. Monitoring of patient's level of consciousness
5. Placement of patient in Trendelenburg position as appropriate
6. High flow supplemental oxygen (100%) with pulse oximetry monitoring
   - *Dose:* 4-10 L/min via a non-rebreather mask such as the Venturi
   - Intubation and mechanical assistance indicated when the $Paco_2$ is greater than or equal to 65 mm Hg
7. Insertion of a short, large bore peripheral IV line as appropriate for age with administration of fluids
   - *IV fluids:* a. **Initial recommendation:**
     - Crystalloid solutions:
       1. 0.9% normal saline or
       2. Lactated ringer's solution
          - Monitor vital signs, pulmonary status, and urine output
          - Keep SBP greater than or equal to 90 mm Hg
          - This may require up to 1 L q15-30min in an adult or 20-30 ml/kg/hr in the pediatric age group for the first several hours
   - b. **Severe or persistent hypotension:**
     - Colloid solutions:
       - i. Dextran—available in 2 forms:
         1. Dextran 70 (6% solution)
         2. Dextran 40 (10% solution)
       - ii. Hetastarch (Hespan)
       - iii. Serum Albumin—available in 2 concentrations:
         1. 5% solution: effective plasma expander
         2. 25% solution: more potent elevator of plasma oncotic pressure
8. For severe or refractory hypotension:
   - a. Also consider use of antishock trousers to increase afterload. (Note: controversial efficacy in the treatment of peripheral shock)
   - b. Lack of efficacy of measures discussed in steps one to seven above, including fluid resuscitation may mandate use of inotropic agents. By this stage, a central line to determine central venous pressure and/or Swan-Ganz catheter insertion is recommended. For unresponsive hypotension due to myocardial depression, an intra-aortic balloon counterpulsation pump may be considered
9. Observation in a monitored setting (i.e., ICU) for at least 24 hours after a moderate-severe anaphylactic reaction; for at least 8-12 hours after a mild reaction

*Exclusive of drug treatment, which is presented in Tables 4 and 5.

oxygenation and cardiac output. Other medications may be administered to supplement the effect of epinephrine. Clinical and experimental evidence suggests that treatment with a combination of H_1- and H_2-receptor antagonists such as diphenhydramine and ranitidine may be more effective than treatment with an H_1-antihistamine alone in preventing histamine-induced hypotension. Patients with severe anaphylaxis or those who have received systemic corticosteroid therapy within the previous 6 months should receive pharmacologic doses of parenteral glucocorticoids given the low but discernible frequency of biphasic and protracted anaphylactic reactions.

For respiratory involvement, patients must be managed aggressively with nebulized and parenteral agents (Tables 4 and 5). Most commonly, nebulized beta-adrenergic agonists are administered for bronchospasm, with nebulized epinephrine or racemic epinephrine given for upper airway edema. Supplemental oxygen should always be administered in the highest concentration possible, with serial arterial blood gas analyses performed to maintain oxygen saturation greater than or equal to 90 percent ($Po_2 < 60$ mm Hg, $Pco_2 > 65$ mm Hg). In recalcitrant cases, endotracheal intubation, cricothyroid membrane puncture (avoid this procedure in children younger than 10 years of age), or tracheostomy may be necessary to ensure adequate airflow.

Hypotension is generally managed initially via administration of crystalloid solutions (Table 3) such as 0.9 percent normal saline or lactated Ringer's solution through a large bore intravenous line at a rate depending on the degree of hypovolemia, status of the vital signs, pulmonary exam, and urine output. The goal of treatment is to maintain the systolic blood pressure (SBP) greater than or equal to 90 mm Hg. Because these isotonic solutions contain small molecules that rapidly escape from the vascular space into the interstitium, their volume expansion effects are short-lived. Nonetheless, crystalloids offer the advantage of being nonallergenic and virus free and having no potential to produce a hypotensive reaction.

Refractory hypotension or frank shock in a patient with anaphylaxis warrants a two fold approach to therapy. First, central venous access should be established for monitoring of the central venous pressure and possible need for Swan-Ganz catheter placement and monitoring of cardiac output and the pulmonary capillary wedge pressure. Concomitantly, colloids or solutions

Table 4 Step-Wise Treatment of Systemic Anaphylaxis: Pharmacologic Therapy in Adults

Medication	*Route*	*Dosage*	*Complications*
A. Indicated for all reactions (urticaria, angioedema, bronchospasm, laryngeal edema, and systemic symptoms)			
1. Epinephrine (drug of first choice)	SC	0.3 ml of a 1:1,000 dilution (usual range 0.2-0.5 ml) q10-15min × 3 doses, if necessary	Tachycardia, tremor, anxiety, arrhythmias
	IM	0.3 ml of a 1:1,000 dilution q10-15 min (**pregnant patient**)	
2. Ephedrine	IV push	10-25 mg (**only to be considered in the pregnant patient**)	
3. Antihistamines			
H_1-Blockers:			
Diphenhydramine	IM or IV	50-75 mg q6h Drip may afford better control of sxs: 5 mg/kg/24h	Large doses: anticholinergic effects, may depress respiration
H_2-Blockers:			
Ranitidine	PO (mild sxs)	150 mg q8-12h	
	IV	50 mg q6-8h	
Cimetidine	PO (mild sxs)	300 mg q6-8h	*Note:* cimetidine is not compatible with IV aminophylline
	IV	300 mg q6-8h	
Famotidine	IV	20 mg q12h	
B. Indicated for laryngeal edema			
1. Epinephrine	Nebulized	1% solution of 1:100 epinephrine via hand bulb nebulizer, 1-3 deep inhalations q3h	
2. Racemic epinephrine	Nebulized	2.25% solution of 1:100 racemic epinephrine via hand bulb nebulizer, 1-3 deep inhalations q3h	*Note:* racemic epinephrine has approximately half the activity of epinephrine
C. Indicated for bronchospasm			
1. Beta-adrenergic bronchodilators:			Nausea, vomiting, arrhythmias
Albuterol	Nebulized	2.5-5.0 mg (0.5 ml of 0.5% solution diluted to a final volume of 3 ml with 0.9% NS) given over 5-15 min. each dose, q20min × 6 doses maximum	
Metaproterenol	Nebulized	0.3 ml of 5% solution diluted in 2.5 ml of 0.45% or 0.9% NS, given over 5-15 min each dose, q4h	
Terbutaline	Metered	400 μg or 2 inhalations (200 μg/metered spray), q4-6h	
2. Steroids:			
Methylprednisolone	IV	60-80 mg × 1 dose, followed by prednisone 60 mg PO q.d. × 2d	*Note:* steroids have no antianaphylactic actions and do not alleviate immediate acute, life-threatening manifestations
Hydrocortisone	IV	100-200 mg q6-8h (up to 5-10 mg/kg q6-8h)	
Prednisone	PO (mild rxns)	20-40 mg q.d. with quick taper	
3. Aminophylline (second-line therapy)	IV	5-6 mg/kg in 20 ml D_5W over 10-15 min (loading dose), 0.5-1.0 mg/kg/h (maintenance dose)	Nausea, vomiting, seizures, arrhythmias

Continued.

containing large macromolecular polymers should be administered intravenously. These solutions allow a greater increase in the plasma oncotic pressure via attraction of water from the interstitium, thereby actually producing intravascular volume expansion in an increment above that which is administered. Example colloid solutions are dextran, hetastarch (Hespan), and serum albumin. Dextran solutions are available in two forms—a high molecular weight form (dextran 70, 6 percent solution) and a low molecular weight form (dextran 40, 10 percent solution)—which have intravascular half-lives of 2 to 3 days and 12 to 18 hours, respectively. Disadvantages of dextran administration include the potential for anaphylaxis and a bleeding diathesis, along with agglutination of red blood cells, thus making subsequent blood cross-matching difficult or impossible. Hetastarch (Hespan), an artificial polymer with a M_r 450 kD, displays a long-lasting volume expansion effect of 24 to 36 hours, is relatively nonallergenic, and doesn't interfere with blood typing and cross-matching. Disadvantages include alteration of the coagulation function. Serum albumin, available in a 5 percent and 25 percent solution, is the most commonly used plasma expander, but it is expensive and occasion-

Table 4 Step-Wise Treatment of Systemic Anaphylaxis: Pharmacologic Therapy in Adults—cont'd

Medication	*Route*	*Dosage*	*Complications*
D. Indicated for cardiovascular collapse (refractory hypotension, shock)			
1. Epinephrine (initial therapy)	Via ETT	1 mg = 10 ml of a 1:10,000 dilution in 5 ml 0.9% NS, given via a long needle or catheter into an ETT, followed by hyperventilation	*Note:* given when response to SC Epi is too slow or adequate vascular access has not been obtained yet
	IV push	0.1-0.2 ml of 1:1,000 dilution in 10 ml 0.9% NS, given over 5′. This may require follow-up administration of an epinephrine IV drip	
	IV drip	0.1 μg/kg/min, use 1 ml of 1:1,000 dilution in 250 ml D_5W (4 μg/ml) at 1 μg/min, increasing to a maximum of 4-10 μg/min	
2. Dopamine	IV drip	2-20 μg/kg/min (2 amps = 400 mg in 500 ml D_5W)	Arrhythmias
3. Dobutamine	IV drip	2-30 μg/kg/min (2 amps = 500 mg in 500 ml D_5W)	Arrhythmias, esp. tachycardia
4. Norepinephrine	IV drip	0.5-1.0 μg/min (initial dose), followed by 2-12 μg/min	Arrhythmias
5. Amrinone	IV drip	0.75 mg/kg IV bolus over 2-3 min, then 2-15 μg/kg/min (maintenance)	
E. Indicated for patients on beta-blockers with refractory shock			
1. Glucagon (first-line therapy)	IV push	1-5 mg over 2-5 minutes IV push	Nausea, vomiting
	IV drip	1 mg in 1 L D_5W at 5-15 μg/min	
2. Isoproterenol	IV drip	2-10 μg/min, start with 0.1 μg/kg/min (1 mg in 500 ml D_5W), doubling dose q15′	Tachycardia, arrhythmias

D_5W, 5% glucose in distilled water; *ETT,* endotracheal tube; *NS,* normal saline; *rxns,* reactions; *sxs,* symptoms.

ally associated with increased pulmonary interstitial edema.

In addition to fluid resuscitative measures, treatment of refractory hypotension and shock may require pharmacologic intervention. Replacement of serial subcutaneous or intramuscular epinephrine injections with an intravenous bolus, followed by a continuous intravenous 1:10,000 epinephrine drip, is generally recommended as first-line therapy. Lack of response to this measure may warrant addition of an intravenous continuous infusion of dopamine or dobutamine, depending on the patient's underlying cardiovascular status, followed by norepinephrine or amrinone. Patients on maintenance beta-blocker therapy may be relatively resistant to epinephrine; in these patients intravenous glucagon should be considered as a treatment for refractory hypotension, followed by isoproterenol. Established dosages of these vasoactive inotropic medications (Tables 4 and 5) are as provided by the American Heart Association (AHA) guidelines. Patients receiving any of these agents must be monitored for development of anginal symptoms and possible arrythmias in an intensive care unit setting, with both reactions being treated according to AHA guidelines with the appropriate agent. Hypertension resulting from unopposed beta-adrenergic and alpha-adrenergic activity may require prompt treatment with nitroprusside (initial dose: 10 μg per minute IV, increasing by 10 μg per minute IV every 4 minutes to 10 to 20 mg per minute IV until BP stabilizes) or phentolamine (initial dose: 0.5 mg per minute IV to a maximum of 10 mg IV, maintenance dose: 25 to 50 mg IV every 3 to 6 hours). Even with close cardiac monitoring and titration, myocardial infarction is a known associated sequelae of systemic anaphylaxis, either from the initial hypotensive insult to the myocardium or from alpha- and/or beta-adrenergic effects on an already compromised cardiovascular system.

Patients with a mild to moderate anaphylactic reaction should have their vital signs and cardiac and respiratory status monitored for at least an additional 8 to 12 hours after clinical signs and symptoms of anaphylaxis abate. For moderate reactions (i.e., bronchospasm, generalized urticaria) antihistamines and steroids may be continued for several days after the initial reaction, and the patient may be given a self-injectable epinephrine device (EpiPen or Ana-Kit) with a prescription for refills and counseled in its proper use before being discharged. Patients with severe reactions may require monitoring for a minimum of 24 hours after stabilization and warrant close outpatient follow-up and allergy evaluation.

PREVENTION AND PROPHYLAXIS

Basic principles in the prevention of anaphylaxis in high-risk individuals are outlined in Table 6. Identification and avoidance of causative agents, if feasible,

Table 5 Step-Wise Treatment of Systemic Anaphylaxis: Pharmacologic Therapy in Children

Medication	*Route*	*Dose*	*Complications*
A. Indicated for all reactions (urticaria, angioedema, bronchospasm, laryngeal edema, and systemic symptoms)			
1. Epinephrine (drug of first choice)	SC	0.01 mg/kg of a 1:1,000 dilution, up to 0.3 ml q10-15min	Tachycardia, tremor, anxiety, arrhythmias
2. Antihistamines			
H_1-Blockers:			
Diphenhydramine	IM or IV	1-2 mg/kg q6h Drip may afford better control of sxs: 5 mg/kg/24h	Large doses: anticholinergic effects, may depress respiration
H_2-Blockers:			
Ranitidine	IV	12.5-50 mg q6-8h	
B. Indicated for laryngeal edema			
1. Epinephrine	Nebulized	For use only in children >4 yrs of age: 1% solution of 1:100 epinephrine via hand bulb nebulizer, 1-3 deep inhalations q3h	
2. Racemic epinephrine	Nebulized	For use only in children >4 yrs of age: 2.25% solution of 1:100 racemic epinephrine via hand bulb nebulizer, 1-3 deep inhalations q3h	*Note:* racemic epinephrine has approximately half the activity of epinephrine
C. Indicated for bronchospasm			
1. Beta-adrenergic bronchodilators:			Nausea, vomiting, arrhythmias
Albuterol	Nebulized	For use only in children >5 yrs of age: 2.5-5.0 mg (0.5 ml of 0.5% solution diluted to a final volume of 3 ml with 0.9% NS) given over 5-15 min each dose, q20min × 6 doses maximum For use in children <5 yrs of age: 1.2-2.5 mg given over 5-15 min each dose, q20min × 6 doses maximum	
Metaproterenol	Nebulized	For use only in children >12 yrs of age: 0.3 ml of 5% solution diluted in 2.5 ml of 0.45% or 0.9% NS, given over 5-15 min each dose, q4h For use in children between 6-12 yrs of age: 0.1 ml of 5% solution diluted in 0.9% NS to a final volume of 3.0 ml, given over 5-15 min each dose, q4h	
Terbutaline	Metered dose inhaler	For use only in children >12 yrs of age: 400 μg or 2 inhalations (200 μg/metered spray), q4-6h	
2. Steroids:			
Methylprednisolone	IV	0.5 mg/kg/24 hr in divided doses	*Note:* same effects as listed in Table 4
Hydrocortisone	IV	4-8 mg/kg q6-8h	
3. Aminophylline (second-line therapy)	IV	5-6 mg/kg in 20 ml D_5W over 10-15 min (loading dose), 0.5-1.0 mg/kg/hr (maintenance dose)	Nausea, vomiting, seizures, arrhythmias

Continued.

remains the most important step in the management of susceptible individuals. Patients should be taught to recognize the clinical signs of impending anaphylaxis (i.e., lump in the throat with difficulty breathing, lightheadedness, feeling of impending doom) and feel comfortable and skilled in the technique of self-administration of subcutaneous epinephrine. An epinephrine autoinjector device should be carried by the patient at all times, with several spares in convenient locations (home, work) and these should be renewed on a yearly basis.

Patients with idiopathic anaphylaxis who experience more frequent attacks should be placed on maintenance therapy with oral antihistamines and perhaps, steroids (i.e., oral prednisone 20 to 40 mg daily), until the episodes abate, with tapering of steroids thereafter. High-risk patients on beta-blocker therapy, including topical medications used in the treatment of glaucoma,

Table 5 Step-Wise Treatment of Systemic Anaphylaxis: Pharmacologic Therapy in Children—cont'd

Medication	*Route*	*Dose*	*Complications*
D. Indicated for cardiovascular collapse (refractory hypotension, shock)			
1. Epinephrine (initial therapy)	Via ETT	0.1 mg/kg of a 1:10,000 dilution in 5 ml 0.9% NS, given via a long needle or catheter into an ETT, followed by hyperventilation	*Note:* given when response to SC Epi is too slow or adequate vascular access has not been obtained yet
	IV drip	0.1 μg/kg/min (use 0.5 mg of a 1:1,000 dilution of epinephrine in 100 ml 0.9% NS to produce a concentration of 5.0 μg/ml)	
2. Dopamine	IV drip	2-20 μg/kg/min (2 amps = 400 mg in 500 ml D_5W)	Arrhythmias
3. Dobutamine	IV drip	2-30 μg/kg/min (2 amps = 500 mg in 500 ml D_5W)	Arrhythmias, esp. tachycardia
4. Norepinephrine	IV drip	0.5-1.0 μg/min (starting dose), followed by 2-12 μg/min (maintenance dose)	Arrhythmias
E. Indicated for patients on beta-blockers with refractory shock*			
1. Glucagon (first-line therapy)	IV push	1-5 mg over 2-5 minutes, IV push	Nausea, vomiting
2. Isoproterenol	IV drip	2-10 μg/min. Start with 0.1 μg/kg/min (1 mg in 500 ml D_5W), doubling dose q15min	Tachycardia, arrhythmias

D_5W, 5% glucose in distilled water; *ETT,* endotracheal tube; *NS,* normal saline; *sxs,* symptoms.
*Beta-blockers less commonly used in children than adults.

Table 6 Strategies to Prevent or Lessen the Severity of Anaphylactic Reactions

I. General Principles:
  A. Obtain accurate and complete patient medical history. Skin tests or RAST are valuable in identifying individuals at risk for anaphylaxis from agents such as penicillin and insect venoms
  B. Patient avoidance of allergens known to precipitate anaphylaxis
  C. Medic-Alert bracelet should be worn by at-risk patients at all times
  D. Patients at risk should carry an Epi Pen or Ana-Kit at all times and be properly skilled in its correct use
    Adults: 0.3 ml of 1:1,000 dilution of Epinephrine (Epi Pen)
    Pediatric: 0.15 ml of 1 :1,000 dilution of Epinephrine (Epi Pen Jr.)
  E. Desensitization may be recommended for patients with Hymenoptera sensitivity
  F. Require a clear indication for drug use. Consider desensitization by oral route
  G. Desensitize patients to any drug known to have caused anaphylaxis if urgently required to treat a life-threatening disease. Prefer oral desensitization, if feasible
  H. Avoid use of beta-blockers, NSAIDs, or aspirin or replace with reasonable alternatives
II. Prophylaxis of Exercise-Induced Anaphylaxis:
  A. Avoid food ingestion for approximately 6 hours before exercise
  B. Avoid intake of NSAIDs or ASA
  C. In general, prophylactic antihistamines (H_1- and H_2-receptor antagonists) and cromolyn are ineffective
III. Prophylaxis (Desensitization procedures, necessary administration of agent known to cause anaphylaxis):
  A. Pretreatment with an H_1-receptor and possibly H_2-receptor antagonist 12 to 24 hr before administration of agent known to cause anaphylaxis
    1. H_1-blocker: **diphenhydramine IV** 5 mg/kg/24 hr **(adult + pediatric)** in divided doses q6h (25-75 mg IV q6h)
    2. H_2-receptor blocker: **ranitidine IV** 1-2 mg/kg/24 hr **(adult + pediatric)** in divided doses q6-8h or **cimetidine IV** 20-40 mg/kg/24 hr **(adult + pediatric)** in divided doses q6-8h
  B. Pretreatment with steroids. **Hydrocortisone 100 mg PO or I.V.** q.d., q8h **(adult)**
  C. Avoid use of beta-blockers
  D. Continue above medications for the duration of the administration of the inciting agent
IV. Radiocontrast Allergy Prophylaxis (Adults):
  A. Switch to low osmolar nonionic contrast agents when possible
  B. Administer steroids before scheduled test:
    1. **Prednisone: 30-50 mg PO q6-8h** (i.e. 13, 7, and 1 hour prior to the study)
    2. **Methylprednisolone: 32 mg PO 12 and 2 hr before study**
  C. H_1-receptor antagonists: **Diphenhydramine: 50 mg PO 7 hr and 1 hr, or 50 mg IM 1 hr before study**
  D. H_2-receptor antagonists: **Ranitidine: 150 mg PO 7 hr and 1 hr, or 50 mg IM 1 hr before study**
  E. **Ephedrine: 25 mg PO 1 hr before study**

should be continued on these medications only if feasible alternatives are unavailable and the drug is medically indicated.

Short-term desensitization to agents such as penicillin or beta-lactam antibiotics, insulin, antithymocyte globulin, or aspirin should be performed if clearly indicated, and then so in a closely monitored setting such as an intensive care unit. Patients may be considered for premedication with H_1- and H_2-antihistamines and steroids. Because this procedure constitutes a form of "controlled anaphylaxis," patients will likely require repeat desensitization in the event of a future requirement for re-administration of the known agent. Immunotherapy is often efficacious and indicated for the prevention of Hymenoptera hypersensitivity.

Radiocontrast allergy, usually due to high osmolar ionic contrast agents, may be significantly decreased via the use of nonionic contrast agents. Pretreatment with oral steroids such as prednisone or methylprednisolone, an H_1-antihistamine such as diphenhydramine, and possibly an H_2-antihistamine such as ranitidine (with or without ephedrine) at least 2 hours before administration of radiocontrast media has been shown to decrease the risk of fatal anaphylaxis.

SUGGESTED READING

AAAI. Position statement: The use of epinephrine in the treatment of anaphylaxis. J Allergy Clin Immunol 1994; 94:666–668.

Cummins RO. Hypotension/shock/acute pulmonary edema. In: Textbook of advanced cardiac life support. Dallas: American Heart Association 1994;1.40–1.47.

Metcalfe DD. Acute anaphylaxis and urticaria in children and adults. In: Schocket AL, ed. Clinical management of urticaria and anaphylaxis. New York: Marcel Dekker, 1992;1–20.

Saryan JA, O'Loughlin JM. Anaphylaxis in children. Pediatr Ann 1992; 21:590–598.

Schatz M, Zeiger RS. Management of asthma, rhinitis, and anaphylaxis during pregnancy. Curr Obstet Gynecol 1991;1:65.

IDIOPATHIC ANAPHYLAXIS

GAILEN D. MARSHALL Jr., M.D., Ph.D.

Anaphylaxis is an untoward systemic reaction characterized by various combinations of cutaneous (urticaria, angioedema), respiratory (bronchospasm, upper airway obstruction), gastrointestinal (nausea, diarrhea, untoward tastes), and/or cardiovascular (hypotension, syncope, cardiac arrhythmias) manifestations. It is mediated by the release of histamine, leukotrienes, and other mediators from activated mast cells and/or basophils. If activation is via antigen-specific IgE bound to the mast cells, it is an *anaphylactic* reaction. In contrast, mast cell activation that is independent of IgE is an *anaphylactoid* reaction. Some agents such as certain foods, drugs, and even infections can precipitate either. However, when no specific etiologic agent can be established in spite of reasonable clinical and laboratory diagnostic efforts, the patient is classified as having *idiopathic anaphylaxis.*

CLINICAL EVALUATION AND DIAGNOSIS

Idiopathic anaphylaxis (IA) is a diagnosis of exclusion. Because of the specific therapy involved, it is important to establish the correct diagnosis by considering other etiologies that can have similar clinical presentations (Table 1). In addition to appropriate physical and laboratory examination, the history is of fundamental importance in establishing the diagnosis. The most important aspects include searching for inciting events in the immediate prodromal period. Such events may include ingestion of a specific food, drink, or medication. Particular attention should be paid to the use of over-the-counter preparations such as aspirin and other nonsteroidal-containing compounds. A history of exposure to stinging insects should be sought. Pre-episodic exercise (often in conjunction with specific ingestants) and acute febrile illnesses should also be considered. It is critical that a current history be documented after *each* episode.

Table 1 Differential Diagnosis for Idiopathic Anaphylaxis

Endocrine
Carcinoid syndrome
Pheochromocytoma
Diabetes mellitus (ketoacidosis)
Physical
Exercise-induced anaphylaxis
Cholinergic urticaria
Cold-induced urticaria (anaphylaxis)
Ingestants
Foods
Food additives
Drugs
Latex
Other Etiologies
Vasovagal syncope
Systemic mastocytosis
Hysterical
Factitious anaphylaxis

Laboratory evaluation is often unrevealing in establishing the diagnosis of IA. A serum tryptase drawn at or within a few hours of the acute event can help to

Table 2 Management of Idiopathic Anaphylaxis

Acute
Emergency resuscitation, including fluids and other cardiovascular support as necessary; supplemental O_2 with airway management as necessary
Epinephrine: Adult: 0.3 ml of a 1:1,000 dilution of epinephrine;
Child: 0.01 ml/kg up to adult dose;
Can be given every 10 minutes as needed × 3
Prednisone: 50 mg po (or 125 mg solumedrol IV) acutely
H_1 antihistamines: Diphenhydramine 25-50 mg po q6h
Hydroxyzine 25-50 mg q6h
H_2-antihistamines: Cimetidine 300 mg po q12h
Ranitidine 150 mg po q12h
Infrequent
Same as acute episodes
Recurrent or Severe, life-threatening
Epinephrine kits (Ana-Kit, Epi Pen): Kept up-to-date with patient at all times until no episodes for 5 years
Prednisone: 60-100 mg po daily for 1 week or until symptoms are fully controlled
Move to every-other-day dose
Gradual taper by 5 mg per week
H_1-antihistamine: Diphenhydramine 25-50 mg po t.i.d. or
Hydroxyzine 25-50 mg po t.i.d. or
Terfenidine 60 mg po b.i.d.
Loratadine 10 mg po daily
Sympathomimetic: Albuterol 2 mg po t.i.d.
Ephedrine 25 mg po t.i.d.

establish a mast cell–mediated mechanism for the symptoms but does nothing to establish the inciting agent or event. Additional acute laboratories include serum complement levels (i.e., CH100, C3, and C4) to look for possible immune complex or vasculitis-induced anaphylatoxin formation. A complete blood count, chemistry profile, and urinalysis should be performed at least once to rule out alternate diagnoses. Immediate hypersensitivity skin testing is seldom definitive in this patient population but should at least include a reasonably significant food battery. In addition, if history warrants (i.e., medical worker, exposure to condoms, balloons, etc.), specific testing for latex sensitivity should also be performed.

Other more specialized tests that may be indicated include 24-hour urinary histamine and serum tryptase to differentiate IA from systemic mastocytosis (SM). In SM, both urinary histamine and serum tryptase are persistently elevated, whereas both levels are normal in IA except during and shortly after an acute episode. If patients present with repeated skin flushing and/or prominent gastrointestinal symptoms, urinary 5-hydroxyindole acetic acid and metanephrines should be obtained to rule out carcinoid and pheochromocytoma. If C1-esterase inhibitor deficiency (congenital or acquired) is suspected, C4 should be obtained during an acute episode as well as plasma C1-esterase activity.

Once anaphylaxis has been established as the reason for the symptoms and no cause for the reaction can be established, the patient is appropriately classified as having idiopathic anaphylaxis.

CLASSIFICATION OF IA AND APPROACHES TO MANAGEMENT

Acute management of IA is no different than other systemic mast cell–mediated reactions (Table 2). Necessary resuscitative techniques to manage acute symptoms (supplemental oxygen, parenteral fluids, and so on) are promptly initiated as needed upon presentation. Use of epinephrine (adult: 0.3 cc of 1:1,000 sc; child: 0.01 ml per kilogram up to adult dose given every 10 minutes up to three times as needed) can be life-saving, particularly if given early in the course of the episode with a portable kit (Ana-Kit, EpiPen), which should be carried by the patient at all times. It is particularly important to emphasize to the affected patient and family members the importance of keeping the epinephrine kits within easy reach since the episode can rapidly progress to a potentially fatal stage in a matter of minutes. Despite these admonitions, a significant proportion of these patients fail to carry epinephrine with them at all times (43 percent in one study). Thus, several epinephrine kits should be kept in strategic locations (i.e., work, car, briefcase, or purse) if there is any question about the patient keeping the epinephrine close. Life-long epinephrine therapy is usually not necessary since spontaneous remission is high in this condition. However, the kits should be kept at hand until 5 years after the last attack.

Antihistamines (both H_1 and H_2) should also be kept at hand to be used immediately at the onset of symptoms. Diphenhydramine or hydroxyzine (50 mg

Table 3 Classification of Idiopathic Anaphylaxis

*Classification**	*Characteristics*
IA-frequent (IA-F)	6 or more episodes per year
IA-infrequent (IA-I)	5 or fewer episodes per year
IA-generalized (IA-G)	Multisystem symptoms including urticaria, bronchospasm, upper airway compromise, hypotension, syncope, and/or gastrointestinal symptoms
IA-angioedema (IA-A)	Urticaria or angioedema with upper airway compromise such as laryngeal edema, severe pharyngeal edema, and/or severe tongue edema without other systemic manifestations
IA-questionable (IA-Q)	Patient referred for presumptive IA, but repeated attempts to document objective clinical findings are unsuccessful and successful response to adequate doses of prednisone does not occur

Modified from Patterson R, Greenberger PA, Grammar LC, et al. Idiopathic anaphylaxis (IA): Suggested theories relative to the pathogenesis and response to therapy. Allergy Proc 1993; 14:365.

*Various combinations (i.e., IA-F-G, IA-I-A, and so on) are possible.

orally every 6 hours) and cimetidine (300 mg) or ranitidine (150 mg) should be given orally every 12 hours, particularly if hypotension is part of the clinical presentation. Prednisone, 50 mg orally, can prevent development of late-phase reactions which occur in up to 50 percent of affected individuals.

Chronic management depends upon the classification of IA (Table 3) as described by Patterson and associates. By frequency, IA can occur more than (IA-F) or fewer than (IA-I) six episodes per year. Further classification is based upon generalized, multisystem reaction (IA-G) or primarily angioedema causing upper airway obstruction (IA-A). Two other classifications include IA-Q, in which the diagnosis is actually in question and the patient continues to have episodes while on systemic corticosteroid therapy, and IA-V, in which the symptoms vary from the classic presentation.

Initial prophylactic management for IA-F (both generalized and angioedema) and severe, life-threatening reaction regardless of frequency includes prednisone 60 mg daily in single morning oral doses for 1 week or until signs and symptoms are controlled. Prednisone is then converted to alternate-day prednisone 60 mg with gradual tapering by 5 mg weekly. When prednisone has been discontinued for 1 year, the patient can be considered in remission.

Continuous antihistamines (e.g., diphenhydramine or hydroxyzine 25 to 50 mg three times daily) should be given until the patient has achieved clinical remission and then should be withdrawn gradually with careful observation for recurrence. Nonsedating antihistamines (e.g., terfenidine 60 mg twice daily or loratadine 10 mg daily) may be given when side effects of other antihistamines are excessive to the level of compromising day-to-day lifestyle. In addition, sympathomimetic agents (e.g., albuterol 2 mg orally three times a day, ephedrine 25 mg orally three times a day) are given continuously if tolerated in particularly recalcitrant cases.

If an exacerbation occurs, acute therapy is reinstituted with maintenance medications restarted and tapered as previously described. In those patients who continue to report episodes while taking adequate doses of prednisone, IA-Q (questionable) should be considered. These patients merely *report* the symptom complex, but physiologic changes are never documented. Such individuals may benefit from psychiatric evaluation and treatment.

PROGNOSIS

Although the natural history of IA may be variable depending upon the individual, the risk of mortality with adequate treatment is exceedingly low. Recurrence is common in undertreated individuals. This appears most commonly in those patients whose physicians do not provide an adequate dose of corticosteroids for a sufficient period of time or who do not take corticosteroids as they were prescribed. The frequency of repeat episodes typically lessens after the first 6 months and eventuates in remission in the vast majority of patients. Thus, since any episode of anaphylaxis poses a significant fatality risk, proper management and precautions must be taken by the patient and physician until clinical remission is obtained with certainty.

SUGGESTED READING

Friedman BS, Germano P, Miletti J, Metcalf DD. A clinicopathologic study of ten patients with recurrent unexplained flushing. J Allergy Clin Immunol 1994; 93:53.

Lieberman PL, Taylor WW. Recurrent idiopathic anaphylaxis. Arch Int Med 1979; 139:1032.

Patterson R, Greenberger PA, Grammar LC, et al. Idiopathic anaphylaxis (IA): Suggested theories relative to the pathogenesis and response to therapy. Allergy Proc 1993; 14:365.

Patterson R, Stoloff RS, Greenberger PA, et al. Algorithms for the diagnosis and management of idiopathic anaphylaxis. Ann Allergy 1993; 71:40.

Tanus T, Mines D, Atkins PC, Levinson AI. Serum tryptase in idiopathic anaphylaxis: a case report and review of the literature. Ann Emer Med 1994; 24:104.

Wong S, Dykewicz MS, Patterson R. Idiopathic anaphylaxis: A clinical summary of 175 patients. Arch Int Med 1990; 150:1323.

INSULIN ALLERGY AND INSULIN RESISTANCE

KRISTI SILVER, M.D.
ALAN R. SHULDINER, M.D.
JESSE ROTH, M.D.

INSULIN ALLERGY

Insulin provides life-sustaining therapy for patients with type I (insulin-dependent) diabetes mellitus and may play an important role in the treatment of many patients with type II (noninsulin-dependent) diabetes. Shortly after the introduction of insulin therapy in the early 1920s, adverse reactions were recognized, some of which involve the immune system. Before the widespread use of highly purified insulins, it had been estimated that as many as 15 to 55 percent of patients manifested allergic reactions during their initial course of insulin therapy. Today, the incidence of local insulin allergy is much less, since highly purified insulins are significantly less allergenic. Systemic insulin allergy or insulin resistance caused by circulating anti-insulin antibodies is even rarer and occurs in only about 0.1 percent of patients receiving insulin. In many developing countries, less pure insulins continue to be used and immune reactions are more prevalent. In the United States, human insulins are currently less expensive than animal insulins, and are widely used.

Insulin allergy usually occurs within weeks to months of initiating therapy. Some patients allergic to insulin give a history of interrupted use of insulin. Interestingly, up to one-third of patients who have an allergy to insulin also report allergy to penicillin. There has been no clear association between insulin allergy and atopic diseases such as allergic rhinitis or asthma. The tendency to develop an immune response to insulin may be genetically determined since patients with certain histocompatibility (HLA) antigens appear to have a greater likelihood of developing insulin allergy than those who do not bear these antigens.

Type I diabetes is characterized by autoimmune-mediated destruction of the beta cells of the endocrine pancreas. Anti-insulin and anti-islet cell antibodies can often be detected before the clinical manifestations of diabetes become apparent and before insulin therapy is initiated. In addition, an insulin autoimmune syndrome has been described in some patients with fasting or postprandial hypoglycemia and circulating anti-insulin antibodies. First reported in Japanese women with hyperthyroidism who were being treated with methimazole, the clinical syndrome and the antibodies are found with a broad range of diseases and drugs. In two reported cases, one with benign monoclonal gammopathy, the second with multiple myeloma, the offending antibody was monoclonal. For a detailed review of these immunologic mechanisms, we refer the reader elsewhere (see Suggested Reading).

The Antigen

Insulin

Insulin is a two-chain polypeptide of molecular weight approximately 5,700, derived from the single-chain peptide precursor proinsulin. Insulins or insulin genes have been studied from more than 50 chordate species from mammals to cyclostome fish and amphioxus. Not surprisingly, the amino acid sequence of the insulin molecule is well conserved throughout this period of evolution. However, there are two regions in which major interspecies variations typically occur: (1) amino acids 8, 9, and 10 of the A chain, and (2) residue 30 of the B chain (Table 1).

Until recently, commercially available insulins have been prepared by extraction of beef and pork pancreatic tissue. Beef insulin differs from human insulin by three amino acids, whereas pork insulin differs from human insulin by only one amino acid (Table 1). Although these closely related insulins have equal biopotency, it has been generally noted that the greater the difference in primary structure from human insulin, the greater the antigenicity in humans. But, even when the structure of the injected insulin is identical to endogenous insulin, it may be antigenic. Overall, human insulin tends to be less antigenic in humans than pork insulin, which tends to be less antigenic than beef insulin.

Species variations within the insulin molecule are not the only determinants of antigenicity. It has been shown, for example, that dimeric and other aggregated forms of insulin are more antigenic than monomeric insulin.

The frequency and route of insulin delivery may play a role in insulin antigenicity. Comparison of antibody levels in conventional insulin therapy, multiple daily injections, and subcutaneous insulin infusion have shown conflicting results; some studies demonstrate similar antibody levels in the three groups while other studies demonstrate higher antibody levels in the multiple daily injection and subcutaneous infusion groups. Several studies involving intraperitoneal insulin administration using 21 PH insulin, which contains glycerol and Genapol as insulin stabilizers, have shown an increase in insulin antibodies. These antibodies did not produce insulin resistance or insulin allergy; however, in three subjects, these antibodies may have contributed to significant nocturnal hypoglycemia.

Peptide Impurities

Commercial insulin preparations in the United States before the early 1970s (USP insulin) contained approximately 8 percent protein impurities. These protein impurities included (1) higher molecular weight species, such as proinsulin, proinsulin derivatives, and

Table 1 Differences in Amino Acids of Commercially Available Insulins

	A Chain			*B Chain*
Species	*A–8*	*A–9*	*A–10*	*B–30*
Human	Thr	Ser	Ile	Thr
Pork	Thr	Ser	Ile	Ala
Beef	Ala	Ser	Val	Ala

multimeric insulins; (2) chemically modified insulins, such as esterified insulins, desamido insulins, or insulins in which the secondary or tertiary structure had been disrupted; and (3) proteins of lower molecular weight, such as glucagon, pancreatic polypeptide, vasoactive intestinal peptide, somatostatin, and possibly other peptides of pancreatic origin (Table 2). In 1974, more extensive purification of commercial insulins in the United States excluded both high and low molecular weight impurities in preparations designated single peak insulins. These preparations were 98 percent pure and were clearly less antigenic than previously available preparations. By 1980, commercial insulin preparations were further purified by chromatography on modified celluloses to yield single component or monocomponent insulins. Monocomponent insulins are more than 99 percent pure and contain less than 10 ppm proinsulin.

Since 1983, human insulin has been commercially available. Human insulin is produced by recombinant DNA technology in which bacteria (Lilly; Humulin) and yeast (Novo Nordisk; Novolin) are genetically engineered to produce human proinsulin, which is then purified and converted enzymatically to insulin. Additional potential impurities in recombinant DNA human insulin are microbial products.

Pharmaceutical Additives

Pharmaceutical additives may also be antigenic. Virtually all commercially available insulin preparations contain small quantities of zinc to promote crystallization during the purification process. Neutral protamine Hagedorn insulin (NPH) and protamine zinc insulin (PZI) contain the positively charged polyanion protamine. Protamine may be antigenic by itself or may enhance an allergic response to insulin (so-called schlepper phenomenon). Indeed, lethal anaphylactic reactions to protamine used for reversal of heparin-induced anticoagulation during vascular surgery have been reported in diabetic patients receiving protamine-containing insulin preparations. Lente insulins lack protamine but contain a higher concentration of zinc and an acetate buffer rather than phosphate. Finally, preservatives present in minute quantities in commercial insulins can be antigenic; the nature and concentrations of preservatives often vary among commercial preparations.

In summary, the greater the similarity in primary structure to human insulin, the less antigenic the insulin tends to be, but all insulins appear to be antigenic to some degree. Allergy associated with the injection of insulin may not specifically involve insulin as the offending antigen. Potential antigens present in commercially available insulins are listed in Table 2. In general, purer preparations tend to be less antigenic than cruder preparations, and short-acting (so-called regular) insulins that contain fewer additives tend to be less antigenic than sustained-action preparations. However, among regular insulins of similar purity from different commercial sources, one cannot predict which preparation will be less antigenic for a particular patient. These points are important when considering insulin therapy for patients with diabetes and when considering treatment options for patients with insulin allergy.

Table 2 Potential Antigens in Commercially Available Insulins

Antigen	*Preparation*
Insulin	All (beef > pork > human)
Peptide impurities	
Proinsulin	USP and single peak
Multimeric insulins	All
Modified insulins	USP and single peak
Glucagon	USP and single peak
Pancreatic polypeptide	USP and single peak
Somatostatin	USP and single peak
Vasoactive intestinal peptide	USP and single peak
Microbial-derived substances	Recombinant DNA, human
Pharmaceutical additives	
Zinc	All
Protamine	NPH, PZI
Preservatives	All
Buffers	All
Genapol	21 PH insulin
Glycerol	21 PH insulin

NPH, Neutral protamine Hagedorn; *PZI,* protamine zinc insulin.

The Immune Response

Insulin may elicit both cellular and humoral immune responses. The triggering of each of these mechanisms may determine the character as well as the severity of the allergic response.

The Gell and Coombs classification applies well to the immunologic mechanisms that cause insulin allergy (Table 3). Most common are type I reactions, which are IgE mediated; the antigen cross-links IgE on the surface of mast cells, causing release of mediators such as histamine and lymphokines, resulting in an immediate local reaction. When severe, a systemic anaphylactic reaction may ensue. Type II reactions have not been described with insulin. Type III immune reactions involve the formation of antigen-antibody complexes that result in complement fixation, leukocyte attraction, and an inflammatory response. These reactions may manifest themselves as local Arthus-like reactions or as systemic serum sickness-like reactions. Alternatively, when an anti-insulin antibody of high capacity is present, insulin

Table 3 Gell and Coombs Classification of Immunologic Reactions to Insulin

Class	*Mechanism*	*Clinical Manifestations*
Type I	IgE→mast cell degranulation	Local immediate; anaphylaxis
Type II	Cytotoxic	None described
Type III	IgG→complement fixation	Local Arthus reaction; serum sickness
	Anti-insulin antibodies	Insulin resistance
Type IV	Lymphocyte mediated	Local delayed hypersensitivity

resistance may result. While IgG predominates, virtually all classes of antibody molecules have been identified in patients with this form of insulin resistance. Finally, type IV reactions are cell mediated and are characterized by local delayed hypersensitivity.

Local Insulin Allergy: Diagnosis and Treatment

Local insulin allergy occurs most commonly within the first few weeks or months after beginning insulin therapy. Complaints include erythema, swelling, itching, burning, or pain as well as induration or wheal formation from 1 to 5 cm in diameter at the site of injection. Local allergy may occur immediately after injection and subside rapidly, or its appearance may be delayed for several hours after injection and persist for as long as 24 to 48 hours. Most often, patients show a biphasic allergic response.

Before making the diagnosis of local insulin allergy, the injection technique should be carefully scrutinized since nonsterile techniques, injection of cold insulin, or excessive trauma can cause an inflammatory response that can mimic cutaneous allergy. Treatment of local insulin allergy that is mild or even moderate may consist simply of reassurance since an overwhelming majority of local allergic reactions are self-limited and cease to occur within 1 to 3 months, despite continuation of insulin therapy. Since the allergy may be the result of one of the pharmaceutical additives, a change in the type or brand of insulin may relieve the reaction.

For severe or intolerable local reactions, intradermal skin testing with various insulin preparations often helps to identify the least antigenic preparation. Alternatively, one might empirically switch insulin preparations in an attempt to find a preparation that is less antigenic, remembering that in general purer preparations are less antigenic than cruder preparations, human insulin is less antigenic than insulins from other species, and short-acting preparations are less antigenic than sustained-action preparations. When a less antigenic insulin preparation cannot be identified, subcutaneous coinjection of hydrocortisone (2 to 10 mg) with insulin may prevent or attenuate the appearance of a local allergic response. In cases in which local allergic reactions are of the delayed type, subcutaneous coinjection of a longer-acting glucocorticoid such as dexamethasone (0.1 to 0.5 mg) is often more efficacious. Oral antihistamines,(i.e., diphenhydramine [Benadryl]), 25 to 50 mg orally every 6 hours, is often helpful in relieving symptoms of local allergy. Since local insulin allergy is almost always a self-limited process, most patients will not require long-term treatment, and periodic attempts should be made to discontinue glucocorticoids or antihistamines. In a minority of cases, local allergy may become generalized; thus, the patient should be instructed on the use of epinephrine for possible emergency use.

Systemic Insulin Allergy: Diagnosis and Treatment

Symptoms of systemic insulin allergy, like local allergy, usually develop within the first weeks or months after initiating therapy. The clinical manifestations of systemic insulin allergy may vary widely in severity and may be clinically indistinguishable from those observed with penicillin allergy.

Systemic allergy usually begins with an immediate localized reaction at the site of injection that spreads into a generalized urticarial pattern with pruritus and angioedema. Skin manifestations may be accompanied by rhinorrhea, nausea, and abdominal or uterine cramps. In more severe cases, laryngeal edema, bronchospasm, hypotension, and death may ensue.

The diagnosis of systemic insulin allergy is usually unambiguous. A thorough drug history should be elicited to exclude other possible offending antigens. Conditions such as idiopathic urticaria and idiopathic anaphylaxis can usually be excluded based on the temporal association of symptoms with insulin injection. Cutaneous skin testing may help to point away from the diagnosis of systemic insulin allergy when a negative test result is elicited. However, since as many as 40 to 50 percent of patients receiving insulin may have a positive skin test result in the absence of clinically significant systemic insulin allergy, a positive skin test result is of limited diagnostic significance.

In patients manifesting mild-to-moderate symptoms of systemic insulin allergy such as pruritus or urticaria, skin testing may be helpful in identifying a less antigenic insulin preparation, which may then be substituted. Alternatively, a less antigenic preparation may be chosen empirically (i.e., regular human insulin). Substitution of a less antigenic insulin preparation can result in improvement in symptoms in up to 70 percent of patients.

Table 4 Typical Rapid Desensitization Schedule*

Time (hr)	*Dose (U)*	*Route*
0.0	0.001	Intradermal
0.5	0.002	Intradermal
1.0	0.004	Subcutaneous
1.5	0.01	Subcutaneous
2.0	0.02	Subcutaneous
2.5	0.04	Subcutaneous
3.0	0.1	Subcutaneous
3.5	0.2	Subcutaneous
4.0	0.5	Subcutaneous
4.5	1.0	Subcutaneous
5.0	2.0	Subcutaneous
5.5	4.0	Subcutaneous
6.0	8.0	Subcutaneous

Modified from Galloway JD, Bressler R. Insulin treatment in diabetes. Med Clin North Am 1978; 62:663.

*Follow by increase of dosage every 4 to 6 hours until desired therapeutic affect is achieved.

Systemic treatment with an antihistamine (e.g., diphenhydramine, 25 to 50 mg orally every 6 hours) is useful in many patients. Again, the patient should have epinephrine available in case symptoms progress.

Severe systemic insulin allergy or anaphylaxis may require immediate lifesaving therapy in an acute care setting. Urticaria and respiratory or hemodynamic compromise characteristic of anaphylaxis should be managed accordingly. Beta-adrenergic agents and glucocorticoids should be used as necessary, temporarily ignoring their metabolic activities that may compromise blood glucose control.

When the severe allergic reaction is under control, a key medical decision needs to be confronted: how essential is insulin for this particular patient? In a large study conducted at the National Institutes of Health, about half of the patients with type II diabetes referred for management of insulin allergy did well after complete withdrawal of insulin.

When insulin is required, it should be continued without interruption; the patient should be hospitalized promptly and closely observed while desensitization is carried out. Cutaneous skin testing may be helpful in identifying the least antigenic insulin preparation that may then be used for the desensitization procedure.

When the patient has received insulin within the previous 24 hours, the first desensitization dose should be 20 percent of the patient's usual dose. Most patients will tolerate this reduced dose without significant adverse effects. Should adverse effects occur, the dose may be decreased further. The insulin dose may be increased by 3 to 5 units each day until the desired therapeutic effect is achieved.

Patients who have not received insulin in the previous 24 hours need to be started at a much lower desensitization dose since unbound IgE titers are much higher, increasing the likelihood of an allergic reaction. A typical rapid desensitization schedule is outlined in Table 4. Successful desensitization can be accomplished in most patients with this schedule.

LOCALIZED LIPOATROPHY AND LIPOHYPERTROPHY

Insulin-induced lipoatrophy, the loss of subcutaneous fat at the site of insulin injection, is a localized adverse effect of insulin therapy. Insulin-induced lipoatrophy occurs more commonly in young women than men and is seen more frequently when less pure insulin preparations are used. With the introduction of highly purified human insulin, the prevalence of lipoatrophy has decreased substantially. Lipoatrophy may occur alone or may be accompanied by localized insulin allergy. It is thought that lipoatrophy is immunologically mediated since skin biopsies of the affected areas indicate abnormal deposition of immunologic components in dermal vessel walls.

Lipoatrophy is a benign process but may be cosmetically unacceptable for some patients. Preventive measures include the use of human insulin. In addition, localized lipoatrophy may be minimized by teaching patients to rotate their injection sites properly. In patients in whom lipoatrophy is already present, human insulin should be substituted for pork or beef preparations. Repeated injection of the purer preparation into and around the affected site can paradoxically result in dramatic resolution of lipoatrophy. Improvement should be noted within 2 to 6 weeks.

In some patients, repeated injection of purer insulin preparations may result in localized lipohypertrophy, which is thought to be due to the direct lipogenic actions of insulin. When injection sites are rotated properly, this complication can usually be prevented as well. In some patients, localized lipoatrophy and lipohypertrophy may coexist.

INSULIN RESISTANCE

Clinical diagnosis of insulin resistance is made in an insulin-treated patient when larger than expected quantities of exogenous insulin are needed to achieve euglycemia. Based on the study of insulin requirements in pancreatectomized adults, and more recently using euglycemic clamp techniques, it has been determined that the average rate of endogenous insulin secretion in normal adults is 20 to 60 units per day. Often, patients require 60 to 200 units of insulin per day and may be considered to have mild-to-moderate insulin resistance. Patients with severe insulin resistance typically require more than 200 units of insulin per day. Fortunately, severe insulin resistance is quite rare and probably accounts for only about 0.01 percent of patients.

Within months to years of commencing insulin therapy, virtually all patients develop circulating anti-insulin antibodies. Since the clinical consequences of such antibodies are usually of little significance, common nonimmune causes of mild or moderate degrees of insulin resistance such as obesity, noninsulin-dependent (type II) diabetes mellitus, uremia, acromegaly, glucocorticoid excess, and numerous other diseases, as well as

Table 5 Causes of Insulin Resistance

Causes
Nonimmunologic causes
Mild to moderate
Type II diabetes
Obesity
Pregnancy
Glucocorticoid excess
Acromegaly
Acidosis
Cirrhosis
Uremia
Excess insulin
Insulinoma
Exogenous insulin
Severe
Subcutaneous insulin resistance syndrome
Genetic syndromes
Type A syndrome of extreme insulin resistance
Leprechaunism
Lipoatrophic diabetes
Rabson-Mendenhall syndrome
Immunologic causes
Mild to moderate
Low-capacity anti-insulin antibodies
Severe
High-capacity anti-insulin antibodies
Type B syndrome of extreme insulin resistance

treatment with excessive doses of insulin, the so-called Somogyi effect, must first be excluded before an immunologic cause can be invoked (Table 5).

Severe insulin resistance points toward a shorter list of etiologies, some of which have an immunologic basis (Table 5). Determination of the cause of extreme insulin resistance often requires special tests, and patients should be referred to an appropriate center for evaluation and treatment.

Immunologic Causes of Insulin Resistance

Insulin Resistance Caused by Circulating Anti-Insulin Antibodies

In virtually all patients treated with insulin, low concentrations of anti-insulin antibodies (i.e., less than 10 units of insulin bound per liter of plasma) can be detected but are of little clinical significance. Rarely, high concentrations of high-affinity circulating anti-insulin antibodies may bind large quantities of exogenously administered insulin (i.e., 100 to 1,000 units of insulin bound per liter of plasma), thus impairing its egress from the plasma and delivery to target tissues. These antibodies, which are usually of the IgG class, are readily measured *in vitro.* The absolute binding capacity of circulating anti-insulin antibodies typically correlates well with the degree of insulin resistance.

Generally, the development of high-affinity anti-insulin antibodies is a transient phenomenon that can be treated by switching to human insulin and increasing the dose as needed. When very large doses of insulin are required (i.e., >500 units per day), U-500 insulin preparations may be useful. In some instances, fish insulin or sulfated insulin may be efficacious substitutes; these insulins retain adequate bioactivity but because they bind to the patient's antibodies much less well than unmodified mammalian insulins, they are more effective *in vitro*. These insulins are available for clinical use only in research settings.

In circumstances in which insulin resistance is severe despite these measures, administration of a systemic glucocorticoid (i.e., prednisone, 40 to 60 mg orally per day) may paradoxically result in a rapid decrease in insulin requirements (even without a change in antibody titer). Since insulin resistance caused by anti-insulin antibodies is typically transient and resolves after several months, glucocorticoid therapy should only be used when necessary, and when instituted, attempts to taper the dose should be made early and repeatedly until successful.

Glycemic control in patients with high titers of circulating anti-insulin antibodies may be difficult since antibody titers vary in unpredictable ways. Caregivers must be aware that in occasional patients, variations in the severity of insulin resistance in combination with very high doses of insulin can lead to rather abrupt onset of severe hypoglycemia that may be quite protracted and life threatening.

Type B Syndrome of Extreme Insulin Resistance

Type B syndrome of extreme insulin resistance occurs predominantly in women who have a well-defined autoimmune disease such as systemic lupus erythematosus or Sjögren's syndrome, or a less well-defined constellation of features that suggest autoimmunity (e.g., elevated erythrocyte sedimentation rate, positive antinuclear antibody, decreased complement, pancytopenia, and proteinuria). Insulin resistance in patients with type B syndrome is caused by polyclonal autoantibodies that bind to insulin receptors at or near the insulin-binding site, thereby impairing their function. Removal of anti-insulin receptor antibodies *in vitro* restores normal insulin binding, implying that the underlying receptors are normal. These anti-receptor antibodies may be readily detected *in vitro* at some diabetes research centers, and the diagnosis is thereby definitively distinguished from type A syndromes (due to genetic defects in the insulin receptor) and from resistance due to anti-insulin antibodies.

Patients with extreme insulin resistance and severe glucose intolerance should be treated with insulin. The goal should be to decrease or prevent the symptoms of hyperglycemia. Large doses of insulin (i.e., up to 100,000 units per day) may be required. U-500 insulin is preferred when such high doses are needed. Since the titer of anti-insulin receptor antibodies tends to change during the course of the disease and spontaneous remission is common, insulin requirements can vary dramatically and glycemic control may be problematic. Patients with type B syndrome of extreme insulin resistance usually have evidence of systemic autoimmunity, problems such as nephritis, cerebritis, and thrombocytopenia, which must be watched for and treated aggressively.

In some patients the circulating titers of anti-insulin receptor antibodies may be insulinomimetic and may lead to hypoglycemia. It appears that the same population of polyclonal antibodies may cause hyperglycemia at high titers but hypoglycemia at lower titers. Clinically, the patient may present initially with hyperglycemia, and in the face of fluctuating titers of anti-insulin receptor antibodies, may later become hypoglycemic. Rarely, patients with anti-insulin receptor antibodies may present initially with hypoglycemia indistinguishable from other causes of fasting hypoglycemia such as insulinoma or sereptitious use of insulin or sulfonylureas. When the anti-insulin receptor antibodies are insulinomimetic, hypoglycemia may be life threatening and should be treated with glucose and high doses of systemic glucocorticoids (prednisone, 60 to 100 mg orally per day).

Like other forms of extreme insulin resistance, type B syndrome of extreme insulin resistance is often associated with acanthosis nigricans, a hyperpigmented hyperkeratotic rash commonly seen in the intertriginous areas of the body as well as over the elbows, base of the neck, and waist. When cosmetically bothersome, treatment with topical retinoic acid (tretinoin) is often efficacious. In addition, sexually mature premenopausal women with type B syndrome of extreme insulin resistance often have high serum testosterone levels; the hormone is produced by cells in the ovary. Hypertestosteronemia is probably a major contributor to the amenorrhea, hirsutism, and polycystic ovaries that are commonly seen in these disorders. Hirsutism may respond to estrogen therapy (e.g., Premarin, 0.625 to 1.25 mg per day).

SUGGESTED READING

Arnquist HJ, Halban PA, Mathiesen UL, et al. Hypoglycemia caused by atypical insulin antibodies in a patient with benign monoclonal gammopathy. J Int Med 1993; 239.

Beck-Nielsen H, Richelsen B, Schwartz-Sorensen N, et al. Insulin pump treatment: effect on glucose homeostasis, metabolites, hormones, insulin antibodies and quality of life. Diabetes Res 1985; 2:37.

Dahl-Jorgensënk, Torjesen P, Hanssen KF, et al. Increase in insulin antibodies during continuous subcutaneous insulin infusion and multiple-injection therapy in contrast to conventional treatment. Diabetes 1987; 36:1.

deShazo RD, Mather P, Grant W, et al. Evaluation of patients with local reactions to insulin with skin tests and *in vitro* techniques. Diabetes Care 1987; 10:330.

Galloway JA, deShazo RD. Insulin chemistry and pharmacology; insulin allergy, resistance, and lipodystrophy. In: Rifkin H. Porte D. eds. Diabetes mellitus, theory and practice. New York: Elsevier, 1990:497.

Kahn CR, Rosenthal AS. Immunologic reactions to insulin: insulin allergy, insulin resistance, and autoimmune insulin syndrome. Diabetes Care 1979; 2:283.

Lassmann-Vague V, Belicar P, Raccah, et al. Immunogenicity of long-term intraperitoneal insulin administration with implantable programmable pumps: metabolic consequences. Diabetes Care 1995; 18:498.

Micossi P, Galimberti G, Librenti MC, et al. Glycerol-insulin raises circulating insulin antibodies in type I diabetic patients treated with permanently implanted devices. Metabolism 1988; 37:1029.

Moller DE, Flier JS. Insulin resistance – mechanisms, syndromes and implications. N Engl J Med 1991; 938.

Olsen CL, Chan E, Turner DS, et al. Insulin antibody responses after long-term intraperitoneal insulin administration via implantable programmable insulin delivery systems. Diabetes Care 1994; 17:169.

Ratner RE, Phillips TM, Steiner M. Persistent cutaneous insulin allergy resulting from high-molecular weight insulin aggregates. Diabetes 1990; 39:728.

Redmon B, Pyzdrowski KL, Elson MK, et al. Hypoglycemia due to a monoclonal insulin-binding antibody in multiple myeloma. N Engl J Med 1992; 326:994.

Shades DS, Duckworth WC. In search of the subcutaneous insulin resistance syndrome. N Engl J Med 1986; 315:147.

Shuldiner AR, Roth J. Insulin allergy and insulin resistance. In: Bardin CW, ed. Current therapy in endocrinology and metabolism. 4th ed. Philadelphia: BC Decker, 1991.

Small P, Lerman S. Human insulin allergy. Ann Allergy 1984; 53:39.

Taylor SI, Dons RF, Hernandez E, et al. Insulin resistance associated with androgen excess in women with autoantibodies to the insulin receptor. Ann Intern Med 1982; 97:851.

Taylor SI, Grunberger G, Marcus-Samuels B, et al. Hypoglycemia associated with antibodies to the insulin receptor. N Engl J Med 1982; 307:1422.

Van Haeften TW. Clinical significance of insulin antibodies in insulin-treated diabetic patients. Diabetes Care 1989; 12:641.

ARTHRITIS

RHEUMATOID ARTHRITIS

JOSEPH M. CASH, M.D.
GARY S. HOFFMAN, M.D.

Inflammatory arthritis is the most prominent symptom of the systemic disease rheumatoid arthritis or, more accurately, rheumatoid disease (RD). RD encompasses a wide spectrum of illness from patients with mild symmetric inflammatory arthritis to those with a serious systemic illness that may also include lethargy, weight loss, pleural-pulmonary inflammation, cardiovascular symptoms, dry mucous membranes, or other systemic complications, including vasculitis. Early clinical and epidemiologic investigations employed the 1958 American Rheumatism Association (ARA) criteria as the primary tool to assess epidemiology and outcomes of RD. Studies that applied the 1958 criteria revealed the incidence of RD to be as high as 3.2 percent. Because many of the patients who were included in studies had "probable" as opposed to "definite" disease, the view that rheumatoid arthritis was a relatively benign disease was frequently reflected in textbooks of medicine and shaded the attitudes of both clinicians and the general public regarding the long-term prognosis.

It is now clear that the 1958 ARA criteria were excessively sensitive and not adequately specific. The 1987 American College of Rheumatology (ACR) (previously known as the American Rheumatism Association [ARA]) criteria for RD are more restrictive and when applied to large American populations, reveal a prevalence of RD of 1 percent, substantially lower than previously thought. In addition, persons who satisfy the revised diagnostic criteria had a much worse prognosis than previously appreciated. The 1987 ACR criteria requires the presence of four of seven criteria for more than 6 weeks (Table 1). The newer criteria do not include categories of possible or probable RD. This revised guide to diagnosis has been found to have 91

Table 1 The American College of Rheumatology 1987 Revised Criteria for the Classification of Rheumatoid Arthritis*

Criterion	*Definition*
1. Morning stiffness	Morning stiffness in and around the joints, lasting at least 1 hour before maximal improvement
2. Arthritis of three or more joint areas	At least 3 joint areas simultaneously have had soft tissues swelling or fluid (not bony overgrowth alone) observed by a physician. The 14 possible areas are right or left PIP, MCP, wrist, elbow, knee, ankle and MTP joints
3. Arthritis of hand joints	At least 1 area, swollen (as defined above) in a wrist, MCP, or PIP joint
4. Symmetric arthritis	Simultaneous involvement of the same joint areas (as defined in no. 2) on both sides of the body (bilateral involvement of PIPs, MCPs, or MTPs is acceptable without absolute symmetry)
5. Rheumatoid nodules	Subcutaneous nodules, over bony prominences, or extensor surfaces, or in juxta-articular regions, observed by a physician
6. Serum rheumatoid factor	Demonstration of abnormal amounts of serum rheumatoid factor by any method for which the results have been positive in $<5\%$ of normal control subjects
7. Radiographic changes	Radiographic changes typical of rheumatoid arthritis on posteroanterior hand and wrist radiographs, which must include erosions or unequivocal bony decalcification localized in or most marked adjacent to the involved joints (osteoarthritis changes alone do not qualify)

MCP, metacarpophalangeal; *MTP,* metatarsophalangeal; *PIP,* proximal intenphalangeal.

*For classification purposes, a patient shall be said to have rheumatoid arthritis if he or she has satisfied at least 4 of these 7 criteria. Criteria 1 through 4 must have been present for at least 6 weeks. Patients with 2 clinical diagnoses are not excluded. Designation as classic, definite, or probable rheumatoid arthritis is *not* to be made.

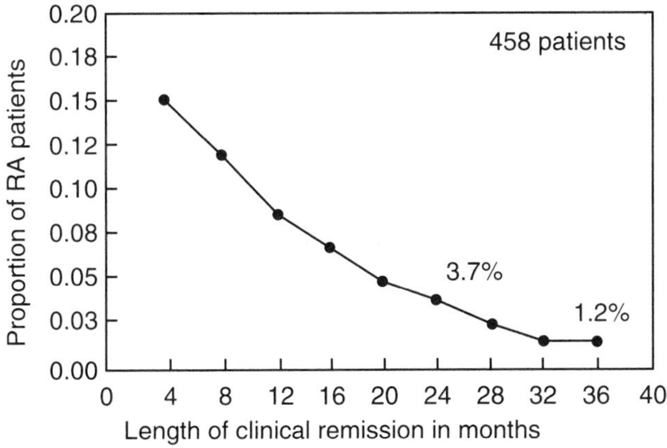

Figure 1 Remission in RD. (From Wolfe F, Hawley DJ. Remission in rheumatoid disease. J Rheumatol 1985; 12: 245–252; with permission.)

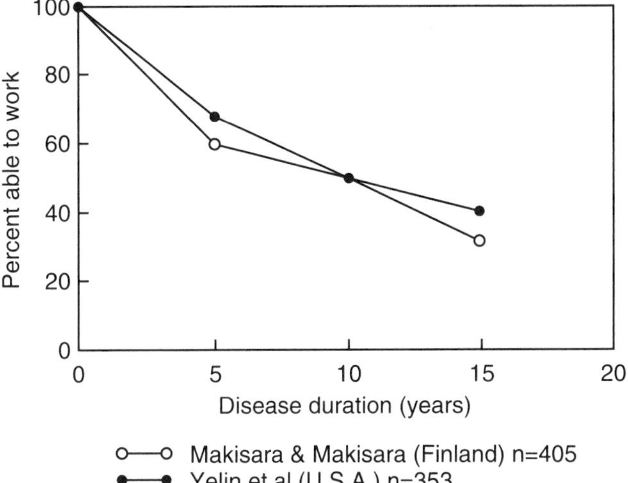

Figure 2 Occupational disability in patients with RD. (From Wolfe F. 50 years of antirheumatic therapy: the prognosis of rheumatoid arthritis. J Rheumatol 1990; 17(suppl):24–32; with permission.)

to 94 percent sensitivity and 89 percent specificity for RD when compared with other rheumatologic disease–control subjects.

Over the past 10 years, numerous studies of long-term outcomes of RD that have included patients with a definite diagnosis by current criteria have raised serious questions about the effectiveness of many anti-RD therapies. In spite of treatment, substantial functional loss occurred in over 50 percent of patients within 5 years. Only about 8 to 10 percent experienced remission that lasted an average of 12 months. The probability of achieving remission of at least 24 months' duration was 3.7 percent (Fig. 1). Analyses of work disability and subsequent unemployment have revealed that within 5, 10, and 15 years of disease onset, 33, 50, and 60 percent of patients, respectively, become occupationally disabled (Fig. 2). Patients with higher levels of education who functioned in decision-making positions and whose work required few physical demands were most likely to remain employed.

Our perspective on prognosis has also been altered by long-term studies that have demonstrated relentlessly progressive joint destruction and increased mortality in RD, contrary to former teaching. Radiographically defined joint damage increases in a linear fashion for the duration of a patient's life. Age of death in RD patients is 4 and 10 years earlier than noted in other American men and women, respectively. Premature deaths compared with those in the remainder of the population occur as the result of infection (9.4 versus 1 percent, renal disease (7.8 versus 1.1 percent), respiratory disease (7.2 versus 3.9 percent), and gastrointestinal abnormalities, particularly hemorrhage (4.2 versus 2.4 percent). In addition, patients with RD commonly undergo joint replacement and other surgical procedures, which place them at risk for infections, deep venous thrombosis, and other surgical complications. Finally, RD extracts a tremendous toll from its victims through economic loss, pain, and suffering.

GENERAL APPROACH TO TREATMENT

It would be inappropriate in a textbook or a clinical practice to provide a set of recommendations for treatment without establishing realistic expectations for both the patient and all members of the health care team. The patient, his or her family, and employer need to know that RD can be helped a great deal by treatment, but it is not curable and complete remission from all symptoms over an extended period of time is infrequent.

RD has medical, psychological, economic, and physiologic implications that extend beyond the direct consequences of joint inflammation. A multidisciplinary approach to treatment is essential to provide optimal care and to aid the patient in adapting to disability. Psychological services and support groups may be extremely valuable in this regard. Social workers may help guide the patient through the myriad of private sector and government programs available to the chronically ill. The Arthritis Foundation is an important resource for educational materials and for information concerning other services available for patients with RD. Because most patients continue to have some degree of discomfort despite medical therapy, physical activities are almost always curtailed. RD in conjunction with a more sedentary lifestyle will contribute to progressive loss of joint motion, muscle atrophy, and osteoporosis. These consequences can be diminished by a team approach, including the medical physician, physical and occupational therapist, and in some instances the orthopedic surgeon. Those joints and muscle groups that are not acutely inflamed should be exercised on a daily basis in an attempt to maintain range of motion, bone density, and muscle tone. The physician should tell the rehabilitation team which sites have been permanently damaged so that normal motion cannot be achieved and for which attempts at full restoration would create excessive pain and discouragement. Advanced joint destruction should be verified by radiograph. If available, physical therapists can assist the patient in the use of mechanical devices, including canes, crutches, or walkers. In the past 25 years, the advent of reconstructive surgery for severely damaged joints has led to major improvements in mobility and quality of life for patients with severe RD.

The many facets of RD and its treatment require a team of individuals with special skills. Although desirable, it is not essential for all team members to be assembled as a formal unit to maximize care benefits. It is crucial for the primary care provider to ensure that the patient has access to each team member in a timely, coordinated fashion.

PHARMACOLOGIC INTERVENTIONS IN RHEUMATOID DISEASE

Salicylates and Nonsteroidal Anti-Inflammatory Drugs

Salicylates and nonsteroidal anti-inflammatory drugs (NSAIDs) are usually the first medications employed in the treatment of RD; they improve joint stiffness and pain in the majority of patients with RD. Salicylates and NSAIDs are most useful as sole agents in patients with extremely mild disease or in those patients in which a clear-cut diagnosis of RD cannot be established. Patients with established RD associated with poor prognostic features, such as elevated rheumatoid factor titer, rheumatoid nodules, and/or erosive changes on radiographs should be strongly considered for second-line treatment as early as possible in the course of their disease.

Much has been written about the efficacy of different NSAIDS. Simply stated, prescription NSAID therapy has not been shown to be more efficacious than aspirin therapy. The main advantage of prescription NSAID therapy is the convenience of fewer tablets per day and, possibly, greater patient compliance. All NSAIDS are associated with a substantial risk of gastric and duodenal ulceration, upper gastrointestinal hemorrhage, and gastric perforation. Patients at highest risk for gastrointestinal complications include the elderly, patients with a previous history of peptic ulcerations or upper gastrointestinal hemorrhage, and persons who are concurrently using glucocorticoids.

Several strategies are available to minimize the risk of gastrointestinal toxicity. Available evidence suggests that enteric-coated aspirin is substantially safer than plain aspirin or prescription NSAIDs. Nonacetylated salicylates are prescription medications that have analgesic and anti-inflammatory properties comparable to NSAIDs but with a significant reduction in the risk of upper gastrointestinal complications. These medications are available only by prescription, are associated with tinnitus at therapeutic doses, and are poorly tolerated by some elderly patients because tablets are large (500 to 1,000 mg). Ibuprofen is the NSAID believed to have the most favorable gastrointestinal toxicity profile. Ibuprofen may be purchased over the counter in 200 mg tablets. It offers a reasonably safe alternative to prescription NSAIDs if patients achieve reasonable benefit at relatively low dosages (< 2,000 mg per day).

In the course of using these agents, it is important that adequate doses be employed before assuming lack of efficacy. In the absence of a therapeutic clinical response, the dose of these agents should be increased as tolerated about once a week until improvement occurs or the maximum recommended dose is reached. Conversely, one should not approach therapy with a preconceived notion of a minimal "therapeutic dose." Patients should be treated with the lowest effective dose possible. Gastrointestinal toxicity is far and away the most important adverse effect of NSAID therapy. Practitioners should be aware that patients treated with NSAIDs and salicylates may rarely develop renal impairment, hepatic inflammation, and allergic reactions.

Systemic Glucocorticoid Therapy

Glucocorticoid therapy, first introduced by Hench and colleagues in 1950, is a commonly used though controversial treatment for RD. Daily oral glucocorticoid therapy is frequently effective at reducing pain, stiffness, and improving constitutional symptoms associated with RD that may be resistant to other pharmacologic interventions. Strong evidence suggests that central hypocortisolism may be a fundamental mechanism in the development of experimental arthritis in animal models. Although indirect evidence suggests that similar mechanisms may be operative in some patients with RD, this hypothesis is far from proven in humans. Nevertheless, daily oral glucocorticoid therapy offers the potential for disease modification in addition to symptomatic improvement.

Given the chronic nature of RD, many clinicians believe that daily prednisone dosages of greater than 7.5 mg likely cause more long-term harm than good. Clinicians using low-dose prednisone for the treatment of RD should always strive to find the lowest effective dose and should not use glucocorticoids as sole therapeutic agents. Because experienced patients are excellent self-evaluators of disease activity, some patients may be candidates for as-needed (ad lib or prn) dosing of prednisone. Using this strategy, patients are given 1 mg prednisone tablets and instructed not to exceed a pre-set upper limit of 7 mg per day. Patients are encouraged to experiment with both the timing of prednisone doses and the total daily prednisone dosage. It has been our experience that many patients with RD are able to taper themselves down to lower effective doses of prednisone than may otherwise be achieved through physician-controlled dosing.

Several potential complications may occur from

daily prednisone treatment. Weight gain is the most common side effect seen. Patients with pre-existing hypertension or diabetes may have an exacerbation of these problems. It is unclear whether low-dose prednisone therapy increases the risk of osteoporosis; evidence to date is contradictory. If low-dose glucocorticoid therapy allows patients to engage in more weight-bearing exercise than they would otherwise be able to do than this effect will likely counteract any tendency of the drug per se to exacerbate osteoporosis. Higher doses of glucocorticoids may be necessary to treat patients with severe disease flares (discussed later in this chapter) and those with acute systemic rheumatoid vasculitis. Patients with associated systemic vasculitis require treatment with prednisone in doses of about 1 mg per kilogram per day. In severe life-threatening situations, glucocorticoid therapy may need to be supplemented by methotrexate or cyclophosphamide.

Second-Line Agents

A number of chemically unrelated medications have been shown to improve the overall level of disease activity in many RD patients (Tables 2 and 3). Although originally considered to be "remission inducing," this clearly is not the case with any of these agents, which have also been termed "slow-acting antirheumatic drugs" because of their delayed onset of action. The term "second-line antirheumatic drugs" may be the best single designation given the fact that these agents are rarely, if ever, the first drugs used in the treatment of RD. All of these agents have been shown in at least one short-term (generally 24 weeks or less) controlled clinical trial to be more effective than placebo. It has not been proven that any of the second-line agents favorably alter the ultimate natural history of RD, though many investigators feel that they do. All second-line antirheumatic drugs have been associated with significant toxicity, and this fact frequently guides treatment decisions.

Hydroxychloroquine

Hydroxychloroquine is an antimalarial agent that has largely replaced chloroquine in the treatment of RD. Two recent placebo-controlled studies have established hydroxychloroquine as a modestly effective drug in RD. The onset of action may not be apparent for 3 to 6 months. Hydroxychloroquine may be particularly useful in patients with mild to moderate disease. However, it is a poor choice as the initial second-line treatment in patients with poor prognostic features or particularly active disease given its slow onset of action and modest efficacy. Hydroxychloroquine is well tolerated and very few patients stop therapy because of perceived side effects. Chloroquine was associated with significant rates of retinal damage, which led to its abandonment by most clinicians. Hydroxychloroquine appears to be much safer at doses of 400 mg per day or less in average-sized adults; nevertheless, it is still recommended that patients undergo ophthalmologic evaluations every 6 to 12 months.

Gold Salts

Gold salts were the first of the "second-line" antirheumatic drugs to be introduced. Gold salts, active in vitro against mycobacterium, were introduced in the late 1920s to eradicate the supposed infectious cause of rheumatoid arthritis. Short-term placebo-controlled trials have, in general, confirmed intramuscular gold to be superior to placebo. However, one well-designed controlled trial sponsored by the Cooperative Clinics of the American Rheumatism Association failed to show benefit of drug over placebo. It has been our experience that treatment with intramuscular gold salts is extremely effective in a minority of treated patients, modestly effective in many patients, and occasionally ineffective. It is very common for patients who initially respond to intramuscular gold therapy to have disease flares despite continuation of the drug after 6 to 18 months.

Gold is among the most toxic of the second-line antirheumatic drugs. The most common adverse effect seen during gold therapy is skin rash, which may be mild or severe. Other common problems include oral ulcerations; thrombocytopenia, which may be severe; and nephritis. The popularity of intramuscular gold therapy has been waning in recent years because of the frequent loss of initial efficacy, relatively high rate of toxicity, and expense. Like intramuscular gold, auranofin, an oral gold preparation that was introduced in the 1980s, has high rates of associated side effects and questionable efficacy.

D-Penicillamine

D-Penicillamine is structurally related to both the amino acid, cysteine, and penicillin. D-penicillamine has a variety of immunomodulatory effects and effects on collagen structure that led to its introduction as a treatment to rheumatoid arthritis, but shares with gold a variety of potentially serious adverse effects, including cytopenias, hematuria and proteinuria; skin rashes; and gastrointestinal complications. In addition, D-penicillamine induces autoimmunity in some patients. The popularity of D-penicillamine is waning because of the increasing conviction that its questionable long-term benefits do not justify the substantial risk of treatment.

Sulfasalazine

Designed specifically as a treatment for RD in the mid-1930s, sulfasalazine is a unique hybrid of sulfa antibiotic (sulfapyradine) and a salicylate (5-aminosalicylic acid). After initially falling into disfavor, controlled clinical trials in the 1970s and 1980s firmly established sulfasalazine as an effective agent for the treatment of rheumatoid arthritis. Sulfasalazine is administrated orally at dosages of 1.5 to 4 g per day. Pa-

Table 2 Second-Line Antirheumatic Drugs: Overview

Agent	*Effective Dosage*	*Time to Onset of Action*	*Relative Efficacy*	*Relative Toxicity*	*Comments*
Methotrexate	5-25 mg/week IM/SC/PO	3-8 weeks	+ + + +	+ +	Best efficacy-toxicity ratio
Azathioprine	75-150 mg/day PO	6-12 weeks	+ + +	+ + +	Reasonably effective Lingering concerns about malignancy limit usefulness
D-Penicillamine	250-1,000 mg/day PO	8-16 weeks	+ +	+ + +	Relatively unfavorable efficacy-toxicity ratio
Cyclosporin A	2-5 mg/kg/day PO	6-16 weeks	+ + +	+ + +	Renal toxicity is universal Expensive
Sulfasalazine	2-4 g/day PO	4-12 weeks	+ + +	+ +	Excellent short-term efficacy Reasonably well tolerated
Cyclophosphamide	75-150 mg/day PO	4-12 weeks	+ + + +	+ + + +	Limited to refractory cases only
Chlorambucil	2-6 mg/day PO	4-12 weeks	+ + + +	+ + + +	Limited to refractory cases only
Intramuscular Gold	25-50 mg/wk IM loading*	12-20 weeks	+ + +	+ + + +	Excellent short-term efficacy Toxicity is common, effect wanes with time
Hydroxychloroquine	200-400 mg/day PO	12-24 weeks	+ +	+	Modest efficacy, minimal toxicity
Auranofin (oral gold)	3-9 mg/wk PO	8-16 weeks	+	+ + +	GI toxicity common, marginal efficacy

+ to + + + + = lesser to greater efficacy or toxicity.
*See text for details.

tients generally respond to therapy in 3 to 8 weeks. Although the short-term efficacy of sulfasalazine appears to be excellent, little is known about its long-term success. Sulfasalazine therapy is associated with high rates of skin rash and allergic phenomenon. In addition, many patients discontinue treatment because of nausea and vomiting. In addition, rare patients experience hepatic and hematologic toxicity (especially thrombocytopenia).

Methotrexate

Methotrexate was first used in the treatment of RD in 1951; however, it did not emerge as a popular treatment until the 1980s. Methotrexate has now been extensively studied in RD and because of numerous favorable reports, it is arguably the single most important second-line agent available for the treatment of moderate to severe RD. Methotrexate is an antimetabolite that inhibits the enzyme dihydrofolate reductase and ultimately the production of purines and DNA. This specific mechanism may be more important in producing toxicity than in providing clinical improvement in RD. Methotrexate has been demonstrated to have a variety of immunologic effects including inhibition of IgM rheumatoid factor synthesis, impairment of cytokine synthesis, impairment of leukotriene synthesis, and interference of cell-to-cell adherence. The specific mechanism of drug effect in RD in unknown. Methotrexate is administered once a week by either the oral, intravenous, intramuscular, or subcutaneous routes. Oral methotrexate is well absorbed by most patients. Methotrexate is eliminated by the kidney, and therefore its half-life and toxicity are enhanced in the presence of renal efficiency.

Treatment is usually started at a dose of about 0.2 mg per kilogram per week (or about 7.5 to 10 mg per week), which can be administered as a single dose. If gastrointestinal symptoms occur, they can be minimized by changing to 2 or 3 divided doses given at 12-hour intervals or by switching from oral administration to subcutaneous or intramuscular injections. If significant improvement is not seen over a 12-week period, the weekly dose can be provided parenterally and/or gradually increased to 0.4 mg per kilogram per week. Some physicians prefer to give methotrexate by the parenteral route because of enhanced bioavailability compared to variable absorption that may occur with oral administration. The use of weekly doses in excess of 30 mg is experimental and is not recommended outside of formal study protocols.

The short-term efficacy of methotrexate has been well established in a number of placebo-controlled and comparative clinical trials. Longitudinal studies suggest

Table 3 Toxic Effect of Second-Line Antirheumatic Drugs

Drug	*Gastrointestinal Effects**	*Effects on Liver**	*Effects on Lung**	*Effects on Renal Function**	*Infection†*	*Teratogenicity†*	*Cancer†*	*Miscellaneous Disorders*
Methotrexate	+ +	+ +	+ +	–	Moderate	Strong	Weak	Weak association: nodulosis, osteoporosis
Azathioprine	+ + +	+ +	–	–	Moderate	Weak	Moderate	–
D-Penicillamine	–	+	+ +	+ +	None	Moderate	None	Weak association: myasthenic syndrome, lupus, myositis
Cyclosporin A	–	+	–	+ + +	Weak	Unknown	Weak	Strong association: hypertension, neuropath
Sulfasalazine	+ +	+	+	–	None	None	None	Weak association: oligospermia
Cyclophosphamide	+	–	–	–	Strong	Strong	Strong	Strong association: hemorrhagic cystitis, ovarian and testicular failure
Chlorambucil	–	–	–	–	Strong	Strong	Strong	Strong association: ovarian and testicular failure
Intramuscular Gold	+	+	+	+ +	None	None	None	–
Hydroxychloroquine	–	–	–	–	None	None	None	Weak association: retinopathy, neuromyopathy
Auranofin (oral gold)	+ + +	–	–	+	None	Weak	None	–

Modified from Cash JM, Klippel JH. Second-line drug therapy in rheumatoid arthritis. N Engl J Med 1994; 330:1368–1375.
*The relative importance of the toxic effect is indicated as follows:
– denotes not reported or extremely rare.
+ denotes rare and an infrequent cause of discontinuing the drug.
+ + denotes common but an infrequent cause of discontinuing the drug.
+ + + denotes common and a frequent cause of discontinuing the drug.
†Degree of association.

that approximately 50 percent of patients will be able to continue low-dose weekly methotrexate beyond two years—a number that is substantially higher than that found for other second-line agents. Approximately 10 to 15 percent will stop treatment because of inadequate efficacy, while 30 percent will stop treatment because of toxicity.

Minor toxic reactions are common during methotrexate therapy; up to 15 percent of patients experience nausea, and other common side effects include stomatitis, elevated liver enzymes, transient fatigue, mild anemia, and macrocytosis. In rare cases, nausea and stomatitis are cause for medication discontinuance. Leucovorin (folinic acid) has been demonstrated to reduce the rate of nausea and liver enzyme abnormalities without reducing efficacy. Because leucovorin is expensive, we do not recommend its routine use. However, if toxicity arises during methotrexate therapy, leucovorin, 2.5 to 5 mg given as a single dose 24 hours after methotrexate administration, may allow patients to continue methotrexate therapy.

The development of cirrhosis of the liver and other life-threatening hepatic complications has been a significant problem in patients treated with methotrexate for psoriasis in the 1970s and early 1980s. This does not appear to be the case in rheumatoid arthritis patients treated since the mid-1980s, probably because of careful prescreening of patients for chronic liver disease and warnings to patients regarding the potential added toxicities of alcohol and methotrexate. Liver biopsies were once recommended before instituting methotrexate therapy, but this practice has now been largely abandoned because of recent studies suggesting that routine liver biopsies in low-risk patients are not cost-effective within at least 5 years of continuous methotrexate therapy. Patients treated with methotrexate for rheumatoid arthritis should have a complete blood count and SGOT, serum albumin, and serum creatinine levels checked every 4 to 12 weeks during therapy to monitor for toxicity. If elevations of SGOT or reductions in serum albumin occur, the dose can be held or reduced. If significant concerns arise regarding the status of the liver, a liver biopsy during the course of treatment may be necessary.

Contraindications of methotrexate use include acute and chronic liver disease, excess ingestion of alcoholic beverages, active peptic ulcer disease, morbid obesity associated with insulin-dependent diabetes mellitus, the presence of malignancy or a history of recent malignancy, pregnancy or potential child bearing, moderate to severe acute or chronic lung disease, and patient unreliability. Methotrexate is teratogenic and fertile women should be thoroughly warned regarding the necessity to practice effective birth control during treatment. Significant impairment of renal function has been well documented to increase a variety of methotrexate-associated side effects and mandates dose reduction. Methotrexate therapy should be generally avoided in patients with serum creatinine levels greater than 2.0 mg per deciliter.

Several patients who developed lymphoma while being treated with methotrexate have been reported, including two patients whose lymphomas resolved spontaneously with withdrawal of the drug. This occurrence appears to be rare and a direct causative role of methotrexate in the development of lymphoma has not been established. Methotrexate has not been shown to be carcinogenic in long-term follow-up studies of patients treated for germ cell cancer and psoriasis.

Because methotrexate is not curative, concern remains about potential relapse following discontinuation of treatment. Very limited efficacy-toxicity data are available in patients who have required more than 5 years of continuous weekly methotrexate therapy. Nevertheless, available data and the author's experience suggest that prolonged treatment with methotrexate is possible in patients who continue to respond to the drug and are monitored carefully for potential toxicity.

Azathioprine

Azathioprine has been studied extensively in RD and has been demonstrated in placebo-controlled trials to have moderate short-term efficacy; however, toxicity limits its usefulness. Azathioprine therapy is associated with relatively high rates of gastrointestinal and minor hematologic problems, as well as occasional occurrences of severe cytopenias, especially leukopenia. In addition, azathioprine-treated patients have an increased risk of herpes, cytomegalovirus, and human papilloma virus infections. Perhaps the most controversial issue regarding azathioprine treatment is that of malignancy. Although rheumatoid arthritis patients are at somewhat higher risk of developing hematologic malignancy than the general population, azathioprine may further increase this risk. Because of these problems, azathioprine treatment has been restricted to patients who have either failed or not tolerated other second-line antirheumatic drugs.

Alkylating Agents

Three alkylating agents have been used in the treatment of rheumatoid arthritis: cyclophosphamide, chlorambucil, and intravenous nitrogen mustard. Most clinicians would agree that alkylating agents are among the most effective drugs available for the treatment of severe rheumatoid arthritis. However, the toxicity of alkylating agents therapy is severe, and they therefore have limited use in RD. The primary problems associated with alkylating agent therapy are severe hematologic toxicity and significant risk of malignancy. All alkylating agents are associated with an increased risk of hematologic malignancies, including lymphoma and leukemia, and the frequency of skin cancer is increased as well. Cyclophosphamide has also been associated with hemorrhagic cystitis and bladder cancer. Alkylating agent therapy is recommended only in cases of RD associated with systemic vasculitis and in rare patients with extremely resistant disease. Physicians using these agents should be thoroughly aware of the associated risks and should monitor patients accordingly.

MANAGEMENT OF RESISTANT RD

Unfortunately, many patients fail to respond to treatment with NSAIDs, low-dose glucocorticoids, and single second-line agent therapy. The first responsibility of a clinician faced with this situation is to recognize and treat co-morbid conditions. Depression and secondary fibromyalgia amplify the common symptoms of fatigue, pain, and restless sleep. Antidepressant treatment may be useful in this patient group. As many as one-third of rheumatoid arthritis patients have hypothyroidism, which may worsen functional status and quality of life. Patients with both overt and subclinical hypothyroidism should benefit symptomatically from thyroid replacement. Septic arthritis, which may be monoarticular or polyarticular, is relatively common in patients with serious RD and may mimic generalized disease flares. Patients at highest risk include debilitated patients and patients who have undergone invasive procedures. Clinicians caring for patients with RD should have a very low threshold for joint aspiration and culture in the patient who is doing poorly or has a monoarticular flare.

The course of RD may be punctuated by flares of arthritis, bursitis, and tendonitis at one or more sites. Once it has been established that such foci are not the sites of complicating infection, it is reasonable to offer patients intra-articular or soft tissue depo-glucocorticoid injections, which can be repeated safely as often as every 3 months. Glucocorticoid injections are extremely safe if sterile technique is used. If injections are done at too frequent intervals, patients may develop osteonecrosis or joint instability caused by soft tissue damage. Cutaneous atrophy is an occasional complication as well, especially when depo-glucocorticoids are used in small joints. When used judiciously, depo-glucocorticoids are among the most palliative treatment options in the patient with severe RD. For some patients they may produce prolonged, though not indefinite, improvement in inflammation. Limited data suggest that local glucocorticoid injection may favorably influence the rate of disease-associated joint destruction. The most rewarding results obtained from glucocorticoid injections occur in inflamed joints that have not already suffered severe mechanical damage. It is unrealistic to expect prolonged improvement when glucocorticoids are injected into a markedly destroyed joint. When improvement occurs for a period of less than a week, repeated injections may only serve to increase the risk of ligamentous instability, osteonecrosis, or infection.

High-dose parental glucocorticoids are frequently used to abate generalized flares of RD. Commonly employed protocols include intramuscular depo-methylprednisolone in doses of up to 320 mg, intramuscular adrenocorticotropic hormone (ACTH), and intravenous methylprednisolone. In general, systemic administration of high-dose corticosteroids or ACTH leads to prompt improvement in the symptoms and signs of RD, though this effect may be short-lived. An over-reliance on this approach may lead to progressive shorter duration of benefit and progressive increases in glucocorticoid-associated toxicity.

Many experts have recommended combinations of second-line agents in patients who do poorly with standard doses of methotrexate or other second-line drugs. Only a few well-designed clinical trials have looked at the usefulness of combination second-line therapy, and results have been disappointing. Nevertheless, there are few remaining options in this patient group. Several authors have noted the success of methotrexate in combination with hydroxychloroquine, sulfasalazine, and azathioprine in uncontrolled studies.

Cyclosporine therapy is another option in patients who are resistant to more traditional second-line drugs. Cyclosporine has been shown in several controlled trials to be effective in patients with otherwise refractory rheumatoid arthritis. Cyclosporine treatment is associated with unacceptable rates of nephrotoxicity in doses greater than 5 mg per kilogram per day. Cyclosporine also should not be used in association with NSAIDs—a fact that significantly limits its applicability. It is recommended that clinicians using cyclosporine to treat refractory rheumatoid arthritis begin at doses of approximately 2.5 mg per kilogram per day. If renal function remains stable for 8 weeks, the dose can be slowly titrated upwards to a maximum of 5 mg per kilogram per day. Patients treated with cyclosporine require close monitoring of renal function and blood pressure and should be fully warned about the potential of cyclosporin to cause permanent renal damage. In addition, the expense of cyclosporin therapy may be substantial and may disuade some patients from its use.

Cyclosporine was recently studied in RD patients who experienced a partial response to methotrexate. Patients were continued on methotrexate with the subsequent addition of cyclosporine (2.5 mg per kilogram per day) or placebo. The cyclosporine-methotrexate group did substantially better than the group who received methotrexate alone. Further confirmation of this observation is needed before this combination is applied widely in clinical practice.

SUGGESTED READING

Arnett FC, Edworthy SM, Bloch DA, et al. The American Rheumatism Association 1987 revised criteria for the classification of rheumatoid arthritis. Arthritis Rheum 1988; 31:315.

Cash JM, Klippel JH. Second-line drug therapy in rheumatoid arthritis. N Engl J Med 1994; 330:1368–1375.

Cash JM, Wilder RL. Refractory rheumatoid arthritis. Therapeutic options. Rheum Dis Clin North Am 1995; 21;1–18.

Epstein WV, Henke CJ, Yelin EH, et al. Effect of parenterally administered gold therapy on the course of adult rheumatoid arthritis. Ann Intern Med 1991; 114:437–444.

Felson DT, Anderson JJ, Meenan RF. Use of short-term efficacy/toxicity tradeoffs to select second-line drugs in rheumatoid arthritis: A meta-analysis of published clinical trials. Arthritis Rheum 1992; 35:1117–1125.

Pincus T, Callahan LF. What is the natural history of rheumatoid arthritis? Rheum Dis Clin North Am 1993; 19:123–152.

Sternberg EM, Young WS, Bernardini R, et al. A central nervous system defect in biosynthesis of corticotropin-releasing hormone is associated with susceptibility to streptococcal cell wall–induced arthritis in Lewis rats. Proc Natl Acad Sci USA 1989; 86:4771–4775.

JUVENILE RHEUMATOID ARTHRITIS

DAVID D. SHERRY, M.D.

Juvenile rheumatoid arthritis (JRA) is a heterogeneous group of conditions divided into three subsets based on clinical finding (Table 1). Spondyloarthropathies in childhood frequently involve peripheral joints; however, they are not discussed in this chapter. The two most common subsets of JRA, pauciarticular and polyarticular, are defined by the number of joints involved during the first 6 months of disease. There is no well-defined biologic reason for this division by number; therefore, children in our clinic who have under seven inflamed joints are treated like those with pauciarticular JRA. Children with systemic onset JRA, the least frequently occurring subset, have a completely different presentation and therefore require an entirely different diagnostic and therapeutic approach.

The etiologies for all forms of JRA are unknown; as a result, definitive treatment has not been established. Current theories hold that immunologic dysregulation is a major aberrant process underlying these conditions. Therefore, suppression of the immune system is the primary medical goal while trying to limit untoward reactions. Early and aggressive control of joint inflammation seems to lead to fewer disease complications, including joint damage and abnormal growth. Unfortunately, there are very few well-controlled studies; therapeutic regimens are mostly empiric, based on collective experience rather than science. Since we cannot fully control the arthritis, physical and occupational therapy is required to maintain normal joint function, strength, activities of daily living, and, at times, basic joint protection. Surgical intervention is reserved for relieving pain in those with severe joint damage. Throughout treatment it is paramount to maintain the psychological health of the child and family. Therapies can neither be overly onerous nor can the participation of the child and family in the treatment process be overlooked. Education and establishment of trust are imperative for a good outcome.

PAUCIARTICULAR JRA

Pauciarticular JRA typically afflicts toddlers or preschool girls. The most frequently involved joints are knees and ankles; less common are fingers, elbows, and wrists. Occasionally a child has temporomandibular joint involvement. Hip involvement is very uncommon, and the shoulder is only rarely involved. One-quarter of these children have painless disease but present because someone notices a swollen joint. More than 70 percent have a positive antinuclear antibody (ANA) test, usually low titer (< 1:320). The presence of ANA is associated with asymptomatic iritis, which is observed in 20 percent of these children.

If an ANA test is positive, it is critical to closely observe the child's iris in a darkened room to determine if synechia are present. If present, or if the pupil is not round, or if there is a hint of precipitate on the posterior cornea, immediate ophthalmologic consultation for slit-lamp examination is indicated. If synechia are not present routine ophthalmologic surveillance should begin (Fig. 1). The iritis is not associated with redness or photophobia, is usually controllable with eye drops, and, if untreated, may lead to blindness. Diligent surveillance is imperative.

Figure 2 shows an outline of a therapy strategy. In many cases the arthritis can be controlled with intra-articular (IA) corticosteroid injection. If marked dysfunction, pain, or a flexion contracture is present, it is usually best to inject the joint sooner rather than later. If those symptoms are not present, or if it is very early in the course of the arthritis, oral nonsteroidal anti-inflammatory drugs (NSAIDs) may be used for a month to determine if the arthritis persists. NSAIDs may be prescribed at any time; they will not mask JRA nor will they obscure a neoplastic or infectious process.

If there is an early recurrence (< 4 months) or no response following administration of IA corticosteroids,

Table 1 Characteristics of the Different Forms of Juvenile Rheumatoid Arthritis

JRA Form	*Pauciarticular*	*Polyarticular*	*Systemic*
Age of Onset	1-3	1-3, adolescence	3-12
Gender: female: male	4:1	3:1	1:1
ANA present	70%	40%	10%
RF positive	1%	10%-50%	1%
Arthritic joints	1-4	5+	Any
Iritis	20%	5%	1%
Prognosis	Good	Good; fair	Good; poor

ANA, Antinuclear antibody; *RF*, rheumatoid factor.

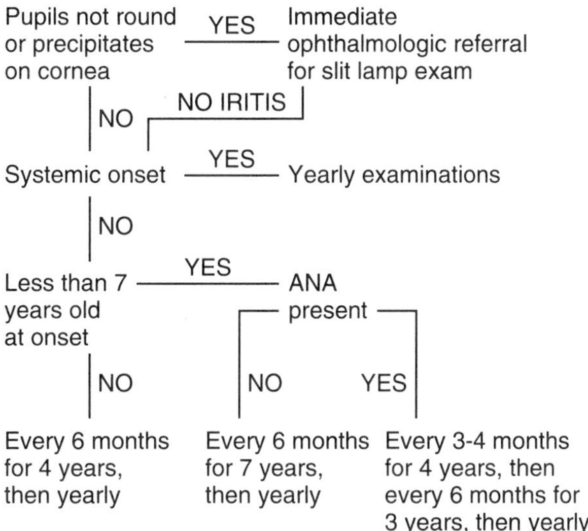

Figure 1 Ophthalmologic screening. These are surveillance recommendations for children without iritis. If iritis develops, more frequent care by the ophthalmologist will be required.

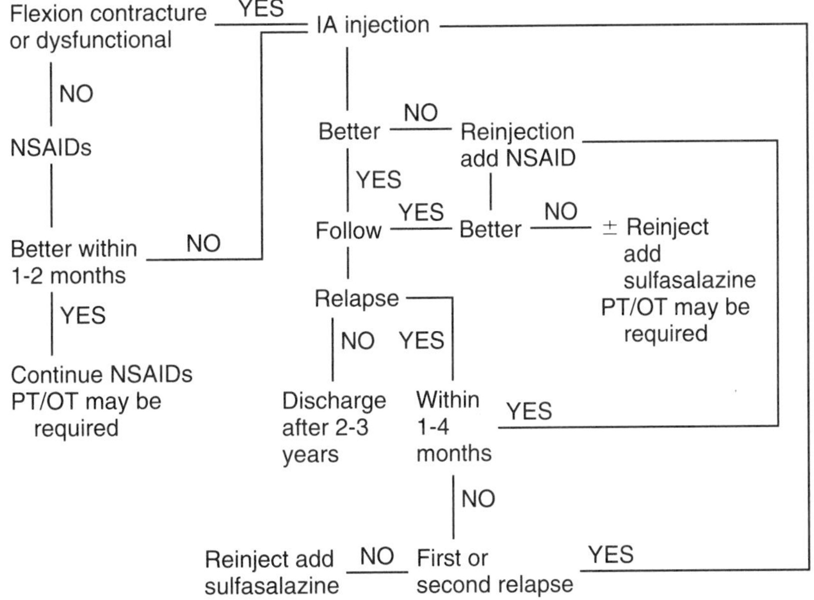

Figure 2 Pauciarticular involvement in juvenile rheumatoid arthritis.

the joint should be reinjected and the child started on an NSAID. If further recurrences occur, sulfasalazine, a slow-acting remittive agent, should be given. Several months may be required for sulfasalazine to have full effect. In children with multiple, widely spaced recurrences, sulfasalazine is given in an attempt to prevent recurrent arthritis without the toxicity of daily NSAIDs.

A few children will have persistent flexion contractures, which are best treated with serial casting. Serial night splinting or a dynamic splint may also be tried. Specific physical therapy will be needed afterward for the child to regain strength, and flexion, and for gait training. Children with unilateral knee disease are at the highest risk for leg length inequality. Those with active disease while young (1 to 8 years of age) will typically have overgrowth. The contralateral shoe should be fitted with a lift if the leg length discrepancy is sufficient to alter gait. Older children are more likely to have early epiphyseal closure and thus a shortened leg. Rarely,

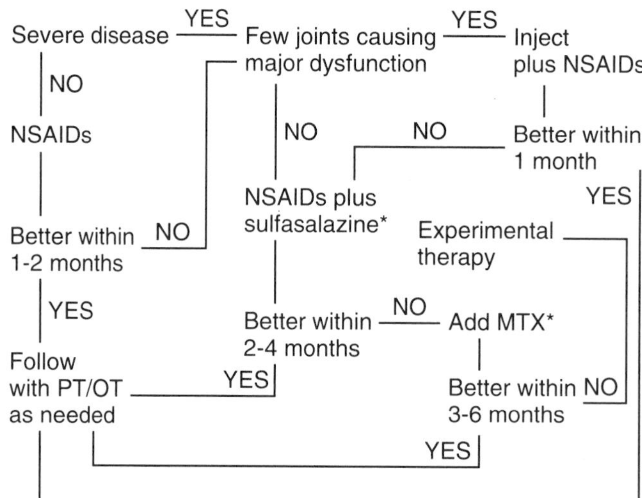

Figure 3 Polyarticular involvement in juvenile rheumatoid arthritis.

surgical intervention is required to obtain reasonably equal leg lengths.

POLYARTICULAR JRA

Children with multiple joint involvement fall into two major categories: (1) younger girls (1 to 5 years of age) who are rheumatoid factor negative and have a better long-term prognosis and (2) adolescent girls who frequently are rheumatoid-factor positive and have a higher risk for long-lasting, erosive arthritis.

The spectrum of disease is broad; degree of involvement and impairment greatly factor into therapeutic decisions. Figure 3 shows one hierarchy of treatment. NSAIDs are begun. If the arthritis proves to be JRA, that is, if it lasts longer than a couple of months, sulfasalazine is added. If the arthritis has not responded by 2 to 6 months after the introduction of sulfasalazine (less time for more severe arthritis), methotrexate is added. Occasionally an older child may respond to hydroxychloroquine before going on to methotrexate. In severely involved children, one may use methotrexate before sulfasalazine and add sulfasalazine if methotrexate alone is insufficient.

The dose of methotrexate, in those less severely involved, is 0.5 mg per kilogram as a single weekly dose, either orally (PO) (on an empty stomach) or subcutaneously (SC). In the more severely involved, the dose is 1 mg per kilogram weekly SC, up to 40 mg per week. Once remission is achieved, the dose should be maintained for a prolonged time before a gradual taper is attempted.

If a few joints are causing particular difficulty (flexion contractures, pain, limiting function) intra-articular injection is helpful. Some children with widespread arthritis may be helped with weekly pulse intravenous methylprednisolone. Oral steroids should be used only after other therapeutic agents have failed, and only at very low dosage, 0.1 mg per kilogram per day as a single daily dose. A single morning dose is preferable, but a few children do better, especially with morning stiffness, with an evening dose.

Other medications can be tried when the above measures inadequately control the arthritis. These include D-penicillamine, gold, azathioprine, and other cytotoxic drugs. Azathioprine is usually the least toxic of these.

Continuing physical and occupational therapy maintains joint function while the arthritis is active. (See Pauciarticular JRA.) Joint protection is particularly important in those with hand and wrist involvement. Environmental changes may be indicated (grab bars for the bath tub, double set of school books, and so on).

SYSTEMIC ONSET JRA (STILL DISEASE)

Systemic onset JRA is defined by the characteristic spiking fever at onset. Frequently associated findings include an evanescent rash, lymphadenopathy, pericarditis, splenomegaly, and leukocytosis. Less frequent complications include frank vasculitis, disseminated intravascular coagulation, and myocarditis. Iritis is rare in this form of JRA.

Systemic onset JRA has the best and worse prognoses. Some children spontaneously resolve all signs and symptoms, whereas others develop aggressive and destructive arthritis. Those with active systemic symptoms and elevated acute phase reactants after the first 6 months are more likely to have a worse outcome.

Initially, indomethacin may control fever and many

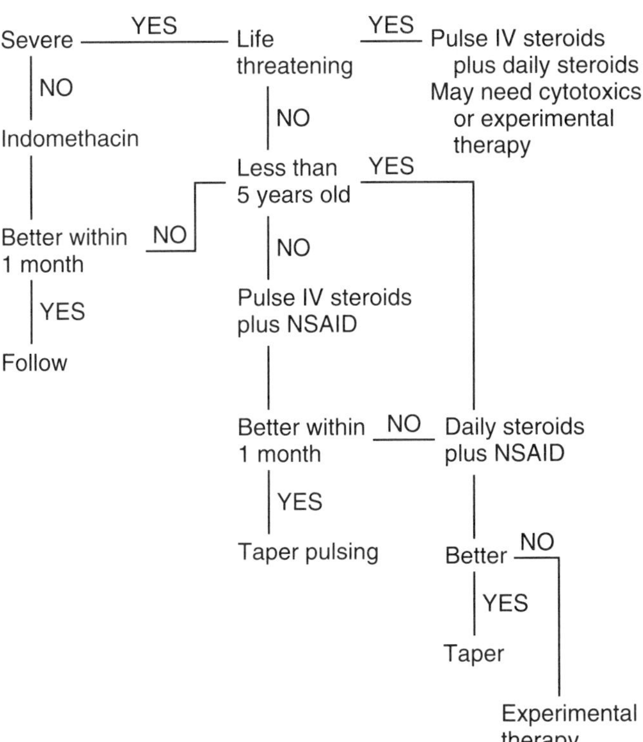

Figure 4 Systemic manifestations of systemic onset juvenile rheumatoid arthritis.

systemic features such as pericarditis. If indomethacin is not effective, or if more severe complications occur, such as myocarditis, pulse intravenous methylprednisolone may ameliorate the symptoms. If methylprednisolone is not effective, daily prednisone should be used. Frequently, the doses required to control symptoms are high enough to cause multiple side effects. The systemic manifestations may be resistant to therapy. In individual patients, intravenous immunoglobulin or cytotoxic agents have been helpful (Figure 4).

Arthritis may follow the onset of systemic symptoms by weeks or months. If the arthritis affects a few joints, treatment with NSAIDs or intra-articular injection may be sufficient. In those patients with widespread arthritis, treatment is similar to that for individuals with polyarticular JRA. Most, however, require high-dose methotrexate initially and at least a few intra-articular joint injections. It is in this group that we have had the most severely affected children and have needed to add other cytotoxic agents such as azathioprine, cyclophosphamide, or chlorambucil. In Europe, amyloidosis occurs in about 5 percent of these children (rare in North America).

Over the past 20 years the majority of children who have become wheelchair dependent or have required joint replacement have had systemic onset JRA, the most infrequent form. Early and aggressive treatment and physical and occupational therapy are required for those who have continuing synovitis.

DRUG COMPLICATIONS AND MONITORING

NSAIDs (Tables 2 and 3)

Choice

Compliance is more of a factor to consider than side effects for most children with one exception—blond, fair-skinned, freckled children are at a higher risk to develop facial scars and pseudoporphyria with naproxen (this may be a concern with oxaprozin also). Many parents fear aspirin but it is an excellent choice for small children who require a chewable medicine. (The teeth should be coated with plastic to prevent enamel damage if the child is chronically chewing aspirin.) For smaller children, liquid ibuprofen or indomethacin is acceptable and is administered three times daily. Naproxen is available as a liquid and is given twice daily. Choline magnesium salicylate is available as a liquid and is given twice daily. Choline magnesium salicylate may be associated with Reye's syndrome as is aspirin, and like aspirin, necessitates influenza immunization annually. For somewhat older children diclofenac and sulindac are given twice daily and piroxicam and oxaprozin are single daily dose medications. Piroxicam capsules can be opened and the contents put directly on a bite of food for those who cannot swallow pills since it has almost no taste. Indomethacin SR capsules are taken twice daily but, initially, regular indomethacin is given at a low dose and increased to the therapeutic dose over 4 to 8 days to prevent side effects, especially headache. Indomethacin is a very good antipyretic.

Cost and palatability are important factors in the choice of NSAIDs. Individual differences in taste are not predictable; a trial sample may save time and money. Few of these drugs are approved for use in children. Adequate discussion with the patient and family and appropriate monitoring are required (see following discussion).

Complications

Although taking NSAIDs with food can usually prevent it, gastrointestinal distress is the most common side effect associated with NSAID therapy. Additional therapy may include antacids, misoprostol, H_2-blockers, or sucralfate. A few children will have significant gastrointestinal blood loss without pain; paleness resulting from anemia is the only sign. Shallow facial scars or blisters with sun exposure (pseudoporphyria) may occur, especially in patients taking naproxen.

Alterations in behavior and headache are not uncommon. Less frequent complications include leukopenia, agranulocytosis, hepatotoxicity, hematuria, papillary necrosis, rashes (urticaria), tinnitus, and exacerbation of asthma, especially if nasal polyps are present.

Switching NSAIDs may promptly relieve side effects since many of these agents are particular to the patient and the individual drug.

Table 2 Selected NSAIDs: Recommended Dosages

Medication (trade name)	*Dose*	*Maximum Daily Dose*
Three-Times-a-Day Medications		
*Aspirin	80-100 mg/kg	5,200 mg
*Ibuprofen	40 mg/kg 45 mg/kg	3,200 mg
Indomethacin (Indocin)	2-3 mg/kg	200 mg
*Tolmetin (Tolectin)	30-40 mg/kg	1,800 mg
Twice-a-Day Medications		
*Naproxen (Naprosyn)	15-20 mg/kg	1,000 mg
*Choline Magnesium Salicylate (Trilisate)	50-65 mg/kg	4,500 mg
Sulindac (Clinoril)	3-4 mg/kg	400 mg
Diclofenac (Voltaren)	2-3 mg/kg	225 mg
Indomethacin SR (Indocin SR)	2-3 mg/kg	150 mg
Once-a-Day Medications		
Piroxicam (Feldene)	0.25-0.4 mg/kg	20 mg
Oxaprozin (Daypro)	10-20 mg/kg	1,200 mg

*Approved for use in young children (Ibuprofen not labeled for arthritis).

Table 3 Selected NSAIDs

Medication	*Supplied (mg)*	*Form*
Aspirin	81, 325, 500, 650, 975	Tablet
Ibuprofen	200, 300, 400, 600, 800	Tablet
	100 mg/5 cc	Liquid
Indomethacin	25, 50	Capsule
	25 mg/5 cc	Liquid
Tolmetin	200, 400, 600	Tablet
Naproxen	250, 375, 500	Tablet
	125 mg/5 cc	Liquid
Choline Magnesium Salicylate	500, 750, 1,000	Tablet
	500 mg/5 cc	Liquid
Sulindac	150, 200	Tablet
Dilofenac	25, 50, 75	Tablet
Indomethacin SR	75	Capsule
Piroxicam	10, 20	Capsule
Oxaprozin	600	Tablet

Monitoring

Monitoring patients on NSAID therapy includes obtaining the following tests after 1 to 2 months, and then every 4 to 12 months (younger children 4 to 6 months, older children 6 to 12 months): complete blood count, creatinine and transaminase levels, urine analysis.

Sulfasalazine

Drug rash is the most common side effect of sulfasalazine therapy, and desensitization over 1 month is usually successful in eliminating this complication. Stevens-Johnson syndrome rarely occurs but may be fatal. Leukopenia, hepatotoxicity, and a serum sickness-like reaction may also occur.

Monitoring

Patients taking sulfasalazine should be monitored after one month, and then every 4 to 6 months by obtaining a complete blood count and transaminase levels.

Methotrexate

Methotrexate (MTX) is perhaps one of the safest drugs used, and although it has not been associated with malignancies or permanent sterility, it is a potent teratogen. Liver toxicity is the most worrisome untoward effect, but it is much less of a problem in those who do not consume alcohol. Nausea is the most frequent troublesome side effect.

Absorption of methotrexate is quite variable so it needs to be given either on an empty stomach or subcutaneously. There may be dramatic improvement in switching to subcutaneous administration if oral methotrexate is not effective. Oral absorption diminishes with increasing dose so patients on higher doses (1 mg per kilogram per week) also receive MTX subcutaneously.

Nausea may be controlled in several ways. Folic acid may become depleted and contribute to side effects. We prescribe a complete daily vitamin (400 μg of folic acid), and Folate, 1 mg per day, may be helpful in adolescents. The NSAID may exacerbate the nausea so withholding it the day MTX is administered (and maybe the night before) should be tried. To prevent nausea from the first pass through the liver, changing to subcutaneous administration frequently helps. This also allows the child to eat right after administration, which helps to avoid hunger pains that the youngster may confuse with nausea. In those with severe nausea, ondansetron, 4 to 8 mg before and, if needed, 4 to 6 hours after the dose, is helpful.

Monitoring

Every month for the first year patients taking MTX need to be monitored by obtaining the following: complete blood count, creatinine and transaminase levels, and urine analysis. If no problems with liver enzyme elevations occur, monitoring can decrease to every other month.

Corticosteroids

Before administering these drugs, neoplastic diseases must be ruled out since even intra-articular steroid injections have masked leukemia.

Intra-articular Corticosteroids

Intra-articular corticosteroids that may be used include triamcinolone hexacetonide (20 mg per cubic centimeter) or triamcinolone acetonide (40 mg per cubic centimeter). In children 1 cc is used in the knee or ankle; proportionally less is used in smaller joints. We frequently administer midazolam, 0.25 mg per kilogram orally, 15 minutes before the procedure to help reduce the child's anxiety. Local anesthesia is obtained by lidocaine and prilocaine cream (if it can be applied 1 hour before), ethyl chloride spray, and buffered lidocaine (0.8 cc lidocaine to 0.2 cc sodium bicarbonate) using a 30 gauge needle. Injection techniques are well described in other texts. Side effects include local hypopigmentation and subcutaneous fat atrophy, which resolves over a few years in most cases, and joint irritation, which starts a few hours after the injection and subsides in a few days. Infection is rare, occurring in approximately 1 out of 50,000 injections. Onset of septic joint symptoms starts a few days postinjection. Pituitary adrenal axis can be affected, especially if multiple joints are injected. Calcification in and around the joint may occur but these deposits are rarely symptomatic.

Monitoring. Our monitoring procedures for patients receiving intra-articular corticosteroids include calling the family 2 to 4 days after each injection to assess response and side effects. We also examine the child within 2 months.

Intravenous Pulse Corticosteroids

IV pulse corticosteroid therapy is administered using methylprednisolone 30 mg per kilogram (up to 1 g) given over 60 to 120 minutes. Usually this is administered 3 days in a row and then as a single weekly dose. Hypotension or hypertension can occur and usually responds to slowing the rate of administration. Children uniformly develop a metallic taste in their mouths; strongly flavored hard candy helps. Abdominal pains or visual symptoms rarely occur and are short lived. Anaphylaxis is rare but has been reported.

Monitoring. Monitoring IV pulse corticosteroid administration includes assessing blood pressure every 15 minutes during the infusion.

Oral Corticosteroids

Oral steroids are only rarely required. In systemic disease, low to high doses may be necessary depending upon the degree of illness. Very rarely, children with polyarticular JRA may be helped by low-dose prednisone (0.1 mg per kilogram per day).

Monitoring. In patients taking oral steroids, growth should be assessed at each follow-up visit. Urine glucose should be assessed every 6 months.

SUGGESTED READING

Herzberger-ten Cate R, De Vries-van der Vlugt BCM, Suijlekom-Smit LWA van, Cats A. Intra-articular steroids in pauciarticular juvenile chronic arthritis, type I. *Eur J Pediatr* 1991; 150:170–172.

Joos R, Veys EM, Mielants H, et al. Sulfasalazine treatment in juvenile chronic arthritis: An open study. *J Rheumatol* 1991; 18:880–884.

Rose CE, Singsen BH, Eichenfield AH, et al. Safety and efficacy of methotrexate therapy for juvenile rheumatoid arthritis. *J Pediatr* 1990; 117:653–659.

Rosenberg AM. Advanced drug therapy of juvenile rheumatoid arthritis. *J Pediatr* 1989; 114:171–178.

Wallace CA, Sherry DD. A practical approach to avoidance of methotrexate toxicity. *J Rheumatol* 1995; 22:1009–1012.

REACTIVE ARTHRITIS

JOHN H. KLIPPEL, M.D.

Reactive arthritis refers to a syndrome of inflammatory monoarticular or oligoarticular arthritis triggered by an infection. The arthritis typically develops 2 to 4 weeks following the infection and, in contrast to septic arthritis, cultures of synovial fluid and synovial tissues are negative at the time of clinical joint inflammation. Recent studies using immunoelectron microscopy or the polymerase chain reaction, however, have shown clear evidence of the triggering infectious agent within the joint tissues. Whether this occurs as a result of the deposition of immune complexes containing antigens of the infecting organism or some other form of nonbiodegradable fragments of the organism within joint tissues is the subject of intensive research.

Although clinical descriptions of reactive arthritis generally emphasize involvement of the musculoskeletal system, most patients often experience profound constitutional symptoms as part of the acute illness and develop extra-articular manifestations during the course of the disease. Fever, anorexia, and fatigue are commonly present early. There is a strong predisposition for patients with reactive arthritis to develop inflammatory disease of the eyes, skin, mucous membranes, and cardiac tissues.

Although the diagnosis of reactive arthritis is currently limited to arthropathies that develop following infections of the genitourinary or gastrointestinal tracts, a number of other postinfectious inflammatory arthropathies clearly belong in this classification. For example, Reiter's syndrome—the tetrad of arthritis, nongonococcal urethritis, conjunctivitis, and mucocutaneous lesions—is generally acknowledged to be a form of a reactive arthritis and on clinical and treatment grounds it is difficult to justify continuing to think of it as a separate entity. Worldwide rheumatic fever is the most common type of reactive arthritis; other examples include Lyme borreliosis, disseminated gonococcal infection, and rheumatic manifestations of subacute bacterial endocarditis. The importance of the concept of reactive arthritis for most of the idiopathic forms of inflammatory joint disease such as the seronegative spondyloarthropathies, psoriatic arthritis, or rheumatoid arthritis is obvious with recently renewed interest in studies to search for evidence of infectious agents in these diseases using molecular approaches.

DIAGNOSIS

The diagnosis of reactive arthritis is readily suggested in patients who present with classic features of an antecedent infection, arthritis, and clinical findings of conjunctivitis, uveitis, or mucocutaneous lesions. Many patients, however, present with an acute arthritis in which only a vague history of infection can be elicited and signs of extra-articular involvement are absent. Conversely, patients may actually present with an infection commonly associated with reactive arthritis such as urethritis with minimal joint symptoms. These types of patients pose much more of a problem in diagnosis. The key steps in the evaluation of patients with suspected reactive arthritis are shown in Table 1.

Table 1 Evaluation of Patients with Suspected Reactive Arthritis

Synovial Fluid Studies
Cell count
Examination for crystals
Gram stain
Culture
Bacterial Cultures
Blood
Pharynx
Cervix
Urethra
Rectum
Serologies
Rheumatoid factor
Antimicrobial antibodies
HIV
Acute phase reactants
Erythrocyte sedimentation rate
C-reactive protein
Electrocardiogram
HLA-B27 typing

In most patients it is important to exclude septic arthritis, and synovial fluid should be aspirated for cell count, gram stain, and cultures. The cell count may be high (10,000 to 50,000 per cubic millimeter). The differential shows predominantly polymorphonuclear leukocytes in the early stages of the illness followed by a lymphocyte predominance late in the disease course. Large macrophages with vacuoles that contain nuclear debris ('Reiter's cells') may be seen and offer a clue to the diagnosis.

In addition to synovial fluid, cultures of all potential sites of infection, including blood and swabs of the cervix, urethra, and rectum should be taken. In patients with genitourinary symptoms, or if disseminated gonococcal infection is suspected on clinical grounds, cultures should be plated on chocolate agar or Thayer Martin medium. In reactive arthritis, Gram stains and routine cultures of the synovial fluid for bacteria, fungi, and mycobacteria are entirely negative. The detection of organisms from other sites, particularly those known to be commonly associated with reactive arthritis, provides confirmation of the diagnosis. However, in many patients even with a clear antecedent infection, all cultures will be negative at the time of the arthritis. In such patients, serologic studies for organisms associated with reactive arthritis (Table 2) may be helpful to document a recent infection. However, these should be ordered on a case-by-case basis directed by clinical findings and not indiscriminately as a panel in all patients. Patients

Table 2 Organisms Associated with the Development of Reactive Arthritis

Enteric
Shigella flexneri, Shigella dysenteriae
Salmonella enteritidis, Salmonella typhimurium
Yersinia enterocolitica, Yersinia pseudotuberculosis
Campylobacter jejuni
Clostridium difficile
Genitourinary
Chylamydia trachomatis
Respiratory
Chylamydia pneumoniae

infected with the HIV virus have been reported to develop a Reiter's-like syndrome, and serologic studies for HIV should be obtained in all patients. In addition, serologic studies for Borrelia burgdorferi should be ordered in patients with a clinical history or findings on physical examination compatible with Lyme disease and antistreptolysin O (ASO) titers in patients with suspected rheumatic fever.

A complete blood count and differential count, rheumatoid factor, and measurement of acute phase reactants should be routinely measured in all patients. A modest leukocytosis is commonly present and patients are seronegative for rheumatoid factor. Acute phase reactants such as the erythrocyte sedimentation rate or the C-reactive protein are usually markedly elevated, a measure that is often used to monitor the "activity" of the arthritis over the course of the disease. Since cardiac conduction defects may develop in patients with reactive arthritis, a baseline electrocardiogram should be obtained as part of the initial evaluation. Typing for HLA-B27 is occasionally helpful when characteristic extra-articular manifestations are absent. Recent studies suggest that HLA-B27 is a marker for a clinical subset of reactive arthritis with axial joint involvement, uveitis, and carditis.

In acute reactive arthritis, radiographic studies are rarely indicated. Standard joint radiographs reveal only soft tissue swelling without abnormalities of bone or cartilage. By scintigraphy with ^{99m} Tc-MDP increased uptake of the isotope may be demonstrated in involved joints, a finding that may on occasion be useful in patients with suspected sacroiliac involvement. In patients with recurrent or chronic reactive arthritis, characteristic radiographic features may be seen, including bone formation at sites of osseous erosions leading to subchondral sclerosis and eburnation, and calcification and ossification of the enthesis causing spur formation.

MUSCULOSKELETAL MANIFESTATIONS

Articular manifestations range from mild arthralgias to severe disabling polyarthritis. Although virtually any joint may be affected, the most common presentation is an asymmetrical monoarthritis or oligoarthritis of the weight-bearing joints—knees, ankles, and hips. Involved joints are typically red, warm, and tender to palpation, and tense synovial effusions may develop overnight. In addition, inflammation and swelling of an entire toe or finger (dactylitis) is a frequent finding. Patients may note stiffness or pain in the lower back, particularly at night, which causes them to sleep poorly. The course of arthritis follows a migratory pattern with physical findings often varying greatly from day to day.

The entheses—areas where tendons, ligaments, and the joint capsule insert into bone—are a prominent site of inflammation in reactive arthritis. The enthesitis causes severe pain when the patient attempts to move the joint and voluntary immobilization of the joint by the patient can lead to rapid loss of muscle mass. On physical examination point tenderness of the insertions of the Achilles tendon or the plantar fascia into the calcaneus or other periarticular sites of ligamentous attachments can often be found.

MANAGEMENT

In the majority of patients reactive arthritis is a self-limited disease process lasting 2 to 4 weeks. The primary goals of therapy of the acute illness are to (1) suppress joint inflammation with the use of anti-inflammatory drugs, (2) provide local management of various extra-articular manifestations, and (3) institute a program of physical therapy to relieve symptoms and prevent or minimize functional impairments. The role of antibiotic therapy is controversial, although recent studies suggest a role for their use particularly in patients with *Chylamydia* urethritis. In 25 to 40 percent of patients, however, reactive arthritis evolves into a recurrent or chronic disease course with lingering extra-articular complications and a seronegative arthropathy that resembles spondyloarthritis or rheumatoid arthritis.

NSAIDs

Nonsteroidal anti-inflammatory drugs (NSAIDs) are the mainstay for the drug treatment of joint symptoms in reactive arthritis; there is a general consensus that systemic corticosteroids have little or no role in the management of acute reactive arthritis. Selection among the many different NSAIDs (Table 3) is largely a matter of physician and patient preference with no convincing evidence that one drug is more effective than any other in reactive arthritis. However, most clinicians recognize that individual patients often respond better to one drug than another. Thus it may be necessary to give courses of several different NSAIDs in maximum doses before settling on optimal therapy with these drugs. Initiation of therapy with indomethacin at 100 mg per day divided into four doses and taken with food is a widely used and an often effective regimen. Increases in the dose of indomethacin beyond these levels often causes intolerable headaches and light-headedness. There are a host of potential adverse

Table 3 Nonsteroidal Antiinflammatory Drugs Available for Treating Reactive Arthritis

	Dose Range (mg/day)	*Doses per Day*
Short Acting (half-life <6 hours)		
Phenylic Acids		
Ibuprofen	1,200-2,400	3-6
Fenoprofen	1,200-2,400	3-4
Ketoprofen	150-300	3-4
Diclofenac	100-200	2-4
Flurbiprofen	100-300	2-4
Pyrrolealkanoic acids		
Tolmetin	600-1,800	2-3
Naphthylalkanone		
Nabumetone	1,000-2,000	1-2
Long Acting (half-life >6 hours)		
Indoleacetic acids		
Indomethacin	50-200	2-4
Sulindac	300-400	2
Etodolac	600-1,200	3-4
Pyrazolidinediones		
Phenylbutazone	200-800	1-4
Oxicams		
Piroxicam	10-20	1
Oxazolepropionic acid		
Oxaprozin	600-1,200	1

reactions associated with NSAID therapy; gastrointestinal symptoms of varying degrees occur with essentially all the available NSAIDs and often limit therapy. In addition, NSAIDs alter metabolism, protein binding, and excretion of a number of drugs; potential interactions with other drugs taken by the patient should be assessed before NSAIDs are prescribed.

Physical Therapy

Physical therapy is an important and often overlooked aspect of management in patients with reactive arthritis. The program should be individualized based on the needs of the individual patient. Most patients benefit from bed rest or immobilization of involved joints by splinting. However, passive range of motion exercises by an experienced therapist must be used during this time to prevent joint contractures and muscle wasting. Local applications of heat or cold are often helpful to relieve joint or periarticular pain. In patients with arthritis of the forefoot, ankle, or subtalar joints, custom-made orthotics may reduce pain and enable the patient to remain ambulatory. Once joint inflammation has subsided the patient should begin active, rehabilitative exercises to restore full motion within the joint.

Intra-Articular Corticosteroids

Intra-articular or periarticular injections of corticosteroids are often beneficial in patients with refractory arthritis limited to a single joint or in patients with severe tendinitis or enthesitis. Long-acting corticosteroid preparations such as triamcinolone hexacetonide are preferred in doses of 5 to 10 mg for small joints and injections into tendon sheaths and doses of 20 to 40 mg for large joints. The corticosteroid preparation is often combined with 1 percent lidocaine, which provides immediate pain relief. Adherance to sterile techniques is required with all injections and OSHA regulations require that gloves be worn during the procedure. In the instance of infiltrations of tendon sheaths or entheses, meticulous care must be taken to avoid injections directly into the tendon itself. No area should be injected more often than three or four times per year. Although joint sepsis is a potential complication of intra-articular injections, this is extremely rare if sterile precautions are followed.

Drug Therapy in Chronic Arthritis

In patients who develop chronic joint inflammation, drug therapy is similar to approaches in rheumatoid arthritis involving the use of disease-modifying or second-line antirheumatic drugs (Table 4). Because of its known efficacy in treating inflammatory bowel disease and its potential antibacterial role, sulfasalazine (500 to 3,000 mg per day) is being increasingly used in patients with chronic forms of reactive arthritis. Low-dose oral methotrexate (7.5 to 15 mg per week) or azathioprine (50 to 150 mg per day) are popular alternative options. However, it is important to exclude HIV infection before starting either of these drugs since reports of precipitation of full-blown AIDS and severe exacerbations of reactive arthritis have been reported in HIV-positive patients treated with these drugs.

OCULAR INVOLVEMENT

Inflammation of various structures within the eye is a common feature in patients with reactive arthritis. An acute, transient sterile conjunctivitis develops early, which may rarely progress to episcleritis, keratitis, or corneal ulcerations. Acute unilateral anterior uveitis (iritis) occurs in 20 to 40 percent of patients and causes redness, photophobia, and increased lacrimation. Attacks of uveitis are frequently recurrent and may involve the contralateral eye.

Patients with ocular symptoms should be referred to an ophthalmologist for a thorough eye examination and treatment recommendations. In general, conjunctivitis resolves spontaneously without specific treatment, whereas topical corticosteroids are usually advised in patients with anterior uveitis. In addition, dilating eyedrops are recommended in patients with uveitis for relief of pain induced by spasm of the ciliary muscles and to prevent synechiae formation. Systemic corticosteroids or immunosuppressive agents may be indicated for patients with very severe uveitis associated with visual loss. The long-term prognosis of eye involvement in patients with reactive arthritis is good; however, cases of

Table 4 Antirheumatic Drugs Used in the Treatment of Recurrent or Chronic Reactive Arthritis

Agent	*Recommended Dosages*
Sulfa compounds	
Sulfasalazine	Oral, 500 mg daily increasing dose to maximum of 3,000 mg daily
Gold compounds	
Gold sodium thiomalate	Intramuscular, single doses of 10 mg followed by 25 mg 1 week later to test for sensitivity; maintenance therapy with 50 mg weekly
Gold sodium thioglucose	Intramuscular, single doses of 10 mg followed by 25 mg 1 week later to test for sensitivity; maintenance therapy with 50 mg weekly
Auranofin	Oral, 3-6 mg daily
Antimalarial drugs	
Hydroxychloroquine	Oral, 400 to 600 mg daily for 4 to 6 weeks followed by 200 to 400 mg daily
Antimetabolite drugs	
Methotrexate sodium	Oral (less commonly intramuscular), 7.5 to 15 mg weekly
Azathioprine	Oral, 50 to 100 mg daily, maximum dose 2.5 mg/kg daily

visual loss from macular degeneration and reduced intraocular pressure have been reported.

GASTROINTESTINAL AND UROGENITAL SYMPTOMS

Infections of the gastrointestinal or genitourinary tracts may cause transient mild abdominal pain, diarrhea, or urethritis in the month preceding the onset of arthritis. Additional urogenital findings may include cystitis, proctitis, and pelvic inflammatory disease. In patients with urogenital involvement, it is very important to exclude infection with *Neisseria gonorrhoeae,* and appropriate cultures need to be obtained. The finding of bloody or prolonged diarrhea is distinctly unusual in reactive arthritis and should suggest the possibility of inflammatory bowel disease, ulcerative colitis, or some other bowel pathology as a cause of the arthritis. In such instances, ileocolonoscopy or radiographic studies may be required to differentiate among these diseases.

The role of antibiotic therapy in patients in whom an infection of the genitourinary or gastrointestinal tract has been documented, either through cultures or serologic studies, is controversial. The value of antibiotic treatment has only been convincingly demonstrated in patients with a *Chlamydia*-triggered reactive arthritis in whom treatment of the acute illness with lymecycline, a lysine conjugated tetracycline, has been shown to shorten the time course of acute arthritis. To date, studies of antibiotic treatment of reactive arthritis associated with enteric infections have been uniformly negative. In addition, the use of long-term antibiotic therapy in patients with reactive arthritis to prevent relapses of the disease has not been established and cannot be recommended.

MUCOCUTANEOUS SYMPTOMS

Mucocutaneous symptoms include a hyperkeratotic skin lesion termed keratoderma blenorrhagicum develops on the soles of the feet and palms, but may involve the toes, scrotum, trunk, and scalp. The keratotic material may accumulate under the finger and lift the nail from the nail bed. The rash resembles pustular psoriasis both clinically and histologically. Shallow painless ulcers may develop on the glans penis (circinate balanitis). Various superficial lesions may also be seen on the oral mucous membranes.

Topical corticosteroids and keratolytic agents such as salicylic acid ointment are useful for the treatment of keratoderma blenorrhagicum. In patients with severe or chronic skin involvement, drug therapies used in advanced psoriasis, including low-dose weekly methotrexate, retinoids, or cyclosporin A, should be considered. Ulcerative lesions of the penis and inflammatory lesions of the oral mucous membrane resolve spontaneously and do not require specific treatment.

VISCERAL INVOLVEMENT

Involvement of major organs in reactive arthritis is distinctly uncommon. Conduction defects may occur early in patients with reactive arthritis, the most common being a prolonged PR interval. Second and third degree atrioventricular blocks have been reported that, in rare instances, have required the use of a cardiac pacemaker. In patients with recurrent or chronic disease, aortic insufficiency may develop as a result of inflammation and scarring of the valvular cusps and aortic wall.

Other very rare complications of reactive arthritis include IgA nephropathy, amyloidosis, thrombophlebitis, cranial and peripheral neuropathies, and choreoathetosis.

SUGGESTED READING

Keat AC, Hughes R. Infectious agents in reactive arthritis. Curr Opin Rheumatol 1993; 5:414–419.

Kvien TK, Glennas A, Melby K, et al. Reactive arthritis: Incidence, triggering agents and clinical presentation. J Rheumatol 1994; 21:115–122.

Lauhio A, Leirisalo-Repo M, Lahdevirta J, et al. Double-blind, placebo-controlled study of three-month treatment with lymecycline in reactive arthritis, with special reference to Chlamydia arthritis. Arthritis Rheum 1991; 34:6–14.

Leirisalo-Repo M. Are antibiotics of any use in reactive arthritis? APMIS 1993; 101:575–581.

Sieper J, Braun J, Reichardt M, et al. The value of specific antibody detection and culture in the diagnosis of reactive arthritis. Clin Rheumatol 1993; 12:245–252.

Toivanen A. Reactive arthritis. In: Klippel JH and Dieppe P, eds. Rheumatology. London, Mosby, 1994:4.9.1.

SJÖGREN'S SYNDROME

JUAN-MANUEL ANAYA, M.D.
NORMAN TALAL, M.D.

Sjögren's syndrome (SS) is a chronic autoimmune disease characterized by a progressive lymphocytic and plasma cell infiltration of the salivary and lachrymal glands leading to xerostomia and xerophthalmia (sicca complex). SS is associated with the production of rheumatoid factor and other autoantibodies including anti-Ro/SSA and anti-La/SSB. The spectrum of the disease extends from an organ specific autoimmune disorder (autoimmune exocrinopathy) to a systemic process. Despite being a "benign" autoimmune process, adult patients with SS are known to have increased risk of developing lymphoma.

SS may occur alone (primary SS) or in association with almost all of the autoimmune diseases (secondary SS). Prevalence of SS in the general population is nearly 2 percent. Although SS can occur in patients of all ages, it affects primarily females during the fourth and fifth decades of life with a female-male ratio of 9:1.

The clinical presentation of SS may be quite variable. Sicca complex is the main clinical presentation in adults, whereas in children swelling of the parotid glands is the most common symptom. Xerostomia, xerophthalmia, and swelling of the parotid glands may be observed in other conditions summarized in Table 1. These conditions must be excluded before a diagnosis of SS is made.

Table 1 Differential Diagnosis of Oral and Ocular Involvement in Sjögren's Syndrome

Parotid Gland Swelling	*Xerostomia*	*Xerophthalmia*
Infectious	**Infectious**	**Drugs**
Viral	**Drugs**	**Ocular diseases**
Mumps	Psychotherapeutic	Chronic conjunctivitis
Influenza	Parasympatholytic	Bullous dermatitis
Epstein-Barr	Beta-blockers	Chronic blepharatis
Coxsackievirus	Phenilbutazone	Blink abnormality
Cytomegalovirus	**Psychogenic**	**Senil xerophthalmia**
HIV	**Dehydration**	**Neurologic diseases**
Bacterial*	**Congenital**	V and VII cranial nerve involvement
Streptococcus	**Senil xerostomia**	**Hypovitaminosis A**
Staphylococcus	**Oral breathing**	**Virus**
Salmonella	**Neurologic diseases**	Epstein-Barr
Actinomyces	Multiple sclerosis	HIV
Tuberculosis	Parkinson's disease	HTLV-1
Sarcoidosis	**Irradiation**	**Graft-vs-host disease**
Amyloidosis		**Cystic fibrosis**
Metabolic/endocrine		**Diabetes mellitus**
Hyperlipoproteinemias		
Chronic pancreatitis/ Cystic fibrosis		
Hepatic cirrhosis		
Diabetes mellitus		
Acromegaly		
Malnutrition		
Hypovitaminosis A, B_6, C		
Recurrent parotitis of childhood*		
Tumors*		

*May be unilateral.

DIAGNOSIS OF SJÖGREN'S SYNDROME

Many diagnostic tests exist to assess salivary and lachrymal involvement in SS. Although there is no worldwide consensus regarding the diagnostic criteria for SS, we use the validated European diagnostic criteria (Table 2). In addition to subjective symptoms of xerostomia and xerophthalmia, an assessment of oral and ocular involvement is considered essential to the diagnosis of SS. The degree of oral and ocular involvement is measured using several parameters, such as the quantity and quality of secretions and morphologic changes in the glands. A test for autoantibodies (rheumatoid factor, antinuclear antibodies, anti-Ro/SSA, and anti-La/SSB) should be performed on every patient suspected of SS. However, some primary SS patients may lack these autoantibodies.

Secretions can be measured quantitatively by Schirmer's test for the eye and by collecting saliva from the mouth. The Schirmer's test, in which a strip of Whatman No. 41 filter paper is folded and placed in the lower conjunctival sac, is a simple measure of tear production. A positive test is considered when patients moistened less than 5 mm of the test paper after 5 minutes of the test. A more reliable diagnostic sign for xerophthalmia is the rose Bengal score (RBS) performed by placing 25 μl rose Bengal solution in the inferior fornix of each eye and asking the patient to make one to two full blinks. The number of red spots formed are counted and scored: 1+ (sparsely scattered), 2+ (densely scattered), or 3+ (confluent) in lateral and nasal conjunctiva and the cornea. The sum of scores from the three regions of one eye form the RBS of that eye and define the presence of keratoconjunctivitis sicca (KCS). A score greater than or equal to 4 in at least one eye is considered abnormal.

Unstimulated whole saliva collection should be performed in the morning. Patients should not be allowed to eat or drink, brush their teeth, rinse their mouth, or smoke tobacco 1 hour prior to the procedure. Saliva is collected in conical calibrated tubes for 15 minutes. The normal limit is greater than 1.5 ml of saliva. Other tests used to evaluate salivary gland involvement in SS are parotid sialography and salivary gland scintigraphy.

Minor salivary gland biopsy is the test most widely used as a specific diagnostic criterion for the salivary component of SS. Site of biopsy (through histologically normal oral mucosa) and size of biopsy (at least four evaluable salivary gland lobules) are essential for analysis to yield interpretable results. The characteristic histopathologic feature in SS labial salivary glands is the presence of focal lymphocytic sialadenitis in all or most of the glands. Focal lymphocytic sialadenitis (FLS) has been defined as multiple, dense aggregates of 50 or more lymphocytes (one focus) in perivascular or periductal locations. The FLS is graded in focus score, meaning the number of foci per 4 mm^2. A focus score of 10 is generally the highest value that can be counted before foci become confluent. A value of 12 is assigned to those

Table 2 European Criteria for the Diagnosis Classification of Sjögren's Syndrome

(Patients must meet 4 of 6 criteria in the absence of pre-existing lymphoma, acquired immunodeficiency, sarcoidosis, or graft-versus-host disease)

1. **Ocular symptoms**
   Definition: A positive response to at least one of the following:
   a. Have you had daily, persistent, troublesome dry eyes for more than 3 months?
   b. Do you have a recurrent sensation of sand or gravel in the eyes?
   c. Do you use tear substitutes more than three times a day?
2. **Oral symptoms**
   Definition: A positive response to at least one of the following:
   a. Have you had a daily feeling of dry mouth for more than 3 months?
   b. Have you had recurrent or persistently swollen salivary glands as an adult?
   c. Do you frequently drink liquids to aid in swallowing dry foods?
3. **Ocular signs**
   Definition: A positive result on at least one of the following two tests:
   a. Schirmer test (<5 mm in 5 minutes)
   b. Rose Bengal score (>4)
4. **Histopathologic features**
   Definition: Focus score >1 on minor salivary gland biopsy
5. **Salivary gland involvement**
   Definition: A positive result on at least one of the following three tests:
   a. Salivary scintigraphy
   b. Parotid sialography
   c. Unstimulated salivary flow (<1.5 ml in 15 minutes)
6. **Autoantibodies**
   Definition: Presence of at least one of the following:
   a. Anti-Ro/SSA or anti-La/SSB
   b. Antinuclear antibodies
   c. Rheumatoid factor

specimens having two or more glands with confluent lymphocytic infiltration. A focus score greater than one focus per 4 mm^2 has a specificity of 95 percent and a sensitivity of 63 percent in the diagnosis of SS. Inaccurate methods in biopsies and failure to record the focus score are common problems with this technique.

No single test measuring oral or ocular involvement is sufficiently sensitive and specific to form the basis for diagnosis of SS. Tear secretion and saliva production may be physiologically reduced in elderly patients. Also, FSL may be observed in other conditions different from SS. Therefore, only the simultaneous positivity of various tests in conjunction with the presence of subjective symptoms and serologic abnormalities allow sufficient accuracy in the diagnosis of SS.

TREATMENT OF SJÖGREN'S SYNDROME

Sjögren's syndrome is often a neglected disease, adding greatly to the distress of the patient. The physician must remember that there is nothing minor about dryness of the eye and mouth, as well as dryness of other mucosal surfaces. Patients with SS should be seen regularly by a rheumatologist, an ophthalmologist, and a dentist. Patients should also be properly informed about the nature of their illness and the goals of therapy. Patients with SS should be followed closely for significant functional deterioration, significant changes in the course of the disease, or the appearance of symptoms attributable to drug side effects or comorbid conditions (i.e., depression, fibromyalgia).

Treatment of Glandular Disease

Dry Eyes

The patient may notice accumulation of thick ropy secretions along the inner canthus owing to a decreased tear film and an abnormal mucous component. Related complaints include erythema, photosensitivity, eye fatigue, decreased visual acuity, and the sensation of a "film" across the field of vision. Desiccation can cause small superficial erosions of the corneal epithelium. In severe cases, slit lamp examination may reveal filamentary keratitis (filaments of corneal epithelium and debris). Other complications may include conjunctivitis caused by *Staphyloccus aureus.*

Low levels of humidity in air-conditioned environments may worsen symptoms. Similar problems arise in windy or dry climates, in patients who either smoke cigarettes or are exposed to cigarette smoke, and in patients taking drugs with anticholinergic side effects. The most implicated drugs are phenothiazines, tricyclic antidepressants, antispasmodics, antiparkinsonian, and decongestant medications.

The mainstay of treatment for dry eyes is lubrication through the use of artificial tear drops, which may be used as often as necessary (generally once every 1 to 3 hours). Varieties of such drops are available without prescription, differing primarily in viscosity and preservative (Table 3). The thicker, more viscous drops require less frequent application, although they may cause blurring and leave a residue on the lashes. Many patients prefer thinner drops, which require more frequent applications. An apparent failure to respond to artificial tears may be indicative of eye irritation caused by the topical application of preservatives such as benzalkonium chloride, chlorbutanol, or thimersol. Also available are lubricating ointments that may produce significant blurring and are best used at night to provide protection over a longer period of time (Table 4).

Other steps may be taken to preserve tears if tear substitutes are insufficient to control symptoms. Watertight swimmer's goggles can be very helpful in creating a moisture chamber effect by preventing evaporation. Goggles also protect against wind and dust particles. The same effect can be achieved with ordinary food plastic wrap taped over the eyes. Commercial "bubble" bandages are also available.

Punctual occlusion is another method of conserving the few tears that SS patients produce. This procedure should be considered only in severe cases. Stents have been devised as nonsurgical means of occlusion; this is a good way to predict the success of surgical occlusion.

Sympathomimetics and parasympathomimetics serve to stimulate tear flow. Pilocarpine administered either orally or topically to the eye has been reported to be successful. In patients with a relative excess of mucin production and formation of filaments, a mucolytic agent such as acetylcysteine has been found to be useful. However, other investigators have failed to confirm this. The use of topical steroids for corneal ulcers of SS was associated with a worsening clinical course and is not recommended.

Dry Mouth

Xerostomia is often the initial symptom of SS. However, it is a common and subjective clinical complaint with a large variety of etiologies (see Table 1). Patients with dry mouths have various complaints. The "cracker sign" describes the difficulties such patients encounter when trying to eat dry foods without sufficient lubrication. Additional features include oral soreness, adherence of food to buccal surfaces, fissuring of the tongue, and dysphagia. Dental caries may also appear, as well as angular cheilitis associated with superimposed candidiasis. Patients may lose their ability to discriminate foods on the basis of taste and smell.

Treatment of xerostomia associated with SS is difficult. Currently, there is no single method that is completely effective. Treatment of oral SS should include (1) methods to increase salivary flow and selective use of saliva substitutes, (2) elimination or replacement of factors contributing to decreased salivary secretions (mouth breathing, heavy smoking, drugs), (3) prevention of dental caries and provision of ongoing dental treatment, and (4) diagnosis and treatment of oral candidiasis (Table 5). Most patients discover that it is

Table 3 Products for Dry Eyes

Major Component	*Trade Name*	*Preservative*
Artificial Tear Preparations (Demulcents)		
Hydroxyethylcellulose	Tear Guard	Sorbic acid + edetate disodium
Hydroxypropylcellulose	Lacrisert (Rx)	Benzalkonium chloride + edetate disodium (water soluble insert)
Hydroxypropyl methylcellulose	Lacril	Chlorobutanol
	Moisture Drops (0.5%)	Benzalkonium chloride
	Tears Renewed	Benzalkonium + edetate disodium
Carboxymethylcellulose	Cellufresh (0.5%)	Preservative free
	Celluvisc (1%) (unit dose)	Preservative free
	Gum cellulose (Rx) (0.3%, 0.625%, 0.9%)	Unpreserved; refrigerate after opening
Polyvinyl alcohol	Liquifilm Tears	Chlorobutanol
	Liquifilm Forte	Thimersol + edetate disodium
	Dakrina	Potassium sorbate + EDTA
	Dwelle	Potassium sorbate + EDTA
	Nutratear	Benzalkonium 0.004% + 0.08% EDTA
Polyvinyl alcohol and povidone	Refresh (unit dose)	Preservative free
Other Polymeric Systems	Comfort Drops	Benzalkonium chloride + edetate disodium
	Hypotears	Benzalkonium chloride + edetate disodium
	Hypotears P.F. (unit dose)	Preservative free
	Tears Naturale	Benzalkonium chloride + edetate disodium
	Tears Naturale II	Polyquad
	Tears Natural Free (unit dose)	Preservative free
Sterile saline	Unisol	Preservative free
Methylcellulose 1%	Murocel	Methylparaben 0.023% + Propylparaben 0.01%

Table 4 Products for Dry Eyes

Trade Name	*Composition*
Occular Emollients	
Akwa-Tears Ointment	Petrolatum, liquid lanolin, mineral oil
Duolube	Sterile ointment containing white petrolatum and mineral oil
Duratears	Sterile ointment containing white petrolatum, liquid lanolin, mineral oil, methylparaben, and polyparaben
Hypotears	Sterile ointment containing white petrolatum and light mineral oil
Acri-Lube S.O.P.	Sterile ointment with 42.5% mineral oil, 55% white petrolatum, lanolin, and chlorobutanol
*Refresh P.M.	White petrolatum, mineral oil, lanolin, purified water, sodium chloride
Special Preparations and Equipment for the Eye	
EV Lid Cleanser II	Mild cleansing formula for eyelid and delicate skin
EV Lid Cleanser Kit	Includes pads and cleaning lotion
EV Lid Cleanser Travel Pak	½ oz cleanser and 10 pads
Clearclenz	Sterile eyelid cleanser
Opticrom (Rx)	Cromolyn sodium solution for allergic manifestations
Vistacrom	Cromolyn sodium solution for allergic manifestations
I-Scrub	Eyelid cleanser
OCuSOFT	Lid scrub lotion and pads
Medicool Medication Protector	Case and holder in which to carry preservative-free eyedrops or other medications that should be kept refrigerated
Moist Eye Moisture Panels	Can be fitted to most configurations of eyewear to create a moisture chamber
Muro-128	Hypertonic sodium chloride 5% and 7% for corneal edema

helpful to carry water, sugarless lemon drops, or chewing gum. Fluids *ad libitum* should be utilized for all meals and snacks. The consumption of large amounts of water during the day, though symptomatically helpful, may produce nocturia that interrupts sleep patterns and leads to fatigue.

Artificial saliva substitutes offer some additional palliation. Mucin-containing saliva substitutes seem to be more effective than substitutes based on carboxymethyl cellulose or polyethylenoxide. Mucins tend to protect against desiccation, provide for lubrication and cleaning, and have some antimicrobial effects. However, saliva substitutes should be used sparingly with only the minimum volume necessary for oral lubrication. This usually consists of no more than 2 ml before and after meals, at bedtime, and following oral hygiene.

Increased salivary flow rates may be induced by potassium iodide or parasympathomimetic agents such as pilocarpine or neostigmine, systemically or as a mouthwash. Varying degrees of success have been noted. Bromhexine, a synthetic alkaloid originally used as a mucolytic agent in cough syrups, has been tested with limited success. A new battery-powered electronic device for stimulating salivary flow (Salitron System) has been shown to be effective in stimulating increased production of saliva and in reducing the symptoms of xerostomia in SS patients.

Increased moisture to the upper airways by use of normal saline sprays and humidifiers at night may reduce respiratory symptoms and alleviate mouth breathing. During surgery, SS patients are at increased risk for corneal abrasions because of use of anticholinergic agents by the anesthesiologist and low humidity in the operating room. Also, a risk of atelectasis and pneumonia exists because of upper airway dryness and inspired mucous secretions. Therefore, the use of ocular lubricants, humidified oxygen, and respiratory therapy should help to minimize these potential complications.

Approximately one-half of all SS patients have parotid or other major salivary gland enlargement, often painless, recurrent, and bilateral. Salivary gland enlargement may be due to cellular infiltration or ductal obstruction. There is no effective treatment for parotid gland swelling related with SS, which is a mild, and usually self-limited condition. Methods to increase salivary flow (see Table 5) and local moist heat may be helpful in preventing ductal obstruction. Corticosteroids have transient efficacy, may favor infection, and therefore are not recommended. Local radiation treatment and/or cytotoxic drugs have no long-term efficacy and may increase the risk of malignancy. If the gland remains tender or enlarged, lymphoma must be ruled out. Superficial parotidectomy could be considered in these cases. Tenderness, fever, or erythema suggest superimposed infection, in which treatment includes penicillinase-resistant penicillins combined with beta-lactamase inhibitors (i.e., amoxicillin 500 mg, plus clavulanic acid 125 mg, every 8 hours orally for 7 days), local moist heat, and nonsteroidal anti-inflammatory drugs (NSAIDs).

Nose, Skin, and Vaginal Dryness

Dry nose may also be taken into consideration. In addition to the use of nasal solutions (Table 6), lavage of the sinus to remove crusted secretions allows the nasal

Table 5 Products for the Dry Mouth

Trade Name	*Composition*
Saliva Substitutes	
Mouthkote	Citrus flavor in spray bottle with Mucroprotective Factor
Oral Balance	Moisturing gel
Orex	Squirt bottle; several flavors
Salivart	Pressurized container; can use with one hand
Xero-Lube	Regular 6 oz pump container; some patients recommend diluting slightly with water. Mint flavor available in ½ oz squirt container
Evian mineral water spray	Other mineral waters can be used the same way
Special Toothpastes and Mouthwashes	
Aquafresh for kids	Contains sodium monofluorophosphate; sugarless (sorbitol main sweetener)
Biotene toothpaste	Contains glucoseoxidase/lactoperoxidase
Biotene mouthwash	Alcohol free
Crest for kids	Contains fluoristat
Saline solution	Mouth rinse; breaks up thick mucus
Alkalol	Mucolytic agent; mouth rinse and nasal douche
Products that Stimulate Salivary Flow	
Biotene chewing gum	Contains glucoseoxidase/lactoperoxidase sweetened with xylitol
Extra sugarless gum	Contains Nutrasweet; several flavors, including peppermint, spearmint, winter fresh, bubble gum
Oralbalance	Soothing gel
Pro-Flow	Stimulates saliva; nonacidic
Sialor (Rx) (Anetholtrithion)	Stimulates salivary flow
Sugarless candies	To be sucked
Trident sugarless gum	Contains sorbitol; in Canada, available with xylitol; several flavors
Xylitol mints	To be sucked, not chewed
Products to Soothe the Oral Mucosa and/or Lips	
Blistex	
Boric Acid Ointment	Does not contain lanolin
Borofax	Contains boric acid ointment and lanolin; also good inside tips of nostrils
Mouthkote	Citric flavor in spray bottle with Mucoprotective Factor
Phen-oris	Medicated lip care
Smile lip moisturizer	
Vaseline	

passages to remain open and the patient to avoid mouth breathing which is a cause of xerostomia.

Dry skin and lips are common complaints in SS patients. Topical treatments with alcohol-free creams and moisturizing lotions are often helpful, as are cosmetics such as lipstick.

Vaginal dryness is often observed in female patients with SS, and may be a cause of dyspareunia. A gynecologic examination is useful to rule out other causes of vaginal dryness. The most frequent cause of vaginal dryness in perimenopausal or postmenopausal women is declining estrogen levels; therefore, vaginal estrogen creams should be advised. Vaginal yeast infection also must be ruled out and treated promptly. When vaginal dryness occurs as a part of SS, sterile lubricants are helpful (Table 7).

Treatment of Extraglandular Disease

In approximately 50 percent of patients with primary SS, an extraglandular manifestation (EGM) may develop during the evolution of the disease (Table 8). In some cases, one EGM may disclose the disease. Systemic manifestations or EGM seen in primary SS patients may lead to confusion regarding its diagnosis. Nevertheless, EGMs in primary SS are usually mild and sometimes subclinical, revealed only by careful examination. Systemic corticosteroids and immunosuppressive drugs are only used to treat potentially life-threatening disease often involving the lung or kidney. They are not recommended for the treatment of dry eyes and dry mouth. No controlled studies have been performed because relatively few patients require immunosuppressive treatment.

Table 6 Products and Devices to Soothe the Dry Nose and Dry Ear

Trade Name	*Composition*
Nasal irrigator	Attaches to Water-Pik; loosens dried up mucus; use with saline solution
Nasal douche	Loosens dried-up mucus; use with Alkalol or saline solution
Saline solution	Helps prevent nosebleeds
NaSal	Saline solution to prevent nosebleeds
Ocean	Saline solution to prevent nosebleeds
Salinex	Saline solution to prevent nosebleeds
AYR	Saline solution to prevent nosebleeds
Mineral oil	Use with Q-tip for dry ear

Musculoskeletal Manifestations

Arthralgia or arthritis may occur in 60 percent of patients with primary SS. The arthropathy of primary SS is essentially an intermittent polyarticular arthropathy affecting mostly small joints, sometimes asymmetrically. In most cases, sicca symptoms precede arthropathy in which course and prognosis are generally good. Joint deformity and mild erosions are unusual. Although myalgias are frequently observed, inflammatory muscle disease is confirmed in less than 10 percent of patients.

Musculoskeletal symptoms associated with primary SS respond well to NSAIDs. In cases in which NSAIDs fail to control arthritis, either hydroxychloroquine (6 mg per kilogram per day) or sulfasalazine (3 to 4 g daily in evenly divided oral doses) may be useful.

Pulmonary Involvement

Interstitial lung disease (ILD) is probably the most common functional abnormality identified in patients with primary SS and lung involvement, particularly in those with other EGMs. Obstructive disease is more prevalent in secondary SS to rheumatoid arthritis. It has been shown that over 30 percent of unselected primary SS patients have ILD, in which the majority of cases is subclinical. Fibrosing alveolitis is rare in SS. Lung involvement in SS may originate from the exocrine tissue at the bronchi and from bronchus-associated lymphoid tissue. However, its natural history and prognosis are not well known. Once the diagnosis of ILD is established, clinical assessment, radiographic, and pulmonary function tests should be performed and monitored twice per year to determine the extent of functional impairment. High resolution computed tomography is useful when open-lung or transbronchial biopsy is planned identifying areas of thickened bronchial walls and alveolitis. These sites often yield more useful histologic information than do areas of fibrotic disease. Lung biopsy should be performed before treatment is started. There is a better chance for therapeutic success if a highly cellular infiltrate is found.

Table 7 Products for Vaginal Dryness

Trade Name	*Composition*
Astroglide	Provides light lubrication
Estrace Vaginal Cream (Rx)	Synthetic human estrogen
H-R lubricating jelly	Lubricating jelly
K-Y lubricating jelly	Lubricating jelly
Lubrin vaginal inserts	Unscented precoital suppositories
Maxilube	Thickest of the vaginal lubricants
Premarin vaginal cream (Rx)	Conjugated estrogens
Replens	Unit dose applicator filled with polycarbophil
Surgilube	Lubricating jelly
Vitamin E oil, cream, or capsules	For topical application to labia (capsules must be pierced, but are the cheapest form)

Table 8 Extraglandular Manifestations of Primary Sjögren's Syndrome

Musculoskeletal (40%-60%)	**Pulmonary (10%-30%)**
Arthralgias/arthritis	Xerothrachea
Myalgias/myositis	Interstitial lung disease
Vascular/Skin (30%)	Obstructive lung disease
Photosensitivity	Lymphoma
Vasculitis:	**Gastrointestinal (5%-10%)**
Cutaneous	Dysphagia
Systemic	Atrophic gastritis
Raynaud's phenomenon	Pancreatitis
Thyroiditis (30%)	Autoimmune hepatitis
Renal (5%-20%)	**Hematologic (5%-20%)**
Interstitial nephritis	Anemia
Renal tubular acidosis	Leukopenia (lymphopenia)
Glomerulonephritis	Hypergammaglobinemia
Neurologic (Rare)	Monoclonal gammopathy
Peripheral and central nervous systems involvement	Cryoglobulinemia
	Lymphadenopathy
	Splenomegaly
	Lymphoma

The therapy of progressive ILD, regardless of the agent used, requires 3 to 6 months before its effectiveness can be assessed. Treatment is usually initiated with corticosteroids in the range of 1 to 2 mg per kilogram per day. High-dose intravenous corticosteroid treatment (pulse therapy) may be used at the beginning of treatment or in patients with aggressive and severe disease in hopes of arresting progression (usually methylprednisolone, 10 to 15 mg per kilogram per day IV for 3 days). The reasons for varied patient response to corticosteroids is still poorly understood. Determining whether treatment is producing the desired effect may be difficult. A composite clinical, roentgenographic, and physiologic score (CRP score) has been developed allowing a quantification of the clinical course and the impact of therapy in individual patients. As a patient improves, the dose of steroids may be tapered to a maintenance level of 50 percent of the starting dose. If there is no apparent response within 3 to 6 months, azathioprine should be added in addition to low-dose prednisone. The recommended dose of azathioprine is 2 mg per kilogram per day. Cyclophosphamide may succeed when azathioprine has been tried first and failed. Monthly bolus (0.5 to 1 g per square meter), instead of daily oral cyclophosphamide (2 mg per kilogram), may be administered to reduce the risk of side effects. The duration of immunosuppressive therapy has not been established, but conventional use is generally over the course of several months. Thereafter, a low oral maintenance dose should be attempted. Cyclophosphamide bolus may be administered quarterly for a period of 1 year. Although the risk of lymphoma is an important consideration, in our experience it has not appeared in SS patients treated with cyclophosphamide.

Vascular Involvement

Raynauds's phenomenon may be observed in nearly 30 percent of patients with primary SS generally associated with other EGMs. The course of Raynauds's phenomenon in SS is usually mild. Treatment includes the use of gloves in colder seasons, and either nifedipine or diltiazem.

Vasculitis may be observed in diseases which SS is associated, such as rheumatoid arthritis and systemic lupus erythematosus. In primary SS, vasculitis may occur in two forms: cutaneous vasculitis or systemic necrotizing vasculitis. Vasculitis limited to the skin may occur in about 30 percent of patients with primary SS, and manifest as purpura (palpable or not) or urticaria-like lesions. Leukocytoclastic vasculitis is the most frequent histologic finding. This form of vasculitis requires no specific therapy. Measures avoiding orthostatism may be helpful. In some patients with longstanding cutaneous vasculitis, low-dose steroids, colchicine, or pentoxyfilline have been used empirically with variable success.

Systemic necrotizing vasculitis is rare in primary SS. It is often associated with mixed cryoglobulinemia. It manifests as ulcerative skin lesions, digital gangrene, mononeuritis multiplex, myositis, and glomerulonephritis. Due to the seriousness of such systemic vasculitis, steroids, cyclophosphamide, and plasmapheresis are the recommended treatment.

Renal Involvement

The renal abnormalities in primary SS arise as a result of either lymphocytic infiltration in the renal parenchyma or immune complex deposition in the glomeruli. Interstitial nephritis in SS is usually mild and subclinical. When clinically detectable, the most common presentations are diminished urinary concentrating ability, and distal (Type 1) renal tubular acidosis (RTA). Proximal (Type 2) RTA can also occur, although less frequently. Hyposthenuria may be treated by hydric restriction (often difficult in SS patients) or low-dose thiazides. Type 1 acidosis is treated with sodium bicarbonate tablets (0.5 to 2.0 mmol per kilogram in 4 to 5 divided doses daily). In addition, low-dose steroids (0.1 mg per kilogram per day) may be useful.

Renal insufficiency resulting from interstitial nephritis is extremely rare in SS. Steroids and cyclophosphamide have been used empirically with good results in almost all cases. However, some patients require prolonged periods of treatment to maintain normal renal function. Glomerulonephritis is rare in primary SS. Its presence should raise the possibility of systemic vasculitis or an associated condition such as systemic lupus erythematosus.

Lymphoma

Benign polyclonal lymphocytic and plasma cell proliferation localized in exocrine glands may progress into monoclonal malignant lymphoma. The term pseudolymphoma has been used to describe an intermediate stage between benign to malignant lymphoproliferation. Histologically tumor-like aggregates of lymphoid cells that do not meet the histologic criteria for malignancy characterize pseudolymphoma. Although monoclonality may occur, lymphocytes eluted from pseudolymphoma biopsies are predominantly polyclonal T cells and contain a small percentage of B cells. When pseudolymphoma is suspected, low-grade B-cell lymphoma, including mucosal-associated lymphoid tissue (MALT) lymphoma, should be ruled out.

Clinical aspects relevant to lymphoma evolution include persistent enlargement of parotid glands, spleen, and lymph nodes. In addition, cough, dyspnea on exertion, mediastinal or hiliar lymph nodes, unilaterally localized nodules in the lungs, and persistent Raynaud's phenomenon may also indicate malignancy evolution. Laboratory findings of the appearance of monoclonal gammopathy and mixed cryoglobulinemia, lowered IgM, high-serum beta$_2$-microglobulin, and negative rheumatoid factor (having been positive), all suggest the presence of underlying malignancy.

Prevalence of clinically identifiable lymphoma in SS patients is nearly 5 percent. Malignant lymphoproliferation may be present initially or may develop later in the illness. Most lymphomas complicating SS belong to the B-cell lineage, are of either low- or intermediate-grade malignancy, and are localized in extranodal areas (gastrointestinal tract, thyroid, lung, kidney, orbit, salivary glands). Recent studies have suggested good prognosis for SS-associated lymphoma and have also implied a less aggressive approach to therapy than in the past. Patients with low-grade lymphomas affecting exocrine glands should be completely evaluated for the extent of the disease and, if the disease is localized, a "wait-and-watch" policy should be undertaken. In the case of histologically high-grade and clinically aggressive malignancy, then combination chemotherapy is recommended, and patients should be assessed by a cooperative team with an oncologist.

Treatment of Associated Conditions

Although hypothyroidism is frequently associated with SS, most of the cases are subclinical. Nevertheless, hypothyroidism may be one of the causes of common fatigue observed in SS patients. Substitution therapy is advised when hormone deficiency is confirmed.

Fibromyalgia is a frequent co-morbid condition observed in patients with SS and in other connective tissue diseases, including systemic lupus erythematosus and rheumatoid arthritis. Why fibromyalgia is becoming the most frequent rheumatologic disease remains poorly understood. Patients with fibromyalgia may also have chronic fatigue syndrome (CFS), irritable bowel syndrome (IBS), sleep disorder, or depression. The presence of fibromyalgia is not associated with the severity nor the activity of SS. On the other hand, some patients with fibromyalgia, IBS, and CFS may present sicca symptoms, Raynaud's phenomenon, and positive antinuclear antibodies. Some of these patients may have hypothyroidism. In the absence of clear evidence of a connective tissue disease, patients must be informed about the absence of "systemic" involvement in "primary" fibromyalgia, IBS, or CFS.

Treatment of fibromyalgia includes patient education, physical therapy, and an appropriate use of analgesic (usually NSAIDs). Ensuring a patient's own responsibility for the treatment may be critical. Possible environmental factors, including occupational, social, economic and psychological and/or psychosomatic factors should be identified. Measures should be taken against poor physiological fitness and sleep disturbances. Patients should work toward a balance between rest and aerobic activity over several months.

When antidepressant medication is indicated, drugs that have no anticholinergic side effects are recommended (e.g., fluxetine, trazodone). Interferon-α (INF-α) has been experimentally used in patients with fibromyalgia. Also, because some patients with hepatitis C virus (HCV) infection may present with sicca symptoms, INF-α has been used in SS patients with positive serology for HCV, regardless of the HCV-associated cryoglobulinemia. However, there is no clear evidence that HCV causes SS, and there is no controlled study using INF-α in SS. Further, since INF-α may induce autoimmune conditions, one should be prudent about its use in SS.

Treatment of secondary SS is usually directed at the associated disease. The treatment of rheumatoid arthritis or systemic lupus erythematosus is not altered because of the concomitant presence of SS. The clinical expression of secondary SS is generally milder and managed as already discussed.

Acknowledgments. We would like to thank our colleagues Drs. Hanna Abboud and Randal Otto for helpful suggestions, and George Tye Liu for his help in the preparation of the manuscript. Funded by the RGK Foundation (Austin, TX).

SUGGESTED READING

Fox PC, Datiles M, Atkinson JC, et al. Prednisone and piroxicam for treatment of primary Sjögren's syndrome. Clin Exp Rheumatol 1993; 11:149–156.

Fox RI. Treatment of the patient with Sjögren's syndrome. Rheum Dis Clin North Am 1992; 18:699–709.

Kruize AA, Hené RJ, Kallenberg CGM, et al. Hydroxychloroquine treatment for primary Sjögren's syndrome: a two-year double-blind crossover trial. Ann Rheum Dis 1993; 52:360–364.

Moutsopoulos HM, Vlachoyiannopoulos PG. What would I do if I had Sjögren's syndrome. Rheumatol Rev 1993; 2:17.

Talal N. Clinical and pathogenetic aspects of Sjögren's syndrome. Semin Clin Immunol 1993; 6:11–20.

Talal N, Quinn JH, Daniels TE. The clinical effects of electrostimulation on salivary function of Sjögren's syndrome patients. A placebo-controlled study. Rheumatol Int 1992; 12:43–45.

ANKYLOSING SPONDYLITIS

DANIEL J. CLAUW, M.D.

Ankylosing spondylitis (AS) falls within a group of inter-related disorders, termed seronegative spondyloarthropathies, that are characterized by similar patterns of joint disease, as well as nonarticular involvement. The other entities within this category include Reiter's syndrome, psoriatic arthritis, and the arthritis associated with inflammatory bowel disease (enteropathic arthritis). In addition to the similar clinical features of these disorders, these entities share a common genetic predisposition and likely pathogenesis.

AS is the prototypical seronegative spondyloarthropathy. In recent years, it has become clear that this disorder is much more common than previously suspected and may affect up to 1 percent of the population. Contrary to previous belief, these studies have also suggested that the incidence of AS is equal between sexes, although females are more likely to have less severe disease, with more frequent peripheral joint and cervical spine involvement. The typical age of symptom onset is in the second or third decade, but the diagnosis may be delayed when symptoms are insidious.

The genetic predisposition to develop AS is conferred by the presence of the HLA-B27 haplotype. The frequency of this haplotype ranges from up to 50 percent in certain Indians to less that 1 percent in African-Americans and Asians, which accounts for the tremendous variability in prevalence of AS in different populations. Over 90 percent of individuals with AS (and over 50 percent of those have other seronegative spondyloarthropathies) will be HLA-B27 positive, but only approximately 20 percent of HLA-B27–positive individuals will have AS. Recent studies using transgenic mice suggest that the HLA-B27 gene is directly involved in the pathogenesis of the seronegative spondyloarthropathies rather than being a surrogate marker, although the precise mechanism remains unclear.

Involvement of the axial skeleton is the hallmark of AS and the other seronegative arthropathies. Thus, back pain is the most common symptom in this condition. Historic features of back pain suggestive of AS include an age of onset of less than 40, insidious onset and chronicity of pain, and stiffness that worsens with rest and improves with exercise. Other symptoms that may help differentiate AS from other disorders involving the back include the presence of pleuritic or chest wall pain, or the absence of radicular pain.

This involvement of the axial skeleton leads to characteristic features on physical examination and radiographs, which confirm the diagnosis of AS. On examination, individuals with AS with lumbar involvement will usually display significant limitation of motion of this region of the spine in all three planes. When the axial involvement has extended cephalad to the thoracic region, diminished chest expansion is noted, usually to 1 in. or less when measured at the level of the fourth thoracic interspace. The radiographic findings of AS are most specific, however, in that most individuals will display bilateral and symmetric sacroiliitis. These changes can be best delineated by performing a Ferguson view of the pelvis, which allows better visualization of the entire joint. Later changes include squaring of the vertebral bodies and formation of syndesmophytes (calcification of the anterior spinal ligament), which form the characteristic "bamboo spine."

As noted, individuals with AS can also develop peripheral articular disease. These manifestations include an inflammatory arthritis involving nearly any peripheral joint, as well as inflammation at sites of tendon insertions (enthesopathy). The most common sites of peripheral joint involvement are the large joints, and the lower extremities may be more commonly affected than the upper. Areas of tendon involvement include the Achilles, plantar fascia, and intercostal region.

Other clinical symptoms may be seen in AS. Because AS is an inflammatory disorder, afflicted individuals may experience malaise, fatigue, and low-grade fever. Inflammatory eye disease (uveitis, iritis) and cardiac conduction defects can occur in AS, and appear to be related to HLA-B27 positivity. Individuals who express this haplotype but do not have AS are still predisposed to develop these manifestations. Other extra-articular manifestations include aortic valve insufficiency, pulmonary disease, prostatitis, and neurologic symptoms.

APPROACH TO THE PATIENT

Diagnosis

The diagnosis of AS is based on the development of clinical and radiographic features previously mentioned. Laboratory tests are generally not helpful for diagnostic purposes, although the sedimentation rate and C-reactive protein may be elevated. Arriving at the correct diagnosis early in the course of AS may be difficult, especially before the development of classic changes on plain radiographs. Some studies have suggested that more advanced imaging modalities (e.g., computed tomography [CT] and magnetic resonance imaging [MRI]) may detect sacroiliitis earlier, but given the nonspecific treatment of AS, it is rarely vital that the correct diagnosis be made at the onset of initial symptoms.

Patient Education

As with any chronic disorder, at the time of diagnosis it is important to counsel patients regarding what they may expect over time. Since there is no therapy that clearly alters the course of this disease, the patient should be advised that the primary goals of treatment are to maintain range of motion and function and reduce discomfort.

Because of the known genetic predisposition to AS, individuals may ask for genetic counseling if diagnosed. It is important to explain that, assuming the patient carries the HLA-B27 haplotype, one-half of their offspring will be HLA-B27 positive, but only 20 percent of those who are B27 positive will develop AS. Thus, the risk of a parent with AS having a child with the same disease is approximately 10 percent.

THERAPY

Physical Modalities

As previously noted, maintenance of range of motion and function is of paramount importance in this disorder. Physical therapists can be extremely beneficial in instructing AS patients on the types of exercises that are beneficial in maintaining range of motion. Special emphasis should be placed on avoiding fusion of the apophyseal joints in the chest wall or cervical spine, which can result in significant functional disability. Even when fusion cannot be avoided, therapists familiar with this disorder can instruct the patient on exercises and activities that can lead to ankylosis in a physiologic position. This is particularly important in the cervical spine, since the natural history of this disorder is to lead to fusion of the neck in a flexed position, which results in an inability to look upward. It is important to emphasize to the patient and therapist that the exercise regimen should include aerobic as well as stretching exercises, since there are some data that suggest that the improvement in respiratory function with exercise may be most strongly related to improved cardiopulmonary fitness.

In addition to physical therapy, there are a number of other physical modalities that can be of benefit in the AS patient. These include measures such as sleeping on a firm mattress, utilizing specially designed furniture or household implements, or being fitted with prism glasses if the cervical spine fuses in flexion. Once again physical and occupational therapists can be of tremendous assistance in these matters.

Nonsteroidal Anti-Inflammatory Drug Therapy

Nonsteroidal anti-inflammatory drugs (NSAIDs) are the mainstay of pharmacologic treatment for AS. Although there are no data suggesting that these agents impede ankylosis or change the natural history of the disease, they are generally effective in improving stiffness, discomfort, and mobility.

Although few studies have compared drugs within this class for relative efficacy, anecdotal experience suggests that phenylbutazone and indomethacin are the most effective, perhaps because they are the most potent inhibitors of prostaglandin synthesis. Because of the rare blood dyscrasias seen with phenylbutazone, this drug should probably be reserved for individuals who are resistant to other NSAIDs. When used, the dosage of this drug is 100 mg taken three times daily. Because of these problems with phenylbutazone, indomethacin is generally employed as the initial agent for the management of AS. It is typically given at a dose of 50 mg three times daily with food, although there is also a slow-release formulation (75 mg) that only needs to be taken twice daily. Indomethacin may have more side effects than other NSAIDs, in particular headaches and cognitive dysfunction. If individuals are intolerant of this medication, any number of other drugs in this class may be effective, although some feel that the other indole NSAIDs may be most efficacious (e.g., sulindac [200 mg twice daily] or tolmetin [400 to 600 mg three times daily]).

Since the goal of therapy is alleviation of pain and stiffness, the most reasonable approach to the use of any NSAID in AS is to begin with the recommended dosage of the drug and if this is effective, slowly decrease the amount until a minimal dose that relieves symptoms is achieved. Intermittently, the NSAID should be tapered or stopped briefly to determine if it is still needed, because the inflammatory component of this disease can wax and wane with time.

All of the NSAIDs have some gastrointestinal toxicity, which can be manifested as symptoms such as dyspepsia and heartburn, and/or the development of peptic ulcer disease (PUD). This latter complication of NSAID therapy is more likely to occur in individuals with a past history of PUD; prior chronic use of antacids or histamine-blockers; concurrent alcohol, corticosteroid, or anticoagulant use; or smoking. In individuals with these risk factors, the practitioner should consider the concurrent use of misoprostol (100 or 200 μg four times daily), a prostaglandin analog. It is important to recognize that most individuals who develop major gastrointestinal bleeding from NSAID use are asymptomatic, so one should not make a decision regarding misoprostol co-administration based on the presence or absence of gastrointestinal symptoms after initiating NSAID therapy. Other side effects seen commonly with NSAIDs are renal dysfunction (which is typically reversible), platelet dysfunction, allergic reactions, and liver function abnormalities.

Corticosteroids

Corticosteroids may be useful for the management of the local manifestations of AS. Ocular steroids are used for the treatment of eye disease, and corticosteroid injections can be beneficial for the treatment of tendinitis. The exception to this is with Achilles tendinitis, in which injections are typically avoided because of anecdotal reports of tendon rupture. Systemic steroids have not generally been utilized for the treatment of AS because anecdotal evidence suggested a relative lack of efficacy of these agents, not only in AS but also in the other seronegative spondyloarthropathies. There have been recent reports, however, suggesting that monthly "pulse" methylprednisolone may be helpful in treating both axial and peripheral joint disease in AS (375 to 1,000 mg given intravenously), and low dose prednisone (e.g., 5 to 10 mg each morning) may be helpful in the treatment of peripheral joint disease.

Second-Line Agents

There have been clinical trials examining the effects of several second-line drugs in AS. The best studied is sulfasalazine (SS). SS is best tolerated when begun at 500 mg daily for 1 to 2 weeks, and the dose is escalated by 500 mg at this interval until a dose of 2,000 mg is achieved. The beneficial effects may not occur for several months, and usually not until the 2,000 mg dose is reached. Although some of these studies suggested that SS was more effective for the peripheral joint disease than the axial joint disease in AS, most studies demonstrated a global improvement in both symptoms and laboratory variables. Gastrointestinal symptoms are by far the most common side effect of SS. These can frequently be avoided by utilizing the enteric-coated form of this medication and ingesting it with food. Other side effects include leukopenia, rash, headache, azoospermia, and liver function disturbances. If 2,000 mg of SS is not effective in alleviating symptoms, the dose can be increased to up to 4,000 mg in divided doses daily.

As rheumatologists have become more comfortable with the safety profile of methotrexate (MTX), this drug likewise has been utilized in severe cases of AS and other seronegative spondyloarthropathies. This drug is given once weekly as a single dose, typically beginning at 7.5 mg (three tablets), and escalated to 15 to 20 mg, if necessary. As with other second-line drugs, the peak beneficial effect may take several months. There are a number of annoying side effects that occur during MTX administration, including a number of gastrointestinal symptoms, fatigue, and dizziness. Some of these side effects may be less frequent when folic acid (1 mg per day) is given concurrently. The two most serious side effects of MTX when used in this manner are a hypersensitivity pneumonitis and cirrhosis, although the latter problem appears quite rare if there are no concurrent liver problems or ingestion of alcohol or other hepatotoxins. Other second-line agents such as gold, penicillamine, cyclophosphamide, and hydroxychloroquine have not received adequate study to evaluate their efficacy.

Other Treatments

Several decades ago there was some enthusiasm regarding the use of low-dose radiation therapy in AS. Although this treatment was in many cases effective, the later risk of myeloproliferative disorders has led to concern about its use. Several surgical options are sometimes used for these patients. Some centers with experience in this condition have had reasonable outcomes in performing vertebral wedge osteotomies to correct the cervical spinal defect in severe cases. In this late stage of disease, individuals with AS are more susceptible to fractures of the lower part of the cervical spine, in some cases caused by relatively minor trauma. Joint arthroplasties appear to have good success in this group of patients. Despite the initial fear that there may be ankylosis or excessive bone formation after these procedures, this does not appear to be the case.

SUGGESTED READING

Calin A. Seronegative spondyloarthropathies. Med Clin North Am 1986; 70:323.

Creemers MCW, van Riel PLCM, Franssen MJAM, et al. Second-line treatment in seronegative spondyloarthropathies. Semin Arthritis Rheum 1994; 24(2):71.

Godfrey RG, Calbro JJ, Mills D, et. al. A double-blind crossover trial of aspirin, indomethacin, and phenylbutazone in ankylosing spondylitis. Arthritis Rheum 1972; 15:110.

Moll JMH, Wright V. New York clinical criteria for ankylosing spondylitis. A statistical evaluation. Ann Rheum Dis 1973; 32:354.

TEMPORAL ARTERITIS

GEORGE F. DUNA, M.D.
LEONARD H. CALABRESE, D.O.

Temporal arteritis (TA) is a medium and large vessel systemic vasculitis, generally affecting persons above 50 years of age (mean age is about 70 years). It is in fact the most common systemic vasculitis in this age group. The clinical features of TA have been well described and are summarized in Table 1. Headache,fever, and polymyalgia rheumatica (PMR) are more common than focal or multifocal ischemic symptoms. However, the latter are more serious and may lead to permanent sequelae such as blindness. PMR is a syndrome characterized by bilateral shoulder and hip girdle aching and stiffness in association with elevated acute phase reactants. The relationship between PMR and TA is complex; PMR occurs in about 50 percent of patients with TA. On the other hand, temporal artery biopsy may reveal arteritis in up to 33 percent of patients presenting with symptoms of PMR. In addition, PMR and TA may share a common genetic background as recently suggested by HLA subtype analysis. Some authors thus argue that PMR and TA are manifestations of the same disease process.

Table 1 Temporal Arteritis: Clinical Features

Abnormality	*Frequency (%)*
Headache	60-90
Fever	21-48
Polymyalgia rheumatica	50
Scalp tenderness	47
Visual signs or symptoms	36-40
Claudication	
Extremity	5-8
Jaw	36-67
Stroke or TIAs	7
Tenderness of temporal artery	55-69
Absent temporal artery pulse	40-51

Although nonspecific, an elevated erythrocyte sedimentation rate (ESR >40 mm per hour) is the most sensitive laboratory abnormality found in untreated patients with TA. The ESR is preferably measured by the Westergren method (WSR) since it is often markedly elevated, averaging 100 mm per hour in most series. Cases of TA with a normal WSR have been reported but are rare. Prior treatment with glucocorticoids for PMR or other conditions may result in a normal or near normal WSR in a patient with TA. When the clinical presentation is compelling (high pretest probability), a normal WSR does not exclude the diagnosis of TA. Measurement of C-reactive protein (CRP), another acute phase reactant, may be useful in such patients.

Temporal artery biopsy remains the standard test for the diagnosis of TA and should be obtained in most circumstances. Prior treatment with glucocorticoids should not dissuade clinicians from seeking histologic proof in patients with features of active TA. Although a positive biopsy is capable of confirming the diagnosis with certainty, false-negative biopsies do occur. Failure to find characteristic histopathology may be due to inadequate sample size and the patchy nature of the vasculitic process. To improve the diagnostic yield, we recommend that a large segment of artery (3 to 5 cm) be obtained. In addition, the specimen should be carefully sectioned to ensure that "skip lesions" have not been overlooked. If thorough examination of an adequate sample is unrevealing, the decision to treat must be based on clinical grounds. If the clinical index of suspicion is high, treatment should be initiated and the therapeutic response carefully assessed. Contralateral temporal artery biopsy is recommended under extreme circumstances (i.e., in critically-ill patients with serious co-morbid conditions) when empiric treatment is associated with unacceptable risks.

THERAPY OF TEMPORAL ARTERITIS

Timing of Therapy and Patient Selection

If the diagnosis of TA is strongly suspected, particularly in the presence of ocular symptoms, the condition should be treated as a medical emergency. Treatment should be initiated immediately to minimize the risks of ischemic complications such as blindness. Diagnostic testing should not delay the prompt institution of therapy, but should rather proceed in parallel. Waiting for the results of temporal artery biopsy before intervening therapeutically is a dangerous approach that is best avoided. Glucocorticoids (GCs) remain the standard treatment for TA and adjunctive therapy with cytotoxic agents continues to be the subject of investigation (see new approaches). In the absence of other therapeutic options, patients who are at high risk for GC toxicity may simply need more frequent and careful monitoring (see following discussion).

Table 2 Mechanisms of Action of Glucocorticoids

Molecular Processes Inhibited
- Enzymatic function: PL-A2, Cox 2, and NOS
- Production of proinflammatory PG, LT, and TX
- Production of proinflammatory cytokines (IL-1, IL-2, and IL-6, TNF-α)

Cellular Processes Inhibited
- Neutrophil adhesion to endothelium and chemotaxis
- Monocyte/macrophage activation, chemotaxis, and ability to recognize and eliminate antigen
- T-lymphocyte proliferative response to antigen and IL-2 mediated expansion

PL-A2, Phospholipase A2; *Cox 2,* cyclooxygenase 2; *NOS,* nitric oxide synthetase; *PG,* prostaglandins; *LT,* leukotrienes; *TX,* thromboxanes; *IL,* interleukin; *TNF-α,* tumor necrosis factor-alpha.

Glucocorticoids: Mechanisms of Action

GCs have diverse mechanisms of action (Table 2), and appear to work in TA by generally suppressing the inflammatory response. Recent studies focusing on the role of proinflammatory cytokines in PMR and TA have demonstrated that increased interleukin-6 (IL-6) production closely correlates with clinical symptoms. Treatment with GCs suppresses IL-6 production, whereas withdrawal of GCs results in an immediate rise in IL-6 levels. Although GCs do not provide a "cure" for TA, they do allow us to minimize morbidity until the disease runs its course, in about 2 years in most patients.

Initial Therapy

Side effects of GCs should be discussed in detail with the patient before initiating therapy. Since high-dose GC therapy invariably leads to some degree of toxicity, an inadequately informed patient may understandably become frustrated. Suboptimal communication may adversely affect both compliance and outcome. We generally initiate therapy with oral prednisone at a dose of 1 mg per kilogram per day (60 mg per day in most patients). A split-dose regimen (e.g., 20 mg three times daily) is more effective than a single morning dose (e.g., 60 mg daily) in the initial control of disease symptomatology and also increases the risks of GC toxicity when maintained for long periods of time. We thus consolidate

Table 3 Initiating Glucocorticoid Therapy: Alternative Approaches

Regimen	*Comments*
Oral Prednisone	
Single morning dose (1 mg/kg/day)	Standard approach
Split dose (20 mg t.i.d.)	More effective, more toxic
Intravenous Methylprednisolone	
For example, 1 gm daily for 3 days, 500 mg q6h for 3 days, 1 gm q12h for 3-5 days	Used by ophthalmologists for the treatment of ischemic eye disease Anecdotal results Optimal dose and frequency unknown No direct comparison with oral prednisone

Table 4 Decision-Making in the Maintenance Phase of TA Therapy

Symptoms/Signs	*WSR*	*Taper GC*	*Comments*
Absent	Normal	Yes	Proceed with tapering regimen
Absent	Elevated	Yes	More frequent and cautious clinical assessment
Present*	Elevated	No	Increase GCs to previous level and subsequently slow rate of tapering
Present*	Normal	No	Increase GCs to previous level and subsequently slow rate of tapering

*If visual or CNS ischemic symptoms are present, treatment should be reinitiated at 1 mg/kg/day.

our regimen to a single morning dose as soon as symptoms are controlled. The high single morning dose (e.g., 60 mg daily) is then maintained for another 4 weeks before tapering is initiated (see next section).

Alternative approaches to initiating GC therapy are summarized in Table 3. Alternate-day GC therapy has been shown to be inferior to daily GCs in the initial treatment of TA and should be avoided. High-dose intravenous methylprednisolone has been recommended by ophthalmologists for the initial treatment of ischemic eye disease in patients with TA (see Table 3). Results have been anecdotal, but improvement in vision has been claimed. The optimal dose and frequency of methylprednisolone administration remains to be determined. No direct comparisons with oral prednisone regimens exist. The risks of high-dose intravenous GCs are discussed later.

Maintenance Therapy

Following initial therapy with high-dose GCs for 4 to 6 weeks, a steroid-tapering regimen needs to be implemented. This is usually the most challenging part of TA management. Relapses occur in up to 30 percent of patients, even with cautious tapering of GCs. Clinicians are encouraged to individualize treatment rather than abide by strict and rigid guidelines. Several principles should apply: (1) GC should not be tapered in the face of active disease, (2) activity of disease should be assessed primarily by clinical parameters, and (3) the WSR is a useful laboratory measure of disease activity; however, when it is discordant with the clinical assessment, tapering of GCs should be guided by the latter, as illustrated in Table 4.

After the disease is controlled, GCs are generally tapered while maintaining daily dosing. An alternate-day regimen can also be used, but it may carry a higher risk of disease breakthrough (Table 5). In addition, predictors of efficacy have not been identified. In patients with a history of visual or CNS ischemic symptoms, we prefer to taper GCs on a daily-dose regimen. In others, with well-controlled disease and without ischemic signs and symptoms, switching to alternate-day dosing may be reasonable.

Regardless of the regimen used, the rate of GC tapering needs to be individualized. In general, doses are reduced every 6 to 14 days and decrements are proportional to the starting dose of GCs: 10 mg decrements for doses greater than 20 mg; 5 mg decrements for doses of 10 to 20 mg; and 1 to 2.5 mg decrements for doses less than 10 mg. Overzealous tapering and discontinuation of GCs over a period of only a few months virtually guarantee disease exacerbation and should be avoided. Rapid withdrawal of GC therapy is the most common reason for "refractory" or "relapsing" cases of TA referred to our institution. Most of our patients require maintenance GCs for a period of about 2 years.

Complications of Treatment

Glucocorticoid-related morbidity is quite common in TA patients. Patient-associated risk factors include

Table 5 Glucocorticoid-Tapering Regimen

Regimen	*Comments*
Daily → alternate-day schedule	Less GC toxicity Not all patients can be switched No clinical predictors for success
Taper on a daily dose schedule	Greater GC toxicity Most frequently utilized regimen Rate of tapering still needs to be individualized

Table 6 Side Effects of Glucocorticoid Therapy

Acute and Chronic Effects
- Fluid overload
- Hypertension
- Cardiac dysfunction
- Impaired glucose metabolism
- Electrolyte imbalance
- Impaired wound healing
- Increased risk of infection
- Neuropsychiatric symptoms

Chronic Effects
- Cushing's syndrome
- Adrenal suppression
- Cataracts, glaucoma
- Myopathy
- Osteonecrosis
- Osteoporosis/fractures
- Hyperlipidemia

age and coexistent medical conditions, while drug-related risk factors include dose, frequency, and duration of GC therapy. In the absence of disease activity, GCs should thus be tapered to the minimum dose required to maintain disease control. Switching to an alternate-day regimen following initial daily therapy reduces the risks of GC toxicity with two exceptions: osteoporosis and cataract formation. Most importantly, acute and chronic side effects of GCs should be recognized early and addressed promptly (Table 6).

Glucocorticoid-induced bone loss is greatest in the first 6 months of therapy and affects trabecular bone (spine, hips, pelvis, distal radius, ribs) to a greater extent than cortical bone. Blacks are as sensitive to GC-induced osteoporosis as are whites, and men are as sensitive as women. The risks are increased in female patients with TA in view of their uniformly postmenopausal status. To minimize the risks of osteoporosis, we suggest the following preventive measures:

1. In the absence of contraindications, hormone replacement therapy is strongly recommended for female patients, postmenopausal for 10 years or less.
2. Vitamin D (800 IU per day) and calcium (1,000 to 1,500 mg elemental per day) is recommended for all patients.
3. Physical activity is encouraged.

Table 7 Relative Associations of Immunosuppressive Drugs and Toxicity

Toxicity	*CPA*	*AZA*	*MTX*
Infection	+ + +	+ +	+ +
Malignancy	+ + +	+ +	+, rare
Cystitis	+ + +	−	−
Hematologic	+ + +	+ +	+
Infertility	+ + +	−	+
Teratogenicity	+ + +	+ +	+ +
Hepatic	−	+	+ + +
Pulmonary	+ +	+	+ +

CPA, Cyclophosphamide; *AZA,* azathioprine; *MTX,* methotrexate; (−) = no association; (+) → (+ + +) = weak → strong association.

Administration of large doses of intravenous methylprednisolone (500 to 2,000 mg per day) has, in extreme situations, been associated with anaphylaxis, seizures, cardiac arrhythmias, myocardial infarction, and sudden death. Less serious but more common side effects have included palpitations, facial flushing and curiously, polyarthralgias associated with noninflammatory joint effusions. When intravenous methylprednisolone is planned for the treatment of ischemic eye or CNS manifestations of TA, patients should be admitted to the hospital and closely monitored.

Cytotoxic Agents

The addition of cytotoxic agents to GCs in TA may be considered in a variety of clinical circumstances, including (1) failure to control disease activity with appropriate doses of GCs, (2) inability to taper GCs below 20 mg daily without facing disease exacerbation, or (3) development of unacceptable GC toxicity. Prospective controlled trials are needed to determine whether de novo treatment of TA with a cytotoxic agent and GCs is more effective than treatment with GCs alone, allowing more rapid tapering of GCs and reducing GC toxicity. Unfortunately, the published experience with the use of cytotoxic agents in TA has been, to this date, anecdotal. Successes have been claimed with azathioprine, cyclophosphamide, and more recently, methotrexate. In the clinical circumstances previously outlined, we generally favor the use of oral weekly methotrexate (maximum dosage of 0.3 mg per kilogram per week) in view of its demonstrated efficacy in other systemic vasculitides (Wegener's granulomatosis and Takayasu's arteritis) and its comparatively low toxicity (Table 7).

Duration of Follow-Up

Once TA is diagnosed and treatment is initiated, the clinician is obligated to provide frequent and regular follow-up. The goals of the periodic evaluation are (1) to assess disease activity, (2) to monitor for drug-related toxicity, and (3) to make the appropriate changes in therapy. As GCs are tapered, clinicians need to be more vigilant about the possibility of disease recrudescence. Most patients do well and are able to discontinue GCs within 2 years. However, clinical follow-up at periodic intervals remains indicated because relapses have been documented up to 11 years after initial treatment.

SUGGESTED READING

Hunder GG. Giant cell (temporal) arteritis. Rheum Dis Clin North Am 1990; 16:399.

Hunder GG. Daily and alternate-day corticosteroid regimens in treatment of giant cell arteritis. Ann Intern Med 1975; 82:613.

Krall PL, Mazanec DJ, Wilke WS. Methotrexate for corticosteroid-resistant polymyalgia rheumatica and giant cell arteritis. Cleve Clin J Med 1989; 56:253.

Kyle V, Hazleman BL. Treatment of polymyalgia rheumatica and giant cell arteritis. I.Steroid regimens in the first two months. Ann Rheum Dis 1989; 48:658.

Kyle V, Hazleman BL. Treatment of polymyalgia rheumatica and giant cell arteritis. II. Relation between steroid dose and steroid associated side effects. Ann Rheum Dis 1989; 48:662.

Myles AB, Perera T, Ridley MG. Prevention of blindness in giant cell arteritis by corticosteroid treatment. Br J Rheumatol 1992; 31:103.

CONNECTIVE TISSUE DISEASE

SYSTEMIC LUPUS ERYTHEMATOSUS

MICHELLE PETRI, M.D., M.P.H.

Lupus occurs in three major forms: systemic, discoid lupus without systemic involvement, and drug-induced (the most common drugs that induce lupus are phenothiazines, isoniazid, and procainamide). Systemic lupus erythematosus (SLE) is one of the most fascinating and challenging of the autoimmune diseases. Although SLE most often presents with cutaneous, arthritis, or renal manifestations, almost any organ system can be involved, in any combination. It occurs in approximately one of 250 African-American women and one of 400 Caucasian women; the female-male ratio is 9:1. The etiology of SLE is not known, but several inciting or enabling factors have been identified, including female hormones, pregnancy, infections, antibiotics (especially sulfas), and ultraviolet light exposure. Genetic predispositions have been identified as HLA-DR2 and HLA-DR3, and null complement alleles. The diagnosis of SLE requires a thorough history and physical examination with laboratory and, in some cases, radiographic tests to ascertain organ system involvement. Serologic tests such as high-titer ANA, lupus-specific autoantibodies (anti-Sm, anti-dsDNA), other autoantibodies (anti-Ro, anti-La, anti-RNP, antiphospholipid antibodies), and low serum complement (C3, C4) levels, can help to confirm the clinical diagnosis.

GENERAL MEDICAL MANAGEMENT

Although the 10- and even 20-year survival of SLE patients after diagnosis is better than 90 percent in most centers, one-half of SLE patients are surviving with damage to one or more major organ systems. The challenge in the treatment of SLE is not only to control the inflammatory component of the disease, but also to recognize the toxicity of some of the major treatments, including corticosteroids and immunosuppressive drugs. Even without immunosuppressive treatment, patients with SLE are at increased risk of infection. Opportunistic infections must be considered in any SLE patient treated with immunosuppressive drugs who presents with fever.

The general medical management of a lupus patient includes routine follow-up visits (usually every 3 months if the patient is doing well) to assess and treat disease activity, complications of lupus and/or its treatment, and co-morbid factors, such as hypertension, hyperlipidemia, and obesity. SLE, however, is frequently characterized by unpredictable "flares" or exacerbations that require urgent outpatient visits or even hospitalization. Pneumococcal vaccination and yearly influenza vaccination are recommended.

CUTANEOUS LUPUS

Sun avoidance and the use of sunscreens that block both UV-A and UV-B are the cornerstone of the treatment of cutaneous lupus, whether it be a malar rash, generalized photosensitive cutaneous lupus, subacute cutaneous lupus, or discoid lupus (Table 1). The antimalarial drug hydroxychloroquine is the first line of pharmacologic treatment. Patients who have G6PD deficiency cannot take hydroxychloroquine. A baseline ophthalmology examination is recommended before starting antimalarial therapy. The frequency of retinal toxicity with hydroxychloroquine (the major antimalarial used in the United States) is less than 1 percent. Follow-up ophthalmologic monitoring can be done on a 6-month basis. The usual dose of hydroxychloroquine in an adult is 400 mg a day. Cutaneous lesions may begin to respond in 2 weeks, but full response may take several months. SLE patients with cutaneous vasculitis or severe cutaneous involvement will require corticosteroids, but every attempt is made to quickly taper the daily dose or to add "steroid-sparing agents" (such as methotrexate or azathioprine) to the regimen. A rare form of cutaneous lupus, bullous lupus, responds to dapsone. Both dapsone and retinoids may be helpful in some patients with cutaneous lupus. Potent topical fluorinated steroids cannot be used on the face, because of the risk of cutaneous atrophy, but can be used on the extremities and trunk. Although thalidomide appears to be a very effective drug for discoid lupus, teratogenicity and toxicity limit its use.

Table 1 Treatment of Cutaneous Lupus

Treatment
Sunblock
Antimalarial drugs (usually hydroxychloroquine)
Check G6PD status. Monitor for retinal toxicity (rare) with a baseline eye examination followed by 6-month follow-ups
Dapsone
Check G6PD status. Monitor hematocrit and liver function tests, and check for peripheral neuropathy
Etretinate or isotretinoin
Retinoids should not be prescribed to women at risk of pregnancy. Monitor serum lipids, which may increase
Methotrexate
Monitor complete blood counts and liver function tests. Methotrexate must be stopped in a woman planning pregnancy
Corticosteroids: topical or oral
Monitor glucose, electrolytes, lipids, and blood pressure in patients on oral corticosteroids

Table 2 Treatment of Lupus Arthritis

Treatment
Nonsteroidal anti-inflammatory drugs (NSAIDs)
Once-daily NSAIDs: piroxicam, nabumetone, oxaprozin
Twice-daily NSAIDs: naproxen, sulindac, diclofenac
Thrice-daily NSAIDs: tolmetin, indomethacin, flurbiprofen, etodolac, ketoprofen
Over-the-counter NSAIDs: ibuprofen, naproxen
Monitor renal function, liver function, hematocrit, and gastrointestinal symptoms
Antimalarial drugs
Hydroxychloroquine
Check G6PD status and monitor for toxicity with 6-month ophthalmology examinations
Corticosteroids
Monitor glucose, electrolytes, lipids, and blood pressure.
Methotrexate
Monitor complete blood counts and liver function tests. Methotrexate must be stopped in a woman planning pregnancy

Table 3 Determining the Activity and Monitoring of Renal Lupus

1. Determine and monitor GFR by a cimetidine-corrected creatinine clearance (because of tubular secretion of creatinine) *or* a nuclear medicine GFR, such as technetium-DTPA or iothalamate
2. Quantitate the 24-hour urine protein excretion
3. Look for RBC casts in a morning urinalysis and quantitate urine RBCs per high-power field
4. Determine serum C3 and C4 (or CH50, total hemolytic complement) and anti-dsDNA
5. Consider a renal biopsy if
   a. the diagnosis of SLE is unclear,
   b. it is necessary to differentiate ongoing active renal lupus from inactive, sclerosed kidneys, or
   c. it will influence the choice of therapy (i.e., the use of alkylating agents)

MUSCULOSKELETAL LUPUS

Over 90 percent of SLE patients have polyarthralgia or polyarthritis at some point in the evolution of their disease. Nonsteroidal anti-inflammatory drugs (NSAIDs) and antimalarial drugs (hydroxychloroquine) are the mainstay of treatment (Table 2). Some unusual reactions to NSAIDs that have occurred in patients with SLE include aseptic meningitis, most commonly reported with ibuprofen, and salicylate hepatitis, most commonly occurring with aspirin (but occasionally occurring with other NSAIDs). NSAIDs are available from multiple classes; a patient who develops an intolerance to one may usually be given an NSAID from another class. However, a patient with a severe allergic reaction (such as urticaria and/or angioedema or anaphylaxis) should not be rechallenged with any NSAID. The major toxicities of NSAIDs in SLE patients are NSAID gastropathy, renal toxicity, or platelet dysfunction and bleeding. Corticosteroids, usually prednisone in doses of 5 to 20 mg daily, may be required for severe polyarthritis. The addition of an immunosuppressive agent (methotrexate or azathioprine) may allow corticosteroid taper.

The major musculoskeletal damage in SLE patients is due to avascular necrosis of bone and to osteoporotic fractures. Both complications are highly associated with corticosteroid use. Every attempt should be made to keep the maintenance prednisone dose below 20 mg daily, the threshold above which the odds ratio of avascular necrosis of bone rises dramatically. Early avascular necrosis of bone may respond to surgical core decompression. Osteoporosis in SLE is multifactorial, with corticosteroids, disease activity, and other risk factors contributing. Preventive measures, including an exercise regimen, calcium and vitamin D supplementation, and smoking cessation are encouraged. Severe premenopausal osteoporosis can be treated with calcium supplementation, vitamin D, calcitonin, and bisphosphonates. In addition to these measures, the postmenopausal SLE patient is a candidate for estrogen replacement therapy (ERT). In established SLE patients, ERT does not appear to increase the risk of disease flare, although this has not been extensively studied.

RENAL LUPUS

Approximately 50 percent of SLE patients will have some renal involvement. Active renal lupus will present as hematuria and/or proteinuria, usually in the setting of active serologic tests (low complement and high anti-dsDNA) (Table 3). The goal of treatment is to reduce inflammation, thereby improving or maintaining the glomerular filtration rate (GFR) and decreasing proteinuria (Table 4). Minor renal involvement may re-

Table 4 Treatment of Renal Lupus

Corticosteroids
- May be the sole agent for mild or moderate renal lupus
- In patients with rapidly progressive glomerulonephritis or diffuse proliferative glomerulonephritis, may be initially given as pulse methylprenisolone, 1,000 mg a day for 3 days, followed by a daily maintenance dose of oral prednisone, in the range of 40 to 60 mg a day

Azathioprine
- May be added to corticosteroids in patients who have a partial, but incomplete response to corticosteroids and are not considered candidates for alkylating agents
- May be added as a "steroid-sparing agent" in a patient who has responded to corticosteroids, but who cannot be tapered to an acceptable maintenance prednisone dose (usually ≤ 20 mg daily)
- Monitor complete blood counts, liver function tests, and amylase

Cyclophosphamide
- May be used initially (with corticosteroids) in patients with rapidly progressive glomerulonephritis or diffuse proliferative glomerulonephritis
- Monthly "pulse" intravenous cyclophosphamide (750 to 1,000 mg/m^2 body surface area) is preferable to daily oral cyclophosphamide, because of lower toxicity (malignancy)
- Monitor complete blood counts. Sodium 2-mercaptoethanesulfonate (MESNA) and hydration are used to prevent hemorrhagic cystitis. Infections must be identified early and treated appropriately. Cyclophosphamide cannot be used during pregnancy because it can cause birth defects. Even IV pulse cyclophosphamide may lead to later malignancy, including leukemia

Plasmapheresis
- Plasmapheresis may be helpful in some patients resistant to corticosteroids and alkylating agents
- Experimental regimens of sequential plasmapheresis followed by cyclophosphamide are currently being tested

Reduce or control co-morbid factors that contribute to renal sclerosis
- Hypertension
- Hyperlipidemia
- Diabetes mellitus

spond to a low (<20 mg prednisone daily) to moderate dose (20 to 40 mg prednisone daily) of corticosteroids. Moderate renal involvement may respond to moderate-dose corticosteroid therapy (20 to 40 mg of prednisone daily) and the addition of azathioprine (100 to 150 mg daily). Attention should always be paid to other factors that hasten renal decline, including hypertension and hyperlipidemia. However, severe or rapidly progressive lupus nephritis will usually require an alkylating agent. Based on clinical trails at the National Institutes of Health, the alkylating agent of choice is intravenous "pulse" cyclophosphamide, 750 to 1,000 mg per square meter of body surface area, monthly for 6 months. Adjustments of dose are made on the basis of clinical response and toxicity (such as cytopenias or serious infections). A maintenance schedule of cyclophosphamide treatment every third month for 2 years may be needed to maintain disease control, or it may be possible to maintain the patient on an agent with lesser toxicity such as azathioprine. Cyclophosphamide has more toxicity (especially in terms of hemorrhagic cystitis and malignancy) when used in a daily oral regimen, but even intravenous pulse cyclophosphamide can have important toxicity, including cytopenias, infection, and premature gonadal failure. SLE patients who develop renal failure do better, in terms of disease activity, with hemodialysis rather than with peritoneal dialysis. SLE patients with renal failure are candidates for renal transplantation.

HEMATOLOGIC LUPUS

Many of the hematologic manifestations of SLE are mild, including leukopenia and mild chronic thrombocytopenia. However, SLE patients can have life-threatening hemolytic anemia and thrombocytopenia, requiring intravenous "pulse" methylprednisolone therapy, 1,000 mg a day for 3 days. Patients who do not respond may require intravenous gammaglobulin (IVIG). Patients who are IgA deficient should not receive IVIG. Induction therapy consists of 0.4 g IVIG per kilogram body weight for 2 to 5 days. If maintenance therapy on a monthly basis is necessary, 0.4 g per kilogram of body weight can be given as a single infusion. For patients who respond to high-dose corticosteroid therapy but relapse when the dose is tapered, the addition of danocrine or an immunosuppressive agent such as azathioprine may be beneficial. A rare patient may require splenectomy and although this procedure may not result in a cure of the hemolytic anemia or thrombocytopenia, it is usually easier to manage the cytopenia after splenectomy.

NEUROLOGIC LUPUS

The neurologic manifestations of lupus are varied and must always be differentiated from infection, thrombotic diathesis secondary to antiphospholipid antibody syndrome, metabolic imbalance, and drug toxicity. Seizures are managed with anti-epileptics and control of any underlying active lupus. Psychosis is treated with major tranquilizers and control of the underlying disease. Severe neurologic lupus, whether presenting as organic brain syndrome, coma, transverse myelitis, or other disorder, is treated aggressively with intravenous pulse methylprednisolone. Patients who do not respond may require the addition of cyclophosphamide or plasmapheresis. SLE patients can rarely develop a syndrome resembling thrombotic thrombocytopenic (TTP) purpura, which will respond to plasmapheresis.

Serositis

SLE can cause pericarditis, pleurisy with pleural effusions, or peritonitis. Mild serositis will respond to NSAIDs and/or low doses of daily prednisone. Severe serositis may require intravenous pulse methylprednisolone therapy and the addition of immunosuppressive therapy. Rare patients require surgical intervention for pericardial "window" or chest tube drainage with later sclerosis.

Antiphospholipid Antibody Syndrome

Between 10 to 15 percent of SLE patients will eventually develop the secondary form of antiphospholipid antibody syndrome (APS). This hypercoagulable state is defined by the presence of venous or arterial thrombosis, pregnancy loss (fetal death or recurrent first trimester spontaneous abortions) or thrombocytopenia, in the presence of the lupus anticoagulant or moderate-to-high titer anticardiolipin (IgG or IgM isotype). SLE patients with the lupus anticoagulant or anticardiolipin antibody, who have not had a clinical criterion for APS, are not currently treated prophylactically (Table 5). It is prudent to remove other factors such as smoking and estrogen-containing oral contraceptives that might further increase the risk of thrombosis. Patients who have had a venous or arterial thrombotic event are preferably anticoagulated with warfarin, aiming for an international normalized ratio (INR) of three. Patients with fetal death or recurrent pregnancy losses can be treated with subcutaneous heparin and low-dose (80 mg) aspirin during a subsequent pregnancy. Warfarin cannot be used during pregnancy because of its teratogenic potential.

Pregnancy

Pregnancy in a woman with SLE is high risk from both the maternal and fetal viewpoint. The woman with SLE is at risk for flare of her disease (occurring in as many as 60 percent of pregnancies) or a renal exacerbation (due to SLE, preeclampsia, or both). We have found, however, that flares are severe in only 11 percent of pregnancies. Corticosteroids are metabolized by the placenta and can be used as needed to control SLE disease activity. NSAIDs are stopped in the first trimester because of their potential adverse effect on fetal cardiac involvement. Azathioprine is continued during pregnancy if its use has been shown to be required to control renal, hematologic, or neurologic lupus. Because of its teratogenic potential, cyclophosphamide must be stopped while the woman with SLE is trying to conceive. Chloroquine, one of the antimalarial drugs, has been shown to cross the placenta. Decisions on the use of hydroxychloroquine must be made on an individual basis, weighing risks and benefits in an informed manner.

Table 5 Treatmentof Antiphospholipid Antibody Syndrome

After a venous or arterial thrombotic event
- *Acute management* with heparin, thrombolytic agent, and/or angioplasty, as appropriate
- *Chronic management* with warfarin (INR 3 to 4); occasional patients require low-dose aspirin in addition

To prevent fetal death
- Heparin: 8,000-10,000 units subcutaneously twice a day AND low-dose aspirin (80 mg)
- Continue therapy for 6 weeks postpartum; low-dose aspirin may be continued indefinitely

Risks to the fetus include fetal death secondary to the antiphospholipid antibody syndrome, preterm birth, and neonatal lupus. We have found that 15 percent of pregnancies end in fetal loss. Preterm birth is a significant problem, occurring in over one-third of pregnancies. Preterm birth is multifactorial, with preeclampsia and/or toxemia, material HELLP syndrome (hemolysis, elevated liver enzymes, and low platelet count), fetal distress, oligohydramnios, and premature rupture of membranes all contributing. Therefore, we recommend that SLE pregnancies be followed by an obstetrician who specializes in high-risk pregnancies. If the pregnant woman with lupus has anti-Ro antibodies, fetal four-chamber cardiac echocardiograms should be performed, starting at the sixteenth week of gestation, to identify fetal heart block and/or myocarditis early ("neonatal lupus") when it is amenable to treatment with dexamethasone and plasmapheresis.

Patient Education

Immediately after the diagnosis of SLE, the patient is often overwhelmed and frightened. Patients with SLE may benefit from the support groups and educational materials offered by the Lupus Foundation of America (4 Research Place, Suite 180, Rockville, MD 20850–3226; telephone: 1–301–670–9292) and their State Lupus Foundation Chapter. The eventual goal is to have the patient be an equal partner with the physician in her care.

SUGGESTED READING

Alarcon-Segovia D, Deleze M, Oria CV, et al. Antiphospholipid antibodies and the antiphospholipid syndrome in systemic lupus erythematosus: a prospective analysis of 500 consecutive patients. Medicine 1989; 68:353–374.

Canadian Hydroxychloroquine Study Group: A randomized study of the effect of withdrawing hydroxychloroquine sulfate in systemic lupus erythematosus. N Engl J Med 1991; 324:150–154.

Felson DT, Anderson JA. Treatment of lupus nephritis. N Engl J Med 1986; 315:458.

McCune WJ, Golbus J, Zeldes W, et al. Clinical and immunologic effects of monthly administration of intravenous cyclophosphamide in severe systemic lupus erythematosus. N Engl J Med 1988; 318:1423–1431.

Petri M. Systemic lupus erythematosus and pregnancy. Rheum Dis Clin North Am 1994; 20:87–116.

SCLERODERMA

FREDRICK M. WIGLEY, M.D.
ALLAN C. GELBER, M.D., M.P.H.

Systemic sclerosis (scleroderma) is a chronic disfiguring disease that is clinically manifested by thick immobile skin (scleroderma); abnormal vascular reactivity (Raynaud's phenomenon); and dysfunction of lungs, heart, gastrointestinal tract, musculoskeletal system, and kidneys. Women are affected more commonly than men (3:1) with a mean age of onset in the fourth or fifth decade. Its prevalence has been estimated at approximately 10 to 25 cases per 1 million. Characteristic pathologic findings include a widespread vasculopathy of capillaries and small arteries with fibrosis of the intima and signs of injury to the endothelium. Excessive fibrosis causes irreversible malfunction of the involved organ. Specific treatment has been hampered not only by our incomplete understanding of the pathogenesis of this disease, but also by its heterogenous expression. Scleroderma is thought to be an autoimmune disease because of the uniform expression of very specific T cell–dependent autoantibodies and the frequent association with other immune-mediated disease such as polymyositis. However, the exact role of the immune system in the pathogenesis of scleroderma is unclear. Immunosuppressive drugs have not proven to be efficacious in its treatment. To date, there is, in fact, no treatment that has been proven uniformly successful in either the prevention or reversal of scleroderma. Therefore, much of conventional therapy is aimed largely at symptomatic relief.

GENERAL COMMENTS

There are several important principles to keep in mind when treating a patient with scleroderma: (1) in the scleroderma-related disorders there are subsets of disease, each with a unique clinical course and a specific autoantibody profile; (2) the course of the disease is quite variable; (3) subclinical organ involvement is usually present in early disease; and (4) early disease may represent a stage of active inflammation that is potentially responsive to drug therapy; whereas (5) late-stage organ failure may be manageable but is likely irreversible.

In addition to the usual comprehensive history and physical examination there are several scleroderma-specific measurements that should be done at the outset and then periodically during follow-up (Table 1). The extent of skin involvement should be carefully assessed by determining the degree and extent of skin thickening and the patient classified into one of two subtypes ("limited" or "diffuse") of scleroderma. Since patients with diffuse skin involvement are more likely than those with limited skin involvement to have significant visceral disease, this classification has important prognostic and therapeutic implications.

The "limited variant" of scleroderma, also called CREST syndrome, is defined by cutaneous thickening that is limited to the fingers or distal extremities, face, and neck, but excludes the trunk. In these patients, Raynaud's phenomenon typically precedes the other manifestations of disease by many years. Anticentromere antibodies are found in 40 to 60 percent of patients with limited scleroderma. This subset follows a relatively benign or indolent course, generally sparing the viscera. Although proximal and/or truncal extension of skin involvement in limited scleroderma is unlikely to occur, other morbid complications may occur as late as 10 or more years after the initial presenting symptom. These include ischemic digital ulcerations with gangrene (resulting in auto or surgical amputation), progressive pulmonary hypertension (often in the absence of pulmonary fibrosis), gastrointestinal manifestations, and subcutaneous calcification.

The second major subset of scleroderma is characterized by diffuse thickening of skin. In addition to the distal extremities, the proximal arms and legs, anterior trunk, and occasionally, the upper back are also involved. The presence of antibody directed against nucleolar antigens such as topoisomerase 1 (Scl 70) or RNA polymerase I, II, or III are very specific for diffuse scleroderma. Unlike limited scleroderma, the onset of skin thickening follows quickly (within several months) after the onset of Raynaud's phenomenon and is more intense, frequently resulting in rapid progression over the body. Joint contractures also commonly occur and are due to fibrosis, not only of skin, but also of tendons and muscles. Major pulmonary, gastrointestinal, renal, and cardiac manifestations of the disease, like the skin,

Table 1 Suggested Evaluation of a Scleroderma Patient

1. All patients should have a complete history and physical examination with special attention to cardiopulmonary and gastrointestinal signs and symptoms
2. Baseline measurements of skin involvement by determination of a total skin score of fingers, hands, arms, face, chest, abdomen, legs and feet. (0 = none, 3 = very thick). Size of oral aperture, presence of tendon friction rub (wrist, ankle), and measurement of hand stretch (tip of fifth to tip of thumb) are helpful parameters to follow. Global assessment of skin involvement by the patient is most important
3. Special laboratory testing should include thyroid function and muscle enzymes—creatinine kinase and aldolase. Autoantibody determination should include antinuclear anticentromere and antitopoisomerase antibodies
4. Chest radiography, electrocardiogram, and complete pulmonary function testing, including diffusion capacity and echocardiogram with Doppler to estimate pulmonary artery pressure

are likely to evolve in a relatively short period of time following the presenting sign or symptom. Therefore, the presence of diffuse involvement of skin, because of its association with visceral involvement, serves as a marker of poor prognosis; indeed the 5-year survival in this subgroup of patients is only 60 to 70 percent.

After 2 or 3 years of disease, thickening of the skin generally fails to progress any further and often improves with skin softening, new hair growth and improved mobility. Visceral involvement, on the other hand, is more likely to slowly progress. However, its course is highly variable and some patients may, in fact, even show improvement in functional parameters. Both diffuse and limited scleroderma may also be found in conjunction with other rheumatic diseases, the most common of which are Sjögren's syndrome, rheumatoid-like polyarthritis, polymyositis, and systemic lupus erythematosus. The lack of response of systemic sclerosis to immunosuppressive therapy does not preclude its use in the treatment of these overlapping diseases.

After categorizing each individual patient with regard to subtype of disease, guidelines for treatment, as outlined below, can then be followed.

Table 2 Approach to Raynaud's Phenomenon in Scleroderma

Nondrug treatment	
Avoid cold exposure	
Dress with loose-fitting warm clothing	
Wear mittens, warm footwear, and a hat	
Reduce emotional stress	
Stop smoking and caffeinated drinks	
Avoid sympathomimetic drugs	
Attempt biofeedback therapy	
Drug therapy	
Calcium channel blocker:*	
Nifedipine	10 to 30 mg PO t.i.d.-q.i.d.
Diltiazem	30 to 120 mg PO t.i.d.
Verapamil	not helpful
Nicardipine	not helpful
Extended dosing calcium channel blockers:	
Nifedipine XL	30-120 mg PO q.d.
Diltiazem SR	60-120 mg PO b.i.d.
Amlodipine	5-15 mg PO q.d.
Other available options:	
Prazosin	1 mg test dose then 5 mg PO t.i.d.
Nitroglycerin	2% ointment (¼-1 in q6h)
Hydralazine	40-50 mg daily
Captopril	25-150 mg t.i.d.
Pentoxifylline	400 mg t.i.d

*An initial test dose in the office is recommended. The slow release calcium channel blocker (single dose capsules) may be better tolerated but have not been studied in Raynaud's phenomenon. Combination vasodilator therapy should be used with caution.

Therapeutic Options for Generalized Treatment

Patients with scleroderma must adjust to a chronic incurable disorder that may lead rapidly to major disability and change in body image. Therefore, emotional support, in the form of patient education, development of coping mechanisms, family counseling, appropriate rest and exercise programs, and involvement in support groups, must supplement any treatment program.

The earliest and most common manifestation of scleroderma is Raynaud's phenomenon. This peripheral vascular phenomenon may mirror similar vasospastic processes in the cardiac, pulmonary, and renal vasculatures. The mainstay of nondrug treatment (Table 2) is focused on the avoidance of abrupt changes in temperature and of emotional stress. Since central body chill is the most effective trigger of Raynaud's phenomenon, keeping the entire body warm, and not just the fingers, is essential. Education and emotional support are also critical.

There is no drug therapy that has been proven to alter the natural history of the vascular disease of scleroderma probably because the insult to the vasculature causes not only functional abnormalities (vasospasm) but also fixed irreversible structural changes. Attempts to improve local blood flow and provide symptomatic relief have been tried with a variety of agents including vasodilators, inhibitors of platelet aggregation, and hemorheologic modifiers. Calcium channel blockers are the best tolerated of the vasodilators (Table 2), and in response to these agents, subjective improvement in the number and intensity Raynaud's attacks has been reported. However, response in patients with scleroderma is less dramatic than in patients with primary Raynaud's phenomenon. Interestingly, rather than enhancing local blood flow, the acute administration of the calcium channel blocker, nifedipine, can induce a drop in digital blood pressure and flow. This appears to be due to shunting of blood from nondistensible digital blood vessels to distensible systemic vessels. Calcium channel blockers may also lower the esophageal sphincter pressure and thus aggravate esophageal reflux. Potential side effects include edema, headache, dizziness, flushing, and hypotension. These agents are contraindicated during pregnancy.

Other classes of vasodilating drugs, including nitrates and sympatholytic agents, are generally of no greater efficacy than the calcium channel blockers and may be less well tolerated. Therefore they are not recommended for the specific treatment of Raynaud's phenomenon in scleroderma, but should be reserved for empiric treatment of unresponsive ischemic lesions. Vasodilating prostaglandins given intravenously (prostacyclin, Iloprost, PGE_1) have been shown to be helpful in reducing Raynaud's episodes and improving digital ischemia. Oral PGE_1 (misoprostol) was not effective in one trial, but other oral prostaglandins are now being developed and may be available in the future. Although clotting and platelet activation occur in the vasculature, anticoagulation is not recommended. Daily aspirin (<365 mg) is recommended for all patients, while dipyridamole is not recommended. Antifibrinolytic therapy has been tried in isolated cases of severe digital ischemia, but we do not recommend it. Pentoxifylline has been used in scleroderma but has been disappointing in clinical trials for Raynaud's phenomenon. Cervical sympathectomy may improve regional blood flow acutely but is not recommended for long-term management of Raynaud's phenomenon.

No drug treatment has been proven definitively to reduce or arrest the excessive deposition of collagen and subsequent tissue fibrosis that occurs in scleroderma. The drugs that have been used are potentially toxic and should only be started in patients with early diffuse disease (of 1 to 3 years' duration) who have demonstrated new areas of active skin involvement in recent months. Although no controlled studies have been done, D-penicillamine (Table 3) is currently the drug of choice since in vitro, it is, a potent inhibitor of production and extracellular cross-linking of collagen. D-penicillamine may also have some immunosuppressive effects. Uncontrolled surveys of patients treated with D-penicillamine have shown a response, but usually skin improvement occurs after 6 months to a year following initiation of treatment. Unfortunately, during these initial months of treatment, skin involvement generally advances, particularly over the hands, distal limbs, and face. The maximal tolerated dose of D-penicillamine should be continued for at least 1 year before determination of treatment failure is made. Response to the drug is measured by softening of the skin, although some studies suggest that improvement in pulmonary function may also occur. Skin over the hand and lower forearm is the most resistant area. Approximately 50 percent of patients will have side effects from D-penicillamine often requiring discontinuation of the drug. It is recommended, therefore, that frequent monitoring for side effects be performed during D-penicillamine therapy (Table 3). There are currently no established guidelines for length or dosage during long-term maintenance treatment with D-penicillamine.

Because of the lack of good evidence that D-penicillamine works and the prolonged lag phase before benefit is seen, many other agents have been used in the treatment of scleroderma. Immunosuppressive and cytotoxic therapy in the treatment of scleroderma has been disappointing. Corticosteroids have not been shown to be of benefit and should not be given to patients with scleroderma except for well-defined, steroid-responsive situations. For example, prednisone should be used for active myositis and may be necessary to treat features of an overlapping, immune-mediated disease such as polyarthritis or systemic lupus erythematosus. Chlorambucil and azathioprine have no role in the treatment of scleroderma. Methotrexate, 5-fluorouracil, cyclosporine, and FK506 have shown some benefit in small or uncontrolled studies and should be considered experimental. Methotrexate is currently the most popular alternative to D-penicillamine for severe diffuse disease.

New strategies of treatment with some potential merit include the use of gamma interferon, PUVA therapy, and photopheresis. Additional therapies that have not been proven to be effective in systemic sclerosis and are not recommended include colchicine, para-aminobenzoic acid (PABA), dimethyl sulfoxide (DMSO), and cyclofenil. In our opinion patients with early diffuse scleroderma should be referred to a research center for consideration into experimental protocols before specific drug treatment is started. Only through cooperative clinical trials will effective therapy for this rare disease be defined.

Table 3 Guidelines for Use of D-Penicillamine in Systemic Sclerosis

1. Use only in patients with early diffuse disease who demonstrate a definite change in skin in the preceding 2 months
2. Start with 250 mg daily and increase at 1- to 3-month intervals (depending on the aggressiveness of the disease), moving to a maximum dosage of 1,000 mg daily
3. Maintain therapy for at least 1 year. If no benefit, discontinue treatment
4. Monitor clinical status, complete blood count, platelet count, and urinalysis every month
5. Recognize that controlled prospective studies are needed to define the role of D-Penicillamine. We may move to experimental therapy in aggressive disease
6. Early (few months) toxicities: dermatitis, altered taste, pemphigus, pruritus, fever
7. Late toxicities: stomatitis, nausea, leukopenia, thrombocytopenia, (1-2 years) proteinuria, autoimmune disease

ORGAN SPECIFIC TREATMENT

Skin Care

In early active scleroderma, the skin, particularly over the forearms, is often intensely pruritic and exhibits mild erythema and nonpitting edema. During this phase, mast cells and other mononuclear cells infiltrate the dermis. A topical corticosteroid cream (1 percent hydrocortisone or 0.1 percent triamcinolone, applied twice daily) can be tried but should be limited to short-term treatment because corticosteroids may cause atrophy of skin. Antihistamines (hydroxyzine, diphenhydramine, chlorpheniramine, promethazine, or terfenadine) may reduce itching and associated local trauma from excoriation. Topical light therapy (PUVA treatments) has been helpful in reducing itching.

Over several weeks the edematous phase disappears and the skin becomes thickened. With this thickening, the patient experiences drying, fissuring, and sometimes ulceration, as well as decreased mobility of fingers, limbs, and even facial movements. Topical care is essential. Drying may be minimized by avoiding sun and excessive water exposure. Emollients such as Theraplex, Aquaphor, Eucerin, Lubriderm, Vaseline Dermatology lotion or Lac-Hydrin 12 percent lotion should be applied to the skin immediately after bathing and frequently during the day. Fissuring and drying of the skin over the fingertips can be minimized by apply petrolatum at nighttime and then covering the hands with cotton gloves.

Ulcerations of the skin over the elbows, dorsal fingers, and ankles are usually traumatic in etiology, in contrast to those on the fingertips, which are ischemic. Treatment with topical antibiotic ointment such as Bacitracin, applied two to three times daily, and cleansing with soap and water between applications, generally results in successful healing within 6 to 8 weeks. Prevention of traumatic ulcers can be accomplished by surgical reduction of finger contractures and by padding of susceptible areas. Vasodilator therapy (see Table 2) is used in an attempt to improve local tissue perfusion.

Large ischemic, or nonhealing, ulcers warrant more aggressive therapy. The patient should be kept in a warm environment and at rest. A local digital block with 2 percent lidocaine can provide transient relief of pain and reversal of vasospasm. The ischemic lesion, particularly a demarcated digit, that is unresponsive to maximum doses of a calcium channel blocker is quite worrisome. Experimental or unconventional treatment such as intravenous prostaglandins can then be used. Iloprost, an analogue of prostacyclin, is available in Europe and is given at a rate of 0.05 to 2.0 ng per kilogram per minute for 6 hours each day for 5 days. PGE^1 can be administered through a central line at 6 to 10 ng per kilogram per minute with appropriate close monitoring. Intra-arterial phentolamine (50 to 150 μg per minute) and oral phenoxybenzamine (10 to 20 mg daily) have also been used with caution to treat acute ischemic digital ulcers. Intra-arterial injections of reserpine or guanethidine are no longer available or recommended.

Bedrest and warmth coupled with the use of maximally tolerated doses of a calcium channel blocker currently provide the most practical and effective treatment of severe digital ischemia. Cervical sympathectomy has been shown to improve local blood flow acutely, but because of significant perioperative morbidity and lack of long-term efficacy, it is not recommended. Individual cases of sympathectomy at the level of the hand or digit have been reported to be successful. Lumbar sympathectomy may be helpful for vasospastic disease of the lower extremities. If the ischemia cannot be reversed by the aggressive use of vasodilators, thrombotic or occlusive etiologies should be considered. Fibrinolytic therapy may be helpful but experience is quite limited. Rarely, surgical removal of an acute arterial thrombus has been successful, but most often the occlusive disease is diffuse, involving both small and medium-sized vessels. In such cases, local surgical excision or amputation is frequently the only option.

The Lung

The most common manifestation of lung disease is a restrictive ventilatory deficit with reduced lung volumes secondary to interstitial fibrosis. A reduction in diffusing capacity also occurs as a consequence of reduced gas exchange caused by both parenchymal fibrosis and widespread intimal disease of the pulmonary vessels. The course of lung involvement is highly variable and difficult to predict, so that therapeutic intervention should target those patients with progressive and nonstable disease. Retrospective uncontrolled studies suggest that treatment with D-penicillamine may result in slight improvement in lung function. It has been suggested that patients who have evidence of an inflammatory alveolitis may be responsive to a combination of corticosteroids and cytotoxic drugs; however, the results are from uncontrolled trials. Our approach is to aggressively evaluate patients for evidence of active alveolitis. All patients regardless of symptoms should have pulmonary function testing done on initial evaluation. Patients who have progressive pulmonary symptoms or greater than a 10 percent decline in pulmonary function on serial testing done at 3-month intervals are suspect for active alveolitis and associated severe lung involvement. These patients should have a high-resolution computed tomogragraphy (CT) scan. If a "ground glass" appearance is seen suggesting alveolitis, bronchoalveolar lavage (BAL) is used to confirm and characterize the lung process. Patients who have evidence of a polymorphonuclear cell dominant alveolitis are considered candidates for aggressive therapy. Patients with negative studies or a mononuclear cell alveolitis can be followed serially with pulmonary function testing (PFT) every 3 months. Subsequent decline in pulmonary function may necessitate either restudy or empiric treatment. Controlled studies utilizing other drugs or immunosuppressive therapies for the treatment of parenchymal lung disease in scleroderma are lacking, and the use of these drugs must be considered empiric and experimental. One approach is to use a combination of corticosteroids (1 month of 1 mg per kilogram then tapered to 5 to 10 mg daily) and cyclophosphamide (1 to 2 mg per kilogram daily). Treatment is reassessed at 3-month intervals and if improvement or stability occurs, discontinuation of immunosuppressive therapy is considered.

Although reversible vasospasm has been postulated to contribute to the pathogenesis of pulmonary hypertension in scleroderma, most evidence suggests that a fixed, nonreactive vascular defect occurs early in the course of lung disease in these patients. All patients with cardiopulmonary symptoms or abnormal pulmonary function testing (particularly an isolated low diffusing capacity) should have an echocardiogram with Doppler. If significant pulmonary hypertension is evident, then a ventilation perfusion scan should be done to rule out pulmonary emboli.

Vasodilator therapy has had little impact on the outcome of pulmonary hypertension. Nonetheless, in patients with life-threatening pulmonary hypertension, potential response to oral vasodilators can be evaluated either by cautious empiric treatment or during catheterization of the right side of the heart, with documentation of the vasodilator effect on pulmonary pressure. All patients with severe pulmonary hypertension secondary to scleroderma require supplemental oxygen, diuretics in those with failure of the right side of the heart, anticoagulation, and vasodilator therapy. Patients with a resting arterial PO_2 of 55 to 60 mm Hg should be given low-flow supplemental oxygen. Vasodilator therapy with calcium channel blockers or intravenous prostacyclin (or its analogue) have been used in scleroderma and primary pulmonary hypertension. We recommend that all patients with severe pulmonary hypertension be hospitalized and appropriately monitored during initiation of vasodilation therapy. Angiotensin-converting enzyme inhibitors may also be helpful but have not been well studied in pulmonary hypertension. Supportive pulmonary care includes pneumococcal and influenza vaccination and early antibiotic treatment for respiratory infections. Lung transplantation is a consideration in scleroderma patients with severe lung disease.

GI Tract

Gastrointestinal disease in scleroderma is usually secondary to motility abnormalities caused by vascular disease and tissue fibrosis. Esophageal dysfunction with reflux is almost universal in scleroderma. Unfortunately, no therapeutic interventions have been shown to alter the muscular disease, and therefore treatment is directed at reduction of symptoms and prevention of Barrett's esophagus and esophageal stricture. Antireflux therapy should be supplemented by instructions to the patient to eat small frequent meals, to avoid late evening meals, and to discontinue smoking and consumption of alcohol. A histamine (H_2) receptor blocker such as cimetidine, ranitidine, or famotidine should be started in patients who have symptomatic reflux. Sucralfate (1 g four times daily) can also be used. If symptoms persist, then endoscopy should be performed to determine if esophagitis and/or ulceration are present. Esophageal disease that is refractory to maximum doses of an H_2-blocker or combination therapy should be treated with omeprazole (20 to 40 mg daily), with subsequent documentation of healing by endoscopy. Maintenance therapy is continued by use of an H_2-blocker. Although it is recommended that patients intermittently refrain from omeprazole use, some patients have severe reflux requiring continual use. In scleroderma, symptoms may not correlate with the degree of reflux or esophagitis. Therefore, clinical judgment should be used to determine the need for gastrointestinal studies.

In early systemic sclerosis, esophageal motility and gastric emptying may be improved by the promotility drugs, metoclopramide and cisapride. However, they are not effective in advanced disease. Efficacy of treatment with promotility drugs is generally assessed in scleroderma patients by improvement in clinical symptoms and signs of good nutrition. Cisapride (10 to 20 mg 30 to 60 minutes before mealtime and at bedtime) is the preferable drug because it has less central nervous system toxicity than metoclopramide; cisapride does not have antidopaminergic properties. Gastric emptying is often delayed in patients with scleroderma. Cisapride or low-dose erythromycin (150 mg), a motilin receptor agonist, may improve gastric motility. Dysphagia that is unresponsive to medical treatment may indicate the presence of a stricture; the treatment for this is intermittent, endoscopic dilation.

Patients who exhibit weight loss in the face of good oral intake should be evaluated for malabsorption. If malabsorption is found, it is likely to be due to dysmotility and bacterial overgrowth and should be treated with broad-spectrum antibiotics. Drugs that are reported to improve small bowel motility have been disappointing in the treatment of this aspect of scleroderma. However, a trial of cisapride or octreotide, a synthetic analog of somatostatin can be used in severe cases. Severe malabsorption that is unresponsive to repeated courses of antibiotics and appropriate dietary manipulation may be treated by long-term parenteral nutrition.

Most patients with colonic involvement in scleroderma are asymptomatic. However, alternating diarrhea and constipation may be a manifestation of colonic dysmotility. Administration of a synthetic fiber such as metamucil to increase stool bulk may be helpful. Low doses of Lomotil or Imodium can be used with caution. Rarely, advanced disease may lead to an atonic colon and pseudo-obstruction.

Kidney

Most patients with renal involvement are asymptomatic until a hypertensive crisis develops that may, in turn, lead to rapid loss of renal function and death in the absence of dialysis. Patients with early diffuse scleroderma are more likely to develop renal crisis than those with limited disease and should be carefully monitored. The belief that the renal crisis of scleroderma is triggered by "Raynaud's phenomenon" of the kidney is supported by the observations that these crises occur primarily in the winter months and that cold exposure can induce transient reduction in blood flow to the kidney. Patients who develop hypertension (> 160/90 mm Hg) or deterioration of renal function should be treated aggressively (Table 4) with an angiotensin-converting enzyme (ACE) inhibitor. Captopril, an ACE inhibitor, has reduced the mortality from renal crisis, which was once nearly universal to 75 percent. Another ACE inhibitor, enalapril, has also been successfully used and produces less bone marrow suppression than captopril. Other antihypertensive drugs such as minoxidil and methyldopa or combinations of antihypertensive drugs have had variable success in the treatment of hypertensive crisis. We recommend the use of a calcium channel blocker in the patient who cannot take an ACE inhibitor. Occasionally, progressive deterioration of renal function occurs despite adequate control of blood pressure. Use of an ACE inhibitor is also recommended in patients who have progressive renal failure despite being normotensive. Outcome is usually poor if serum creatinine is greater than 3 mg per deciliter at the initiation of treatment. Long-term dialysis may be necessary.

Cardiac

Although cardiac involvement is common in scleroderma, it is usually asymptomatic until late in the disease. Microvascular disease, vasospasm of the myocardial vessels, and patchy myocardial fibrosis are thought to be the primary mechanisms of cardiac

Table 4 Treatment of Renal Crisis in Systemic Sclerosis

1. Definition of renal crisis
   Diastolic pressure of 110 mm Hg or greater with at least two of the following: Grade III or IV Kimmelstiel-Wilson fundoscopic changes, seizures, proteinuria, hematuria, azotemia, microangiopathic hemolytic anemia, or rapidly changing renal function
2. Patient should be hospitalized and monitored closely
3. Start an ACE inhibitor
   Captopril 25 mg every 8 hours, increasing by 25 mg every 8-12 hours to control blood pressure; the maximal dose is 450 mg daily. Or Enalapril 5 mg daily, to be increased as needed to maximum of 40 mg daily
   Toxicity: Captopril and Enalapril should be adjusted for renal insufficiency. Hypotension, proteinuria, neutropenia, agranulocytosis, anemia, pancytopenia, dysgeusia, dermatitis, cough, and angioedema
4. Other options include use of a calcium channel blocker or Minoxidil or aggressive combination anti-hypertensive therapy
   Dialysis may be necessary

dysfunction. Cor pulmonale can complicate pulmonary disease with signs and symptoms of right-sided heart failure. Pericarditis is common but usually asymptomatic; therefore, large effusions need to be investigated by pericardiocentesis. Since cardiac involvement is generally underestimated in patients with scleroderma, periodic objective testing to determine cardiac rhythm and cardiac function is prudent. Arrhythmias and heart failure are best treated by conventional means in consultation with a cardiologist.

Musculoskeletal System

Contractures of joints, atrophy of muscle, and fibrosis of tendons are common causes of discomfort and disability in scleroderma. Nonspecific musculoskeletal pain is often refractory to anti-inflammatory drugs, including corticosteroids, and is best treated with periods of rest and gentle physical and occupational therapy. However, nonsteroidal anti-inflammatory drugs may be helpful in patients who have signs of an inflammatory arthritis. Muscle weakness can occur in scleroderma for many reasons, including decreased use of muscles, malnutrition, and the effects of a chronic inflammatory illness (likely cytokine-mediated muscle wasting). Occasionally polymyositis occurs in association with scleroderma and is best treated with corticosteroids and/or other immunosuppressive therapy (see chapter on polymyositis).

Other

Hypothyroidism may occur secondary to fibrosis of the thyroid gland; therefore, periodic thyroid function testing is advised. Dryness of the membranes of the mouth and eyes is common and often is secondary to Sjögren's syndrome. Frequent use of artificial tears can prevent ocular damage. Periodontal disease due to poor oral hygiene results from a decrease in oral aperture and poor hand function. Entrapment neuropathies can lead to problems such as carpal tunnel syndrome and trigeminal neuralgia. In males, impotence is very common and thought to be secondary to abnormal regional blood flow. Once recognized, effective management of impotence can be achieved in consultation with a urologist. Although solid data are lacking, pregnancy should be considered high risk. Finally, depression, poor self-esteem, anxiety, abnormal sexual function, fear, and difficulty in coping are issues that must be dealt with in patients with this life-threatening, disfiguring chronic disease.

SUGGESTED READING

Clements PJ, Furst DE. Systemic sclerosis. Baltimore: Williams & Wilkins, 1996.

LeRoy EC. Rheumatic disease clinics of North America. Vol 16. Philadelphia: WB Saunders, 1990.

Seibold J. Scleroderma. In: Kelley WN, Harris ED, Ruddy S, Sledge CB, eds. Textbook of rheumatology. 4th ed. Philadelphia: WB Saunders, 1993.

Steen VD. Systemic sclerosis: Management. In: Klippel JH, Dieppe PA, eds. Rheumatology, 1st ed. London UK: Mosby, 1994.

Wigley FM, Matsumoto AK. Scleroderma. In: Weisman MH, Weinblatt ME, eds. Treatment of rheumatic diseases. Philadelphia: WB Saunders, 1995.

Wigley FM, Matsumoto AK. Raynaud's phenomenon. In: Weisman MH, Weinblatt ME, eds. Treatment of rheumatic diseases. Philadelphia: WB Saunders, 1995.

Wigley FM, Wise RA. Systemic sclerosis: The evaluation of pulmonary involvement. In: Klippel JH, Dieppe PA, eds. Rheumatology, 1st ed. London UK: Mosby, 1994.

DERMATOMYOSITIS AND POLYMYOSITIS

ELIZABETH M. ADAMS, M.D.
PAUL H. PLOTZ, M.D.

Dermatomyositis (DM) and polymyositis (PM) are the two major syndromes that constitute the idiopathic inflammatory myopathies (IIM). Although relatively rare (5 to 10 new cases per million per year), these diseases are increasingly recognized as a cause of significant long-term morbidity. Other IIM not covered in detail here include juvenile dermatomyositis (JDM), inclusion body myositis (IBM), myositis associated with other connective tissue diseases, focal inflammatory myopathies, and granulomatous and eosinophilic myopathies.

DIAGNOSIS

The diagnosis of myositis is usually suggested when a patient complains of new onset proximal muscle weakness often with myalgias. These symptoms may be accompanied or preceded by a rash, Raynaud's phenomenon, arthritis, or dyspnea on exertion. Of the rashes, only Gottron's papules are specific for DM, although a heliotrope eruption of the eyelids, a flat red rash over the knuckles, erythema of the upper back (shawl rash) and upper chest (V rash) also suggest DM. Serum creatine kinase (CK), aldolase and liver transaminases (SGOT and SGPT) are usually elevated. The finding of interstitial lung disease or myositis-specific autoantibodies (e.g., antibodies to aminoacyl-tRNA synthetases such as anti–Jo-1, anti-signal recognition particle antibodies [anti-SRP], and anti–Mi-2 antibodies) strongly support a diagnosis of DM or PM as the cause of myopathy. With the possible exception of JDM, a muscle biopsy is necessary to confirm a diagnosis of myositis and rule out other causes of a myopathy. For example, mitochondrial myopathy may masquerade as PM, and lymphoma may present as focal myositis.

Abnormal findings on electromyogram such as increased irritability (e.g., insertional activity, fibrillations) and changes in motor unit potentials (e.g., decreased amplitude and duration, increased polyphasic potentials, asynchronicity) are helpful in the diagnosis and management of IIM. In addition, observance of increased signal on magnetic resonance imaging (MRI) of muscle with either T2 or fat-suppressive sequence (e.g., STIR) is helpful in defining the extent of active disease (Fig. 1).

If patients are given a diagnosis of myositis within 3 months of the onset of their proximal muscle weakness and are treated promptly, they have greater than an 80 percent chance of completely responding to their first trial of therapy. If their diagnosis is delayed by greater than 18 months from onset of proximal muscle weakness, they have little chance of a complete response to medication. Recent studies show DM-PM patients have significant long-term disabilities related to their disease and glucocorticoid therapy; therefore, the importance of

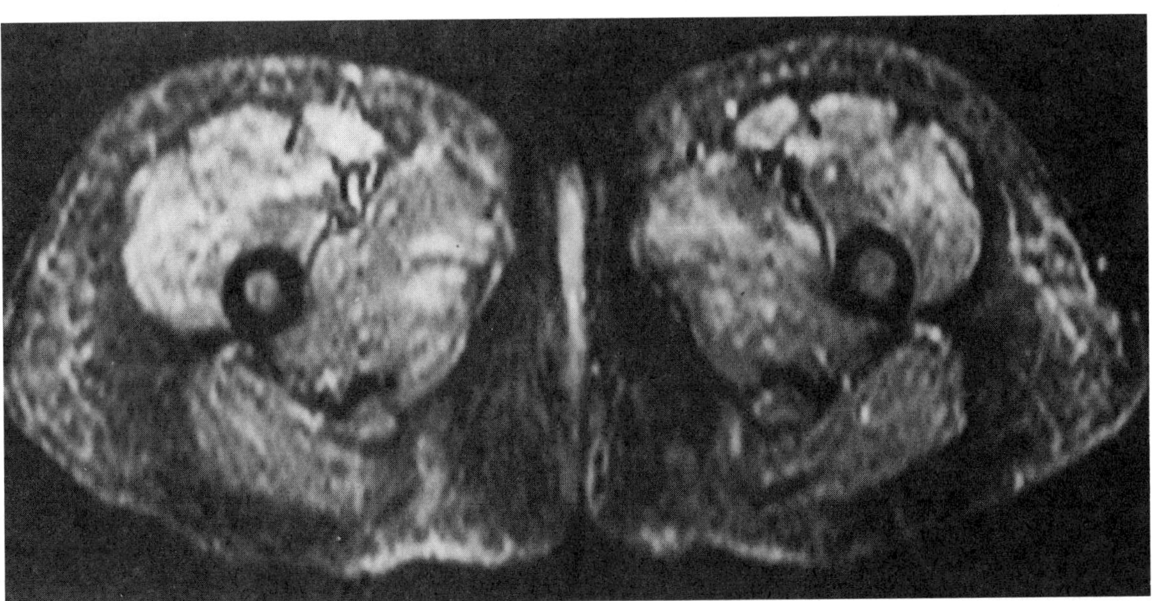

Figure 1 STIR image of the proximal thigh from a 29-year-old female with DM. She had arthralgias, myalgias, proximal muscle weakness, and Gottron's and heliotrope rashes. Her CK was minimally elevated at 305, but her muscle biopsy pathology showed myofiber necrosis and regeneration. Increased signal indicating edema from inflammation and/or necrosis is seen predominately in the anterior muscles and also in the subcutaneous tissue.

Table 1 Syndromes Associated with Myositis-Specific Antibodies

Antigen	*Clinical Features*	*Course*
Mi-2	V and shawl sign rashes; cuticular overgrowth	Acute onset; good response to therapy
Jo-1 or other aminoacyl-tRNA synthetases	Raynaud's phenomenon; arthritis; fevers; interstitial lung disease; "mechanics hands," with or without rash	Moderate response to therapy, but persistent disease
SRP	Severe myopathy; palpitations; female > male	Very acute onset; poor response to therapy

establishing a diagnosis of DM or PM and initiating therapy should be obvious.

For prognostic and therapeutic considerations, myositis syndromes are categorized further based on several possible associations: a concurrent diagnosis of cancer, an associated connective tissue disease, or the presence of myositis-specific autoantibodies. The exact association of myositis with cancer continues to be debated, but a more intensive evaluation for an underlying cancer is warranted if findings unusual for myositis such as anemia are discovered during initial evaluation. Because cancer-associated myositis may respond quickly and completely to glucocorticoid therapy (GC), response to treatment should not be used as a diagnostic maneuver in the management of PM-DM. In several studies with small numbers of patients, myositis associated with another connective tissue disease is reported to usually respond completely to prednisone treatment alone.

Myositis-specific autoantibodies are helpful not only in confirming a diagnosis of DM or PM but also in anticipating the patient's response to medications (Table 1). Patients with anti–Mi-2 autoantibodies often respond completely to medication, which may be withdrawn. Patients with antisynthetase antibodies may partially respond to medication, but they frequently require a protracted course of therapy. If those patients also have interstitial lung disease, their prognosis is poorer. Patients with anti-SRP antibodies have a rapidly progressive course of myositis, which may lead to considerable irreversible weakness before therapy has any effect.

MANAGEMENT OF DM AND PM

Glucocorticoid Therapy

Oral glucocorticoid (GC) therapy is the accepted first line of treatment. Retrospective studies have shown that high-dose prednisone started shortly after disease onset has decreased overall morbidity. One recent retrospective analysis showed that the total dose of GC received during the first 3 months of treatment correlated with the degree of the patients clinical improvement.

Two empiric regimens commonly used for myositis both start with prednisone 1 to 2 mg per kilogram per day (at least 60 mg per day). This dosage is continued for at least 1 month or until the CK is normal, which may take up to several months. The more widely used regimen involves a gradual decrease in daily divided dose prednisone every 4 weeks by no more than 20 percent of the existing dose provided the CK remains normal. The other common approach is to gradually lower prednisone on alternate days over a 6-month to 1-year period.

If myositis is acute and/or severe, a brief course of high-dose intravenous methylprednisolone (1 g per day for one to three doses) may be used as a temporizing measure before slower acting immunosuppressants take effect. Also, pulse GCs may help to reduce the need for prolonged daily corticosteroid therapy.

The patient's response to therapy should be monitored by following his or her ability to perform activities of daily living, CK levels, and strength on manual muscle testing. Frequently the CK will normalize before strength improves and rise before a loss of muscle strength occurs. In some patients, the CK may normalize, but the patient continues to weaken. Steroid myopathy should be considered, particularly in elderly patients who are more at risk for this complication. If the contribution of steroid myopathy to continuing weakness is unclear, the dose of GCs should be reduced.

Patients who do not improve with either GC therapy or later dosage reduction should be reassessed as to whether or not they have idiopathic myositis or another reason for progressive muscle weakness (Table 2) before they are committed to a trial of an additional immunosuppressive agent. An MRI with fat-suppressive sequences is helpful in assessing whether a patient's weakness is from ongoing inflammation in addition to atrophy and/or fatty replacement of muscle. A muscle biopsy should probably be repeated and an ischemic forearm test performed after confounding factors such as hypokalemia are ruled out (see Table 2). Often, several muscle biopsies are needed before a diagnosis of inclusion body myositis is made.

Other Immunosuppressive Therapy

At the time of diagnosis, some myositis patients may be predicted to respond poorly or incompletely to GCs and to be at increased risk for GC toxicity and/or long-term disability from their disease. For these patients, a case can be made for starting additional immunosuppressive or GC-sparing therapy at the time of diagnosis, although data supporting this choice are limited. Even for those patients who have not done well on GC alone, data in support of a second-line agent are limited because reported trials have small numbers of patients.

The two most commonly used second-line therapies are azathioprine and methotrexate. In an older prospec-

Table 2 Differential Diagnosis of Myositis

Endocrine and Electrolyte Disorders
Hypokalemia, hypo- and hypercalcemia, hypomagnesemia
Hypothyroidism, hyperthyroidism
Cushing's syndrome, Addison's disease
Toxic Myopathies
Alcohol, cocaine, emetine/Ipecac
Corticosteroids, chloroquine and hydroxychloroquine
Colchicine; D-penicillamine, cyclosporin, danazol
Lipid-lowering agents such as lovastatin, clofibrate
L-dopa, phenytoin, procainamide, vincristine, amiodorone
Cimetidine
Zidovudine, sulfas, penicillins, rifampin, quinolones
Beta-blockers, minoxidil, hydralazine, enalapril
Eosinophilia myalgia syndrome (l-tryptophan)
Infections
HIV, HTLV I
Coxsackievirus, Epstein-Barr virus, influenza, echovirus, rubella
Staphylococci, streptococci, clostridia, legionella
Leprosy, tuberculosis
Toxoplasmosis, trichinosis, schistosomiasis, cysticercosis
Neuromuscular Disorders
Amyotrophic lateral sclerosis
Myasthenia gravis
Genetic muscular dystrophies:
Fascioscapulohumeral dystrophy
Oculopharyngeal dystrophy
Duchenne and Becker dystrophies
Spinal muscular atrophies
Neuropathies
Guillain-Barré and other autoimmune polyradiculopathies
Porphyria
Diabetic polyradiculopathy
Myotonias
Familial periodic paralysis
Stiff man syndrome
Metabolic Myopathies
Carbohydrate disorder/deficiencies:
Myophosphorylase deficiency (McArdle's)
Phosphofructokinase deficiency
Acid maltase deficiency
Purine disorders:
Myoadenylate (AMP) deaminase deficiency
Mitochondrial myopathies including lipid disorders-deficiencies:
Carnitine palmitoyl transferase deficiency
Miscellaneous
Paraneoplastic syndromes (Eaton-Lambert)
Sarcoidosis, Crohn's disease
Polymyalgia rheumatica
Vasculitis: PAN, Wegener's, Behçet's
Overlaps: SLE, Sjögrens, PSS, RA, MCTD
Celiac disease, jejunoileal bypass
Acne fulminans
Functional disorders

tive trial, azathioprine plus GCs was shown to be more effective than placebo plus GCs; a small number of patients on azathioprine were able to take lower doses of GCs when they were followed for longer than 3 months. A retrospective analysis by Henriksson and Sandstedt showed that 40 percent of patients who did not respond to prednisone alone did respond to a combination of methotrexate or azathioprine and GCs.

Azathioprine is used at doses up to 2 to 3 mg per kilogram per day, provided the white blood cell count (WBC) does not fall below 3,500 per cubic millimeter. It causes less nausea if the dose is gradually increased by 50 mg every 4 weeks. Toxicities other than nausea and bone marrow suppression include hepatitis, pancreatitis, rash, and infection.

Retrospective analyses have clearly shown that methotrexate has at least short-term benefit in the treatment of myositis. Methotrexate is started at 7.5 mg per week and, if necessary, may be increased gradually to 25 to 30 mg per week orally. When patients complain of nausea, it may be given intravenously or as a divided oral dose over 24 hours. A small number of patients are reported to respond to methotrexate at doses of up to 60 mg per week given subcutaneously or intravenously. Whether or not increasing doses of methotrexate improves the rate and level of response in refractory patients has not been established.

In addition to stomatitis, hair thinning, teratogenicity, reversible suppression of WBC, and acute pneumonitis, patients should be warned of long-term liver toxicity with methotrexate. Alcohol clearly potentiates this side effect. Because liver transaminases are frequently elevated in myositis, alkaline phosphate, bilirubin, albumin, and gamma glutamyl transferase (GGT) should be monitored during methotrexate therapy. If the GGT increases to three times normal while the transaminases are falling, methotrexate should be withheld. If the albumin decreases during chronic methotrexate therapy and other confounding factors (e.g., infection) are not present, a liver biopsy should be considered. Methotrexate has been used with some success for myositis associated with pneumonitis, so pneumonitis is only a relative contraindication to its use.

If a patient has partially responded or been unresponsive to either methotrexate or azathioprine, another approach is to combine the two therapies before attempting treatment with more toxic therapies such as cyclophosphamide. Some refractory patients will improve on this combination, thereby enabling a prednisone taper. Azathioprine is started at 50 mg daily and increased to 100 mg, then 150 mg every 4 weeks. At the same time, methotrexate is started at 7.5 mg per week and increased to 15 mg, then 25 mg per week every 4 weeks. The gradual increase in dose appears to improve tolerance to this combination, and little toxicity has been seen.

Several retrospective studies and a recent placebo-controlled randomized trial have reported that intravenous gammaglobulin (IVIG) has controlled myositis, in particular DM. In the controlled trial, IVIG was used at 2 g per kilogram every 4 weeks for a total of three treatments. All of the patients who showed improvement were on steroids and most were on azathioprine, methotrexate, or cyclophosphamide. Disease often worsened when IVIG was discontinued. Thus IVIG may serve as a temporizing therapy before slower-acting agents such as azathioprine take effect. Infrequent problems with IVIG include postinfusion fever, headache, myalgias, nausea and vomiting, increased risk of thrombosis, and an anaphalatic reaction in people with immunoglobulin deficiencies.

Cyclophosphamide and chlorambucil may also be used to treat refractory cases of myositis. High-dose intravenous cyclophosphamide (0.5 to 1.0 g per square meter every 4 weeks) has not proved to be generally successful, but several groups in Europe report some success in small numbers of patients with a lower dose, 0.5 g administered intravenously every 1 to 3 weeks. Daily oral cyclophosphamide (1 to 4 mg per kilogram per day), as used for vasculitis, may have a role in treating interstitial lung disease associated with myositis, but its use has not been carefully studied.

Chlorambucil is also useful for refractory cases of myositis. The medication is started at 1 to 2 mg per day orally and increased to 4 to 6 mg per day. The drop in WBC is less predictable than with cyclophosphamide. Usually, patients successfully taper prednisone. The drug may be discontinued or switched to less toxic therapy after a 6-month plateau in the improvement of muscle strength.

There are many case reports of both success and failure of cyclosporin in treating DM-PM, but results of a large controlled trial have never been published. The drug is reported to be successful when it was used to treat JDM or soon after disease onset in DM. It has shown some impressive control of the rash associated with DM. Doses commonly range from 2.5 to 7.5 mg per kilogram per day. The predominant adverse effect of cyclosporin is nephrotoxicity, which is greatest if the drug is used for any duration at doses greater than 5 mg per kilogram per day. If concomitant GCs are rapidly lowered, hypertension and decreased glomerular filtration rate may be less of a problem. Other side effects include hypertrichosis, tremor, myopathy, and gingival hyperplasia. The drug should not be used when a drug level assay is not available because of irregular gastrointestinal absorption.

A randomized controlled trial of 39 patients showed that plasmapheresis and leukopheresis did not provide even temporary improvement in control of myositis. No group has reported long-term beneficial responses of myositis to total body irradiation.

The reoccurrence of the rash in DM during GC lowering, in spite of topical steroids and sunscreens, is a relatively common problem. Chloroquine compounds (e.g., hydroxychloroquine) are usually tried first and may have a better result in controlling any photosensitive component of the rash. Occasionally, azathioprine may control a rash better than methotrexate during a steroid taper. Pulse methylprednisolone, IVIG, cyclosporin, and chlorambucil have all been reported to improve the rash associated with DM in some refractory patients.

Physical Therapy

The importance of a physical therapy program for myositis patients cannot be overemphasized. Programs should be aimed at preventing contracture, disuse atrophy, and osteoporosis. Maintenance of existing muscle function should be attempted with limited active static and isometric exercises during active disease followed by active isotonic and some resistance exercises when the disease is quiescent.

Evaluation of swallowing function by a trained speech therapist is also useful, even when dysphagia and/or aspiration are not obvious problems. Patients may need advice on how to sustain a high-protein diet, how to take reflux precautions, and how to perform swallowing techniques to avoid aspiration. In some patients, cricopharyngeal myotomy or gastroscopy tube placement may be needed.

Summary

With early diagnosis, initiation of high-dose steroids and appropriate physical therapy, DM/PM patients can be expected to have a significant decrease in long-term morbidity. Any time the diagnosis of myositis is in question, a repeat complete evaluation should be done which may include another muscle biopsy and a forearm ischemia test. Patients who are at significant risk from GC therapy or who can be predicted to have ongoing or relatively refractory disease by autoantibody status should be started on a potentially steroid-sparing immunosuppressant. Initiation of an aggressive immunosuppressive regimen to gain quick control of disease and then gradual lowering of medication may most benefit patients by increasing their chances of returning closer to their former functioning baseline. For some patients whose myositis may be predicted to relapse with discontinuation of therapy, it is probably advantageous to continue therapy for at least 1 to 2 years during remission because each flare produces some irreversible loss of strength.

SUGGESTED READING

Adams EM, Chow C, Premkumar A, Plotz P. The idiopathic inflammatory myopathies: spectrum of MRI findings. Radiographics 1995; 15:563–574.

Dalakas MC, Illa I, Dambrosia JM, et al. A controlled trial of high-dose intravenous immune globulin infusions as treatment for dermatomyositis. N Engl J Med 1993; 329:1993–2000.

Henriksson KG, Lindvall B. Polymyositis and dermatomyositis 1990—diagnosis, treatment and prognosis. Prog Neurobiol 1990; 35: 181–193.

Love LA, Leff RL, Fraser DD, et al. A new approach to the classification of idiopathic inflammatory myopathy: Myositis-specific autoantibodies define useful homogeneous patient groups. Medicine (Baltimore) 1991; 70:360–374.

Marguerie C, Bunn CC, Beynon HL, et al. Polymyositis, pulmonary fibrosis and autoantibodies to aminoacyl-tRNA synthetase enzymes. Q J Med 1990; 77:1019–1038.

Sigurgeirsson B, Lindelof B, Edhag O, Allander E. Risk of cancer in patients with dermatomyositis or polymyositis. A population-based study. N Engl J Med 1992; 326:363–367.

Sinoway P, Callen J. Chlorambucil: An effective corticosteroid-sparing agent for patients with recalcitrant dermatomyositis. Arthritis Rheum 1993; 36:319–324.

MIXED CONNECTIVE TISSUE DISEASE (UNDIFFERENTIATED CONNECTIVE TISSUE DISEASE)

MARCEL-FRANCIS KAHN, M.D.

In 1972 Sharp and coworkers described mixed connective tissue disease (MCTD) as "an apparently distinct rheumatic disease syndrome associated with a specific antibody to an extractable nuclear antigen." The term "mixed" was related to the observation that the patients suffered manifestations of several major connective tissue diseases, including systemic lupus erythematosus (SLE), systemic sclerosis (SS), polymyositis (PM), and rheumatoid arthritis (RA). Patients with MCTD also frequently develop Sjögren's syndrome and their sera have high titers of an autoantibody reacting with an extractable nuclear antigen. This antigen was ultimately demonstrated as being a small ribonucleoprotein (RNP) having U1-RNA involved in the splicing of nucleic acids. Although some are still of the opinion that this condition is merely a variant of any of a number of well-established connective tissue diseases and does not deserve a separate categorization, this syndrome is considered as a distinct entity by the majority of authors.

Since 1974 my group has suggested a different approach to this condition which has gained increasing support. Within a variable period of time, patients with high titers of U1-RNP antibody present with a limited syndrome that includes Raynaud's phenomenon, puffy hands, mild myositis, and no destructive arthritis. Some of the patients manifest the same symptoms indefinitely. Many authors, including Sharp, use the term undifferentiated connective tissue disease (UCTD) to describe this type of presentation. Other patients will ultimately develop an overlapping CTD, the diagnosis of which is definite in the majority of the cases. The "mixed" presentation is therefore due to overlapping features of the UCTD with those of the subsequent CTD. Thus, instead of considering the treatment of each associated CTD, the reader is referred to other chapters in this text. This chapter addresses only the therapy and care of clinical manifestations associated with the U1-RNP antibody.

SYSTEMIC TREATMENT

From a theoretical point of view, the goals of systemic treatment are two-fold. The first objective is to control the general evolution of the UCTD. Treatment to achieve this goal has included the use of various drugs, ranging from antimalarial to immunosuppressive agents, but no prospective controlled study has been carried out to confirm the efficacy of this therapy. Since UCTD itself does not imply a serious prognosis and since systemic manifestations are usually absent or minimal, we do not advise using potentially harmful drugs such as immunosuppressive agents. In most cases, antimalarials may be used, with the usual ophthalmologic precautions associated with long-term therapy.

The second objective is to avoid, if possible, the delayed occurrence of the subsequent CTD. Again, we are unaware of any such clinical trial, a situation probably related to the discrepancies in both the definition and understanding of MCTD. It should be of utmost theoretical and practical importance to set up a prospective controlled study to determine if the occurrence of manifestations of SLE, SS, PM, or RA can be prevented or delayed.

Because of the painful joint tendon, sheaths, and muscle associated with MCTD, many patients have received corticosteroids. With UCTD, low or medium daily doses are sufficient (0.1 to 0.2 mg per kilogram per day of prednisone). This treatment is helpful in controlling locomotor symptoms. In a minority of patients complaining of systemic symptoms such as fatigue and anemia, the results of corticosteroid therapy are satisfactory. Yet one must balance the advantages of corticosteroid therapy with the side effects of such prolonged treatment. There is no evidence demonstrating that corticosteroids achieve the goal of preventing the evolution of an overlapping syndrome. Thus, many authors prefer to use nonsteroidal anti-inflammatory drugs (NSAIDs) in such situations.

SYMPTOMATIC TREATMENT

The majority of patients with UCTD predominantly complain of Raynaud's phenomenon. This symptom is not easy to relieve with well-tolerated drugs that have minimal adverse effects. For this reason, emphasis should be put on simple, supportive measures such as the avoidance of exposure to cold and the use of warm gloves. Classical vasodilators are, in our opinion, ineffective and should be avoided. Pentoxifylline, an anti-TNF-drug, is a logical choice for treatment; however, no clinical trial has been performed thus far to determine efficacy. Calcium channel blockers, nifedipine (10 to 20 mg three times a day), and diltiazem (120 mg three times a day) are effective but are not without side effects. The balance between efficacy and tolerance is to be considered and discussed with the patient, particularly in situations where treatment is not absolutely essential.

In our experience with UCTD, it is quite unusual to be faced with patients experiencing episodes of severe ischemia, which are the hallmark of the evolution to scleroderma. Should such situations occur, vasoactive prostacyclin (Iloprost) in slow, carefully monitored intravenous administration (0.05 to 0.1 mg diluted in serum) has been quite useful in our experience. This treatment can be repeated if the situation requires.

Again, it must be stressed that this treatment is rarely indicated in UCTD.

Musculoskeletal symptoms are also troublesome in UCTD. Nondeforming arthritis and mild myositis should first be treated with NSAIDs. Yet, this treatment is not sufficient in many cases, and patients may ask for more active control of their symptoms.

In certain patients, swollen hands may be related to carpal tunnel syndrome. Local injections of hydrocortisone are effective in some cases of tenosynovitis, and make the systemic use of corticosteroids unnecessary. In other cases, small amounts of prednisone are required to efficiently control symptoms. Patients must be aware that once started on prednisone, it is often difficult to discontinue the drug, particularly in situations where divided doses are needed to control symptoms. Single daily or every-other-day dosage regimens are usually unsuccessful. In most cases, the minimum tolerated prednisone dose, which is often between 6 and 10 mg per day, is sufficient to control symptoms. Additional use of NSAIDs may help to maintain this low dose.

In pure UCTD, it is usually not recommended to use cytotoxic drugs to control musculoskeletal symptoms. In these situations, antimalarials are indicated as disease modifying treatment. If daily doses of prednisone exceed 10 mg per day, small weekly administrations of methotrexate can be tried. In our experience, dosages of 7.5 to 10 mg per week of this drug have proved efficacious, with minimal side effects.

SPECIFIC PROBLEMS

As mentioned earlier, we do not consider the specific problems raised by the added association of UCTD with SLE, PSS, PM, RA, and Sjögren's syndrome. These are discussed in the individual chapters dealing with the respective diseases.

It is often difficult to distinguish the occurrence of symptoms that indicate the presence of the overlapping condition. Also, as previously mentioned, it is still unclear if aggressive early treatment with corticosteroids and/or immunosuppressive agents given as soon as symptoms of major CTD occur can prevent further deterioration and development of the full-blown condition. Worsening of Raynaud's syndrome with tip ulcerations and esophageal and pulmonary symptoms are hallmarks of overlapping scleroderma. Light sensitivity, renal problems, and detection of anti-DNA and/or Sm antibodies with low C3 and C4 levels strongly suggest that SLE will occur. Worsening of muscle symptoms with frank elevation of CPK indicates the development of PM. Radiographic detection of destructive lesions, sometimes associated with subcutaneous nodules and rheumatoid factor make RA likely. If only joint deformation is present, it may be insufficient to indicate the presence of RA, since Jaccoud's hand has been described in isolated UCTD. Sjögren's syndrome should be looked for in every case, and its association with UCTD is not infrequent, even when no other CTD is present. It requires the usual local treatment.

Certain specific systemic signs and symptoms can, however, be associated with pure, nonoverlapping UCTD. Acute, transient pericarditis has been observed in 15 percent of our cases. It should be treated with 30 to 60 mg per day of prednisone for 2 to 4 weeks. Usually, it disappears without recurrence or sequelae.

Pulmonary arteritis, in the absence of other manifestations of PSS, is a much more severe situation representing the only potentially lethal complication of UCTD. Vasoactive drugs and cytotoxic (cyclophosphamide) treatment can be tried with variable results. Trigeminal neuralgia is relatively common in UCTD. It requires the intermittent use of high doses of corticosteroids, together with specific drugs such as carbamazepine.

A peculiar manifestation of UCTD is a febrile acute or subacute enlargement of lymph nodes. Sometimes, histology reveals the so-called necrotizing Kikuchi lesion. It could be related to a superimposed viral infection such as B19 parvovirus, and usually disappears within weeks.

SPECIAL CONSIDERATIONS

UCTD may be seen in infancy. Most of the reported cases put emphasis on the poor prognosis observed in children. Rapid evolution to SLE seems frequent and severe. Special attention is needed in early cases to detect such an evolution so that aggressive management can be instituted promptly.

Pregnancy illustrates quite well the problem of the true definition of MCTD. In the pertinent literature, one can find totally contradictory data. Some authors have found an excellent prognosis, with no complications and normal outcome of pregnancy, whereas others have described severe situations with renal impairment, as seen in SLE. It is quite likely that the former have seen mostly patients with pure UCTD, whereas the latter have followed patients whose disease had already overlapped with full-blown SLE.

DISCUSSION

Controversies in understanding the nature of MCTD have resulted in inconsistencies in the development of proper therapeutic strategies. Such problems may be alleviated if one considers, as we do, that UCTD is the initial, unique, and benign presentation of a spectrum of symptoms that require only mild treatment. In contrast, the multiple manifestations of the so-called MCTD are in reality overlaps with major individual CTDs that require more aggressive management for the respective syndromes. It is of interest to observe that, in our experience, UCTD virtually always precedes the occurrence of the overlapping major CTDs. We have never observed, in our large cohort of patients with SLE,

PM, and RA, the secondary occurrence of clinical (Raynaud's phenomenon, swollen hands) and biologic (anti–U1-RNP antibody) signs of UCTD. The unresolved issue is whether or not it is possible to prevent the evolution of the benign condition to a major and potentially lethal CTD. In this regard, prospective, controlled clinical trials are required to answer this question.

SUGGESTED READING

Alarcon GS, Williams GV, Singer JZ, et al. Early undifferentiated connective tissue disease. Early clinical manifestation in a large cohort of patients with undifferentiated connective tissue diseases compared with cohorts of well established connective tissue disease. J Rheumatol 1991; 18:1332–1339.

Black C, Isenberg DA. Mixed connective tissue disease. Goodby to all that. Br J Rheumatol 1992; 31:695–700.

Kahn MF, Kolsi R, Elleuch M. MCTD: Sharp's syndrome. Clinical and biological consideration. In: Kasukawa R, Sharp GC. Mixed connective tissue disease and antinuclear antibodies. Excerpta Medica, Amsterdam, 1987, pp 249–260.

Mairesse N, Kahn MF, Appelboom T. Antibodies to the constitutive 73 kd heat shock protein. A new marker of mixed connective tissue disease? Am J Med 1993; 95:595–600.

Sharp GC, Irvin WS, Tan EM, et al. Mixed connective tissue disease. An apparently distinct rheumatic disease syndrome associated with a specific antibody to an extractable nuclear antigen, (ENA). Am J Med 1972; 52:148–158.

Sharp GC, Hoffman RW. Mixed connective tissue disease. In: Belch J, Zurier R, eds. Connective tissue diseases. London: Chapman & Hall 1995.

Van den Hoogen FHJ, Spronk PE, Boerbooms ART, et al. Long-term follow up of 46 patients with anti–U1-RNP antibodies. Br J Rheumatol 1994; 33:117–120.

AMYLOIDOSIS

MARTHA SKINNER, M.D.

Amyloidosis is a broad term for a number of diseases that have in common the extracellular deposition of insoluble fibrillar proteins. The deposited fibrillar proteins and the pathogenetic mechanisms of disease are unique in each systemic amyloid type, but all share a beta-pleated sheet conformation and green birefringence on polarization microscopy after Congo red staining. Systemic amyloidosis is classified into four types according to the chemical composition of the fibrillar deposits. These generally correspond to defined clinical patterns termed primary (AL, fibrils composed of immunoglobulin light chains or fragments thereof), secondary (AA, associated with chronic inflammation and fibrils composed of a portion of the acute phase serum amyloid A, SAA protein), hereditary (ATTR or amyloid associated with mutant TTR is most common, but other hereditary forms associated with mutant apolipoprotein A1, mutant gelsolin, mutant fibrinogen, and mutant lysozyme have been described), and dialysis-associated (A$\beta_{2\text{-m}}$, fibrils composed of beta$_2$-microglobulin) (Table 1). In addition to the systemic types, a number of localized amyloidoses exist including Alzheimer's disease (Aβ, fibrils composed of beta-protein in the brain), endocrine-associated amyloidoses (ACal, calcitonin-related in medullary carcinoma of the thyroid; IAPP, islet amyloid polypeptide), localized amyloid tumors of the nasopharynx and the skin (recently found to be of light chain origin and associated with plasmacytomas), and localized amyloid tumors of the urinary bladder (of unknown biochemical type).

Supported by grants from the National Institutes of Health: U.S. Public Health Service, AR 40414; the Multipurpose Arthritis Center, AR 20613; and the Division of Research Resources, RR533.

DIAGNOSIS

A tissue biopsy is necessary to make the diagnosis of amyloidosis. The least invasive biopsy is the abdominal fat aspirate, which is positive in 80 to 90 percent of patients with either AL or ATTR amyloidosis and in 60 to 70 percent of patients with AA amyloidosis. It is easy to perform, does not require a specialty consultation, and can be done in patients who have coagulation abnormalities without concern for a bleeding site that cannot be observed. The result of the aspirate can be available within an hour because the aspirate needs only to be stained with Congo red and viewed in a polarized microscope, without the long process of fixing and embedding that tissue biopsies must undergo. If the fat aspirate is negative, but clinical suspicion for disease persists, a more invasive tissue biopsy must be done. In that case recommended biopsy sites are those suspected of disease involvement. Almost any tissue biopsy is likely to be positive if the patient has systemic amyloidosis. In a recent series of 100 patients with AL amyloidosis, 85 percent of 249 tissues biopsied were positive, including 100 percent of biopsies from the kidney, heart, and liver.

Once a diagnosis of amyloidosis has been confirmed by biopsy, the type must be determined before definitive treatment can be recommended. It is best to make the determination by biochemical analysis of the deposited fibrils, but this is not always possible. In some cases the clinician must rely on clinical features and laboratory testing (see Table 1). Many clinical features are present in more than one type of amyloidosis and thus, the following guidelines are recommended.

Table 1 Types of Systemic Amyloidosis

Type	*Fibril Composition*	*Clinical Features*	*Laboratory Studies*
AL, primary	Immunoglobulin light chain (kappa or lambda)	Multisystem disease including proteinuria, cardiomyopathy, hepatomegaly, macroglossia, orthostatic hypotension, peripheral neuropathy, cutaneous ecchymoses	Monoclonal protein in serum and/or urine; bone marrow plasmacytosis, mild, and showing monoclonality on immunohistochemical staining
AA, secondary	Amyloid A protein	Underlying inflammatory disease; multisystem disease including proteinuria, renal insufficiency, hepatomegaly, splenomegaly, orthostatic hypotension	Elevated serum amyloid A protein (SAA); sensitive reaction of tissue biopsy on KMnO4/Congo red staining; positive immunohistochemical staining of tissue biopsy with anti-AA antiserum*
ATTR, familial	Transthyretin	Midlife onset of peripheral and autonomic neuropathy, cardiomyopathy, vitreous opacities,* family history	Positive test for mutant transthyretin protein in serum or mutant gene in DNA of type known associated with disease*
Aβ2-m, dialysis associated	β_2-microglobulin	Long-term hemodialysis or chronic ambulatory peritoneal dialysis; carpal tunnel syndrome or musculoskeletal disorders of shoulder or hip	Elevated serum β_2-microglobulin; positive immunohistochemical staining of tissue biopsy with anti$-\beta_{2\text{-m}}$ antiserum*

*Definitive features or tests for diagnosis.

AL amyloidosis is the most common type of systemic amyloidosis and frequently the most difficult to diagnose with surety. It usually has an onset after the age of 40 years and is associated with rapid progression, multisystem involvement, and short survival. The most relied on test is the serum protein electrophoresis. Eighty-five to ninety percent of the patients have a serum or urine monoclonal immunoglobulin protein, and this should be looked for by serum and urine protein electrophoresis and typed by immunoelectrophoresis. In addition, the bone marrow usually has some increase in plasma cells. A bone marrow test must be done to rule out multiple myeloma and the plasma cells may show monoclonality on immunohistochemical staining. A monoclonal protein, by itself, is not diagnostic of amyloidosis. However, when it is present in a patient with biopsy proven amyloidosis, the AL type is strongly suspected. If one has enough tissue to isolate amyloid fibrils and find them composed of immunoglobulin light chain, the AL type is confirmed. Since this is rarely possible, typical clinical findings are an acceptable confirmation. Clinical findings in patients with this type of amyloidosis include involvement of two or more systems, with features of cardiomyopathy, proteinuria, sensory or autonomic neuropathy, hepatomegaly, macroglossia, and ecchymoses. The only pathognomonic feature is macroglossia, which occurs in 10 percent of patients with AL amyloidosis.

AA amyloidosis is rare in the United States, occurring in less than 1 percent of individuals with chronic inflammatory diseases, but it is more common in Europe, occurring in 5 to 10 percent of persons with chronic inflammatory disease. It may begin within a year after the underlying inflammatory disease or many years later. It is the only type of amyloidosis that has occurred in children. To positively identify a biopsy as AA amyloid, the first step is the potassium permanganate/Congo red staining of the tissue. In the AA type of amyloidosis, treatment with potassium permanganate prior to Congo red staining abolishes the typical amyloid pattern of green birefringence ("sensitive reaction"). If a "sensitive reaction" occurs, AA amyloid deposits in tissue can be confirmed by more specific immunohistochemical staining with antisera to AA protein. The clinical features in patients with this type of amyloidosis are nearly always proteinuria and/or renal insufficiency, and disease progression is slow. Cardiac involvement and autonomic neuropathy occur only late in the disease. Survival is often more than 10 years, particularly with treatment for end-stage renal disease.

Familial amyloidotic polyneuropathy due to a mutant transthyretin (TTR) protein is a rare disease, but it is now known to be present in persons of nearly every ethnic background. This type of amyloidosis must be excluded in every patient who presents with amyloidosis and does not have either a serum monoclonal immunoglobulin protein or the AA type of amyloidosis. Although the disease has an autosomal dominant transmission, family history may not be apparent when the disease presents later in life. There are now more than 40 different TTR mutations associated with ATTR amyloidosis, as well as a few that are not associated with disease. The simplest way to test for this type of amyloidosis is by isoelectric focusing of the patient's serum TTR protein to determine whether a mutant protein exists. The patient's DNA must then be tested for the precise TTR mutation to definitively confirm ATTR amyloidosis. Clinically, patients present in midlife with peripheral and autonomic neuropathy, cardiomyopathy, vitreous opacities, and renal disease. A pathognomonic feature is vitreous opacities, which have occurred with approximately 25 percent of the TTR mutations associated with ATTR amyloidosis. Without intervention, survival after disease onset is 7 to 15 years.

MAJOR TREATMENT

Treatment for most types of amyloidosis has been unsatisfactory until the present time. The option of liver

Table 2 Major Treatment Options for Amyloidosis

AL (Primary) Amyloidosis
1. Cyclic oral melphalan and prednisone
   Melphalan* 0.15-0.25 mg/kg/day × 4 days
   Prednisone 1.5-2.0 mg/kg/day × 4 days
   Repeat administration every 6 weeks for 1 year for a total of 600 mg of melphalan
2. Colchicine 0.6 mg b.i.d.
   Not recommended as the major therapy alone. May be given with cyclic melphalan and prednisone, but should be omitted on the 4 days other medications are given
3. Newer treatment: High or intermediate dose melphalan with stem cell rescue
   G-CSF primed stem cell harvest from peripheral blood
   IV melphalan: high dose 200 mg/m^2 over 2 days; or intermediate dose 100 mg/m^2 over 2 days
   Autologous stem cell infusion after melphalan treatment

AA (Secondary) Amyloidosis
1. Aggressive treatment of underlying inflammatory disease with monitoring of the SAA level on a regular basis
2. Surgical excision of infectious process when feasible (i.e., lung lobectomy for bronchiectasis, bone resection for osteomyelitis, colectomy for chronic ulcerative colitis)
3. Colchicine 0.6 mg b.i.d. for AA amyloidosis secondary to familial Mediterranean fever

ATTR (Familial) Amyloidosis
Orthotopic liver transplantation

*White blood cell and platelet counts must be determined every 3 weeks and the dosage of melphalan adjusted so that some leukopenia or thrombocytopenia occurs at midcycle.

transplantation for familial amyloidosis has provided the first successful therapy for patients with this disease. Likewise, high-dose melphalan and autologous stem cell rescue is an encouraging new therapy for AL amyloidosis. Once the diagnosis of amyloidosis has been established by positive biopsy and the type defined by biochemical and/or clinical examination, a treatment plan can be formulated. For all types of amyloidosis, the treatment plan comprises two parts: first, major therapy is prescribed with the intent to decrease the precursor protein of the particular amyloid type (Table 2), and secondly, supportive therapy is directed at the specific organ system involvement, resulting from amyloid fibril deposition (Table 3).

AL (Primary) Amyloidosis

AL amyloidosis is a plasma cell dyscrasia with a monoclonal production of an immunoglobulin light chain. The structural properties of the light chain most likely dictate its propensity to form amyloid fibrils, which occur throughout the body. Extensive multisystem involvement typifies this form of amyloidosis and survival with no treatment is generally only a few months. Studies have shown that chemotherapy with oral melphalan and prednisone to decrease the clonal plasma cells has increased survival of patients with this disease. Newer therapies with intravenous high-dose or intermediate-dose melphalan followed by stem cell rescue are being investigated with promising results.

Clinical trials suggest a combination of melphalan and prednisone given cyclically over at least a 1-year time period is the treatment of choice for patients with AL amyloidosis who do not have multiple myeloma (see Table 2). We have just completed a trial of melphalan, prednisone, and colchicine versus colchicine alone in 100 patients with AL amyloidosis and found a median survival of 12.2 months from study entry for those treated with melphalan, prednisone, and colchicine and 6.7 months for those treated with colchicine alone. The overall results were not statistically significant ($p = 0.087$). However, an advantage to the melphalan and prednisone treatment was noted for patients who presented with neuropathy ($p = 0.037$) or hepatomegaly and soft tissue involvement ($p = 0.007$). Patients presenting with cardiomyopathy as the major symptom had a median survival of 4.4 months from study entry and probably did not live long enough to benefit from medication. Patients presenting with renal disease as their major symptom had a median survival of 18.7 months and appeared to benefit from supportive therapy such as dialysis when organ failure occurred regardless of their major medication. In another study of 101 patients with AL amyloidosis treated with melphalan and prednisone versus colchicine alone, survival also tended to favor the melphalan treatment group. Treatment should be started as soon as the diagnosis of AL amyloidosis is sure. Survival curves showed that differences in survival favoring melphalan did not occur until after 4 months of treatment.

A newer form of therapy is currently being evaluated. Patients who are 60 years of age or under and have cardiac and renal function that meets eligibility criteria are being offered high-dose intravenous melphalan therapy and autologous mobilized stem cell rescue (see Table 2). This treatment has been used with success in patients with multiple myeloma, and initial results of a Phase I trial suggest it may be quite successful for treatment of AL amyloidosis. Stem cells are collected from the peripheral blood after mobilization with granulocyte colony-stimulating factor (G-CSF). Then high-dose melphalan is given, and the patient's cryopreserved stem cells are thawed and reinfused. The value of this treatment depends on the technologic advances that will provide ways to ensure removal of any of the clonal plasma cell precursors from the autologous stem cells. When that is possible, this will be a potentially curable treatment. For now at least, it is expected to markedly reduce the tumor burden. If favorable results continue, this will become the treatment of choice for patients well enough to undergo the treatment. Patients with heart or renal system compromise may be able to undergo intermediate-dose melphalan and have greater benefit than with cyclic oral melphalan.

The risks associated with oral melphalan are the development of acute nonlymphocytic leukemia or a myelodysplastic syndrome. It is not expected that this will be a risk for patients receiving intravenous melphalan, but that is yet to be determined. Pancytopenia can also occur with side effects related to anemia, low

Table 3 Supportive Treatment for All Types of Amyloidosis

Organ System	*Symptom*	*Treatment*
Cardiac	Congestive failure	Salt restriction of 1-2 g/day (unless patient has orthostatic hypotension)
		Diuretics: furosamide or zaroxolyn
		Captopril in small doses 2 or 3 times daily
	Heart block	Pacemaker
Renal	Nephrotic syndrome	Salt restriction of 1-2 g/day
		Elastic stockings for edema
		Dietary increase of protein to 1.5 g/kg/day
	Renal failure	Dialysis (chronic ambulatory peritoneal dialysis or hemodialysis)
Autonomic nervous	Orthostatic hypotension	Increase salt to at least 6 g/day (need to evaluate cardiac and renal systems first)
		Elastic stockings
		Fludrocortisone (Florinef)
	Gastric atony	Small frequent feedings (6/day) low in fat
		Metoclopramide hydrochloride (Reglan) or Propulcid; use with caution if patient has orthostatic hypotension
		Jejunostomy tube for commercially prepared formula feeding
Gastrointestinal	Diarrhea	Dietary changes
		Low fat diet of 40 g or less
		Medium chain triglyceride oil supplements of 60 ml/day
		Medications
		Tetracycline
		Psyllium hydrophilic muciloid (Metamucil)
		Loperamide hydrochloride (Imodium)
		Total parenteral nutrition
	Macroglossia	Maintain airway
		Hemiglossectomy
Peripheral nervous	Sensory neuropathy	Avoid trauma
		Medications for pain
		Amitriptyline 25-50 mg at bedtime
		Carbamazepine (Tegretol)
	Motor neuropathy	Shoe braces for foot drop
		Physical therapy
Hematologic	Intracutaneous bleeding	Avoid trauma
	Factor 10 deficiency	Factor replacement before surgery
		Splenectomy, if massively enlarged spleen

white blood cell count, or thrombocytopenia. Since leukemic side effects appear to be dose related, we recommend only 1 year (or 600 mg total) of oral melphalan therapy.

Colchicine has been given for all types of amyloidosis since it was found to be a treatment for familial Mediterranean fever that prevented inflammatory serositis and as a result patients did not develop AA amyloidosis. In a large clinical trial using untreated retrospective controls, colchicine was found to improve the median survival of patients with AL amyloidosis (17 months versus 6 months). We recommend colchicine in a dose of 0.6 mg twice daily or once daily if gastrointestinal side effects occur or if the patient has renal insufficiency. It may be beneficial in slowing disease progression in AL and AA amyloidosis and may even delay onset of familial amyloidosis due to mutant TTR; however, measurable improvements in disease have not been noted with colchicine therapy.

AA Amyloidosis

In AA (secondary) amyloidosis the major therapy is directed towards treatment of the underlying inflammatory or infectious disease (see Table 2). Treatment that suppresses or eliminates the inflammation or infection will also decrease the serum amyloid A (SAA) protein and slow the progression of AA amyloidosis. SAA is an acute phase protein produced by the liver in response to inflammation or cell necrosis and is the precursor protein of AA amyloidosis. Optimal treatment of some inflammatory diseases (chronic rheumatoid arthritis, ankylosing spondylitis, inflammatory bowel disease, and so on) is often difficult, and fortunately the complication of AA amyloidosis occurs only rarely. When AA amyloidosis is found, usually in the course of an evaluation for proteinuria, it is recommended that the treatment of the underlying disease be even more diligent and aggressive. The treatment can be monitored by periodic SAA serum levels (normal $< 1 \mu g$ per milliliter). When the inflammatory disease is familial Mediterranean fever, the appropriate treatment is colchicine 1.2 to 1.8 mg per day.

The course of AA amyloidosis is usually slow when the underlying disease is a chronic inflammatory condition, but more rapid when the underlying disease is an infection (osteomyelitis, tuberculosis, leprosy, and so on). However, infectious diseases can often be treated definitively with antibiotics or surgical resection of the infectious process. The AA amyloidosis does not progress after the infection is treated, although it is not known if the deposited amyloid fibrils ever completely disappear.

ATTR Amyloidosis

The most exciting therapeutic advance in the treatment of amyloidosis has been orthotopic liver transplantation in ATTR (familial) amyloidosis, a condition for which there was no definitive treatment. In 1990, investigators in Sweden proposed liver transplantation to remove the major source of mutant transthyretin production and replace it with normal transthyretin. The surgical procedure is technically easier than for patients with chronic liver failure because patients with familial amyloidosis do not have cirrhosis or portal hypertensive collateral circulation. However, a major risk is hemodynamic instability at the time of transplant due to cardiomyopathy and autonomic dysfunction. The brief follow-up of transplanted patients suggests that the disease progression is arrested and some autonomic and peripheral nervous system improvement has occurred. No changes have been noted in cardiomyopathy. In a report of the First International Workshop on Liver Transplantation for FAP, 11 of 64 transplant recipients from 10 countries died within the first few months after surgery and the risk of death was greater for those with more advanced disease.

It is currently recommended that a patient have biopsy proof of amyloid deposition and DNA analysis to define the mutant transthyretin before considering liver transplantation. Most patients have had objective evidence of at least one organ system involved before being listed for transplantation. The increased risk in patients with more advanced disease and the lack of complete recovery after surgery have suggested the need for earlier transplant intervention in less symptomatic patients. Because of the nature of ATTR amyloidosis and the need to remove a deleterious gene product, it is unlikely that a simpler treatment with a gene therapy option will be available in the near future.

Aβ2-m Amyloidosis

Amyloidosis due to beta$_2$-microglobulin fibril deposition occurs in patients on dialysis for many years. Amyloid deposits tend to occur around synovial membranes and in bone such as the carpal synovium, cartilage of the glenohumeral joint, and femoral head, but they are not exclusive to these tissues and have been found in all tissues, including the heart and gastrointestinal tract. Symptoms are carpal tunnel syndrome and bone pain from cystic lesions, which sometimes lead to fracture. Since the beta$_2$-microglobulin molecule at 11,000 daltons is too large to pass through a dialysis membrane, the treatment is a dilemma. The prevalence of the disease approaches 100 percent of individuals on dialysis for more than 10 years. Patients who have received kidney transplants after developing $A\beta_{2\text{-m}}$ have noted an improvement in symptoms.

SUPPORTIVE TREATMENT

Supportive treatment for all forms of amyloidosis is of the utmost importance (see Table 3). It will enhance the outcome of major treatments and can be offered to patients with extensive organ system involvement for whom it would not be safe to undergo some of the more aggressive treatments. Supportive treatments are measures relating to the therapy for an involved organ system and can be characterized as life saving when they provide treatment for end-organ failure or as general supportive when they assist organ function.

Life-Saving Supportive Treatments

Life-saving supportive treatments include major organ transplantation, renal dialysis, cardiac pacemaker, and nutritional support. In our clinical treatment trial of 100 patients with AL amyloidosis, two patients had heart transplants, two had kidney transplants, 19 were treated with dialysis, seven with pacemakers, seven with jejunostomy tubes, and seven had total parenteral nutrition. Three of the four organ transplant recipients were among those who survived 5 years or longer, while the median survival of these patients with AL amyloidosis was 10 to 14 months. These life-saving supportive treatments significantly improved survival regardless of major treatment assignment (melphalan, prednisone and colchicine, or colchicine alone). In our experience with 74 patients with AA amyloidosis, 25 received dialysis or a kidney transplant. The survival of patients with AA amyloidosis in this series varied with the underlying disease; a median survival for the whole group was 8.9 years.

We recommend organ transplantation in AL amyloidosis if the organ is end stage and the patient has minimal other major organ system involvement. If this form of life-saving supportive treatment can be provided with major treatment that reduces the precursor amyloid protein, an even greater impact on long survival can be expected. In AA amyloidosis the kidneys are frequently the only apparent organ involved and kidney transplantation should be considered.

General Supportive

General supportive measures reflecting high quality medical care individualized for the special needs of each patient with amyloidosis will optimize survival and allow a more comfortable living for the patient with a debilitating illness (see Table 3).

Cardiomyopathy is a common feature of patients with AL and ATTR amyloidosis. Congestive heart failure due to cardiomyopathy is best treated with moderate salt restriction and vigorous diuretic therapy. The use of digitalis is not indicated. In fact, both digitalis and calcium channel blocking drugs have been associated with sudden death and should be avoided. The use of small doses of captopril three times daily may be helpful, but must be used with care if the patient also has orthostatic hypotension.

Renal involvement often results in nephrotic syndrome with massive proteinuria, edema, and a low serum albumin. Patients are encouraged to increase dietary protein (1.5 g per kilogram body weight) in an attempt to replace urinary losses and raise the serum albumin concentration. The salt restriction may need to be liberalized to make the diet palatable. Rest periods during the day with the legs elevated and elastic stockings decrease peripheral edema.

Symptoms of the autonomic nervous system are difficult to treat. Orthostatic hypotension is treated by increasing salt in the diet and the use of elastic stockings of the fitted antigravity type. Patients are encouraged to do some isometric exercises before arising and to get up slowly. Fludrocortisone (Florinef) may be useful, but often causes fluid retention. Gastric atony due to autonomic neuropathy may produce a continuous full feeling, nausea, or vomiting. Its presence should be confirmed by a gastric emptying scan and treatment started with small frequent feedings low in fat. Metaclopramide (Reglan) or Propulcid may be helpful to increase gastric motility or tetracycline to treat the complication of a blind loop syndrome. Gastrointestinal symptoms of diarrhea may also reflect autonomic neuropathy. It sometimes responds to dietary changes limiting fat, medications to decrease bowel motility (Lomotil, Imodium), or to increase bowel contents (Metamucil). Peripheral neuropathy may be helped with tranquilizing of mild antiseizure medications. Physical therapy is important in maintaining muscle mass and preventing contractures.

Symptoms associated with bleeding may be mild or may constitute a serious hematologic emergency. Ecchymoses or intracutaneous bleeding is common, but a mild problem for which there is no specific therapy other than avoiding trauma. Serious bleeding can result from blood clotting factor deficiencies, most commonly factor X, but all calcium-dependent clotting factors can be deficient. It is important to assess the clotting status prior to all surgical procedures. In a few patients splenectomy has corrected clotting factor deficiencies, perhaps by removing large deposits of amyloid fibrils.

SUGGESTED READING

Cohen AS, Rubinow A, Anderson JJ, et al. Survival of patients with primary (AL) amyloidosis and the effect of colchicine treatment: Cases treated with colchicine from 1976–1983 compared with cases seen in previous years. Am J Med 1987; 82:1182–1190.

Kyle RA, Greipp PR, Garton JP, Gertz MA. Primary systemic amyloidosis: Comparison of melphalan/prednisone versus colchicine. Am J Med 1985; 79:708–716.

Skinner M, Anderson J, Simms R, et al. Treatment of 100 patients with primary amyloidosis: a randomized trial of melphalan, prednisone, and colchicine versus colchicine only. Am J Med 1996; 100:290–298.

Skinner M, Lewis WD, Jones LA, et al. Liver transplantation as a treatment for familial amyloidotic polyneuropathy. Ann Int Med 1994; 120:133–134.

Steen L, Holmgren G, Suhr O, et al. Worldwide survey of liver transplantations in patients with familial amyloidotic polyneuropathy. Amyloid 1994; 1:138–142.

VASCULITIS

SYSTEMIC NECROTIZING VASCULITIS

REX M. McCALLUM, M.D.
BARTON F. HAYNES, M.D.

Systemic necrotizing vasculitis comprises a group of clinical syndromes characterized by blood vessel inflammation with resultant vessel injury and organ ischemia. Since inflammation may affect any vessel in the body, the clinical manifestations of the systemic vasculitides are varied and frequently confusing. Systemic necrotizing vasculitis also has a broad range of manifestations from isolated mild cutaneous disease to life-threatening multisystem organ failure. Making a diagnosis of systemic necrotizing vasculitis requires a high degree of clinical suspicion and, frequently, invasive procedures such as angiography and/or tissue biopsy. Ideally, such procedures should be performed before instituting immunosuppressive therapy, which may alter histologic and angiographic patterns.

Despite the heterogeneous nature of systemic necrotizing vasculitis syndromes, several well-characterized clinical entities have been described by studying the histologic pattern of the vessel inflammation, size of the involved vessels, pattern of organ system involvement, and associated clinical abnormalities. With the diagnosis of systemic necrotizing vasculitis, attempted classification into a specific vasculitic syndrome should follow. While the nosology of systemic necrotizing vasculitis continues to evolve, the present classification scheme does have prognostic significance, provides information on preferred therapy, suggests therapeutic alternatives, and suggests associated clinical concerns (Table 1). In addition, defining the extent of vasculitic involvement (severity and number of organ systems involved) and understanding the tempo of the illness is important in clarifying the appropriate intensity of therapeutic intervention, defining the timeliness of treatment, and minimizing treatment-associated morbidity.

The primary focus of this chapter is the treatment of the systemic necrotizing vasculitides of the polyarteritis nodosa (PAN) group, Wegener's granulomatosis, and primary (isolated) angiitis of the central nervous system (CNS). The giant cell arteritides are discussed in the chapters *Temporal Arteritis* and *Takayasu's Arteritis*. Hypersensitivity vasculitides are discussed in the chapter *Cutaneous Vasculitis*.

Table 1 Classification of the Major Systemic Necrotizing Vasculitides

Polyarteritis nodosa group
Classic polyarteritis nodosa
Allergic angiitis and granulomatosis (Churg-Strauss disease)
Polyangiitis overlap syndrome
Wegener's granulomatosis
Giant cell arteritis
Temporal arteritis
Takayasu's arteritis
Primary (isolated) angiitis of the central nervous system
Associated with underlying disease process
Collagen vascular disease
Infections
Neoplasms
Behçet's disease
Other autoimmune illnesses
Hypersensitivity vasculitis
Henoch-Schönlein purpura
Serum sickness—like reaction
Cryoglobulinemic vasculitis

PREFERRED THERAPY

Corticosteroids

A major component of the primary therapy of the polyarteritis nodosa group syndromes, Wegener's granulomatosis, and primary angiitis of the central nervous system is corticosteroids. Corticosteroids should be instituted as soon as the diagnosis of systemic necrotizing vasculitis is made and other differential diagnostic considerations such as infection and neoplasm are excluded. Objective signs of systemic necrotizing vasculitis (Table 2) should be identified in order to monitor response to therapy. Corticosteroids should be started at 1 to 2 mg per kilogram body weight per day of prednisone or equivalent therapy in divided dose, administered either intravenously or orally. The absorption of corticosteroids is identical for oral and intravenous dosing;

Table 2 Objective Signs of Systemic Necrotizing Vasculitis

- Eye
  - Episcleritis/scleritis
  - Retinal vasculitis
  - Ischemic optic neuropathy
  - Retro-ocular inflammatory mass lesion
- Nervous system
  - Mononeuritis multiplex
  - Strokes
- Renal
  - Active sediment with proteinuria and hematuria
  - Renal insufficiency
  - Hypertension of recent onset or exacerbation
- Pulmonary
  - Nodules with or without cavitation
  - Infiltrates
  - Pulmonary hemorrhage
  - Cough
  - Hypoxia
- Skin
  - Palpable purpura
  - Subcutaneous nodules
  - Livedo reticularis
- Upper respiratory tract
  - Opacification of sinuses on imaging study
  - Rhinorrhea and nasal congestion
  - Nasal ulceration
  - Saddle nose deformity
  - Serous otitis media
- Associated clinical features
  - Elevated erythrocyte sedimentation rate
  - Anemia of chronic disease
  - Leukocytosis
  - Thrombocytosis
  - Eosinophilia
  - Cryoglobulinemia
- Other
  - Arthritis
  - Intestinal ulceration, perforation, and infarction
  - Myositis
  - Abnormal angiography

however, intravenous administration is indicated if a question of gastrointestinal malabsorption exists or if the patient is unable to take oral medications.

All patients with PAN group syndromes, Wegener's granulomatosis, and primary angiitis of the CNS require corticosteroid therapy for the control of the vasculitic syndrome. Corticosteroids are used to down regulate proinflammatory effector mechanisms, such as the influx of inflammatory cells into tissues and cytokine production (Table 3). Divided-dose corticosteroids should be continued until manifestations of the disease cease progression and are reduced. The time required to accomplish this varies for each patient and syndrome, with an average range from 5 to 30 days. Pulse methylprednisolone therapy of 0.5 to 1.0 g per day for 3 days can be used initially in patients with rapidly progressive and life-threatening vasculitic syndromes, although there are no controlled trials comparing this regimen to standard corticosteroid dosing. Divided-dose corticosteroid therapy profoundly suppresses the hypothalamic-pituitary-adrenal axis and causes a high incidence of toxic side effects if continued more than a few weeks; therefore, attempts to consolidate treatment

Table 3 Mechanisms of Corticosteroid Immunosuppressive and Anti-Inflammatory Effects

- Inhibition of accumulation of monocytic macrophages at inflammatory sites
- Blockage of accumulation of neutrophils at inflammatory sites
- Selective depletion of T lymphocytes more than B lymphocytes
- Suppression of lymphocytic function in
  - Delayed hypersensitivity skin testing by inhibiting monocyte recruitment
  - Lymphocytic proliferation to antigens
  - Mixed lymphocytic proliferation
  - Spontaneous (natural) cytotoxicity
- Suppression of monocytic-macrophage function in
  - Cutaneous delayed hypersensitivity by inhibition of lymphokine effect on macrophages
  - Blockage of Fc–receptor binding and function
  - Bactericidal activity
  - Inhibition of interleukin-1 production
- Decreased reticuloendothelial clearance of antibody-coated cells
- Decreased synthesis of prostaglandin and leukotrienes
- Inhibition of plasminogen activator release
- Antagonism of histamine-induced vasodilation
- Effect on cytokines
  - Decreased production of interleukin-1

to a single morning dose should be undertaken as soon as early clinical response is evident. A single morning dose of corticosteroid coincides with the normal diurnal variation of plasma cortisone levels and is less toxic. If divided-dose therapy is required less than 10 days, then the dose can be consolidated to a single morning dose rapidly, over 1 to 5 days. If divided-dose therapy is required for more than 14 days, then a more gradual taper over 7 to 10 days to a single morning dose is necessary. The consolidated morning dose of corticosteroids is continued until further clinical improvement is evident in the patient's subjective symptoms, and the objective signs of disease activity chosen for monitoring resolve, usually within 1 to 3 months (Table 4).

Once a clinical response occurs and clinical signs and symptoms of active disease abate, attempts should be made to taper the corticosteroid dose to alternate-day therapy. The therapeutic principle to be followed is that the patient should be on the lowest, least toxic corticosteroid regimen that will control signs and symptoms of the vasculitic syndrome. Most patients with a systemic necrotizing vasculitis syndrome can be tapered to alternate-day corticosteroid therapy (see Table 4), but an occasional patient may be refractory. In this case, tapering of corticosteroids to the least effective daily dose of corticosteroid must be undertaken. The protocol in Table 4 shows a taper from 60 mg of prednisone each day to 60 mg on alternate days over approximately 8 weeks. The actual tempo of steroid taper must be dictated by patient signs and symptoms. Since corticosteroid therapy in patients with hepatitis B virus–associated PAN may enhance viral replication in the liver, corticosteroid taper to alternate-day therapy should be attempted more rapidly and discontinued, if clinical parameters allow.

Once corticosteroids are administered on alternate days and signs and symptoms of the systemic necrotizing

Table 4 Example of Corticosteroid Therapy in Systemic Necrotizing Vasculitis

At the time of diagnosis begin prednisone therapy:

Dose	*Frequency*	*Length of Therapy*
15 mg	Four times per day	10 days
20 mg	Three times per day	2 days
30 mg	Two times per day	2 days
60 mg	Once a day in the AM	30 days

At this time the taper to alternate-day therapy begins:

"High-Day" Dose	*"Low-Day" Dose*	*Length of Therapy*
60 mg	50 mg	6 days
60 mg	40 mg	6 days
60 mg	30 mg	6 days
60 mg	20 mg	6 days
60 mg	15 mg	6 days
60 mg	10 mg	6 days
60 mg	7.5 mg	6 days
60 mg	5 mg	6 days
60 mg	2.5 mg	6 days
60 mg	0 mg	6 days

The alternate-day dose can be tapered after the patient has been stable for 1 month on alternate-day therapy. The above regimen is only an example of a corticosteroid taper scheme. The design and tempo of a regimen for individual patients must rely on each patient's clinical signs and symptoms and their response to therapy

vasculitis remain stable or quiescent for at least 4 weeks, the alternate-day therapy can gradually be tapered to the least effective dose or discontinued, at a rate of 10 mg every 2 weeks or slower. The taper should continue as long as signs and symptoms of the systemic necrotizing vasculitis remain stable or quiescent. If signs or symptoms of the vasculitis recur or worsen, the corticosteroid dose should be increased or the taper should be halted or slowed, depending upon the degree and severity of the recurrent or worsening signs and symptoms.

Alternate-day corticosteroid therapy has a significantly lower incidence of side effects compared to daily oral divided dose therapy. Conversion from daily to alternate-day corticosteroid therapy should routinely be attempted in all patients with forms of systemic necrotizing vasculitis (except temporal arteritis, see the chapter *Temporal Arteritis.* Corticosteroid dose is clearly a factor in the toxic and infectious complications of corticosteroid therapy, and thus the dose should continually be tapered to achieve the lowest effective dose. Calcium supplementation at a dose of 1,200 to 1,500 mg of elemental calcium daily in divided dose combined with 400 IU of vitamin D per day may delay or attenuate the development of corticosteroid-related osteopenia. Monitoring for the development of glucose intolerance, hypertension, steroid myopathy, and increased intraocular pressure is also recommended in

Table 5 Complications of Corticosteroid Therapy

- Central nervous system difficulties
  - Altered morale/personality
  - Steroid psychosis
  - Pseudotumor cerebri
- Cutaneous difficulties
  - Violaceous striae
  - Subcutaneous tissue atrophy
  - Cushingoid habitus
  - Purpura and ecchymosis
  - Acne
  - Hirsutism
  - Facial erythema
- Deposition of fatty tissue
  - Moon facies
  - Buffalo hump
  - Mediastinal lipomatosis
  - Hepatomegaly
- Delayed wound healing (including peptic ulceration)
- Endocrine and metabolic difficulties
  - Hyperglycemia
  - Osteoporosis
  - Suppression of the hypothalamic-pituitary-adrenal axis
  - Hypokalemic alkalosis
  - Fluid retention
  - Hypertension
  - Growth retardation
  - Proximal myopathy
  - Hyperlipoproteinemia
  - Menstrual irregularity
- Immunosuppression
- Ocular difficulties
  - Cataracts
  - Glaucoma
  - Exophthalmos
- Opportunistic infection
- Osteonecrosis
- Pancreatitis
- Weight gain

patients receiving corticosteroid therapy for more than 2 weeks (Table 5).

A few patients with a very mild or slowly progressive PAN group disease, Wegener's granulomatosis limited to the upper respiratory tract, or primary angiitis of the CNS without focal CNS difficulties may be treated with corticosteroids alone. Such patients are rare and must be chosen very carefully and monitored for response to therapy and progression of disease. If response is not documented or disease progression is evident, a second drug must then be added to the regimen.

Cyclophosphamide

Many patients with systemic necrotizing vasculitis as well as the majority of patients with PAN group syndromes, Wegener's granulomatosis, and primary angiitis of the CNS require combination therapy with corticosteroid and another immunosuppressive agent. The most commonly recommended and used second drug is the alkylating agent, cyclophosphamide (Table 6). Patients who fail treatment with corticosteroids alone and patients with renal, pulmonary, neurologic, and gastrointestinal manifestations of PAN group syndromes and Wegener's granulomatosis require treatment with

Table 6 Mechanisms of Immunosuppressive Properties of Cyclophosphamide

Lymphocytopenia of both T and B lymphocytes
Suppression of in vitro lymphocyte blastogenic response to specific antigens
Suppression of antibody response and cutaneous delayed hypersensitivity to new antigen
Selective suppression of in vitro B lymphocytic function with decrease in immunoglobulin production and suppression of mitogen-induced immunoglobulin production
Reduction in serum immunoglobulin levels

cyclophosphamide and corticosteroids, as do patients with primary angiitis of the CNS with focal neurologic findings and/or rapid tempo of progression.

Patients should be started on cyclophosphamide at a dose of 2 mg per kilogram body weight per day given orally or intravenously. The absorption of cyclophosphamide is identical when given orally or intravenously; therefore, the indications to give the drug intravenously are concerns regarding gastrointestinal absorption secondary to gut malabsorption or inability to swallow oral medication. Cyclophosphamide at 2 mg per kilogram body weight per day is maintained for 2 weeks. If evidence of favorable clinical response is noted, this dose is maintained with subsequent dose level adjustments to keep the peripheral white blood cell (WBC) count at greater than 3,000 cells per cubic millimeter^3. Suppressing the WBC to a level of 3,000 to 4,000 cells per cubic millimeter^3 represents the most aggressive level of immunosuppression, but many patients will achieve clinical remission with WBCs in the absence of leukopenia. If there is no evidence of favorable clinical response in 2 weeks, daily dose should be increased by 25 mg every 2 weeks until a clinical response occurs or until a WBC count of less than 3,000 cells per cubic millimeter^3 is reached. The complete blood count (CBC) should be monitored 2 to 3 times per week for the first 2 weeks of therapy and with any increase in cyclophosphamide dose. Subsequently, the CBC can be monitored weekly. It is important to remember that the dose of cyclophosphamide given has the maximum effect on the WBC count 7 to 10 days after administration. Thus, a rapid change in WBCs over 1 week (e.g., from 10,000 per cubic millimeter^3 to 5,000 per cubic millimeter^3) is an indication to temporarily discontinue the cyclophosphamide until the WBC count stabilizes.

In patients with fulminant systemic necrotizing vasculitis involving the kidneys, heart, brain, or lungs, the disease is life threatening and can lead to rapid and irreversible organ damage. Such patients include those with CNS vasculitis and multiple rapid strokes, severe pulmonary involvement with hypoxia, rapidly progressive peripheral neuropathy, and/or rapidly progressive renal insufficiency. Renal failure is the most common clinical manifestation of fulminant vasculitis and constitutes a medical emergency. In patients with fulminant vasculitis, cyclophosphamide is begun at 4 mg per kilogram body weight per day orally or intravenously for 3 days with taper over the subsequent 3 days to a dose of 1 to 2 mg per kilogram body weight per day. This dose is maintained with careful attention to the WBC count and its rate of change because waiting until the WBC count is 3,000 cells per cubic millimeter before modifying the dose of cyclophosphamide may result in clinically significant neutropenia when the nadir is finally reached.

Cyclophosphamide should be continued with careful monitoring of disease activity and potential toxicity for 1 year after remission of the systemic necrotizing vasculitis is believed to have been achieved. As the corticosteroid dose is tapered, the cyclophosphamide dose may have to be tapered because corticosteroid protects the patient from some of cyclophosphamide's effect on lowering the WBC count. A taper to alternate-day corticosteroid often requires a 25 to 50 mg decrease in the cyclophosphamide dose. Prolonged cyclophosphamide therapy may be associated with diminished drug tolerance, calling for further reductions in the cyclophosphamide dose. Finally, decreased renal function also requires modification of the cyclophosphamide dose after the initial 5 to 7 days of therapy because active cyclophosphamide metabolites are renally cleared; therefore, peak drug-induced effects on WBCs may be prolonged. In the setting of a persistent creatinine clearance of less than 15 ml per minute, the dose of cyclophosphamide may be less than or equal to 1 mg per kilogram body weight per day after the first week, depending on the WBC count. After 1 year of therapy in remission, the cyclophosphamide should be reduced 25 mg per day every 1 to 2 months until it is discontinued, provided that disease remains quiescent.

Monitoring of primary angiitis of the CNS is much more difficult than PAN group syndromes and Wegener's granulomatosis. Generally, repeat angiography at 3 to 4 months of therapy is necessary to document a response to therapy. If the angiogram is markedly improved or normal and no new symptoms of cerebral ischemia are present, then it may be possible to say that the patient is clinically in remission.

Cyclophosphamide therapy has many potential complications (Table 7). Patients receiving cyclophosphamide should be told to drink adequate fluids to maintain 3 liters urine output per day to decrease drug-induced bladder toxicity. A careful history of bladder function should be obtained and suggestions of bladder-outlet obstruction and neurogenic bladder should be appropriately evaluated and treated. The failure to empty the bladder may increase the risk of developing cyclophosphamide-related bladder toxicity. Patients treated with daily oral cyclophosphamide require lifelong follow-up regarding their increased risk of bladder cancer. All hematuria (gross and microscopic) should be evaluated with cystoscopy to investigate the possibility of bladder cancer. Yearly urine cytologies should also be performed. If hemorrhagic cystitis complicates a course of cyclophosphamide therapy, methotrexate (20 to 25 mg per week) is the first choice to replace the cyclophosphamide. Methotrexate should not be considered unless the serum creatinine is less than 2.5 mg per deciliter.

Table 7 Complications of Cyclophosphamide Therapy

Alopecia
Antidiuretic hormone effect at higher doses
Bladder Toxicity
Hemorrhagic cystitis
Bladder fibrosis
Bladder cancer
Hypogammaglobulinemia
Lymphoma/leukemia
Marrow toxicity
Neutropenia/leukopenia
Thrombocytopenia
Anemia, often macrocytic
Leukemia
Nausea and emesis
Opportunistic infection
Pulmonary interstitial fibrosis
Reproductive system
Premature ovarian failure
Infertility
Sterility
Teratogenesis

Azathioprine, chlorambucil, and cyclosporine are alternatives to the use of methotrexate in this situation. Azathioprine seems incapable of inducing a remission in most systemic vasculitides, but it seems to work well for maintaining remission in those patients with cyclophosphamide toxicity. The use of cyclic estrogen birth control may decrease immunosuppressive drug–induced toxicity to the ovary. The possibility of sperm banking should be discussed with male patients prior to institution of immunosuppressive therapy.

THERAPEUTIC ALTERNATIVES

Methotrexate

Given the toxicity of cyclophosphamide in the treatment of systemic necrotizing vasculitides, other immunosuppressive alternatives have been actively sought. Methotrexate may be an effective and less toxic alternative for many patients with systemic necrotizing vasculitis. The mechanism of action of methotrexate in systemic necrotizing vasculitis is not known. The therapeutic effect of methotrexate may be secondary to antifolate activity, immunomodulating effects, immunosuppressive effects, or anti-inflammatory effects on leukocytes. The most reported experience with methotrexate as a second drug has been in the treatment of Wegener's granulomatosis, but anecdotal experience also exists with PAN group syndromes and Takayasu's arteritis (see the chapter *Takayasu's Arteritis*).

Methotrexate should be used in combination with corticosteroids to treat patients with PAN group syndromes and Wegener's granulomatosis that do not have rapidly progressive multisystem disease, life-threatening manifestations, or a serum creatinine of greater than 2.5 mg per deciliter. This regimen should be considered in patients with PAN group diseases and Wegener's granulomatosis who have mild to moderate renal disease, mild to moderate pulmonary disease, mild to moderate disease tempo, and the lack of CNS or severe gastrointestinal difficulties. The patient's concerns regarding fertility may also influence the decision to use methotrexate.

Baseline blood counts, liver function tests, and serum creatinine should be obtained prior to methotrexate therapy. If the hemoglobin (Hgb) level is greater than 10 and liver function tests reveal total bilirubin to be less than 1.5 mg per deciliter, alkaline phosphatase less than 50 percent above upper limits of normal, creatinine less than 2.5 mg per deciliter and SGOT/SGPT less than two times normal, methotrexate therapy can be instituted provided that the patient ceases alcohol intake, is not pregnant, and is not breast feeding. Methotrexate is instituted orally as a single weekly dose of 15 mg. If gastrointestinal symptoms occur, the next dose is given in two divided equal doses at 12-hour intervals once a week. If the gastrointestinal symptoms persist with divided-dose oral methotrexate, it should subsequently be given intramuscularly once a week. If well tolerated for 1 to 2 weeks, the dose is increased by 2.5 mg every week until a dose of 20 to 25 mg per week is reached. This dose is maintained unless there are significant side effects or toxicity of the methotrexate. If renal function is not normal, great care should be exercised as higher dose methotrexate is reached because the major route of methotrexate excretion is the kidneys. Complete blood counts, SGOT, SGPT, and albumin should be monitored every 4 to 6 weeks. If WBC is less than 3,000, SGOT or SGPT rise higher than three times normal, platelets fall to less than 100,000, or Hgb falls to less than 10 mg per deciliter, skipping a dose of methotrexate and downward adjustment by 2.5 to 5 mg per week may be necessary. If SGOT is abnormal, five of nine determinations within a given 12-month interval (six of twelve, if performed monthly), then liver biopsy is indicated to make sure that significant methotrexate hepatotoxicity is not occurring.

If significant improvement in vasculitis clinical activity occurs in the first 4 to 6 weeks, prednisone taper should be begun, as previously described. If remission occurs and is sustained for 1 year of methotrexate therapy, methotrexate taper is begun at the rate of 2.5 mg every 2 to 4 weeks until discontinuation or recurrence of vasculitis disease activity is noted. Potential methotrexate side effects are noted in Table 8. Patients who fail to respond to the combination of corticosteroid and methotrexate within 2 to 3 months or have a significant relapse on the regimen should be treated with the combination of corticosteroids and cyclophosphamide.

Vasculitis Associated with Other Diseases

When vasculitis is associated with other well-defined illnesses, such as collagen-vascular diseases or neoplasms, only the underlying disease should be treated unless the vasculitis is multisystem, rapidly progressive, and life-threatening. In such cases, the vasculitis should

Table 8 Complications of Methotrexate Therapy

Alopecia
Drug-induced pneumonitis
Hepatic toxicity
Abnormal SGOT/SGPT
Fatty liver
Fibrosis
Cirrhosis
Marrow toxicity
Leukopenia
Thrombocytopenia
Anemia, often macrocytic
Nausea, emesis, and weight loss
Oligospermia
Opportunistic infections
Skin rash and photosensitivity
Stomatitis
Teratogenic effects

be treated as a PAN group syndrome with corticosteroids and possibly an immunosuppressive agent.

Conclusion

Systemic vasculitides are often serious and life-threatening illnesses that require aggressive diagnostic and therapeutic approaches. Careful monitoring of treatment with regard to side-effects and efficacy gives these challenging patients the best chance for remission without significant toxicity. Unfortunately, recent studies have shown that relapses are common in patients with a systemic necrotizing vasculitis. This, combined with the potential complications of present therapies, lead to the requirement of life-long and informed monitoring of these patients.

SUGGESTED READING

Gross WL. New developments in the treatment of systemic necrotizing vasculitis. Curr Opin Rheumatol 1994; 6:11–19.

Haynes BF, Allen NB, Fauci AS: Diagnostic and therapeutic approach to the patient with vasculitis. Med Clin North Am 1986; 70:355–368.

Hoffman GS, Kerr GS, Leavitt RY, et al. Wegener's granulomatosis: An Analysis of 158 Patients. Ann Int Med 1992; 116:488–498.

Hoffman GS, Leavitt RY, Kerr GS, Fauci AS. The treatment of Wegener's granulomatosis with glucocorticoids and methotrexate. Arthritis Rheum 1992; 35:1322–1329.

Langford CS, McCallum RM. Idiopathic Vasculitis. In: Belch J, Zurier R, eds. Connective tissue diseases. London: Chapman & Hall, 1995.

CUTANEOUS VASCULITIS

JONATHAN L. COOK, M.D.
THOMAS J. LAWLEY, M.D.

CAUSE AND CLINICAL FEATURES

The clinical hallmark of cutaneous necrotizing (leukocytoclastic) vasculitis is palpable purpura. This usually is most prominent on the distal portion of the lower extremities, but also can occur on thighs, buttocks, trunk, and upper extremities. Other clinical presentations of necrotizing vasculitis can include urticaria-like lesions, hemorrhagic pustules and vesicles, ulcers, and infarcts. The proximate cause of cutaneous vasculitis, no matter what the clinical features, is almost always the deposition of circulating immune complexes in the walls of postcapillary venules. This is followed by local activation of the complement system through the classical pathway and the subsequent generation of the anaphylatoxins C3a, C4a, and C5a. These molecules serve to degranulate periendothelial mast cells, releasing proinflammatory substances such as histamine that can dilate blood vessels causing blood flow to slow and endothelial cells lining the postcapillary venules to rapidly express the cell adhesion molecule P-selectin. C5a is a potent chemoattractant for polymorphonuclear neutrophils that can bind to the microvascular endothelial cells initially via P-selectin and subsequently via LFA-1–ICAM-1 interactions. They then exit the postcapillary venule and release lysosomal enzymes while phagocytosing immune complexes. The lysosomal enzymes act to cause tissue damage.

Cutaneous lesions of necrotizing vasculitis may be a manifestation of a process wholly limited to the skin or, conversely, of a systemic process involving multiple other organ systems. Unfortunately, the clinical presentation is usually not helpful in this regard, although several prominent exceptions exist. For example, palpable purpura or infarcts on the upper extremities, especially involving fingertips, may signal the existence of circulating cryoglobulins. Involvement of these same regions and mucosal surfaces suggests showers of complexes in subacute bacterial endocarditis. Urticarial lesions that last more than 24 hours and show leukocytoclastic vasculitis on biopsy are often indicative of an underlying connective tissue disease such as lupus erythematosus. Prominent livedo reticularis in association with palpable purpura can be seen in various connective tissue diseases, Wegener's granulomatosus, polyarteritis nodosa, and Waldenstrom's hypergammaglobulinemic purpura.

A thorough history and guided laboratory evaluation are important factors in determining whether cutaneous necrotizing vasculitis is a localized or a systemic process. It is especially important to determine whether there is renal or gastrointestinal involvement. This can be screened for by a urinalysis and by testing stools for occult blood. A complete blood count with differential analysis, erythrocyte sedimentation rate, and an SMA18 should be obtained in all instances. Further laboratory testing (e.g., ANA, hepatitis B_sA_g, and so on) can be guided by the history, physical examination, and initial screening laboratory test results.

THERAPY

Most patients with cutaneous vasculitis have a benign clinical course. Resolution of the eruption without cutaneous sequelae is common within the first several months. The cornerstone of therapy for cutaneous vasculitis rests on identification of a presumed trigger for vascular inflammation. When an infectious or hypersensitivity source can be found, removal of this stimulus can produce gratifying improvement.

In cases where no definitive stimulus can be identified and subsequently removed, initial therapy for cutaneous vasculitis should be conservative and directed toward symptomatic relief. Rest, compression, antihistamines, and nonsteroidal anti-inflammatory drugs often relieve patient discomfort. In cases where cutaneous vasculitis has an unusually long duration or is complicated by extensive involvement or ulceration, more aggressive therapy may be required. Above all else, it should be remembered that cutaneous vasculitis is typically a benign process. Treatment should not produce effects more worrisome than those of the underlying disease.

Before aggressive therapy with immunosuppressants is instituted, there are several alternative medications that may produce acceptable results. In some cases, colchicine has been effective in controlling disease activity. Colchicine probably blocks the inflammatory vascular response by interfering with the motility, chemotaxis, phagocytosis, and lysosomal degranulation of neutrophils. In addition, colchicine also has been shown to block histamine and kinin release. In chronic cutaneous vasculitis, colchicine is often given in relatively low doses (0.5 to 1.0 mg per day in divided doses). The drug can be titrated depending on patient response and adverse effects. The most common side effects of colchicine are gastrointestinal; abdominal pain, diarrhea, nausea, and vomiting may limit dosing in some patients. Significantly less frequent side effects of colchicine include bone marrow suppression, CNS toxicity, hepatic failure, and alopecia. Toxic effects are more common in patients with significant hepatic, renal, or bone marrow disease.

Dapsone (diaminodiphenylsulfone) is also useful in some cases of cutaneous vasculitis. Dapsone's mechanism of action is not fully understood, but it may interfere with polymorphonuclear chemotaxis as well as expression of cell adhesion molecules. Although many of the disease processes that respond to dapsone involve neutrophils or immune complexes in their pathogenesis, the precise role of dapsone in modulating the inflammatory response remains speculative. Before dapsone therapy is undertaken, the clinician should evaluate patients for G6PD deficiency, because deficient patients may have profound hemolysis on therapeutic doses of dapsone. Initial doses of dapsone typically range from 50 to 100 mg orally per day. Dapsone doses can also be titrated in response to disease activity. The patient on long-term dapsone should be monitored closely for anemia, methemoglobinemia, and leukopenia, especially during the first 12 weeks of therapy. Some degree of hemolysis is inevitable when taking dapsone. Less frequent side effects of dapsone include peripheral neuropathy, agranulocytosis, renal damage, cholestasis, hypoalbuminemia, and psychosis.

Some cases of cutaneous vasculitis are unusually chronic, recurrent, or severe. In patients with such significant disease, aggressive immunosuppressive therapy is occasionally warranted. Prednisone is the standard therapy for difficult cases of cutaneous vasculitis that fail to respond to more innocuous treatments. Before instituting corticosteroid therapy, the clinician must carefully consider the acute and chronic effects of prednisone on intravascular volume, blood pressure control, glucose metabolism, muscular strength, vision, wound healing, bone retention, and immunologic surveillance. This consideration is particularly relevant in patients with coexisting hypertension, cardiac disease, psychiatric disease, diabetes mellitus, or underlying immunosuppression. Rarely does vasculitis with isolated cutaneous involvement require such potentially toxic therapy. Corticosteroids inhibit the chemotactic response of neutrophils and monocytes/macrophages. They also have important effects on the trafficking of these cells as well as on T and B lymphocytes. In addition, corticosteroids may inhibit the binding of effector inflammatory cells to vascular endothelium at the sites of vascular inflammation. When required, initial prednisone doses are often in the range of 0.5 to 1 mg per kilogram orally per day. This initial dose should be maintained until disease activity is well controlled. While observing for a disease flare, the clinician should strive to lower the corticosteroid dose as much as possible over the course of 4 to 8 weeks. Tapering the prednisone therapy to alternate-day dosing may reduce the chance of some iatrogenic complications. Because the long-term adverse effects of prednisone therapy are significant, this medication should not be continued unless the benefits clearly outweigh the potential toxicities. While tapering the corticosteroid, it may be useful to add other therapeutic agents (e.g., colchicine, dapsone) to attempt to control disease activity on progressively smaller doses of prednisone.

SUGGESTED READING

Hoffman GS, Fauci AS. Emerging concepts in the management of vasculitic disease. Adv Intern Med 1994; 39:277–303.
Jennette CJ, Milling DM, Falk RJ. Vasculitis affecting the skin: A review. Arch Dermatol 1994; 130:899–906.
Swerlick RA, Lawley TJ. Cutaneous vasculitis: Its relationship to systemic disease. Med Clin North Am 1987; 73:1221–1235.
Taylor HG, Samanta A. Treatment of vasculitis. Br J Clin Pharmacol 1993; 35:93–104.

TAKAYASU'S ARTERITIS

CAROL A. LANGFORD, M.D., M.H.S
MICHAEL C. SNELLER, M.D.

Takayasu's arteritis is an idiopathic obliterative vasculitis that affects the aorta, its main branches, and the pulmonary arteries. It is differentiated from other forms of systemic vasculitis not only by its involvement of the great vessels but also by its marked predilection to affect younger women. The clinical spectrum of Takayasu's arteritis has historically been viewed as a triphasic process characterized by an initial systemic or preinflammatory phase, an active vessel inflammatory phase, and a final "burnt-out" or pulseless phase. This classification scheme has limited application to therapeutic management because patients often do not exhibit the classic triphasic pattern of disease and clinical manifestations may not accurately reflect the activity of the inflammatory process taking place within the vessel wall.

CLINICAL FEATURES

The clinical manifestations of Takayasu's arteritis may be of a systemic nature or specifically related to blood vessel stenosis or both. Systemic symptoms are nonspecific and frequently include fatigue, malaise, weight loss, night sweats, fever, arthralgias, or myalgias. Although the presence of systemic symptoms is suggestive of active disease, 13 to 63 percent of patients never experience these features. The possibility of ongoing vascular inflammation cannot be excluded despite the absence of systemic manifestations. The nature of ischemic symptoms is directly related to the anatomic location of stenotic lesion(s), the degree of vessel stenosis, and the availability of collateral blood flow (Table 1). Although new or progressive ischemic symptoms should always prompt an assessment of disease activity, they are not diagnostic of active disease because they may occur in the setting of active vasculitis or be the result of noninflammatory stenosis related to vessel healing. Tenderness over the major arteries may be present and, in particular, carotodynia occurs in 32 percent of patients. When present, this sign is very suggestive of active inflammatory disease. Other important findings on examination that may be useful for diagnosis and disease monitoring include the presence of vascular bruits, diminished pulses, asymmetrical blood pressure measurements in the four extremities, hypertension, and evidence of aortic valvular insufficiency.

No laboratory test is diagnostic or specific for Takayasu's arteritis and findings are often reflective of a generalized inflammatory process. The erythrocyte sedimentation rate (ESR) can be a useful marker of active inflammatory disease, although several studies have not found it to be uniformly reliable. For example, one study demonstrated normal ESR values in one-third of patients felt to have clinically active disease and an elevated ESR in up to 56 percent of patients in remission.

Since pathologic confirmation of vasculitis is usually not possible, arteriography is essential in establishing the diagnosis of Takayasu's arteritis. Other studies such as ultrasound and magnetic resonance imaging are currently being investigated but remain unproven to date. A complete aortic arteriogram with visualization of all its major branches is important in determining the extent of disease since multiple lesions typically occur (see Table 1). In the absence of clinical symptoms or signs, pulmonary and cardiac arteriography does not need to be routinely performed. Interpretation of arteriographic progression is complicated by the fact that vessel stenosis or dilatation may result from either acute vasculitis or noninflammatory fibrosis of healing lesions. Although 88 percent of patients with active disease have been found to have new lesions on follow-up arteriography, 61 percent of patients believed to be in clinical remission also had progressive changes. Thus, arteriography demonstrates luminal patency but does not necessarily provide information on the degree of inflammation present in the arterial wall. Despite this limitation, arteriography remains the best way to follow arterial anatomy and is a valuable tool for following the course of this disease. Repeat arteriographic studies should be obtained for new or progressive ischemic symptoms. In the absence of new symptoms, the frequency of obtaining arteriograms must be determined on an individual basis. Repeat studies at 3- to 12-month intervals may be valuable in guiding therapeutic decisions or in following disease at critical locations. Patients with multiple lesions affecting cerebral blood flow may require more frequent arteriography since the availability of collateral

Table 1 Frequency of Arteriographic Abnormalities and Potential Symptomatic Manifestations of Arterial Involvement in Takayasu's Arteritis

Artery	*Frequency of Arteriographic Abnormalities*	*Potential Symptomatic Manifestations*
Subclavian	93%	Arm claudication, Raynaud's
Common carotid	58%	Visual changes, syncope, transient ischemic attacks, stroke
Abdominal aorta*	47%	Abdominal pain, nausea, vomiting
Renal	38%	Hypertension, renal failure
Aortic arch or root	35%	Aortic insufficiency, congestive heart failure
Vertebral	35%	Visual changes, dizziness
Coeliac axis*	18%	Abdominal pain, nausea, vomiting
Superior mesenteric*	18%	Abdominal pain, nausea, vomiting
Iliac	17%	Leg claudication
Pulmonary	10-40%	Atypical chest pain, dyspnea
Coronary	<10%	Chest pain, myocardial infarction

*Arteriographic lesions at these locations are usually asymptomatic but may potentially cause these symptoms.

circulation may be limited and resultant ischemia potentially catastrophic.

Takayasu's arteritis should be viewed as a chronic and relapsing disease in which 45 percent of patients experience at least one disease relapse and 23 percent of patients never achieve a remission, regardless of medical therapy. In spite of this, Takayasu's arteritis has a low mortality rate, which is primarily influenced by the presence and severity of hypertension, Takayasu's retinopathy, aortic valve insufficiency, aneurysms, and a progressive disease course. In the absence of these manifestations, patients with Takayasu's arteritis have a 5- to 10-year eventless survival rate of 97 percent. Disease-related mortality in patients with Takayasu's is usually due to congestive heart failure, cerebrovascular events, myocardial infarction, and aneurysm rupture.

GENERAL THERAPEUTIC APPROACH

Although medical therapy is usually effective in treating the systemic symptoms of Takayasu's arteritis, its role in the preservation of organ function and improvement of survival has been difficult to assess. Information regarding the natural history of this disease suggests that interruption of active inflammation before the development of significant vessel stenosis may lessen the development of ischemic complications and ultimately improve prognosis. Unfortunately, the limitation in this approach comes from our current inability to accurately assess disease activity. In one series where arterial bypass procedures were performed, 44 percent of patients were found to have histologically active vasculitis in the setting of clinically quiescent disease as judged by our current methods of estimating inflammatory activity.

The four criteria that are most often used to assess inflammatory activity in Takayasu's arteritis are listed in Table 2. As discussed earlier, each of these parameters has its limitations and exceptions when used to assess disease activity. For this reason, we have found it useful to consider these parameters collectively, in which having two or more features is suggestive of active disease. Although these guidelines are helpful, they should not be applied too stringently and other factors need to be considered when making therapeutic decisions in individual patients. These factors include the location and severity of lesions, availability of collateral blood flow, nature and intensity of patient's symptoms, past correlation of an individual patient's laboratory parameters and symptoms with disease activity, and the risks of medication toxicity. Until more sensitive and specific markers of disease activity become available, therapeutic decisions will need to be based on the parameters we currently have available tempered by individual considerations.

Table 2 Criteria for Active Disease in Patients with Takayasu's Arteritis

Elevated erythrocyte sedimentation rate
Systemic symptoms
New or progressive features of vascular ischemia
New or progressive arteriographic changes

Modified from Kerr GS, Hallahan CW, Giordano J, et al. Takayasu arteritis. Ann Intern Med 1994; 120:919–929.

SPECIFIC THERAPEUTIC APPROACH

The inability to assess disease activity has complicated not only individual patient management but the ability to assess the efficacy of therapeutic agents in investigational studies. For this reason, the guidelines for the treatment of Takayasu's are less clearly established than with other forms of systemic vasculitis.

At the time of diagnosis, approximately 20 percent of Takayasu's patients will present with "burnt-out" disease having arterial stenoses with no other evidence of active inflammation. In most instances these individuals do not require medical treatment and can be observed closely. The remaining 80 percent of individuals will have active disease and should receive medical therapy. The goals of treatment include the improvement of symptoms, control of inflammation, and achievement of remission. Remission in Takayasu's arteritis would be defined as that point where there is felt to be no evidence of active disease as best determined by the parameters listed in Table 2.

Glucocorticoids

Glucocorticoids are the foundation of treatment in Takayasu's arteritis. The effectiveness of glucocorticoid therapy has varied greatly in the literature with a range of 20 to 100 percent of patients achieving remission on glucocorticoids alone. Previous studies have suggested that glucocorticoids may halt the arteriographic progression of disease and bring about the return of pulses in some instances. Prednisone is the glucocorticoid of choice because it has a shorter half-life and thus causes less suppression of the hypothalamic-pituitary-adrenal axis than other longer-acting preparations. The starting dosage for prednisone is 1 mg per kilogram per day. Initial divided-dose administration may be more efficacious but carries a higher risk of glucocorticoid-associated toxicity and should therefore be consolidated to a single morning dose as soon as possible. The starting dose is maintained for the first 3 months with careful observation for adverse effects and response. If after that time there is decreased disease activity, the prednisone dose should be tapered to an alternate-day regimen of 1 mg per kilogram per day alternating with 0 mg over the next 2 to 3 months. Once alternate-day therapy is achieved, the glucocorticoids can be slowly tapered and discontinued over the next 3 to 6 months. Although these time estimates should be optimally pursued, it is often necessary to temporarily halt or slow the prednisone taper because signs of active disease develop. One recent study found the median time to remission in glucocorticoid treated patients to be 22 months. Prolonged daily glucocorticoid therapy is associated with many potential complications. Adverse effects include weight gain, acne, osteoporosis, avascular necrosis of bone, myopathy, hyperglycemia, hypertension, cataracts, psychiatric disorders, and increased incidence of infection.

Cytotoxic Therapy

The addition of a cytotoxic agent to glucocorticoids is of less proven benefit in Takayasu's arteritis than in other forms of systemic vasculitis. Cytotoxic therapy should be considered in patients who have evidence of persistent disease activity despite daily glucocorticoid treatment for a 3-month period or when remission cannot be maintained on alternate-day glucocorticoids. Using these criteria, a recent study found that 52 percent of patients required the addition of a cytotoxic agent during the course of their disease with about 40 percent of these patients achieving remission at least once. In considering the choice of cytotoxic agent, methotrexate and cyclophosphamide have both been studied in the treatment of Takayasu's arteritis.

Methotrexate is an inhibitor of folic acid metabolism that has recently been found to be of benefit in the treatment of Takayasu's arteritis. In an open label study of 18 Takayasu's patients, 81 percent achieved remission on methotrexate combined with glucocorticoids. The initial dose for methotrexate is 0.3 mg per kilogram given orally once a week (not to exceed 15 mg a week). This is increased at 1- to 2-week intervals until a final dose of 0.5 mg per kilogram per week is reached (not to exceed 25 mg weekly). Methotrexate should be continued for 1 full year past the disease remission point after which time it is tapered by 2.5 mg increments per month until discontinuation.

Contraindications to methotrexate treatment include pre-existing liver disease, ongoing use of alcoholic beverages, and pregnancy. Caution should also be used when considering methotrexate in patients with severe underlying lung disease. The adverse effects include bone marrow toxicity, pneumonitis, hepatotoxicity, teratogenicity, rash, mucositis, and nausea. Techniques to lessen nausea caused by methotrexate include taking the medication at bedtime, splitting the dose into thirds such that it is still taken over a 24-hour period once a week, use of a mild antiemetic, or intramuscular administration at the same dose. The use of folic acid 1 mg per day may also lessen the potential for adverse effects.

Monitoring studies of complete blood count (CBC) and liver function tests (LFTs) should be obtained every 1 to 2 weeks during dosage titration and every 4 weeks thereafter. Methotrexate should be dose reduced by 2.5 mg increments for an abnormal serum aspartate aminotransferase (AST) on two consecutive determinations. Medication should be held for leukopenia less than 3,000 cells per cubic millimeter, thrombocytopenia less than 80,000 per cubic millimeter, or hematocrit less than 20 percent (in the absence of bleeding or hemolytic anemia) and restarted with the dose reduced by 2.5 mg once the parameters normalize. We do not routinely obtain liver biopsies to monitor for hepatic toxicity, but instead follow the guidelines for biopsy set forth by the American College of Rheumatology in 1994 for the monitoring of methotrexate in rheumatoid arthritis. Reasons for indefinite discontinuation of methotrexate include hemocytopenia or elevated LFTs unresponsive to dosage reduction, active ethanol consumption, pneumonitis, and high-grade fibrosis seen on liver biopsy.

Cyclophosphamide is an alkylating drug that has been of proven benefit in decreasing mortality in other forms of systemic vasculitis. Its use in Takayasu's has been less clearly established although evidence would suggest that it is effective in lessening disease activity, halting the progression of vascular lesions, and decreasing glucocorticoid dosage for some individuals. Therapeutic experience in other forms of systemic vasculitis would suggest that daily oral cyclophosphamide is more efficacious at maintaining remission than monthly pulse intravenous administration. A dose of 2 mg per kilogram per day is the initial starting dose after which the dose is adjusted to maintain the leukocyte count greater than 3,500 per cubic millimeter. Cyclophosphamide should be continued for 1 full year after the disease has entered remission and then slowly tapered and discontinued, decreasing by 25 mg increments each month.

Although potentially effective, cyclophosphamide is a toxic drug with multiple adverse effects. Bone marrow suppression, specifically leukopenia, is seen beginning 7 to 21 days after the initiation of therapy. Blood counts should be monitored every 1 to 3 days during this period and every 1 to 2 weeks thereafter. The dosage of cyclophosphamide should be decreased for signs of decreasing white count and temporarily held for leukocyte counts less than 3,000 per cubic millimeter. When assessing dosage adjustments, it is important to recognize that changes in leukocyte count lag behind changes in cyclophosphamide dosing and generally follow the rule that "this week's counts reflect last week's dose." Leukopenia frequently occurs as glucocorticoids are tapered, and the CBC must be closely monitored during this time.

Other adverse effects of cyclophosphamide include hemorrhagic cystitis and a 5 percent incidence of bladder cancer. To lessen the risk of bladder toxicity, it is crucial that the medication be taken in the morning with large quantities of fluid. If gross hematuria develops, cyclophosphamide should be withheld until this is fully evaluated by cystoscopy. All microscopic hematuria that cannot be readily explained should also be cystoscopically evaluated. We consider bladder carcinoma to be a lifelong risk for all patients treated with cyclophosphamide and currently monitor urine cytology specimens every 6 months. Gonadal dysfunction with permanent sterility and teratogenicity can also occur with cyclophosphamide and are of particular concern in Takayasu's patients given the young female prevalence of this disease. Other adverse effects of cyclophosphamide include an increased incidence of herpes zoster infection, pulmonary fibrosis, hypogammaglobulinemia, myelodysplasia, nausea, and alopecia. Significant hemorrhagic cystitis, dysplastic cytologic changes, hemocytopenia unresponsive to dose reduction, and pulmonary fibrosis are indications for permanent discontinuation of cyclophosphamide.

Although a randomized trial has not been performed, methotrexate appears to be as efficacious as cyclophosphamide in Takayasu's and has substantially less toxicity. Thus, in instances where the addition of a cytotoxic agent is indicated, we favor the initial use of methotrexate rather than cyclophosphamide. Cyclophosphamide should be reserved for patients who have clear evidence of active inflammatory disease in which glucocorticoids are effective but cannot be tapered and where the patient is unresponsive, intolerant, or unable to take methotrexate.

There is little or no information on the use of other cytotoxic agents for the treatment of Takayasu's arteritis. Azathioprine, a purine analogue, has been used in some patients who cannot tolerate cyclophosphamide. It is given at a dose of 2 mg per kilogram per day with the toxicities including bone marrow suppression, hepatotoxicity, nausea, teratogenicity, and a possible increased risk of hematologic malignancies.

In addition to their individual toxicities, there is an increased risk of infection in patients treated concurrently with glucocorticoids and a cytotoxic agent. The majority of these infections occur when patients are on daily glucocorticoids and the risk significantly decreases once the patient is tapered to alternate-day glucocorticoid therapy. Because of the relatively high rate of *Pneumocystis carinii* pneumonia that we and others have observed, we now routinely provide prophylaxis to all patients treated with daily glucocorticoids in combination with a cytotoxic agent. Such prophylaxis consists of low-dose trimethoprim/sulfamethoxazole (trimethoprim 160 mg/sulfamethoxazole 800 mg, three times a week) or monthly inhaled pentamidine, which is continued until the glucocorticoid can be converted to an alternate-day schedule. In our experience, the concomitant use of methotrexate and low-dose trimethoprim/sulfamethoxazole has not been associated with increased bone marrow toxicity.

Other Medical Therapies

Hypertension is seen in 33 percent of Takayasu's patients and frequently occurs secondary to renal artery stenosis. In many individuals, blood pressure monitoring can be inaccurate because of extremity vessel stenoses. Renovascular hypertension can be treated with either medical or nonmedical management. In either setting, the level of blood pressure control must be balanced against the risk of worsening ischemia across stenotic sites that require high pressure to maintain blood flow. Thrombosis of vessels is uncommon in Takayasu's and the routine use of anticoagulants is not recommended. Antiplatelet agents such as aspirin and dipyridamole have been used in some treatment protocols, but their potential benefit has not been studied.

Surgical Therapy

Surgical therapy can be extremely useful for revascularization of stenosed or occluded vessels that are producing significant ischemia. The most frequent indications for surgery include cerebral hypoperfusion, renal vascular hypertension, limb claudication, repair of aneurysms, or valvular insufficiency. In carefully selected patients, the safety and potential benefits of surgery have been favorable although the patency and complication rates have varied greatly. It is recommended that vascular reconstruction be deferred until acute inflammation is medically controlled since aneurysm formation, graft dehiscence, or graft occlusion may be more likely in the setting of active arteritis. However, surgery to prevent imminent ischemia of a vital organ should not be delayed for this reason or because of ongoing immunosuppressive therapy. Aortic valvular insufficiency can occur in Takayasu's patients secondary to aortic root dilatation. Although the indications for valve replacement are similar to those used for patients with aortic insufficiency of other etiologies, anatomical changes unique to Takayasu's can make this surgery more complex. The postoperative results from valvular surgery appear to be good and associated with improvement in clinical status and cardiac function.

Percutaneous transluminal angioplasty (PTCA) can be an effective first-line procedure in facilitating the control of hypertension related to renal artery stenosis. In one series of 48 patients, improved blood pressure control was achieved in 85 percent of patients. The risk of restenosis is highest within the first year and for that reason PTCA is primarily a palliative procedure. PTCA has also recently been used with beneficial results in treating short stenotic segments of the subclavian and coronary arteries as well as the aorta, although less is known about its use in these settings.

SUGGESTED READING

Hoffman GS, Leavitt RY, Kerr GS, et al. Treatment of glucocorticoid-resistant or relapsing Takayasu arteritis with methotrexate. Arthritis Rheum 1994; 37:578–582.

Kerr GS, Hallahan CW, Giordano J, et al. Takayasu arteritis. Ann Intern Med 1994; 120:919–929.

Shelhamer JH, Volkman DJ, Parrillo JE, et al. Takayasu's arteritis and its therapy. Ann Intern Med 1985; 103:121–126.

Tada Y, Sato O, Ohshima A, et al. Surgical treatment of Takayasu arteritis. Heart Vessels 1992; 7(suppl):159–167.

Tyagi S, Singh B, Kaul UA, et al. Balloon angioplasty for renovascular hypertension in Takayasu's arteritis. Am Heart J 1993; 125: 1386–1393.

BEHÇET'S DISEASE

JEFFREY P. CALLEN, M.D.

Behçet's disease is a systemic inflammatory disorder characterized by recurrent aphthous ulcerations of the mouth and/or genitalia; uveitis; vascular lesions; arthritis; and/or central nervous system, pulmonary, and/or gastrointestinal involvement. Vessels of all sizes may be affected in Behçet's disease, and vascular occlusion frequently accompanies vessel wall inflammation. In addition, aneurysms may complicate vascular involvement. Perhaps all of the manifestations of Behçet's disease can be accounted for by inflammation of vessels.

The diagnosis of Behçet's disease is made by exclusion of other disorders that may share common features. There is no test available to confirm or exclude the diagnosis of Behçet's disease with any sensitivity or specificity. Exclusion of systemic lupus erythematosus, inflammatory bowel disease, Reiter's syndrome, and infectious diseases should occur before initiation of therapy.

The cause of Behçet's disease is not known; however, it does appear that there is a genetic predisposition linked to HLA-B51. The mechanism of lesion formation is thought to involve a disorder of the immune system initiated by environmental factors such as bacterial or viral antigens or trace chemicals in a genetically predisposed individual. A delayed hypersensitivity reaction ensues with the eventual release of proinflammatory cytokines such as interleukin-1, interleukin-6, and tumor necrosis factor (TNF). These cytokines can lead to neutrophil hyperfunction and vascular inflammation. The ensuing neutrophilic vascular reaction causes tissue damage to vessels of all sizes. It is believed that the vessel wall damage is responsible for the clinical lesions.

TREATMENT

Before selecting a treatment it is necessary to assess the extent of the disease. This often involves several subspecialists, including dermatologists, rheumatologists, ophthalmologists, neurologists, gastroenterologists, infectious disease specialists, and others. Selection of the appropriate therapy must be based on the organ systems involved and the severity of the involvement. Therapeutic agents routinely used in patients with Behçet's disease along with their indications, dosage, and potential toxicity are presented in Table 1. A discussion of approaches to treatment by organ system follows.

It is possible to simplify the therapeutic approach to the patient with Behçet's disease. For patients with non–life-threatening disease, the therapy involves topical agents, nonsteroidal anti-inflammatory drugs, antihistamines, dapsone, colchicine, and occasionally low-dose weekly methotrexate, or low doses of oral prednisone. In patients with ocular disease that can lead to blindness, CNS disease, or involvement of large vessels, high doses of prednisone with or without an immunosuppressive agent can control the disease. Newer agents such as recombinant interferon-alpha 2a, interleukin-2R antagonist, or interleukin-10 may be effective and less toxic than agents such as chlorambucil, cyclosporin, tacrolimus, or cyclophosphamide. Unfortunately data on cytokine therapy have not yet demonstrated its effectiveness or safety.

Table 1 Systemic Medications in the Treatment of Behçet's Disease

Drug	*Indications*	*Dosage*	*Increased Risk Factors*	*Toxicity*
Colchicine	Aphthae Cutaneous pustular vasculitis	0.6 mg b.i.d.-t.i.d.		Diarrhea, nausea Bone marrow suppression Teratogenicity
Dapsone	Aphthae Cutaneous pustular vasculitis	50-200 mg/day	G6PD deficiency	Hemolytic anemia Peripheral neuropathy
Sulfonamides	Aphthae Cutaneous pustular vasculitis	Varies by agent		Drug eruption
Prednisone	Severe mucocutaneous disease Severe arthritis Ocular involvement Central nervous system disease	0.5-1 mg/kg/day		Osteoporosis Cataracts Hypertension Cushing's syndrome Immunosuppression
Methotrexate	Severe mucocutaneous disease Severe arthritis	5-25 mg/week	Reduced renal function Alcoholism	Hepatotoxicity Diarrhea, nausea Bone marrow suppression Pneumonitis
Azathioprine	Posterior uveitis CNS involvement	1-2.5 mg/kg/day	Thiopurine methyltransferase deficiency	Bone marrow suppression Nausea, vomiting Drug-induced fever Pancreatitis
Chlorambucil	Posterior uveitis CNS involvement Severe vascular involvement	Initial: 2 mg/day Maximum: To control or toxicity		Bone marrow suppression Nausea, vomiting Risk of malignancy Sterility
Cyclophosphamide	Posterior uveitis CNS involvement Severe vascular involvement	1-2 mg/kg/day		Bone marrow suppression Nausea, vomiting Risk of malignancy Sterility Hemorrhagic cystitis
Cyclosporine	Posterior uveitis	5 mg/kg/day	Hypertension Reduced renal function	Nephrotoxicity Immunosuppression Possible subsequent neoplasia
Interferon-α 2a	Mucocutaneous disease	3-12 million units, 3 times/week		Fever Flulike symptoms

Mucocutaneous Disease

The therapy of oral and genital aphthae as well as cutaneous pustular lesions is similar. These lesions rarely respond to topical therapy with corticosteroids. Intralesional triamcinolone acetonide is at times temporarily beneficial, but its administration can be traumatic and can result in a spread of the lesion via the phenomenon of pathergy. When adequate relief is not obtained with topical or intralesional corticosteroid therapy, oral colchicine 0.6 mg twice daily may be tried. This drug results in an improvement within days to weeks. If it is not effective within 2 weeks, the dosage may be increased or the drug abandoned. Oral dapsone is a second-line systemic agent. After an appropriate pretherapy evaluation, dapsone is begun at a dosage of 25 mg per day. The dosage can gradually be raised to 200 mg per day if laboratory and/or clinical evidence of toxicity does not occur. Lastly, a recent open trial has demonstrated benefits from oral pentoxyfylline for oral aphthae.

Although oral corticosteroids are effective for the mucocutaneous manifestations of Behçet's disease, their long-term administration is associated with multiple side effects. If dapsone and/or colchicine are ineffective as steroid-sparing agents, the use of low-dose weekly methotrexate should be considered. Methotrexate may be given in doses of 5 to 25 mg per week. After a complete assessment, methotrexate can be begun at a low dose that is raised weekly or biweekly following determinations of complete blood counts and liver function tests. Long-term usage may be required, but whether or not a liver biopsy should be used to monitor Behçet's disease patients has not been determined. The guidelines of the American College of Rheumatology for methotrexate usage in patients with rheumatoid arthritis should be followed.

Other agents that can be considered for mucocutaneous disease include thalidomide and interferon-alpha 2a. A study by Jorizzo and colleagues, found that thalidomide was extremely effective and postulated that the mechanism of action may be via its ability to inhibit immune-complex–mediated vessel wall damage. Unfortunately, this agent is difficult, if not impossible, to obtain for use in the United States because of its well known teratogenicity.

Interferon-alpha 2a was studied in an open-label trial by Alpsoy and associates. They initially administered 3 million units of subcutaneous interferon-alpha 2a three times per week, but gradually increased the dose to 12 million units three times per week. The study period was 2 months, but treatment with 9 million units three times per week was continued in 7 of the 14 patients for 6 months. All patients became symptom-free by the end of the 2-month treatment period, and in some this symptom-free period was maintained even after the cessation of therapy. The most dramatic response was noted for the oral and genital ulcerations, as well as the pustular vasculitis, but positive effects on arthritic complaints and eye disease were also noted. There were too few patients with serious vascular or central nervous system involvement to study the use of interferon in this subset. The usual toxic reaction of a flulike syndrome was noted in the early phases of the treatment, but was controlled with the administration of oral acetominophen.

Synovitis

Arthritis occurs in approximately one-half of the patients with Behçet's disease. Joint involvement is typically oligoarthritic and nonerosive and the disease may affect large or small joints. Therapy is similar to that for other seronegative arthritides; however, agents used to treat the mucocutaneous disease are frequently effective for therapy of the arthritis.

Uveitis

Uveitis occurs in about one-half of the patients with Behçet's disease, and the potential for blindness is the most important morbidity that occurs from the disease. Uveitis may affect the anterior or posterior segment. Anterior uveitis may be treated with topical applications of corticosteroids and, if necessary, agents to reduce ocular pressure. Posterior uveitis is believed to be the result of a retinal vasculitis and tends to be closely linked to disease in the central nervous system. Posterior uveal involvement is the primary cause of blindness. The ability to reduce the risk of blindness is justification for the use of therapeutic agents associated with potential toxicity.

Systemic corticosteroids, such as high-dose prednisone (1 to 2 mg per kilogram per day), have traditionally been the initial treatment of choice for patients with Behçet's disease. However, corticosteroids often are not sufficient to adequately suppress retinal disease, and immunosuppressive/cytotoxic agents are usually recommended early in the course of the disease. Azathioprine, chlorambucil, cyclophosphamide, cyclosporine, and tacrolimus are available and have been suggested as disease-altering, steroid-sparing agents for serious ocular and/or central nervous system involvement. Unfortunately, there are few adequately controlled trials that compare these agents. Thus, recommendations are largely empiric and are often based on familiarity with the drug, dependent upon the institution within which the treating physician trained.

Azathioprine is given in a single morning dose of 2 to 3 mg per kilogram per day. In a recent double-blind, placebo-controlled trial, azathioprine was demonstrated to prevent the development of ocular disease in patients without ocular involvement, and to prevent the development of involvement of the second eye in patients with unilateral involvement. However, the drug was not effective in improving the visual acuity in treated patients. Furthermore, there is little if any data that indicate that azathioprine can effect a long-term remission. Therefore, although azathioprine is less toxic than the other available agents, it is apparently less efficacious.

Chlorambucil is administered in a dosage of 2 mg per day initially and raised by 2 mg per day weekly until the disease becomes quiescent, or there is evidence of toxicity. This therapy is usually effective within 3 to 9 months and has been associated with improvement of visual acuity and long-term remissions. After ocular disease is controlled, chlorambucil dosage can be reduced and often stopped. Relapses generally will respond to readministration of the drug. Chlorambucil may be used with corticosteroids, in which case the corticosteroids are usually tapered and stopped prior to tapering the chlorambucil, or it can be used as the sole therapy in selected patients. Long-term low-dose therapy is at times necessary. The unfortunate risks of neoplasia (leukemia or lymphoma) and permanent sterility (azospermia or anovulation) must be considered and discussed with the patient at the onset of therapy.

Cyclophosphamide, another alkylating agent, has also been demonstrated to be effective in some patients with Behçet's disease. It has been less well studied than chlorambucil, but would be predicted to carry roughly the same benefits based upon its pharmacology. However, in addition to the risks of subsequent malignancy and sterility, hemorrhagic cystitis is also associated with its administration. Recently, cyclophosphamide has been administered via an intermittent high-dose pulse therapy, and it has demonstrated benefits for severe uveitis and central nervous system disease.

Cyclosporine has also been used for treatment of patients with uveitis due to Behçet's disease. It has been demonstrated to reduce the number of ocular attacks and improve visual acuity, but its use has not resulted in long-term remissions. In addition, cyclosporine has seemingly not been effective for therapy of central nervous system involvement, intestinal involvement, or vascular lesions.

Tacrolimus (FK-506) is the newest immunosuppressive agent used for the prevention of transplant rejection. To date there have not been reports documenting efficacious use in Behçet's disease patients.

Central Nervous Disease and Systemic Vascular Involvement

Treatment of central nervous disease and systemic vascular involvement is identical to that for posterior uveal tract involvement. Therapy involves the use of an immunosuppressive/cytotoxic agent with or without high-dose corticosteroids.

SUGGESTED READING

Alpsoy E, Yilmaz E, Basaran E. Interferon therapy for Behçet's disease. J Am Acad Dermatol 1994; 31:617–619.

Hashimoto T, Takeuchi A. Treatment of Behçet's disease. Curr Opin Rheumatol 1992; 4:31–34.

Jorizzo JL, Rogers RS. Behçet's disease: An update on the International Conference held in Rochester, Minnesota, September 14 and 15, 1989. J Am Acad Dermatol 1990; 23:738–740.

Jorizzo JL, Schmalsteig FC, Solomon AR, et al. Thalidomide effects in Behçet's syndrome and pustular vasculitis. Arch Intern Med 1986; 146:878–881.

Jorizzo JL, White WL, Wise CM, et al. Low-dose weekly methotrexate for unusual neutrophilic vascular reactions: Cutaneous polyarteritis nodosa and Behçet's disease. J Am Acad Dermatol 1991; 24: 973–978.

Katz J, Langevitz P, Shemer J, et al. Prevention of recurrent aphthous stomatitis with colchicine: An open trial. J Am Acad Dermatol 1994; 31:459–461.

O'Duffy JD, Kokmen E, eds. Behçet's disease: Basic and clinical aspects. New York: Marcel Dekker, 1991.

Stratigos AJ, Laskaris G, Stratigos JD: Behçet's disease. Semin Neurol 1992; 12:346–357.

COGAN'S SYNDROME

REX M. McCALLUM, M.D.

First described by Dr. David Cogan in 1945, Cogan's syndrome is a rare clinical entity of unknown etiology, occurring primarily in young adults but described in patients of all ages. The syndrome is characterized by inflammatory eye disease, typically nonsyphilitic interstitial keratitis, and vestibuloauditory dysfunction, typically Meniere's-like. Interstitial keratitis is either acute and recurrent or chronic and may vary in intensity from day to day and from eye to eye. Presenting ocular symptoms are ocular discomfort (90 percent), redness (79 percent), and photophobia (68 percent). Examination of the eyes of patients with Cogan's syndrome reveals interstitial keratitis in 72 percent, conjunctivitis in 34 percent, iritis in 32 percent, and episcleritis/scleritis in 28 percent. Presenting vestibuloauditory symptoms are vertigo (85 percent), sudden hearing loss (79 percent), sudden nausea and vomiting (70 percent), tinnitus (53 percent), ataxia (45 percent), and gradual decrease in hearing (17 percent). In addition to these Meniere's-like presenting symptoms, vestibuloauditory features eventually include hearing loss in 92 percent, nystagmus in 32 percent, oscillopsia in 15 percent, Meniere's-like symptoms without hearing loss in 4 percent, and hearing loss without Meniere's-like symptoms in 4 percent of patients. Initial symptoms and signs are ocular in 50 percent of patients, vestibuloauditory in 25 percent, and both ocular and vestibuloauditory within 1 month of one another in 25 percent.

Fifty percent of patients with Cogan's syndrome have an antecedent upper respiratory illness. The most important systemic complication is the development of aortitis and/or systemic necrotizing vasculitis in 10 to 12 percent of patients. Vascular complications may be more frequent in patients with ocular manifestations other than interstitial keratitis, conjunctivitis, and iritis. Previous literature has divided these patients into "typical" and "atypical" subsets based upon the presence of only interstitial keratitis, conjunctivitis, and/or iritis (typical) versus other types of ocular inflammation (atypical). Given that "typical" patients can subsequently develop "atypical" features, these clinical subsets have been found to be less clinically useful than once thought.

PREFERRED APPROACH AND THERAPEUTIC ALTERNATIVES

Ocular

Topical Corticosteroids

Topical corticosteroids are indicated for the control of corneal and anterior ocular inflammation. Therapy should be begun as soon as the diagnosis of interstitial keratitis and/or anterior ocular inflammation is confirmed and differential diagnostic possibilities with contraindications to isolated topical corticosteroids such as herpes keratitis are dismissed. Of course, this requires careful slit lamp and ocular evaluation by an ophthalmologist. One percent prednisolone is a frequently used topical corticosteroid, although a number of alternatives exist and weaker topical corticosteroids (e.g., fluorometholone) may be sufficient to treat moderate interstitial keratitis. Topical corticosteroids may be required every 1 to 2 hours during the acute stages of inflammation. Topical mydriatic solution or ointment such as homatropine is indicated if iritis is present, to prevent synechia formation. Oral nonsteroidal drugs such as indomethacin can be used alone or in combination with topical corticosteroids to treat episcleritis/scleritis.

Once appropriate response is noted, ocular therapies can be tapered over 3 to 6 weeks with careful monitoring for recurrent ocular inflammation. Between flares of ocular inflammation, no topical or other ophthalmic therapy is necessary. Topical corticosteroid therapy improves ocular inflammation by preventing the egress of inflammatory cells into ocular tissues (Table 1). The most common adverse effects of topical ocular corticosteroid therapy are elevation in intraocular pressure, conjunctival irritation, and (with chronic use) cataract formation.

Systemic corticosteroids are rarely required to

Table 1 Mechanisms of Corticosteroid Immunosuppressive and Anti-Inflammatory Effects

Inhibition of accumulation of monocytic macrophages at inflammatory sites
Blockage of accumulation of neutrophils at inflammatory sites
Selective depletion of T lymphocytes more than B lymphocytes
Suppression of lymphocytic function in
  Delayed hypersensitivity skin testing by inhibiting monocyte recruitment
  Lymphocytic proliferation to antigens
  Mixed lymphocytic proliferation
  Spontaneous (natural) cytotoxicity
Suppression of monocytic-macrophage function in
  Cutaneous delayed hypersensitivity by inhibition of lymphokine effect on macrophages
  Blockage of Fc–receptor binding and function
  Bactericidal activity
  Inhibition of interleukin-1 production
Decreased reticuloendothelial clearance of antibody-coated cells
Decreased synthesis of prostaglandin and leukotrienes
Inhibition of plasminogen activator release
Antagonism of histamine-induced vasodilation
Effect on cytokines
  Decreased production of interleukin-1

control ocular inflammation in Cogan's syndrome, except in the uncommon patient with posterior ocular inflammation (papillitis, posterior scleritis, retinochoroiditis have all been described). The rare patient with progressive visual loss on systemic corticosteroids should be considered for a trial of additional immunosuppressive therapy, such as cyclophosphamide or cyclosporin A (for details regarding the use of these drugs see following discussion).

Table 2 Example of Corticosteroid Therapy for Hearing Loss in Cogan's Syndrome

At the time of diagnosis begin prednisone therapy:

Dose	*Frequency*	*Length of Therapy*
15 mg	Four times per day	5 days
20 mg	Three times per day	2 days
30 mg	Two times per day	2 days
60 mg	Once a day in the AM	15 days

At this time the taper to alternate-day therapy begins:

"High-Day" Dose	*"Low-Day" Dose*	*Length of Therapy*
60 mg	50 mg	4 days
60 mg	40 mg	4 days
60 mg	30 mg	4 days
60 mg	20 mg	4 days
60 mg	15 mg	4 days
60 mg	10 mg	4 days
60 mg	7.5 mg	4 days
60 mg	5 mg	4 days
60 mg	2.5 mg	4 days
60 mg	0 mg	4 days

The alternate-day dose can be tapered after the patient has been stable for 2 to 4 weeks on alternate-day therapy. The above regimen is only an example of a corticosteroid taper scheme. The design and tempo of a regimen for individual patients must rely on each patient's clinical signs and symptoms and their response to therapy

Vestibuloauditory

Corticosteroids

Acute hearing loss associated with Cogan's syndrome may be significantly improved by systemic corticosteroid therapy. The initial trial of corticosteroids may be given orally or intravenously in a divided dose of 1 to 2 mg per kilogram body weight per day prednisone or equivalent therapy. The major indication for intravenous treatment is the inability to take oral medication. Depending upon the response and severity of symptoms, divided dose therapy is continued for 3 to 10 days with subsequent consolidation to a single daily morning dose. If hearing improves, a taper to alternate-day corticosteroid therapy is begun after 2 to 4 weeks of treatment. Taper to alternative-day therapy can be accomplished in 6 weeks by following the protocol outlined in Table 2. If clinical parameters such as auditory symptoms, erythrocyte sedimentation rate, ocular inflammation, and audiogram reveal continued evidence of therapeutic response, the corticosteroids can then be tapered from alternate-day 60 mg to 0 mg over the subsequent 6 to 8 weeks. An occasional patient with Cogan's syndrome will not tolerate taper to alternate-day corticosteroid therapy. Such individuals should be tapered to the least effective daily dose of corticosteroids. The mechanisms of action of corticosteroids are reviewed in Table 1. The adverse effects of systemic corticosteroid therapy are noted in Table 3.

If no response is noted after 2 to 3 weeks of corticosteroid treatment, therapeutic options include accepting corticosteroid failure and helping patients to cope with their hearing loss or a trial of other immunosuppressive therapy. The efficacy of additional immunosuppressive therapy in the face of primary corticosteroid failure has never been established. If no additional immunosuppressive therapy is started, corticosteroids should be tapered to discontinuation as rapidly as is possible (i.e., over 2 to 4 weeks). If an additional immunosuppressive drug trial is instituted, corticosteroids should be tapered more slowly to allow the new immunosuppressive agent to become effective before the corticosteroids are discontinued (i.e., over 4 to 6 weeks). Alternative immunosuppressive therapies are discussed in detail in the following discussion.

If the patient notices that auditory acuity persistently decreases (longer than 3 to 5 days), with attempted corticosteroid taper, an increase in corticosteroid dose by a factor of two (up to 1 mg per kilogram body weight per day) is indicated. If subsequent attempts to taper the corticosteroids are also associated with decreased auditory acuity, a trial of other immunosuppressive therapy should be considered, unless the effective dose of

Table 3 Adverse Effects of Systemic Corticosteroid Therapy

Central nervous system difficulties
Altered morale/personality
Steroid psychosis
Pseudotumor cerebri
Cutaneous difficulties
Violaceous striae
Subcutaneous tissue atrophy
Cushingoid habitus
Purpura and ecchymosis
Acne
Hirsutism
Facial erythema
Deposition of fatty tissue
Moon facies
Buffalo hump
Mediastinal lipomatosis
Hepatomegaly
Delayed wound healing (including peptic ulceration)
Endocrine and metabolic difficulties
Hyperglycemia
Osteoporosis
Suppression of the hypothalamic-pituitary-adrenal axis
Hypokalemic alkalosis
Fluid retention
Hypertension
Growth retardation
Proximal myopathy
Hyperlipoproteinemia
Menstrual irregularity
Immunosuppression
Ocular difficulties
Cataracts
Glaucoma
Exophthalmos
Opportunistic infection
Osteonecrosis
Pancreatitis
Weight gain

prednisone is 10 mg per day or less. Other immunosuppressive therapies appear to be effective in "steroid sparing" for some patients whose hearing responds to corticosteroid therapy, but they cannot be tapered to an acceptably low dose in patients who suffer unacceptable side effects. Criteria for response and length of treatment should be established before instituting any other immunosuppressive therapy. Such criteria might include stabilized or improved hearing on a lesser dose of corticosteroid (ideally 10 mg per day or less) after 3 months of additional immunosuppressive therapy. Immunosuppressive alternatives include cyclophosphamide, methotrexate, azathioprine, cyclosporin A, and FK-506.

Cyclophosphamide

Cyclophosphamide is the drug of choice for patients who fail to respond to corticosteroid therapy, who require corticosteroid doses for auditory stability that are unacceptable in the long term (e.g., > 10 mg per day), and those who continue to experience auditory decline despite their corticosteroid therapy. Cyclophosphamide is begun at 2 mg per kilogram body weight per day. This dose is maintained for 2 to 4 weeks. If evidence of favorable clinical response is noted, the dose is maintained at this level with subsequent adjustments to keep the white blood cell (WBC) count at greater than 3,000 cells per cubic millimeter. Suppressing the WBCs to a level of 3,000 cells per cubic millimeter represents the most aggressive level of immunosuppression, but many patients will note improvement with WBCs in the range of 4,000 to 5,000 cells per cubic millimeter. If there is no evidence of favorable clinical response in 2 to 4 weeks, the daily cyclophosphamide dose should be increased by 25 mg every 2 weeks until appropriate response is noted or until drug toxicity occurs (Table 4). The complete blood count (CBC) should be monitored 1 to 2 times per week for the first 2 weeks of therapy and with any increase in cyclophosphamide dose. Subsequently, the CBC can be monitored weekly. The physician must remember that the dose of cyclophosphamide taken each day has the maximum effect on the WBC count 7 to 10 days later; therefore, changes in the cyclophosphamide dose must anticipate the general trend in the WBCs to avoid counts of less than 3,000 cells per cubic millimeter. Cyclophosphamide should be continued with careful monitoring of disease activity and potential adverse drug effects (see Table 4) for 6 to 12 months after auditory acuity is believed to have been stabilized. Subsequently, the cyclophosphamide should be reduced 25 mg per day every 1 to 2 months until it is discontinued, provided that auditory acuity and clinical status remain stable. The mechanisms of immunosuppressive properties for cyclophosphamide are reviewed in Table 5.

Table 4 Adverse Effects of Cyclophosphamide Therapy

Alopecia
Antidiuretic hormone effect at higher doses
Bladder Toxicity
Hemorrhagic cystitis
Bladder fibrosis
Bladder cancer
Hypogammaglobulinemia
Lymphoma/leukemia
Marrow toxicity
Neutropenia/leukopenia
Thrombocytopenia
Anemia, often macrocytic
Leukemia
Nausea and emesis
Opportunistic infection
Pulmonary interstitial fibrosis
Reproductive system
Premature ovarian failure
Infertility
Sterility
Teratogenesis

As the corticosteroid dose is tapered, the cyclophosphamide dose may have to be tapered because corticosteroids protect the patient's bone marrow from some of cyclophosphamide's effect on lowering the WBC count. A taper to alternate-day corticosteroids often requires a 25 to 50 mg decrease in the cyclophosphamide daily

Table 5 Mechanisms of Immunosuppressive Properties of Cyclophosphamide

Lymphocytopenia of both T and B lymphocytes
Suppression of in vitro lymphocyte blastogenic response to specific antigens
Suppression of antibody response and cutaneous delayed hypersensitivity to new antigen
Selective suppression of in vitro B lymphocytic function with decrease in immunoglobulin production and suppression of mitogen-induced immunoglobulin production
Reduction in serum immunoglobulin levels

dose. Prolonged cyclophosphamide therapy may be associated with diminished drug tolerance, necessitating further reductions in the daily cyclophosphamide dose. Finally, decreased renal function also requires modification of the cyclophosphamide dose because active cyclophosphamide metabolites are cleared renally; therefore, peak drug-induced effects on WBCs may be prolonged. In the setting of a creatinine clearance of less than 15 ml per minute the dose of cyclophosphamide should be reduced to 1 mg per kilogram body weight per day.

Patients receiving cyclophosphamide should be told to drink fluids to maintain 3 liters of urine output per day to decrease the drug-induced toxicity to the bladder. A careful history of bladder function should be obtained and suggestions of bladder-outlet obstruction and neurogenic bladder should be appropriately evaluated and treated. The failure to empty the bladder may increase the risk of developing cyclophosphamide-related bladder toxicity. Patients treated with daily oral cyclophosphamide require lifelong follow-up regarding their increased risk of bladder cancer. All hematuria (gross and microscopic) should be evaluated with cystoscopy to investigate the possibility of bladder cancer. Yearly urine cystoscopies should also be performed. If hemorrhagic cystitis complicates a course of cyclophosphamide therapy, methotrexate or azathioprine (see below) should be used to replace the cyclophosphamide.

Methotrexate and Azathioprine

Methotrexate and azathioprine are the principal therapeutic alternatives to cyclophosphamide in the treatment of hearing loss in patients with Cogan's syndrome. Methotrexate is used in doses of 12.5 to 25 mg per week. Methotrexate's dosing, contraindications, monitoring, potential side effects, and possible mechanisms of action are discussed under the Therapeutic Alternatives section of the chapter *Systemic Necrotizing Vasculitis.*

Azathioprine is begun at a dose of 2 mg per kilogram body weight per day in a single morning dose. If gastrointestinal intolerance is noted, the dose may be divided into two or three doses per day. If no response is noted within 3 to 4 weeks, the dose should be increased by 25 mg every 2 to 3 weeks until the desired response is noted, toxicity ensues, a dose of 3 mg per kilogram body weight per day is reached, or the WBC count falls to 3,000 cells per cubic millimeter. Initially, the CBC is monitored weekly with a decrease to every other week after 3 to 4 weeks. Weekly monitoring is resumed with an increase in the azathioprine dose. The mechanisms of immunosuppressive properties of azathioprine are reviewed in Table 6 and the adverse effects are noted in Table 7. If azathioprine is not effective within 3 to 4 months of treatment, it should be discontinued as ineffective. Other alternatives, such as methotrexate, cyclosporin A, and FK-506 could be considered at that time. Cyclosporin A is discussed in detail in the following discussion and FK-506 presently has limited availability.

Table 6 Mechanisms of Immunosuppressive Properties of Azathioprine

Decrease the total number of T and B lymphocytes
Suppression of gamma globulin synthesis
Suppression of antibody response to vaccination, particularly the secondary response
Suppression of B-lymphocyte proliferation
Inhibition of the production of monocytes

Table 7 Adverse Effects of Azathioprine Therapy

Alopecia
Drug interactions
Allopurinol
Angiotensin-converting enzyme inhibitors
Exaggerated effect in other drugs that affect myelopoesis
Gastrointestinal intolerance
Nausea and emesis
Diarrhea
Hepatotoxicity
Marrow suppression
Leukopenia
Thrombocytopenia and anemia rare
Neoplasia
Lymphoma
Skin cancer
Others
Opportunistic infections
Skin rash
Teratogenicity

Patients with Cogan's syndrome can develop cochlear hydrops, a swollen, fluid-filled, damaged cochlea, after a period of persistent or recurrent inflammation. Cochlear hydrops can be associated with hearing fluctuations that are not inflammatory in origin and are generally short lived (hours to 3 to 5 days). Hearing fluctuations secondary to cochlear hydrops may be precipitated by the menstrual cycle in women, eating salty foods, allergies, or upper respiratory illnesses. Absolute distinction between hearing fluctuation due to cochlear hydrops and the inflammation that is Cogan's syndrome is impossible, but hearing fluctuation associated with elevated erythrocyte sedimentation rate, recurrent ocular inflammation, and increased vestibular symptoms suggests recurrent inflammation. Hearing down fluctuations believed to be secondary to inflammation should be documented with audiology and treated with increased doses of corticosteroids to 0.3 to 1.0 mg per kilogram body weight per day, depending on the degree of the hearing fluctuation and the previous dose of corticosteroid therapy. Corticosteroid tapering can be instituted soon after a response, if the response is rapid, or more slowly if the response requires many days or weeks to occur. An elevated dose of corticosteroids and tapering over only 10 to 14 days may be effective for mild to moderate hearing fluctuations that respond rapidly to an increase in the corticosteroid dose, whereas a taper over 6 to 12 weeks may be necessary for a hearing fluctuation that is more severe and requires many days to weeks to respond. If the hearing fluctuation is not believed to be inflammatory in origin, monitoring of auditory status without change in corticosteroid or immunosuppressive therapy, institution of diuretic therapy (e.g., hydrochlorothiazide 25 to 50 mg each morning) for presumed cochlear hydrops, and time may lead to resolution of the downward change in auditory status. If no improvement is appreciated in 3 to 5 days, a trial of corticosteroid therapy should be considered.

All patients with Cogan's syndrome and hearing loss should be directed to classes in lip reading and sign language and encouraged to enroll, since the response to therapy is not predictable. Patients find it easier to learn these skills while they can hear, and lip reading skills help to compensate for moderate loss of auditory acuity.

Inflammatory Vascular Manifestations

The inflammatory vascular complications of Cogan's syndrome assume two forms, a proximal aortitis and a systemic necrotizing vasculitis. The development of aortic insufficiency in a patient with Cogan's syndrome implies aortitis, unless another clear-cut etiology is evident. Two dimensional echocardiography is indicated to assess the degree of regurgitate flow, search for vegetations, and assess left ventricular function. Four to six blood cultures should be performed to rule out infective endocarditis, and corticosteroid therapy is started in divided dose at 1 mg per kilogram body weight per day. When cultures are negative at 3 to 5 days, cyclophosphamide should be instituted at a dose of 2 mg per kilogram body weight per day. Corticosteroids and cyclophosphamide should be continued and tapered in the manner used to treat systemic necrotizing vasculitis (see the chapter *Systemic Necrotizing Vasculitis*), while monitoring the patient's cardiac status by clinical examination and follow-up echocardiography. Many patients who develop aortitis have required aortic valve replacement subacutely because of congestive heart failure. The development of angina in the face of aortitis is an indication for coronary angiography, given the frequent association of coronary ostial stenosis with aortitis. Methotrexate, also used in the manner described for the treatment of systemic necrotizing vasculitis, is an alternative to the use of cyclophosphamide.

Table 8 Adverse Effects of Cyclosporin A Therapy

Gastrointestinal
- Nausea and emesis
- Hepatotoxicity
- Diarrhea

Gum hypertrophy
Hirsutism
Hyperkalemia
Hypertension
Hypomagnesemia
Neoplasms
- Lymphoreticular
- Others

Nephrotoxicity
Nervous system
- Tremor
- Headache
- Paresthesias

Opportunistic infections

Cyclosporin A

Systemic necrotizing vasculitis associated with Cogan's syndrome is most frequently large vessel vasculitis (Takayasu's-like), although medium vessel vasculitis (polyarteritis nodosa–like) has been described. Large vessel vasculitis (Takayasu's-like) associated with Cogan's syndrome is treated with cyclosporin A, beginning with doses of 5 mg per kilogram body weight per day in two equal doses and corticosteroids at a dose of 1 to 2 mg per kilogram body weight per day in divided doses. Cyclosporin A is begun only if baseline creatinine is within normal limits and the patient's blood pressure is well controlled. With a clinical response noted by decrease in erythrocyte sedimentation rate, improved ischemic symptoms (if present), improved pulses, lack of new pulse abnormalities, and improved associated symptoms (e.g., myalgias and arthralgias), the corticosteroids can be consolidated to a single morning dose. As long as the clinical situation is stable, the corticosteroids can be tapered to alternate-day therapy and subsequently discontinued, as is discussed in regard to the use of corticosteroids in the treatment of systemic necrotizing vasculitis.

While using cyclosporin A therapy, CBC, electrolytes, creatinine, liver function tests, magnesium, and blood pressure are monitored every 2 weeks initially, with a change to once a month if no difficulties arise after 4 to 6 weeks. If blood pressure rises, this should be aggressively treated with beta-blockers, nifedipine, and/or angiotensin converting enzyme inhibitors. Diuretics should be avoided. If blood pressure does not come into the normal range within 2 to 4 weeks, decreasing the cyclosporin A dose by 25 to 50 mg per day may be necessary. A rise in the serum creatinine of greater than 30 percent over baseline also requires a decrease in the cyclosporin A dose by 25 to 50 mg per day with repeat studies in 2 to 3 weeks. If creatinine is no longer greater than 30 percent over the baseline, the new dose of cyclosporin A can be continued. If the repeat creatinine remains greater than 30 percent above

Table 9 Partial Listing of Drug Interactions with Cyclosporin A

Nephrotoxic synergy
Gentamicin
Tobramycin
Vancomycin
Cimetidine
Ranitidine
Diclofenac
Amphotericin B
Ketoconazole
Melphalan
Trimethoprim/sulfamethoxazole
Azapropazone
Increase cyclosporin A levels
Diltiazem
Nicardipine
Verapamil
Danazol
Bromocriptine
Metoclopramide
Ketoconazole
Fluconazole
Itraconazole
Erythromycin
Methylprednisolone
Decrease cyclosporin A levels
Rifampin
Phenobarbital
Phenytoin
Carbamazepine
Miscellaneous
Prednisolone
Digoxin
Lovastatin
Potassium-sparing diuretics

baseline, further adjustment in cyclosporin A dose is necessary.

Hypomagnesemia may be noted and require replacement therapy. Persistently elevated SGOT and/or SGPT levels of greater than two times normal and 4 to 6 weeks' duration also require a decrease in the cyclosporin A dose with careful monitoring for appropriate response.

The immunosuppressive effects of cyclosporin A occur via the potent inhibition of T-lymphocyte activation mediated through inhibition of early T lymphocyte actvation genes and cytokine production. The adverse effects of cyclosporin A treatment are reviewed in Table 8. A partial listing of drug interactions with cyclosporin A is found in Table 9. Cyclosporin A is continued for 9 to 12 months beyond the time the large vessel vasculitis is believed to be in remission with a subsequent taper by 25 to 50 mg per month to 0 mg over 3 to 6 months, while carefully monitoring the patient for signs of recurrent vascular inflammation. Alternative treatments for large vessel vasculitis are discussed in detail in the chapter *Takayasu's Arteritis.*

Medium vessel vasculitis (polyarteritis nodosa–like) associated with Cogan's syndrome is treated in a manner identical to that described for polyarteritis nodosa group vasculitides in the chapter *Systemic Necrotizing Vasculitis.* The preferred approach and therapeutic alternatives are also reviewed in this chapter.

DISCUSSION

Ocular outcomes in patients with Cogan's syndrome are good. In the Duke/National Institutes of Health series, only 2 of 31 (6 percent) patients with available follow-up data manifested visual acuity of worse than 20/30 in either eye. In the literature, blindness and severe visual loss are associated with ocular inflammation beyond the anterior segment of the eye. Progression to deafness is common and is clearly the most frequent serious and debilitating consequence of Cogan's syndrome. Twenty-one of 78 (27 percent) ears with available data were deaf in the Duke/National Institutes of Health series. Aggressive and early treatment of hearing loss likely provides the best long-term results for these patients. Inflammatory vascular symptoms generally respond to the therapeutic endeavors discussed here. Aortitis and/or systemic necrotizing vasculitis have stabilized or gone into clinical remission in four of the five patients in the Duke/National Institutes of Health series manifesting these difficulties.

SUGGESTED READING

Allen NB, Cox CC, Cobo LM, et al. Use of immunosuppressive agents in the treatment of severe ocular and vascular manifestation of Cogan's syndrome. Am J Med 1990; 88:296–301.

Haynes BF, Kaiser-Kupfer MI, Mason P, Fauci AS. Studies in thirteen patients, long-term follow-up, and a review of the literature. Medicine 1980; 59:426–440.

Haynes BF, Pikus A, Kaiser-Kupfer MI, Fauci AS. Successful treatment of sudden hearing loss in Cogan's syndrome with corticosteroids. Arthritis Rheum 1981; 24:501–503.

McCallum RM, Allen NB, Cobo LM, et al: Cogan's syndrome: Clinical features and outcomes. Arthritis Rheum 1992; 35(suppl 9):S51.

McCallum RM, Haynes BF: Cogan's Syndrome. In: Pepose JS, Holland GN, Wilhemus KR, eds. Ocular Infection and Immunity. St. Louis: Mosby, 1996.

Vollertsen RS, McDonald TJ, Younge BR, et al. Cogan's syndrome: 18 cases and a review of the literature. Mayo Clinic Proc 1981; 61:344–361.

HEART AND LUNG DISEASE

HYPERSENSITIVITY PNEUMONITIS

RAYMOND G. SLAVIN, M.D.

Hypersensitivity pneumonitis is also referred to as pulmonary hypersensitivity syndrome or extrinsic allergic alveolitis. The latter term is perhaps the most appropriate because it is so descriptive. "Extrinsic" refers to an exogenous allergen as the cause of the problem. "Allergic" refers to the hypersensitivity basis for the disease. "Alveolitis" refers to the part of the lung that is most affected. Despite the different terms, they all refer to the same underlying pathogenetic entity, namely, a disease process that is caused by sensitivity to an organic dust that is inhaled. The clinical presentation of the disease depends on the circumstances and degree of exposure. In the more common acute form associated with intermittent intense exposure to the organic dust, the individual responds 4 to 6 hours after exposure with low grade fever, chills, chest pain, cough, and dyspnea. In the chronic form associated with prolonged low grade exposure, the clinical presentation is much more insidious, with progressively increasing cough, dyspnea, weakness, malaise, and weight loss.

The causative antigens responsible for hypersensitivity pneumonitis can be divided into several categories. This list, with examples, includes thermophilic *Actinomycetes (Micropolyspora faeni),* fungi *(Aspergillus clavatus),* amoeba *(Naegleria gruberi),* animal products (bird droppings), and small molecular weight chemicals (toluene diisocyanate). The majority of cases are associated with occupational exposure, such as farming, mushroom packing, or grain loading. However, offending antigens may contaminate home heating or humidification units or be associated with hobbies such as pigeon breeding.

The diagnosis of hypersensitivity pneumonitis should be suspected in any patient presenting with interstitial pneumonitis or pulmonary fibrosis. Pulmonary function testing reveals a largely restrictive dysfunction, including decreases in pulmonary compliance and in carbon monoxide diffusion capacity. A careful history eliciting the onset of symptoms following exposure with remission on avoidance, together with positive serum precipitins to the appropriate antigen, is presumptive evidence of hypersensitivity pneumonitis. In rare instances further confirmation may have to be made by inhalation challenge with the suspected antigen.

THERAPEUTIC APPROACH

Avoidance

Clearly the most important aspect in the management of hypersensitivity pneumonitis is recognition and avoidance of the causative antigen. The physician's diagnostic index of suspicion must be high, and in every case of interstitial pneumonitis or pulmonary fibrosis a careful environmental survey of the patient's occupational, home, and avocational life must be carried out, searching for the presence of offending antigens. Once the disease is diagnosed and the antigen recognized, early avoidance is the definitive therapy. Hypersensitivity pneumonitis ultimately may be a fatal disease because of progressive respiratory insufficiency. While it is not known how long or what level of exposure is required to produce irreversible pulmonary changes, it is estimated that five acute episodes will be followed by pulmonary damage and progressive disease. Therefore, it is vital to make the diagnosis early and institute proper environmental precautions to prevent the inexorable consequences of pulmonary fibrosis and irreparable tissue damage. Factors that favor a worse prognosis are repeated acute episodes, abnormalities on chest radiographs or pulmonary function tests that last more than 6 weeks, and clubbing.

Table 1 shows a general approach to the prevention of hypersensitivity pneumonitis. A number of interventions will decrease the formation of antigens in conducive environments. For example, the growth of thermophilic *Actinomycetes* spores in compost can be suppressed by treatment with a 1 percent solution of propionic acid. Water that remains for long periods of time in older air conditioning or humidification units may become a fertile source for the growth of thermophilic organisms. Therefore, the water needs to be changed and the unit cleaned on a regular basis. Contaminated ventilation systems have to be thoroughly

Table 1 Prevention of Hypersensitivity Pneumonitis

Decrease formation of antigens
Add chemicals such as 1% propionic acid to prevent growth
Change water frequently in humidification or air conditioning units and clean units regularly
Use storage dryers on hay and straw
Harvest crops when moisture content is low
Decrease exposure to organic dust
Mechanically handle dusty materials within closed spaces
Remove dusts from ambient air
Use personal respirators or masks
Remove worker from disease producing environment

Modified from Terho EO. Extrinsic allergic alveolitis-management of established cases. Eur J Respir Dis 1982; 123:101.

Table 2 Treatment of Hypersensitivity Pneumonitis

Acute form
Remove patient from exposure; may entail hospitalization
Administer oxygen
Prednisone 40-60 mg/day with slow tapering over 10-12 days
Supportive measures-rest, antitussives, antipyretics
Repeated acute or subacute form
Decrease exposure as much as possible
Long term corticosteroid therapy emphasizing alternate day therapy
Chronic form
Trial with corticosteroids but continue only if radiographic findings and physiologic testing indicate a response

cleaned or replaced. Blowing cool air through stored hay helps to prevent the growth of mold. Harvesting crops when the moisture content is low also results in less exposure to organic dusts.

In occupational situations in which organic dust generation is inevitable, every effort should be made to reduce the workers' exposure. In enclosed spaces extremely dusty material should be handled mechanically. The use of particular types of silos may allow for automated feeding of cattle. Materials such as sugar cane should be stored outside and cattle fed outside as much as possible so that the associated organic dusts can be diluted by the ambient air.

In terms of removal of dusts from the air, improved ventilation may aid considerably. Electrostatic air purifiers may be of help when the concentration of dust is not too great. They would be overwhelmed in an area where moldy hay is being handled in which it is estimated that there are 1,600 million spores per cubic meter of air. A person doing light work with moldy hay inhales 10 liters of air per minute, which would deposit 750,000 spores per minute in the lung.

The use of personal dust respirators or masks is limited because of inconvenience. A type 2B filter is effective in filtering small particles but causes so much resistance to the flow of air that people hard at work are unable to wear them. An air stream helmet in which an electrical pump blows air through a filter and into the breathing zone is heavy and uncomfortable to wear. Even the best device has a maximal filtering capacity of 99 percent for fine particles. The remaining 1 percent can produce new attacks in a highly sensitive individual. If the disease is not yet manifest, even a filter with 95 percent filtering capacity is adequate. Good results have been reported with a 3M disposable mask model 8710 or reusable model 7200.

When the foregoing environmental control measures cannot be carried out or are inadequate, the patient should be removed from that work area. This may entail a change in the work place or type of work or, in extreme cases, a change in occupation. If the diffusing capacity has not returned to normal in three months, the individual should be advised to leave that particular workplace permanently. It should be stated that many bird breeders and farmers are unwilling or unable to avoid exposure. One should do as much as possible to educate the patient as to disease pathogenesis and the importance of avoidance.

Drug Therapy (Table 2)

In many cases no treatment is necessary other than avoidance of the causative antigen. Corticosteroid therapy, however, can greatly accelerate clinical improvement and should be considered in very ill patients with gross radiographic or physiologic abnormalities, such as hypoxemia. Oral therapy with prednisone in an initial daily dosage of 40 to 60 mg is usually adequate and should be continued until there is significant clinical, radiographic, and pulmonary function test evidence of improvement. The prednisone dosage then may be tapered slowly until resolution of clinical and radiologic signs is complete, generally in 10 to 12 days. The total duration of therapy should be no more than 4 to 6 weeks provided exposure to the antigen is prevented. Inhaled corticosteroids are of no value in the treatment of hypersensitivity pneumonitis, nor are bronchodilators or cromolyn unless bronchospasm is also present.

The dramatic response of hypersensitivity pneumonitis to corticosteroids may be a two-edged sword. The rapid relief afforded by steroids may result in a false sense of security, so much so that the patient may return to the same work environment. Re-exposure will result in progression of the lung disease. It therefore must be emphasized and re-emphasized to the patient that corticosteroids are not a substitute for antigen identification and avoidance.

In cases of severe hypoxemia in the acute stage, oxygen should be administered in amounts sufficient to keep the PO_2 level between 60 and 100 mm Hg. Other supportive measures include rest, antitussives, and antipyretics.

On occasion, despite the physician's best efforts, the patient may elect to return to the same work place or occupation. This seems to be especially true of farmers, who find it particularly difficult to leave farming because of age, a large financial investment, and a lack of training and skills in other occupations. In these instances long-term continuous corticosteroid therapy may have to be administered. One should strive for an alternate-day program utilizing the lowest dosage that still controls the patient's symptoms.

The chronic form of hypersensitivity pneumonitis develops insidiously and occurs either following repeated acute episodes or as a result of long-term, low-grade exposure. A therapeutic trial of steroids can be given but there are no controlled studies showing benefit. If there is clear evidence that the disease is progressive, corticosteroids can be administered but should be continued only if radiographic findings and physiologic testing indicate a beneficial response.

Appropriate treatment of the acute episode of hypersensitivity pneumonitis with avoidance of further antigen exposure results in an uneventful recovery with no progression to chronic untreatable disease.

SUGGESTED READING

Fink JN. Hypersensitivity pneumonitis. In: Middleton EJ Jr, Reed CE, Ellis EF, et al, eds. Allergy: Principles and practice. St Louis: Mosby, 1993.

Stankus RP, DeShazo RD. Hypersensitivity pneumonitis. In: Schwartz M, King TE Jr, eds. Interstitial lung disease. Toronto: BC Decker, 1988.

Terho EO. Extrinsic allergic alveolitis-management of stable cases. Eur J Respir Dis 1982; 123(suppl):101.

IDIOPATHIC PULMONARY FIBROSIS

GERALD S. DAVIS, M.D.

Idiopathic pulmonary fibrosis (IPF) is a chronic diffuse interstitial lung disease most prevalent in adults 40 to 70 years of age. The name accurately reflects both the condition and our understanding of it – lung scarring of unknown cause. The disease is labeled cryptogenic fibrosing alveolitis (CFA) in the United Kingdom. In Canada and the United States the name IPF has now largely replaced usual interstitial pneumonitis, diffuse fibrosing alveolitis, chronic interstitial pneumonia, and other terms. It is not clear whether IPF represents a unique reaction to a single agent or a stereotypical response to variety of environmental, infectious, or endogenous insults. A familial pattern can be found in approximately 10 percent of cases. It is likely that a combination of genetic susceptibility and several exogenous factors must coincide in order to produce the disease. The clinical syndrome of IPF is quite distinct, and it is not a diagnosis of exclusion. The specific features permit definitive diagnosis, estimates of prognosis, and selection among several choices of therapy.

The clinical and radiologic features (Fig. 1) of IPF are summarized in Tables 1 and 2. Blood laboratory tests are entirely nonspecific and usually not helpful in either diagnosis or management. Bronchoalveolar lavage (BAL) fluid analysis is not specific, but may tip the balance of clinical judgment in selected cases. The cells recovered by BAL from patients with IPF show increased total numbers of alveolar macrophages (AM), neutrophils (PMN), eosinophils (EOS), basophils (BAS), and lymphocytes (LYS); the percentages of PMN, EOS, BAS, and sometimes LYS are increased, thus depressing the relative percentage of AM calculated. Some patients may show normal BAL cell profiles. Analysis of soluble constituents reveals increased albumin and immunoglobulins, increased high molecular weight proteins of serum origin (suggesting altered permeability), elevated procollagen peptide fragments (reflecting newly synthesized collagen), and the presence of a wide variety of proinflammatory cytokines and mediators. Although many investigators have sought distinctive patterns or constituents to help provide diagnosis or prognosis, great variation among patients defeats a simple interpretation of BAL results in IPF.

Lung tissue biopsy provides a specific diagnosis in conjunction with the other clinical features. The tissue reveals a diffuse but patchy pattern described as "usual interstitial pneumonitis." The mildest microscopic changes show diffuse alveolar damage with collections of inflammatory cells, cellular debris, and proteinaceous exudates filling alveolar airspaces. More advanced IPF reveals derangement of alveolar walls with septal edema, interstitial cell accumulations, proliferation of type II epithelial cells lining airspaces, and fibroblast proliferation. There is extensive destruction of the alveolar architecture because some airspaces collapse within the fibrotic process, while others dilate or disrupt to produce enlarged cystic airspaces. The alveolar capillary bed may be obliterated, and small airways become filled with exudate, cells, and new connective tissue. Locations of severe fibrosis may appear nearly acellular, with dilated airspaces, dense bands of connective tissue, and greatly deranged architecture.

A key feature is that the lesions appear as foci isolated in time and space, with areas that appear normal or nearly normal, other foci of inflammation with alveolar remodeling and cell proliferation, and other sites of relatively acellular scar. These three zones are believed to represent an ongoing disease process with sites of current inflammation and fibrosis (alveolitis), past sites of activity (honeycombing), and future sites not yet involved (normal lung). The relative proportions of

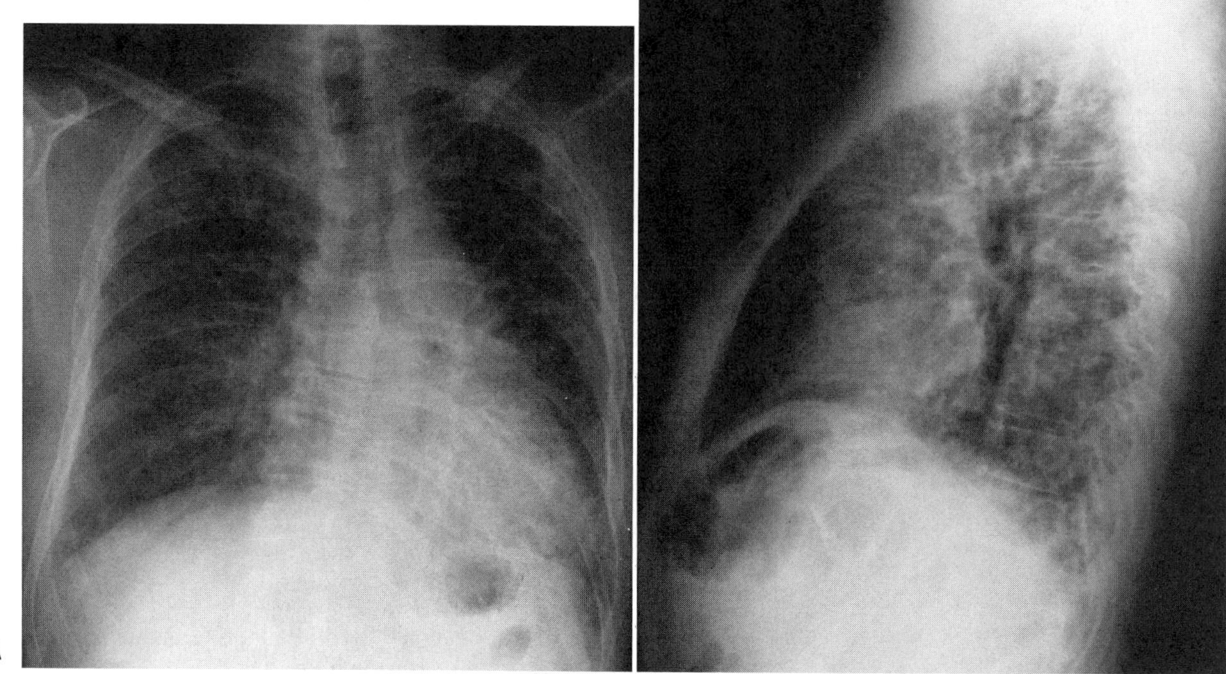

Figure 1 Idiopathic pulmonary fibrosis. Posteroanterior (**A**) and lateral (**B**) chest radiographs of a 58-year-old man with biopsy-proven idiopathic pulmonary fibrosis demonstrate a pattern of small irregular opacities in moderate profusion with a peripheral and lower lung zone predominance. The lung fields appear small and the diaphragms somewhat elevated. The normal vascular markings and cardiac borders are blurred by the adjacent lung tissue opacities.

Table 1 Clinical Features of Idiopathic Pulmonary Fibrosis

Symptoms
Dyspnea with exertion
Cough, usually without sputum
Malaise, reduced energy and endurance
Physical Findings
Bibasilar end-inspiratory crackles
Digital clubbing
Pulmonary Physiology
Reduced vital capacity
Normal or accelerated airflow rates
Small lung volumes
Reduced pulmonary compliance
Decreased gas transfer (diffusing capacity)
Hypoxemia without hypercarbia
Hypoxemia that worsens with exertion

Table 2 Radiographic Features of Idiopathic Pulmonary Fibrosis

Chest Radiograph
Small irregular shadows
Diffuse symmetrical pattern
Predominance in lower lung zones
Normal plain radiograph (5%-10%, early disease)
Peripheral "honeycomb" pattern (end-stage disease)
High-Resolution Computed Tomography
Ground-glass alveolar filling pattern (possibly early disease)
Small irregular shadows, interlobular septal lines
Peripheral sub-pleural pattern
Peripheral "honeycomb" pattern
Mild hilar lymph node enlargement
Traction emphysema
Traction on airways (traction bronchiectasis)

these patterns is an important predictor of response to therapy.

COURSE AND PROGNOSIS

Patients who prove ultimately to have IPF usually present with the gradual onset of cough and dyspnea, a chest radiograph that shows diffuse abnormalities, and spirometry that demonstrates volume reduction without airflow obstruction. These findings point to chronic diffuse interstitial lung disease (ILD), but do not allow a specific choice among the many diagnoses that would be included under this rubric. The great variation in etiology, prognosis, choice of therapy, and response to treatment among the many types of ILD, and the serious prognosis for IPF, require a definitive diagnosis for most patients. A diagnosis of IPF may be strongly suspected after detailed history excludes occupational exposure to asbestos or other pneumotoxins, physical exam demonstrates digital clubbing, and high-resolution computed tomography (HRCT) shows characteristic abnormalities. A lung tissue biopsy is usually required to establish the diagnosis specifically, to exclude other possible diseases, and to estimate disease activity in order to guide treatment.

Most patients report insidious symptoms for 6 months or more before seeking medical attention, and in some cases the disease may have been present for several years before diagnosis. It is important to carefully categorize patients as individuals since both their course and response to therapy may vary greatly. The prognosis for IPF is serious. Overall, approximately 50 percent of patients with IPF survive 5 years after diagnosis, with most deaths attributable to respiratory failure. Even with aggressive therapy, many patients experience an arrest of progression rather than reversal of their impairment, and a substantial fraction fail to respond to treatment.

Table 3 Drug Therapy Options for Idiopathic Pulmonary Fibrosis

Methylprednisolone
Combination: 12-20 mg every other day
Alone: 1-2 mg/kg/day for 6 weeks, then taper to 0.5-1 mg/kg/day
Cyclophosphamide
1-2 mg/kg/day
Monitor urinalysis and WBC count every 2-4 weeks
Adjust dosage to keep WBCs at 3,500-5,000/mm^3
Azathioprine
1-2.5 mg/kg/day
Monitor WBC count and platelet estimate every 2-4 weeks
Colchicine
0.6-1.2 mg twice per day

THERAPEUTIC ALTERNATIVES (TABLE 3)

There is no excellent, always successful, easily tolerated treatment for IPF. Therapeutic alternatives fall into three major categories: cytotoxic and immunosuppressive therapy, general supportive care, and lung transplantation. The physician and the patient must choose carefully among these options to select an appropriate balance between the likelihood of success and the rigors of treatment for each individual.

Cytotoxic Drug Therapy

The pharmacologic therapy of IPF is aimed at suppression of the chronic immune-inflammatory response. The agents that have proved useful in the treatment of IPF are believed to work by combating the proinflammatory actions of activated macrophages and lymphocytes, reducing neutrophil chemotaxis and adherence, and selectively reducing the number of these cells in the lung and in the circulation. It is believed that treatment should be instituted as early as possible to intervene before tissue destruction and fibrosis become extensive. Several specific treatment programs using corticosteroids alone or combinations of these drugs with cyclophosphamide or azathioprine have been tested in limited clinical trials. No large, multicenter treatment trials have been reported, although it is widely agreed that such a trial is required to obtain adequate patient numbers to assess accurately the effect of any therapy on the natural history of the disease and to compare the outcomes of different treatment protocols.

Corticosteroids

Corticosteroids have been used widely for the treatment of IPF, but studies supporting their effectiveness are not available. Oral prednisone or methylprednisolone, taken in moderate to high doses (1 to 2 mg per kilogram per day) on a daily or alternate-day basis, has been used as a comparison regimen in treatment trials. The glucocorticoids are believed to work in IPF by suppressing inflammation and impairing activated lymphocyte function and by their lympholytic effects. No benefit has been reported from low doses of steroids alone. If corticosteroids are used alone as initial therapy, adequate dosage should be employed to assure a clear-cut response. Corticosteroids alone lead to improvement in less than one-half of the IPF patients treated. Objective improvement in pulmonary function or chest radiograph with steroid treatment alone occurs in approximately 12 to 20 percent of patients, but arresting the progress of deterioration may also be considered a useful treatment benefit. Some beneficial effect from steroids may be seen in 30 to 50 percent of patients, but 50 to 70 percent will deteriorate despite treatment. In trails where corticosteroids alone were compared with other cytotoxic agents plus steroids, usually in lower dose, no treatment advantage was found with lone steroids.

The incidence of complications with corticosteroids is substantial and related directly to the dose; minor side effects are usual and significant ones are not rare. Facial rounding, weight gain, and cosmetic changes are virtually universal at higher doses used for 3 to 6 months or longer. Osteoporosis, myopathy, posterior cataracts, and opportunistic infection are not unusual side effects of prolonged corticosteroid therapy. Initial treatment of IPF with a combination of a cytotoxic agent and low alternative-day doses of corticosteroids appears preferable to high daily doses of steroids alone.

There is tremendous variability in the responses of individual patients to corticosteroids. The predictors of a more favorable response to steroid therapy include a cellular biopsy, younger age at presentation, and elevated BAL lymphocyte fractions. Advanced age, a fibrotic biopsy, and the presence of eosinophils and/or neutrophils in BAL fluid may be predictive of a poor response to therapy. Patients who show an initial response to steroids have a significantly better prognosis than those who fail initial therapy—62 percent survival versus 25 percent survival at 5 years.

Cyclophosphamide

Cyclophosphamide (Cytoxan) is an alkylating agent of the nitrogen mustard group that has been used as therapy for IPF in several published trials. It is believed that the drug works by depleting and suppressing the function of lymphocytes. Cyclophosphamide has been administered in daily oral maintenance dosage for IPF, although not specifically approved by the Food and Drug Administration for use in this disease. Weekly or monthly high-dose pulse therapy with cyclophosphamide has been successful in systemic lupus erythematosus with renal disease and in other chronic immune-inflammatory conditions, but this treatment scheme has not been reported for IPF. In a randomized controlled trial to compare prednisolone alone (60 mg per day) with cyclophosphamide plus prednisolone (100 to 120 mg per day plus prednisolone 20 mg every other day) in treating IPF, a slight benefit of stability or improvement at 3 years was found for the cyclophosphamide group (8 of 21) compared to the steroids alone group (5 of 22). A significant benefit with cyclophosphamide was found in survival among patients with moderately severe pulmonary function impairment (total lung capacity 60 to 79 percent predicted), but not among patients with mild or very severe dysfunction. Many patients failed to respond to either treatment.

Cyclophosphamide is expensive, and the adverse effects can be substantial. Many patients experience gastric irritation, nausea, or anorexia, although these symptoms can sometimes be avoided by night-time dosing. Hair loss is common, but it is usually partial, mild, and reversible when treatment is stopped. Bladder irritation and microscopic hematuria can be minimized with a large daily fluid intake volume, and frank hemorrhagic cystitis is rare with oral dosing. Bone marrow suppression and opportunistic infection are the major serious complications of cyclophosphamide therapy. Although all formed elements may be affected, the blood leukocyte count is usually the most sensitive indicator of drug effects. Patients receiving cyclophosphamide should have their white blood cell (WBC) count monitored frequently, and their dosage reduced or discontinued if excessive reduction in total WBCs occurs.

Therapy with cyclophosphamide can be started at oral doses of 1.0 to 1.5 mg per kilogram per day, or 50 to 100 mg (1 to 2 tablets) daily for the average patient. The urinalysis (for hematuria) and the WBC count should be followed every 1 to 2 weeks initially. If the WBC count does not fall after 3 weeks of treatment, dosage can be increased by 25 mg per day at 3-week intervals until mild suppression of total WBC is observed. The dose should then be held steady or reduced slightly. A maximum dosage would be 150 to 200 mg per day. Some physicians choose to assure a maximum drug effect by trying to keep the total WBC in a target range of 3,500 to 5,000 cells per cubic millimeter. Many patients require a slight decrease in dosage after 3 to 6 months because of gradual marrow toxicity. It is imperative to continue to monitor the WBC count on a biweekly or monthly basis throughout treatment, since severe marrow depression can occur even after a prolonged period of stable dosage.

Azathioprine

Azathioprine (Imuran) is a purine analogue that is slowly converted to mercaptopurine in body tissues. It appears to act both by substitution for purines in DNA synthesis and as an inhibitor of adenine deaminase. It is given daily by mouth, but has not been approved by the Food and Drug Administration for use in the treatment of IPF. In a prospective, double-blind randomized trial of 27 patients with IPF who received treatment with azathioprine plus prednisone or with placebo plus prednisone, therapy was tolerated well in both groups. Pulmonary function at 1 year was slightly better in the azathioprine group. There was a substantial survival advantage beyond 3 years for the azathioprine group, but this difference reached significance only when adjusted for age. The overall 5-year survival was 48 percent.

Azathioprine is given in oral daily doses of 1 to 2.5 mg per kilogram per day. It is usually tolerated well, and causes less gastrointestinal intolerance and bone marrow depression than cyclophosphamide. Opportunistic infection remains a risk. The total WBC count, hemoglobin level, and platelets should be monitored periodically because significant bone marrow toxicity can occur. Treatment may be started with 1 mg per kilogram (50 to 75 mg total, 1 to 1.5 tablets) each day, and then increased gradually as tolerance permits.

Alternative Treatment Options

Cyclosporin A has been used to treat IPF in several small groups of patients who had failed other treatment modalities. A favorable response was seen in the majority of patients described, but these reports emphasize a steroid-sparing, temporary, or delaying effect that could be useful for patients awaiting transplantation. D-penicillamine has been considered for use in IPF because of its effectiveness in the treatment of several of the rheumatologic diseases. Although the trials have been small, the results were not encouraging and its use does not appear warranted. Colchicine has been suggested as an adjunct to other therapy because of *in vitro* studies on fibroblast function; it has not been evaluated objectively in patients with IPF.

Supportive Care

Oxygen, exercise, diet, cough suppression, control of intercurrent infection, and psychosocial support offer helpful care for IPF patients. For many patients, as for their physicians, the disease appears to be a rare mystery. Establishing a specific diagnosis, knowing that the disease is clearly recognized and not uncommon, understanding that prognosis can be estimated, and presenting realistic treatment options are of great value and reassurance for most patients.

Oxygen therapy during exertion is a key treatment for many patients. Arterial blood oxygen saturation (O_2 sat percent) and tension (pO_2) remain normal or nearly normal in most patients until quite late in the course of IPF. Conversely, many patients will desaturate considerably with modest exertion quite early in the course of disease. All patients should be tested regularly with digital oximetry while walking in a hallway, climbing several steps, or in other activities of daily living. Some patients may require periodic formal incremental exercise testing to follow their progress. If arterial oxygen desaturation below 88 percent is observed with routine walking or similar activities, therapy with portable devices for liquid or compressed oxygen should be initiated. Portable oxygen therapy can be liberating for patients who are unable to socialize, shop, or exercise without this modality. For patients who desaturate only with more intense exertion, oxygen therapy during a planned exercise program may be helpful. Patients with desaturation at rest who meet the usual criteria for continuous oxygen therapy (O_2 sat <88 percent, pO_2 <56 torr) should be offered this treatment.

Cough may be disabling for IPF patients, interrupting conversation and limiting exertion. Unfortunately, this symptom is often refractory to therapy. Narcotic-based cough preparations may be helpful for short intervals or occasionally at night, but patients soon become tolerant of the cough suppressant effects. Anecdotal experience suggests that cough improves along with pulmonary function if patients respond to cytotoxic drug therapy. Some patients may gain an improvement in cough with low doses of steroids even if pulmonary function has not changed.

Lung Transplantation

Lung transplantation is a useful, life-saving treatment for patients with severe, progressive IPF who are otherwise healthy and have failed to respond to medical therapy. The scarce availability of donor lungs for transplantation is the major limitation on the widespread use of this modality. Candidates must be highly motivated, able to participate in a vigorous exercise and rehabilitation program, willing to work closely with a local or distant transplant program, and have adequate financial and social support resources. For most programs, IPF patients must be younger than 60 to 65 years of age, and not have significant diseases involving other organ systems. They should be receiving no corticosteroids, or only low doses, before transplantation. A prolonged waiting period (6 to 18 months) before transplantation requires early enrollment and preparation of suitable patients.

Single-lung transplantation has become the most common approach for patients with IPF, replacing double-lung or combined heart-lung transplants in most programs. Since the native lung is not infected, it can remain in place. Within a short time after surgery almost all of both the blood flow and the ventilation are diverted to the graft lung. Many patients achieve nearly normal levels of exercise performance, at least for routine activities of daily living.

Patients with IPF who are candidates for transplantation typically will have failed medical therapy, require high levels of continuous oxygen supplementation, are severely limited in their ability to dress, eat, and move about their homes, and may be expected to live 18 months or less without intervention. Current transplant methodology provides favorable odds for those who are able to receive this treatment, and a greatly improved quality of life. About 70 percent of patients will survive 1 year after transplant and 60 percent will survive 3 years or longer, with most of the mortality occurring in the period immediately after transplantation.

APPROACH TO DIAGNOSIS AND TREATMENT

The approach to both diagnosis and treatment of IPF must be tailored to suit each patient. The features of each individual should guide a relatively aggressive or more conservative approach, as summarized in Table 4. Most patients will fall into one of three broad categories: progressive, active disease in a younger patient, active disease in an older patient and/or one with complicating illnesses, or patients without evidence of disease progression.

Patients who are relatively young ($<$ 65 years), who do not have complicating chronic diseases in other organ systems, who do not show end-stage IPF (severe impairment, honeycomb radiographic pattern, cor pulmonale), and who demonstrate evidence of progressive pulmonary impairment should receive detailed evaluation (complete pulmonary function testing, HRCT scan) and definitive diagnosis. In most instances this diagnosis will require lung tissue biopsy by video-assisted thoracoscopic surgery (VATS) or open thoracotomy technique. Transbronchial (bronchoscopic) biopsy generally provides too small a sample of tissue to assess accurately the predominant pattern of disease (cellular or fibrotic) or to establish diagnosis with certainty. If the biopsy reveals a significant component of inflammation and cellularity, a better response to anti-

Table 4 Diagnostic and Therapeutic Approaches to Chronic Diffuse Interstitial Lung Disease

Aggressive Approach	*Conservative Approach*
Patient Features	*Patient Features*
Young age	Old age
Good general health	Co-morbid disease
Rapid progression	Gradual onset of symptoms
Early IPF findings	Advanced IPF findings
Diagnosis and Treatment	*Diagnosis and Treatment*
Definitive lung biopsy (VATS)	Limited or no lung biopsy
Comprehensive evaluation	Limited evaluation
Multiple drug therapy	No specific therapy
Lung transplantation	Palliative therapy

VATS, video-assisted thoracoscopic surgery.

inflammatory therapy may be expected. These patients should be offered initial therapy with cyclophosphamide or azathioprine combined with low doses of alternate-day corticosteroids.

A treatment trial of at least 3 to 6 months should be undertaken, with objective documentation of pulmonary function and radiography at the beginning and the end of the trial. If the patient has clearly improved, then therapy should be continued for at least 1 and possibly 2 years. Some patients will demonstrate a response to therapy by stabilizing their function without further deterioration. One might imagine that the IPF disease process has been arrested, but physiologic impairment persists because of lung zones already scarred by previous injury and fibrosis. After several years of apparent stability, the cytotoxic agent can be stopped and the corticosteroids tapered to discontinuation. Many patients will not demonstrate reactivation of disease, but some may require prompt reinitiation of treatment. If the patient has clearly deteriorated in the initial trial despite aggressive therapy, then treatment should be discontinued. The risks of cytotoxic therapy are significant, and should not be incurred without the balance of reasonable benefit. Referral for transplantation should be initiated at this time, if the patient is an appropriate candidate.

Patients who are elderly, who have complicating diseases in other organ systems, or who appear to have far advanced IPF at the time of presentation suggest a conservative, less invasive, approach to diagnosis and treatment. A transbronchial lung biopsy may be adequate to exclude other more treatable diseases, even if the full spectrum of IPF cannot be assessed. Supportive therapy alone or low-dose corticosteroid therapy to suppress cough and constitutional symptoms may be more appropriate than the risks and discomfort of cytotoxic therapy or high doses of steroids. These patients may require early consideration for a supportive living environment or hospice care.

Occasional patients present for evaluation of IPF because of an abnormal chest radiograph without clear evidence of symptoms or of progressive disease. These patients may not report any impairment of activities and may not have had a previous radiograph for comparison. If there is doubt regarding the activity of their presumed diffuse interstitial lung disease, it is appropriate to follow lung function and radiographs at 3-month intervals to determine if the impairment progresses before obtaining a definitive biopsy diagnosis or beginning treatment. Lung tissue in these instances may reveal modest fibrosis without active inflammation. Presumably, these patients have experienced a subclinical self-limited disease process at some time in the past and have been left with residual lung scarring. It is not known whether these events represent a true variant of IPF or if they are a nonspecific endpoint for healed infections or other pulmonary insults.

PROS AND CONS OF TREATMENT

IPF presents a distinctive constellation of symptoms and signs with a well-defined prognosis, even if the precise cause or causes of this disease are not known. Treatment with cytotoxic or immunosuppressive agents offers the hope of stabilization or partial improvement for two-thirds to three-quarters of patients with active disease. It is believed that early intervention provides a better outcome than treatment for advanced disease. Lung transplantation offers near-total normalization of lifestyle and lung function for more than one-half of the patients with severe drug-resistant IPF who are able to receive this therapy. The disadvantages of either cytotoxic drug treatment or transplantation include high cost, substantial adverse effects, and the need for frequent medical care. Therefore these modalities are appropriate only for otherwise healthy patients with IPF who have a reasonable expectation of benefiting from them.

All patients with IPF can be expected to benefit from general supportive care, supplemental oxygen when indicated during exertion or at rest, and from measures to suppress cough and dyspnea during the final, terminal stages of their disease if it is refractory to other therapies. All patients will benefit from a well-informed, concerned, and attentive team of health care providers to help them through this difficult illness.

SUGGESTED READING

Johnson MA, Kwan S, Snell NJ, et al. Randomised controlled trial comparing prednisolone alone with cyclophosphamide and low dose prednisolone in combination in cryptogenic fibrosing alveolitis. Thorax 1989; 44:280–288.

Kaiser LR, Cooper JD. The current status of lung transplantation. Adv Surg 1992; 25:259–307.

Peters SG, McDougall JC, Douglas WW, et al. Colchicine in the treatment of pulmonary fibrosis. Chest 1993; 103:101–104.

Raghu G, Depaso WJ, Cain K, et al. Azathioprine combined with prednisone in the treatment of idiopathic pulmonary fibrosis: A prospective double-blind, randomized, placebo-controlled clinical trial. Am Rev Respir Dis 1991; 144:291–296.

Schwartz DA, Helmers RA, Galvin JR, et al. Determinants of survival in idiopathic pulmonary fibrosis. Am J Respir Crit Care Med 1994; 149:450–454.

Watters LC, King TE, Schwarz MI, et al. A clinical, radiographic, and physiologic scoring system for the longitudinal assessment of patients with idiopathic pulmonary fibrosis. Am Rev Respir Dis 1986; 133:97–103.

ALLERGIC BRONCHOPULMONARY ASPERGILLOSIS

PAUL A. GREENBERGER, M.D.

Allergic bronchopulmonary aspergillosis is a cause of chest roentgenographic infiltrates in patients with asthma or "pulmonary infiltrates with eosinophilia." The radiographic pattern usually involves upper lobes or the middle lobe and, in contrast to patients experiencing a bacterial pneumonia, symptoms are less intense. Untreated pulmonary infiltrates have been demonstrated to cause bronchiectasis, which can become symptomatic in the future. Early recognition and treatment can prevent emergence of end-stage irreversible fibrocavitary lung disease. Allergic bronchopulmonary aspergillosis complicates some cases of cystic fibrosis, but it is unknown whether the natural history of cystic fibrosis is altered.

GOALS OF THERAPY

After the diagnosis of allergic bronchopulmonary aspergillosis is secured or suspected, the goals of therapy include (1) clearing of the acute roentgenographic infiltrate(s); (2) improving respiratory status (eliminating or reducing sputum production, improving asthma control); (3) determining post-treatment respiratory status, including pulmonary function parameters and baseline chest roentgenogram; (4) establishing a shared relationship with the patient because subsequent monitoring of total serum IgE concentrations will be required; and (5) treating concurrent conditions such as sinusitis, allergic rhinitis, or other atopic conditions that may be present.

PATIENT EDUCATION

Patients should be informed that oral corticosteroids (prednisone) are the most important treatment for allergic bronchopulmonary aspergillosis and that failure to diagnose and treat this condition has resulted in extensive bronchiectasis and pulmonary fibrosis. The oral corticosteroid is used in an alternate-day regimen for the most part, which avoids the serious side effects of prednisone. The patient may be reassured that prednisone may not be required indefinitely because the need for systemic corticosteroids will become apparent after the initial 3-month treatment course is carried out. Specifically, patients should be warned about overeating, smoking, and sources in their home or workplace containing high numbers of fungal spores.

DIAGNOSTIC CRITERIA AND STAGES OF ALLERGIC BRONCHOPULMONARY ASPERGILLOSIS

Diagnostic criteria for allergic bronchopulmonary aspergillosis are listed in Table 1. If patients with asthma have chest roentgenographic infiltrates thought to be consistent with mucoid impactions and peripheral blood eosinophilia, a tentative diagnosis of allergic bronchopulmonary aspergillosis may be made and prednisone started. Pretreatment sera should be obtained and stored. If serologic test results, sputum or bronchoscopy specimens suggest a fungus different from *Aspergillus,* an allergic bronchopulmonary fungosis may be present. The

Table 1 Diagnostic Criteria for Allergic Bronchopulmonary Aspergillosis

Classic Presentation
- Asthma
- Chest roentgenographic infiltrates
- Immediate cutaneous reactivity to *Aspergillus fumigatus* or *Aspergillus* species
- Elevated total serum IgE concentration
- Precipitating antibodies to *A. fumigatus*
- Peripheral blood eosinophilia
- Increased serum IgE and or IgG antibodies to *A. fumigatus*
- Proximal bronchiectasis*

Presentation with Normal Chest Roentgenogram
- Asthma
- History of chest roentgenographic infiltrates
- Immediate cutaneous reactivity to *A. fumigatus* or *Aspergillus* species
- Elevated total serum IgE concentration
- Increased serum IgE and or IgG antibodies to *A. fumigatus*
- Proximal bronchiectasis*

*Proximal bronchiectasis in the absence of cystic fibrosis is pathognomonic for allergic bronchopulmonary aspergillosis or fungosis. If absent, the patient who meets other criteria has seropositive allergic bronchopulmonary aspergillosis and can be classified into stages I-IV but not Stage V disease.

Table 2 Therapeutic Strategies for Allergic Bronchopulmonary Aspergillosis

Stage	*Suggested Regimen*
I. Acute	Prednisone 0.5 mg/kg/day for 2 weeks then q.o.d. for 2½ months. Inhaled corticosteroids and beta-adrenergic agonists if needed. Monitor decline of total serum IgE concentration
II. Remission	No prednisone. Asthma therapy as indicated. Establish baseline total serum IgE range
III. Recurrent exacerbation	Same prednisone regimen as for stage I. Monitor decline in total serum IgE concentration
IV. Corticosteroid-dependent asthma	Prednisone, usually alternate day. Inhaled corticosteroids, beta-adrenergic agonists. Optional therapy depending on severity: nedocromil, theophylline (controversial)
V. End-stage fibrotic	Prednisone alternate day or low dose daily. Beta-adrenergic agonists; inhaled corticosteroids if tolerated Optional therapy: antibiotics, bronchial hygiene, DNase, possibly antifungals

therapeutic approach remains the same. The stages of allergic bronchopulmonary aspergillosis and typical regimens are listed in Table 2.

THERAPEUTIC MANAGEMENT

Stage I: Acute and Stage III: Recurrent Exacerbation

For patients with stage I or stage III allergic bronchopulmonary aspergillosis, prednisone is the mainstay of therapy because it controls the immunologic response precipitated by *Aspergillus fumigatus,* improves respiratory function, helps resolve the chest roentgenographic infiltrates, and reduces or eliminates excessive sputum production. The initial therapy of prednisone is 0.5 mg per kilogram given as a single morning dose for 2 weeks. It is acceptable to give a larger dosage if there is collapse of a lobe or lung caused by mucoid impactions. At the end of 2 weeks of prednisone, the patient can be re-examined and a chest roentgenogram obtained. Typically, the upper lobe infiltrates have cleared either completely or are reduced in size. The patient has less sputum production if any was present initially and reduced symptoms of dyspnea or cough. Prednisone can be converted to alternate-day therapy at the same dosage to be continued for 2½ months. A chest roentgenogram can be obtained to verify a return to baseline.

The total serum IgE concentration should be repeated at 4 to 6 weeks time and then prospectively every 4 to 8 weeks for 6 months to document the decline in total serum IgE. The purpose of collecting these samples is to establish a baseline range of total serum IgE to use as a marker of subsequent exacerbations of allergic bronchopulmonary aspergillosis. As an example, at the time of an acute or recurrent exacerbation when "pulmonary infiltrates with eosinophilia" are present, the total serum IgE concentration is 10,000 ng per milliliter (or 4,166 IU/ml). At least a 33 percent decline in concentration will occur in the first 4 to 6 weeks of prednisone treatment, reflecting concurrent clearing of chest roentgenographic infiltrates. Continued declines in total serum IgE occur to approximately 2,000 to 4,000 ng per milliliter. It is important to avoid continued prednisone administration in an attempt to reduce the total serum IgE concentration to normal concentrations because patients with allergic bronchopulmonary aspergillosis continue to synthesize high amounts of IgE, nearly all of which is not directed at *A. fumigatus.*

Inhaled corticosteroids and beta-adrenergic agonists or other pharmacotherapy for asthma can be used in addition to appropriate treatment for coexisting allergic rhinitis, if necessary. Inhaled corticosteroids have not been demonstrated to be effective for treatment of pulmonary infiltrates. In the Chicago area over a 5-year period, 75 percent of exacerbations of allergic bronchopulmonary aspergillosis were recorded from June to November when outdoor fungal counts are the greatest. However, there is insufficient information to state that exacerbations are associated with higher ambient concentrations of *Aspergillus* because the contributing factors that cause new pulmonary infiltrates are not understood.

Stage II: Remission

After the initial 3 months of treatment, an attempt is made to discontinue prednisone. Stage II, remission of allergic bronchopulmonary aspergillosis, implies the absence of oral corticosteroids and new chest roentgenographic infiltrates for a minimum of 6 months. Some remissions are permanent, but patients likely have ongoing asthma but are not prednisone-dependent. The total serum IgE can be measured less frequently in patients with stage II allergic bronchopulmonary aspergillosis, but IgE concentrations should be obtained if asthma worsens, new sputum plugs are produced, or symptoms suggest a new pulmonary infiltrate. An increase of at least 100 percent over the established baseline total serum IgE concentrations is consistent with a recurrent exacerbation, and a chest roentgenogram should be obtained. New infiltrates, in the absence of other causes, change the patient's stage to III (recurrent exacerbation).

Stage IV: Corticosteroid-Dependent Asthma

If it is impossible to manage the patient's asthma without oral corticosteriods, then stage IV is present. Prior to the diagnosis of allergic bronchopulmonary aspergillosis, the asthma may not have required alternate-day prednisone, so in some cases, the asthma itself has become more severe. Patients with corticosteroid-dependent asthma require maximum dosages of inhaled corticosteroids and prednisone from 10 to 40 mg on alternate days. New chest roentgenographic infiltrates with markedly elevated total serum IgE concentrations still may occur, especially when the prednisone dose is less than 30 mg on alternate days. Nevertheless, stage IV patients may not have radiologic exacerbations. In such patients, total serum IgE concentrations can be obtained infrequently such as every 6 months. The total serum IgE concentrations in stage IV range from 165 to 15,000 ng per milliliter, which may or may not be illustrative of patients having new infiltrates.

There are little data to support the use of itraconazole; however, such antifungal medication can be considered as adjunctive therapy. Curiously, many patients who produce sputum plugs containing *A. fumigatus* will no longer expectorate fungi after treatment of the acute (stage I) or exacerbation (stage III) infiltrates. Prednisone alters the immune response, decreases sputum volume, facilitates a decline in total serum IgE, and resolves pulmonary infiltrates, yet is not directly antifungal. For patients who have persistently positive sputum cultures for *Aspergillus* species, a trial of itraconazole could be considered. There is no experience of treating stage IV allergic bronchopulmonary aspergillosis patients without repeated sputum cultures of aspergilli with antifungal therapy. I favor using maximum dosages of inhaled corticosteroids and alternate-day prednisone with beta-adrenergic agonists. If additional medication is needed for corticosteroid-dependent asthma, nedocromil can be added as an additional anti-inflammatory medication. I have not found that theophylline has prednisone-sparing effects in stage IV patients.

Stage V: Irreversible Fibrotic

The goal of early diagnosis and treatment of allergic bronchopulmonary aspergillosis is to avoid the emergence of end-stage irreversible fibrotic lung disease. Such patients have either extensive bronchiectasis (resembling end-stage cystic fibrosis) or pulmonary fibrosis. Some patients have both processes, which creates obvious management challenges. In patients with end-stage bronchiectasis, clubbing and arterial hypoxemia will occur and supplemental oxygen will be required. Lung transplantation is an alternative but experience is very limited. Some centers will not transplant patients with bronchiectasis. Sputum is typically voluminous in some stage V patients. However, new chest roentgenographic infiltrates are usually attributable to bacterial rather than fungal causes. One patient had the atypical mycobacterium *Mycobacterium chelonei* in sputum saprophytically for 10 years without tissue invasion.

Exacerbations of allergic bronchopulmonary aspergillosis are very rare when the patient has irreversible fibrotic-cavitary lung disease. In a group of 17 patients managed for a total of 83 patient-years, only 1 new infiltrate with elevation of total serum IgE concentration was documented.

Increases in respiratory symptoms may consist of increased sputum production, fever, or wheezing dyspnea. Bronchial hygiene, judicious use of antibiotics, temporary increases in prednisone, and nebulized DNase can be utilized depending on the severity. After the diagnosis of end-stage allergic bronchopulmonary aspergillosis, which occurred in patients from 17 to 67 years of age, if the FEV_1 was less than 0.8 L after 6 months of therapy, respiratory failure and death was likely. Stage V patients whose best FEV_1 was a mean of 1.2 L have remained on a stable clinical level. The latter findings suggest a place for intensive management even though the patients have a significant amount of irreversible obstructive and restrictive pulmonary function abnormalities.

Serial monitoring of total serum IgE concentrations in stage V patients is of little help in that the prednisone dose is usually sufficient to prevent radiographic exacerbations and immunologic pulmonary infiltrates. The rare asymptomatic infiltrate would be detected by a sharply elevated concentration of total IgE. In management of stage V patients, it is not necessary to administer 40 to 60 mg of prednisone daily for months to lower the total serum IgE to less than 1,000 ng per milliliter. Patients in stage V may require 40 to 60 mg prednisone on alternate days or 10 to 20 mg daily. The former regimen is preferable. End points of therapy include stabilizing respiratory function, improving the chest roentgenogram and the patients symptoms, but not the total serum IgE concentration.

MISCELLANEOUS THERAPIES

Many patients with allergic bronchopulmonary aspergillosis have concomitant allergic rhinitis, atopic dermatitis, or drug allergies and develop episodes of acute purulent bronchitis or rhinitis. Allergic management, including allergen avoidance therapy and occasionally allergen immunotherapy, may be recommended. It seems obvious that patients living in homes with repeated flooding of crawl spaces or basements may experience worse allergic symptoms and additional pulmonary infiltrates in such an environment. Attempts should be made to minimize exposure to areas where fungi grow prolifically.

After stabilization of pulmonary symptoms whether from asthma or allergic bronchopulmonary aspergillosis, some patients will experience sinusitis. While management will include topical corticosteroids, antibiotics, and possibly surgery, the presence of nasal "plugs" or refractory symptoms and opacified sinuses should suggest fungal sinusitis. The rare allergic fungal (*Aspergillus*) sinusitis typically occurs in immunocompetent patients with nasal polyps and no asthma. Several patients with both allergic *Aspergillus* sinusitis and allergic bronchopulmonary aspergillosis have been identified. Topical nasal corticosteroids and prednisone have been tried, but until adequate sinus debridement has been performed, sinusitis persists. The "concrete debris" of mucoid impaction, eosinophilic mucin, and *Aspergillus* hyphae in closed sinus cavities requires surgical removal because, in contrast to allergic bronchopulmonary aspergillosis, this debris cannot be expectorated.

Annual influenza immunization is recommended for patients with allergic bronchopulmonary aspergillosis. Pneumococcal immunization can be given although *Streptococcus pneumoniae* pneumonia is extremely unlikely.

SUGGESTED READING

Denning DW, Van Wye JE, Lewiston NJ, Stevens DA. Adjunctive therapy of allergic bronchopulmonary aspergillosis with itraconazole. Chest 1991; 100:813–819.

Greenberger PA, Miller TP, Roberts M, Smith LL. Allergic bronchopulmonary aspergillosis in patients with and without evidence of bronchiectasis. Ann Allergy 1993; 70:333–338.

Lee TM, Greenberger PA, Patterson R, et al. Stage V (Fibrotic) allergic bronchopulmonary aspergillosis: A review of 17 cases followed from diagnosis. Arch Intern Med 1987; 147:319–323.

Lydiatt WM, Sobba-Higley A, Huerter JV Jr, Leibrock LG. Allergic fungal sinusitis with intracranial extension and frontal lobe symptoms: A case report. ENT Journal 1994; 73:402–404.

Miller MA, Greenberger PA, Amerian R, et al. Allergic bronchopulmonary mycosis caused by *Pseudallescheria boydii.* Am Rev Respir Dis 1993; 148:810–812.

Neeld DA, Goodman LR, Gurney JW, et al. Computerized tomography in the evaluation of allergic bronchopulmonary aspergillosis. Am Rev Respir Dis 1990; 142:1200–1205.

SARCOIDOSIS

RICHARD H. WINTERBAUER, M.D.

CLINICAL DECISIONS IN THE MANAGEMENT OF SARCOIDOSIS

Selection of the Patient Who Benefits from Therapy

The clinician's initial therapeutic decision regarding the patient with sarcoid is whether to treat or not. The decision process begins by recognizing subgroups with different patterns of disease progression. Approximately 75 percent of patients with sarcoidosis will have spontaneous remission or mild, stable disease not requiring steroid therapy. Indications for treatment in 10 percent will be involvement of a critical extrapulmonary organ such as the eye, brain, or heart, while only 15 percent will require treatment for progressive pulmonary disease. Recognition of the latter subgroup is important, for clinicians can then avoid giving corticosteroids to a patient who ultimately would have spontaneous resolution, and they can provide early therapy for those patients destined to have progressive pulmonary disease.

Roentgenographic patterns, sequential pulmonary function testing, and clinical patterns of disease have all been used to predict the outcome of sarcoidosis. Although loose correlations exist, none of these techniques has been reliable enough to become clinical dogma. For example, patients with stage 1 roentgenographic disease (bilateral hilar lymphadenopathy, normal lung fields) have an 80 percent frequency of spontaneous remission within 2 years of onset; patients with stage 2 (bilateral hilar lymphadenopathy with lung parenchymal disease) disease have a 65 percent chance of spontaneous remission; and those with stage 3 (lung parenchymal disease and no hilar lymphadenopathy) have a 30 percent chance. Erythema nodosum and acute arthritis indicate an excellent prognosis with an approximate 85 percent frequency of spontaneous remission. At the opposite extreme, patients with hepatomegaly, central nervous system involvement, upper airway disease, lupus pernio, bone lesions, nephrocalcinosis, or cor pulmonale all have less than a 25 percent chance of remission within 2 years, either with or without therapy. Severely symptomatic patients are more likely to have persistent disease. Persistence of symptoms for more than 2 years markedly reduces the chance of spontaneous remission. Racial factors are important since black patients are more likely to develop chronic, progressive disease. While admittedly imperfect, these clinical criteria are still the best data base on which to base treatment decisions. Laboratory tests such as serum angiotensin converting enzyme (SACE), bronchoalveolar lavage (BAL) cell populations, and gallium-67 (Ga^{67}) scans do not add significantly to treatment decisions.

Since clinical patterns, roentgenographic appearance, and serologic measures are imperfect in predicting the natural course of sarcoidosis, decisions regarding whom to treat remain murky. Suggested guidelines for initiation of treatment in pulmonary sarcoidosis are listed in Table 1. The suggestions are based on personal experience and patient symptoms and are offered as a general guide in patient management. Until therapy becomes available that results in cure, symptom control is a reasonable goal. Treating chest radiograph or pulmonary function abnormalities alone in the absence of symptoms is discouraged.

A caveat: A small group of patients with sarcoidosis have severe chest pain. The mechanism of the discomfort is unclear and it does not correlate with either the roentgenographic stage or the degree of abnormality. In my experience, the patient's pain responds better to

Table 1 Guidelines for Initiation of Treatment in Patients with Pulmonary Sarcoidosis

1. Asymptomatic patients with pulmonary sarcoidosis should not receive corticosteroids
2. Patients with significant respiratory symptoms, abnormal pulmonary function tests, and a diffuse abnormality on chest radiograph should receive treatment
3. Patients with minimal symptoms might best be managed by serial evaluations at 2- to 3-month intervals and treatment reserved until there is evidence of disease progression
4. Patients with disease of more than 2 years' duration with deterioration in pulmonary function (FVC decrease $\geq 10\%$, DL_{CO} decrease $\geq 20\%$, increase in D[A-a] $O_2 \geq 5$ mm Hg) over time are candidates for steroid therapy

analgesics than steroids, and chest pain is not an indication for initiation of or an increase in steroids.

TREATMENT

Effect of Corticosteroids

Corticosteroids are the first-line treatment in sarcoidosis. The majority of patients with sarcoidosis receiving corticosteroids show a beneficial response, usually within the first 2 weeks of treatment. Clinical experience, however, has proven that the response represents suppression, not cure. There is no indication that corticosteroid therapy increases the frequency of permanent remission of disease.

The optimal dose of corticosteroids for sarcoidosis has never been accurately defined. Generally, 30 to 40 mg of prednisone daily is adequate to start. Higher doses are rarely required. Symptomatic improvement is usually rapid, with maximum improvement frequently present at 2 weeks. Patients with acute disease (<6 months' duration) show the greatest evidence of therapeutic benefit. Improvement in vital capacity is noted more frequently than changes in the diffusing capacity. Alternate-day therapy can be very effective in maintaining improvement and may decrease side effects.

Complications of corticosteroid therapy include excessive weight gain, diabetes mellitus, aseptic necrosis, peptic ulcer, and cataracts. Tuberculosis has not been observed in more recent series as the disease has become less prevalent. Nevertheless, patients with sarcoidosis and a positive PPD who are treated with corticosteroids should receive 300 mg of isoniazid for 6 months for prophylaxis. Anergic controls are an unnecessary adjunct to tuberculin skin testing in patients with sarcoidosis.

Dose Adjustment and Duration of Therapy

In sarcoidosis, recognition of the time when the treated patient goes into remission that does not require maintenance therapy would allow therapy to be stopped. Unfortunately, there are neither clinical nor laboratory signs that identify this moment. The clinician must pick an arbitrary duration of treatment, stop the medication, and then monitor the patient's symptoms, chest roentgenogram, and pulmonary function tests for signs of relapse. Over 90 percent of patients treated for symptomatic pulmonary sarcoidosis will show improvement in all three parameters during corticosteroid therapy, but only one-third will remain improved after a year of treatment. The duration of therapy is tailored to the disease presentation and natural history of the illness. Some patients presenting with arthritis and/or erythema nodosum will require steroids to control their joint or skin disease. Typically, both arthritis and erythema nodosum will resolve spontaneously within 3 months, and thus steroids to control these syndromes should be stopped at 3 months. Patients with symptomatic pulmonary sarcoidosis of 2 years or longer duration will have only a 20 to 25 percent chance of spontaneous remission within a year, and steroids are continued through 1 year and then stopped to see if remission has occurred.

Some clinicians worry that patients with sarcoidosis who have demonstrated a beneficial response to steroids with symptomatic, roentgenographic, and/or physiologic improvement may have dampened but not extinguished pulmonary inflammation. In this scenario, an unrecognized smoldering inflammatory reaction is viewed as a threat that may either spread to neighboring alveolar units and/or stimulate irreversible pulmonary fibrosis. This leads to the supposition that a measure of persistent inflammation would allow selection of a steroid dose capable of optimal disease suppression and prevent disease extension and fibrosis. It is here that BAL, Ga^{67} scanning. and SACE studies have created much heat but little light. In patients with sarcoidosis, for example, clinical improvement may occur with steroids, with SACE levels and gallium index reduced but not normal, and with BAL evidence of persistent lymphocytosis. The clinical relevance of persistent abnormalities of SACE level, gallium scan, and BAL findings in treated patients is unknown, and there is no basis for regarding persistent abnormalities of these tests as dictates of therapy at this time. SACE levels, gallium scan, and BAL have not been shown to be superior to symptoms, chest roentgenogram, and pulmonary function tests in following the patient with sarcoidosis.

When the Patient Fails

Lack of improvement with corticosteroid therapy should first raise the possibility of incorrect diagnosis. Multiple diseases mimic sarcoidosis, many of which are accompanied by granuloma and yet are refractory to corticosteroid treatment. Examples include histiocytosis X, Wegener's granulomatosis, fungal infection, mycobacterial infection, and neoplasm with paraneoplastic granuloma. When the patient does not improve, the diagnostic evaluation must be reviewed and the possibility of an incorrect diagnosis strongly entertained. Therapeutic failure with 30 to 40 mg of prednisone for 2 weeks is by no means incompatible with sarcoid. Patients with long-standing disease, cystic degeneration or honeycombing on chest roentgenogram, or striking endobronchial involvement all have a blunted response to steroids.

A second explanation for a patient's failure to show symptomatic improvement is steroid side effects negating the improvement from granuloma suppression. This patient typically shows improvement in symptoms, chest roentgenogram, and pulmonary function tests early but has a later recurrence of dyspnea with decreased exercise tolerance despite the improved chest roentgenogram. In such patients, some combination of steroid-induced weight gain, myopathy, sleep deprivation, and/or depression offset the symptomatic improvement obtained from granuloma suppression. If reduction in steroid dose does not improve the patient's symptoms, alternative therapy for steroid-sparing effect should be considered. The use of alternative therapy will almost always be dictated by the necessity to control steroid side effects. In only rare circumstances will alternative therapy offer an enhanced therapeutic effect over that of corticosteroids.

Alternative Therapies

There are only four alternative treatments for sarcoidosis that are considered adequately substantiated to incorporate into current clinical practice. These are nonsteroidal anti-inflammatory drugs for the treatment of acute arthritis and/or erythema nodosum; chloroquine, which has been especially effective in the treatment of skin disease; oral methotrexate for multisystem sarcoidosis; and inhaled budesonide for pulmonary sarcoidosis. Budesonide is not yet available in the United States, but its use in Europe and Canada has been substantial. Table 2 lists a number of other alternative therapies that are supported by anecdotal information. Kirtland and Winterbauer offer a recent indepth discussion of alternative therapy for sarcoidosis (see reference 2 of the suggested reading list).

Nonsteroidal Anti-Inflammatory Drugs

Nonsteroidal anti-inflammatory drugs (NSAIDs) (indomethacin, ibuprofen, salicylates) may ameliorate the acute inflammatory symptoms of sarcoidosis presenting with arthritis and/or erythema nodosum. Anti-inflammatory agents are effective in approximately one-third of cases of acute sarcoid arthritis. Therapy should begin with a brief trial of a single agent such as indomethacin, 25 to 50 mg three times a day. If prompt symptomatic relief does not occur within 7 days, a course of systemic corticosteroids should be given. Trying a variety of NSAIDs for patients with arthritis and/or erythema nodosum who do not get adequate symptomatic improvement from a single agent is discouraged.

Table 2 Alternative Therapies to Corticosteroids in the Treatment of Sarcoidosis

Nonsteroidal anti-inflammatory drugs	Cyclosporine
Chloroquine	Azathioprine
Methotrexate	Cyclophosphamide
Inhaled budesonide	Ketoconazole
Chlorambucil	

Chloroquine

There are 26 investigations in the medical literature in English on the efficacy of chloroquine, hydroxychloroquine, and quinacrine in the treatment of sarcoidosis. Most studies have involved patients with cutaneous sarcoidosis or combined cutaneous and pulmonary lesions and many of these studies involve patients who have previously failed a trial of corticosteroids. All but one of the studies has shown at least temporary improvement in cutaneous lesions. Pulmonary lesions have tended to show less consistent improvement. Relapse after cessation of drug treatment is typical in chloroquine treatment as with corticosteroids, confirming that chloroquine also suppresses but does not cure. Chloroquine's effectiveness in the treatment of hypercalcemia has also been demonstrated.

Chloroquine therapy has not enjoyed wide popularity, partly because of the concern over retinal toxicity. However, in comparison with corticosteroids, the side-effect profile of chloroquine may be preferable. Complications of chloroquine therapy occur relatively infrequently, and most are transient and reversible with discontinuation of therapy. In patients with rheumatoid arthritis, chloroquine side effects occur in 3 percent to 7 percent of patients, with the most common complaints being nausea and diarrhea.

The most common ocular changes associated with chloroquine therapy are corneal deposition and retinopathy. Corneal deposits occur in about 95 percent of patients receiving long-term therapy of 250 mg per day of chloroquine, but over 90 percent of these patients are asymptomatic. Corneal deposition has no direct relationship to the development of retinopathy and is entirely reversible, disappearing within 6 to 8 weeks after discontinuation of therapy. The incidence of retinopathy in patients receiving chloroquine therapy is estimated to be 0.5 to 2 percent. The size of the daily dose rather than total drug exposure correlates with the development of eye disease. Daily dose must be calculated based on ideal body weight, not the actual weight of the patient. In reports in which chloroquine-induced retinopathy has occurred in patients receiving 250 mg per day or less of chloroquine, dosages usually have exceeded 4 mg per kilogram per day. Late onset chloroquine-induced retinopathy is believed by many to be less of a threat than previously suspected. However, it remains very important to have regular ocular examinations and frequent screenings to detect and prevent retinal toxicity. Ophthalmologic examination should be performed before therapy is initiated in all patients and repeated approximately every 6 months during therapy.

Chloroquine is especially effective in treating lupus pernio and cutaneous plaques, or nodules. An initial 14-day course of 500 mg per day of chloroquine phosphate followed by the smaller of either 250 mg per day or 4 mg per kilogram per day of ideal body weight as maintenance therapy is recommended. Before initiating chloroquine therapy, baseline liver function tests are recommended to assure adequate liver function necessary for normal metabolism and excretion of chloroquine. Acute toxic hepatitis can occur in patients with porphyria cutanea tarda who receive high doses of chloroquine.

Methotrexate

The most promising alternative to corticosteroids in the treatment of pulmonary sarcoidosis is low-dose methotrexate. Although its exact mechanism of action is unclear, it is unlikely that the beneficial effects of low-dose methotrexate are related to its immunosuppressive effects, which are relatively mild. Objective improvement defined as improvement on chest roentgenogram, greater than 15 percent improvement in vital capacity, greater than 50 percent reduction in skin lesions, or improvement in liver function tests has been demonstrated in several studies using methotrexate for multisystem sarcoidosis.

It appears that the risk-benefit ratio of methotrexate is quite low in comparison to prednisone. Liver disease, including cirrhosis, can be seen with methotrexate but the incidence is low and dose related. Concern has been voiced over the potential for malignancy associated with long-term use of methotrexate; however, several studies have shown no increased risk in patients followed for more than 7 years after completion of methotrexate treatment. Unfortunately, the drug has the potential to induce an allergic pneumonitis, which may complicate its use in sarcoidosis. This reaction is characterized by dyspnea, nonproductive cough, fever, and hypoxemia in association with diffuse pulmonary infiltrates. Hilar adenopathy and pleural effusions may be seen. Most patients recover with discontinuation of the drug.

Inhaled Corticosteroids

Inhaled corticosteroids became available in 1978 for the treatment of patients with bronchial asthma. Early attempts to use inhaled beclomethasone dipropionate for the treatment of pulmonary sarcoidosis were unsuccessful. However, budesonide, available since 1982 for asthma, is part of a newer generation of more potent inhaled corticosteroids. This agent has revived the enthusiasm for aerosol corticosteroid treatment in sarcoidosis. Animal studies have shown that local installation of inhaled steroids into the bronchial tree have resulted in higher tissue concentrations than systemic administration. Concentrations of budesonide are great enough to cause receptor binding and exert local anti-inflammatory effect. Budesonide is rapidly inactivated in the liver after systemic absorption, systemic bio-availability is low, and high doses can be used by inhalation with a low risk of systemic side effects.

Table 3 Educational Goals for the Patient with Sarcoidosis Who Is to Start Corticosteroids

1. Patients must be warned of an increase in appetite and possible weight gain. Attention to caloric restriction should begin on the first day of therapy
2. Patients should be warned of the potential for water retention and instructed in dietary salt reduction
3. Patients should be urged to exercise as much as they feel comfortable with to help reduce the potential for myopathy and osteoporosis
4. Other side effects such as mood changes, including euphoria, sleep deprivation, epigastric distress, and elevation of blood sugar with polyuria and polydypsia, should be explained

A number of clinical trials have demonstrated improvement in the chest roentgenograms of patients with pulmonary sarcoidosis given budesonide 800 to 1,600 μg daily for 3 to 6 months. Improvement in pulmonary function, however, has been difficult to establish. Additional studies have indicated that patients initially treated with oral glucocorticosteroids who have relapsed after stopping treatment could be successfully treated with inhaled budesonide alone at a dose of 1,200 to 1,600 μg daily. Inhaled corticosteroids have also been shown to have a systemic steroid-sparing effect in patients with symptomatic pulmonary sarcoidosis treated with prednisone. The rate of improvement with aerosol therapy is slow compared to that seen with systemic steroids; frequently it takes 2 months or longer for improvement with the inhaled product. An initial combination of systemic and inhaled corticosteroids for rapid initial improvement and continuation on maintenance therapy with inhaled corticosteroids alone may prove to be best.

Patient Education

Optimal management of the sarcoid patient includes an earnest effort by the physician to educate the patient of the details of his or her illness and its management. Although written material and support groups are helpful, nothing replaces the efforts of a concerned physician speaking directly to the patient and his family. Patients should be told of their prognosis, the reasoning behind the decision to treat or not to treat, anticipated benefit of therapy, complications of therapy, and danger signals to watch for. The untreated patient must watch for cough and/or increasing dyspnea. All patients should be alerted to symptoms of ocular involvement and urged to contact their physicians immediately if they occur.

Similarly, patients should be counseled about the potential ill effects from use of vitamin D and calcium supplements. The educational goals for patients receiving corticosteroids are listed in Table 3.

SUGGESTED READING

Johns CJ, Zachary JB, Ball WC Jr. A 10-year study of corticosteroid treatment of pulmonary sarcoidosis. Johns Hopkins Med J 1974; 134:271–283.

Kirtland SH, Winterbauer RH. Selected aspects of sarcoidosis. In: Tierney D ed. Current Pulmonology. Vol 15. Chicago: Mosby, 1994:399.

Lower EE, Baughman RP. The use of low-dose methotrexate in refractory sarcoidosis. Am J Med Sci 1990; 299:153–157.

Neville E, Walker AN, James DG. Prognostic factors predicting the outcome of sarcoidosis: An analysis of 818 patient. Q J Med 1983; 52:525–533.

Winterbauer RH, Hammar SP. Sarcoidosis and idiopathic pulmonary fibrosis: A review of recent events. In: Simmons DH ed. Current Pulmonology. Vol 7. Chicago: Yearbook Medical Publishers, 1986:117.

Zic JA, Horowitz DH, Arzubiaga C, et al. Treatment of cutaneous sarcoidosis with chloroquine: Review of the literature. Arch Dermatol 1991; 127:1034–1041.

ACUTE RHEUMATIC FEVER

GIANNI MARONE, M.D.
MASSIMO TRIGGIANI, M.D., Ph.D.

Acute rheumatic fever is an autoimmune disease caused by an untreated infection caused by group A beta-hemolytic streptococcus whose pathogenetic mechanisms are still largely unknown. The incidence of acute rheumatic fever has decreased in industrialized nations since the early years of this century. Beginning in 1985, however, occasional epidemics of rheumatic fever have been reported in different areas of the United States. Even though at least eight outbreaks have been described so far, they appear to reflect a focal rather than a generalized increased activity of the disease. In contrast, acute rheumatic fever continues to be a major health problem in third world countries where the most recent studies indicate a prevalence of 2.2 cases of acute rheumatic fever per 1,000 schoolchildren.

The diagnosis of rheumatic fever is based on the presence of the Jones Criteria revised by the American Medical Association in 1992 (Table 1). The presence of two major criteria or one major and two minor criteria, if supported by evidence of previous group A streptococcal infection, indicates a high probability of acute rheumatic fever. Adequate treatment of streptococcal infections should prevent rheumatic fever in all patients (primary prevention). In those who had an attack of rheumatic fever and are, therefore, at high risk of recurrences, prophylaxis against streptococcal infections will prevent new episodes of the disease (secondary prevention).

Table 1 Jones Criteria for the Diagnosis of Acute Rheumatic Fever (1992 Update)

Major Manifestations
- Carditis
- Polyarthritis
- Chorea
- Erythema marginatum
- Subcutaneous nodules

Minor Manifestations
- Clinical Findings
  - Arthralgia
  - Fever
- Laboratory Findings
  - Elevated acute phase reactants
    - Erythrocyte sedimentation rate
    - C-reactive protein
  - Prolonged PR interval
- Supporting Evidence of Antecedent Group A Streptococcal Infection
  - Positive throat cultures
  - Positive rapid streptococcal antigen test
  - Elevated or rising streptococcal antibody titers (ASLO, anti–DNase B, and so on)

Modified from Anonymous. Guidelines for the diagnosis of rheumatic fever. Jones Criteria, 1990 update. JAMA 1992; 268:2069-2073.

PRIMARY PREVENTION

The precipitating cause of rheumatic fever is an upper respiratory tract infection by group A streptococcus including not only pharyngitis but also otitis, sinusitis and, mastoiditis. Skin infections (impetigo and pyoderma) do not lead to acute rheumatic fever. Primary prevention of rheumatic fever consists of prompt eradication of acute streptococcal infection, which is based on both early identification of group A streptococcus and adequate treatment of the infection.

Acute pharyngitis is more often caused by a virus rather than streptococci. Patients with fever, erythematous pharyngitis with exudate, and tender anterior cervical lymph nodes are more likely than others to have streptococcal pharyngitis, but even this "classic" picture may be caused by other bacterial or viral agents. Conversely, some mild sore throats may be of streptococcal origin and may be followed by rheumatic fever or glomerulonephritis. Therefore, a throat culture should be done in all patients with acute pharyngitis, and all those with a positive culture should be treated with appropriate antibiotics.

Antistreptococcal treatment may be started before knowing the results of the throat culture in patients with severe pharyngitis. In milder cases it is safe to wait for the results of the throat culture since a few days' delay in initiating treatment does not compromise rheumatic fever prevention. Rapid antigen detection tests for diagnosis of group A streptococcal pharyngitis are now available and can provide results much faster than the conventional throat culture. These tests are in general very specific, but they may not be very sensitive. Thus, a negative result on a rapid detection test should always be confirmed by a throat culture.

When cultures are positive for group A streptococci in a patient with a sore throat, the appropriate treatment should be given. Studies in military populations, that have a high frequency of streptococcal pharyngitis, demonstrated that penicillin therapy reduced the incidence of rheumatic fever from 3 to 0.3 percent. Such an effective prevention has been more difficult to achieve in civilian populations and, particularly, in children living in endemic areas. Part of this problem may be due, in part, to the high frequency of streptococcal "carriers" defined as individuals with positive throat cultures without clinical evidence of infection. Asymptomatic carriers and children chronically exposed to streptococcus also frequently have a persistent elevation of serum titers of antistreptococcal antibodies. The question of whether or not streptococcal carriers should be treated still remains open. In certain cases, such as the relatives of patients with rheumatic fever or individuals with a high number of streptococcal colonies, a course of antibiotics to eradicate streptococci is advisable.

Current antibiotic treatment for streptococcal pharyngitis is shown in Table 2. Penicillin is still the drug of choice since group A streptococci have remained highly susceptible to this antibiotic. Prevention of acute rheumatic fever depends upon eradication of the infecting organisms from the pharynx, an effect that requires prolonged exposure to the antibiotic. A single intramuscular injection of benzathine penicillin G (600,000 units for patients weighing less than 27 kg [60 lb] and 1,200,000 units for all others) provides the necessary therapeutic dose of penicillin and is the most effective means of primary prevention. If oral penicillin therapy is elected, penicillin V in a dosage of 250 mg four times daily should be administered 30 minutes before or 1 hour after meals. Patients should be instructed to continue this therapy for 10 days even if symptoms have subsided. Oral cephalosporins may be used as an alternative to penicillins, but obviously they should be avoided in patients allergic to penicillin. These patients should be treated with erythromycin for 10 days (250 mg four times a day or 50 mg per kilogram per day, up to 1 g per day, in divided doses). It should be kept in mind, however, that the rate of resistance to erythromycin of group A streptococci isolated from throat cultures has risen from 7 to 20 percent in the last few years.

Table 2 Antibiotic Treatment for Streptococcus Eradication (Primary Prevention of Acute Rheumatic Fever)

Antibiotic	*Dose*	*Route*	*Duration*
Benzathine Penicillin G	1,200,000 U	Intramuscular	Once
Penicillin V	250 mg q.i.d.	Oral	10 days
Erythromycin	250 mg q.i.d. or 50 mg/kg (max 1 g/day)	Oral	10 days

Modified from Dajani AS, Bisno AL, Chung KJ, et al. Prevention of rheumatic fever. A statement for health professionals by the committee on rheumatic fever, endocarditis and Kawasaki disease of the Council on Cardiovascular Diseases in the Young. Circulation 1988; 78:1082–1086.

Tetracyclines are not recommended, because streptococci resistant to them are prevalent in certain geographic regions. Sulfonamides, which are effective in the prophylaxis of acute rheumatic fever, do not eradicate streptococci from the pharynx and therefore should not be used for primary prevention. No conclusive data are available on the use of new antibiotics such as roxithromycin (150 mg once a day for 10 days) in the primary prevention of rheumatic fever.

Family members of a patient with symptomatic streptococcal pharyngitis are at a high risk of being infected. Therefore, it is advisable to obtain throat swabs from all family contacts with recent upper respiratory symptoms and to treat those with positive cultures.

Follow-up visits are necessary to ascertain whether the infection has cleared, to stimulate compliance in patients taking oral medications, and to investigate for streptococcal sequelae. Streptococcal relapses can be clinical and bacteriologic (sore throat with a positive throat culture) or bacteriologic only (a positive throat culture without sore throat). The recommended practice is to treat both kinds of recurrence with a second course of intramuscular benzathine penicillin or erythromycin.

TREATMENT

General Concepts

The management of acute rheumatic fever depends upon the manifestations and severity of the attack that can be judged on the basis of clinical, laboratory, and instrumental findings. In afebrile patients the presence of tachycardia during sleep is usually indicative of carditis. Initial laboratory studies should include a hematocrit determination, white blood cell count, C-reactive protein level, erythrocyte sedimentation rate, one or more throat cultures taken before beginning penicillin treatment, and the determination of serum titers of antistreptococcal antibodies (e.g., ASLO or anti–DNase B). In addition, a chest roentgenogram, an electrocardiogram, and an echocardiogram with Doppler evaluation should be performed. In young children, however, Doppler evidence of minimal mitral regurgitation should not be considered a diagnostic criteria in the absence of a clinically evident murmur.

It is important to avoid the use of anti-inflammatory drugs until the disease process is clearly expressed. Aspirin or corticosteroids administered prematurely to a patient with arthralgia or early monoarticular arthritis and fever may mask the disease process and cause diagnostic confusion. Once the diagnosis of acute rheumatic fever is established, penicillin therapy in doses sufficient to eradicate residual group A streptococci should be initiated. Although prompt treatment of streptococcal pharyngitis prevents initial attacks of acute rheumatic fever (primary prophylaxis), several studies have shown that administration of antibiotics after the onset of rheumatic fever does not influence the course of the rheumatic attack. Nevertheless, the current recommendation is to administer antibiotics that will eradicate streptococci in pharyngeal and tonsillar tissue and, at the same time, will set the course for subsequent prophylaxis. Thus, the preferred therapy consists of an intramuscular injection of 1,200,000 U of benzathine penicillin G. An alternative regimen is to give oral doses of penicillin, 250 mg four times daily for 10 days. Patients with a history of allergy to penicillin should receive erythromycin, 50 mg per kilogram (maximal dosage, 1 g per day divided into four doses for 10 days). In any event, the initial course of therapy should be followed by a regimen for prophylaxis against subsequent streptococcal infections (secondary prophylaxis).

It is now almost unanimously agreed that selection of the antirheumatic drug is not critical to the outcome of most attacks of rheumatic fever. Both corticosteroids and salicylates control the acute manifestations of the disease, but neither of them is curative.

Arthritis

The arthritis of acute rheumatic fever is very responsive to salicylate therapy. Patients with arthritis only should be treated orally with 75 to 100 mg per kilogram per day of aspirin, divided into four doses. Taking aspirin with a meal or with milk reduces gastric irritation. Buffered or gastric-coated aspirin preparations are thought to reduce gastric damage and to be better tolerated. Omeprazole or prostaglandin analogs (e.g., misoprostol) are often used to prevent peptic ulcer during aspirin treatment but their efficacy has not been conclusively proven. Most patients with rheumatic polyarthritis respond to aspirin in less than 72 hours. If a response is not evident, the dosage may be increased; however, it should not exceed 100 mg per kilogram per day. Since the absorption of salicylate varies considerably from patient to patient, determination of salicylate blood levels is useful if the patient does not appear to respond well to treatment. The serum level at which patients respond best is between 20 and 30 mg per deciliter. A lack of response to this dosage of salicylates should raise doubts about the diagnosis of acute rheumatic fever. The therapeutic dosage is continued for 2 to 4 weeks and gradually reduced over the next 4 to 6 weeks. Determinations of the acute phase reactants (i.e., erythrocyte sedimentation rate and C-reactive protein level), twice weekly initially and then once weekly, are helpful in gauging the response to therapy. Corticosteroids should not be used in patients with arthritis without carditis.

Side effects (gastric, hepatic, or hematologic) are common with the use of large doses of salicylates, and hence the dosage may have to be reduced before an optimal response is achieved. If control of the inflammatory state is not adequate with nontoxic dosages, substitution or addition of another nonsteroidal anti-inflammatory drug should be considered. Furthermore, the possibility of aspirin intolerance should always be considered when beginning the treatment. Aspirin intolerance may be a problem in rheumatic patients because of the cross-reactivity between most nonsteroidal anti-inflammatory drugs. In aspirin-intolerant patients, acetaminophen is less likely to induce adverse reactions.

Confinement to bed is limited to the duration of the acute arthritis. Once the arthritis subsides, ambulation should be allowed, with a gradual return to full activity at the end of aspirin treatment. Despite the form of therapy used, about 5 percent of the attacks of rheumatic fever persist with clinically overt rheumatic manifestations for more than 6 months.

Carditis

The management of carditis is related to the severity of cardiac involvement. Many physicians believe that corticosteroids should be used whenever a patient has acute rheumatic carditis. However, the majority reserve this form of therapy for patients with severe carditis with congestive failure. Despite the lack of definitive evidence, clinical experience suggests that the use of corticosteroids in patients with pancarditis may be lifesaving. Patients with mild carditis without significant cardiomegaly can be given salicylate therapy according to the regimen previously outlined. Many physicians prefer to prolong the treatment period to 9 or 12 weeks. Should a good clinical response and a return of acute phase reactant levels toward normal be obtained, anti-inflammatory therapy may be gradually withdrawn.

In patients with severe carditis with marked cardiomegaly with or without congestive failure, and particularly in those with pancarditis as manifested by the presence of pericarditis, corticosteroids are the drugs of choice. Prednisone at a dosage of 40 to 60 mg per day for both adults and children should be administered for 2 to 4 weeks, depending on the clinical response, followed by gradual withdrawal over 2 to 3 weeks. Corticosteroids can be administered initially in divided doses to obtain the maximal pharmacologic effect, and after the initial clinical response, they should be administered in a single morning dose. One week before withdrawing corticosteroids a salicylate regimen should be started, as already described. This regimen minimizes the occurrence of rebound episodes.

Digitalis should be reserved for patients with severe carditis or congestive failure. Digoxin is preferred for children; a total digitalizing dosage of 0.02 to 0.03 mg per kilogram should be given (maximum dosage 1.5 mg). Some patients with rheumatic myocarditis appear to be sensitive to digitalis and it is always preferable to start at a lower dosage and then increase the dosage as needed to avoid digitalis toxicity. The daily maintenance dosage is about one-fourth of the total digitalizing dosage, given in two equal doses. Therapy with other inotropic drugs or diuretics should be instituted if digoxin alone does not control the congestive failure.

Sydenham's Chorea

The manifestations of Sydenham's chorea are self-limited in the majority of patients. In mild cases treatment may be not necessary. In more severe cases bed rest in a quiet room and avoidance of stress are helpful. There is no unanimity as to the value of sedatives. Some patients appear to benefit from phenobarbital given in doses of 15 to 30 mg every 6 to 8 hours. Haloperidol may be effective in controlling choreiform activity. The dose required varies greatly from patient to patient; a low dose (0.5 mg) given every 8 hours may be initiated and increased to 2.0 mg every 8 hours. Thus, the therapy for Sydenham's chorea should be individualized. Corticosteroids and anti-inflammatory drugs have no role in the treatment of isolated Sydenham's chorea.

SECONDARY PREVENTION

The extreme susceptibility of rheumatic hosts to recurrent attacks of acute rheumatic fever makes it crucial to protect such individuals from streptococcal infections (secondary prevention). This is accomplished by continuous antimicrobial prophylaxis that should be started as soon as the attack of rheumatic fever is diagnosed. The most effective regimen is benzathine penicillin G, which should be administered in a single intramuscular dose of 1,200,000 U every 3 weeks. The rate of recurrence of rheumatic fever is lower in patients treated with intramuscular benzathine penicillin every 3 weeks than in those treated every 4 weeks. Penicillin allergy is often a concern in establishing an effective secondary prophylaxis. Approximately 3 percent of patients are expected to have an allergic reaction during the treatment with intramuscular benzathine penicillin G. More than 50 percent of these reactions occur 1 to 72 hours after the injection mostly as urticaria, arthralgia, or dyspnea. Reactions occurring within 30 minutes of the injection are rare (0.2 percent of patients) and are generally severe (systemic anaphylaxis). Physicians should be aware that anaphylaxis can occur even in patients who have been treated with penicillin for several years with no previous episodes of allergy.

Oral prophylaxis endorsed by the American Heart Association may include (1) sulfadiazine, 1 g once daily for patients over 27 kg (60 lb) and 0.5 g once daily for those under 27 kg (60 lb); (2) penicillin G, 200,000 or 250,000 U twice a day; and (3) erythromycin, 250 mg twice daily for patients who are allergic to both penicillin and sulfonamides. Patients taking sulfadiazine should have a blood count after 2 weeks or if they develop a rash in association with fever or sore throat. Therapy with the drug should be stopped if the white cell count falls below 4,000 and the neutrophil level falls below 35 percent.

It should be recognized that the oral regimens are clearly inferior to benzathine penicillin G in protecting against intercurrent streptococcal infections and acute rheumatic fever recurrences. The overall incidences of rheumatic fever recurrence per 100 patient-years in the Irvington House studies were as follows: benzathine penicillin G group, 0.5; oral penicillin, 5.5; oral sulfadiazine, 2.8. Oral prophylaxis should be given only in patients with minimal or no residual cardiac disease who have had a single rheumatic attack and who have a relatively low risk of exposure to streptococcal infection.

There is still no general consensus as to the duration of secondary prophylaxis. Patients with rheumatic carditis have a high risk of recurrences and require a lifelong antibiotic prophylaxis even if they had valvular surgery. Patients who did not have carditis during the initial attack are less likely to develop carditis if they suffer a recurrence of acute rheumatic fever. Furthermore, the risk of rheumatic fever recurrence declines with age and increasing interval since the previous attack. These facts, together with the relative rarity of severe forms of streptococcal pharyngitis and of acute rheumatic fever in certain areas, suggest that rheumatic prophylaxis might be discontinued in patients at low risk. In these patients, antibiotic prophylaxis is usually stopped 5 years after the last attack or at age 18, whichever comes first. In discontinuing prophylaxis, the physician must carefully weigh a number of factors, including the patient's risk of acquiring a streptococcal infection, the anticipated recurrence rate per infection, and the consequences of recurrence. Adults with a high risk of exposure to streptococcal infection include parents of young children, school teachers, physicians, nurses and allied medical personnel, and those in military service. High risk patients are those with a recent previous attack (3 years or less) or with multiple attacks, or those unlikely to take diligently a daily medication. Additional risk factors are young age (childhood and adolescence), exposure to young people, and crowding in the home. Exceptions to maintaining prophylaxis should be considered only in patients who do not fall into the aforementioned categories.

Rheumatic heart disease predisposes to infective endocarditis. Therefore, patients with rheumatic valvular disease must be protected from bacterial endocarditis whenever they undergo dental, surgical, or diagnostic procedures likely to evoke bacteremia. The dosage and time schedule of antibiotic prophylaxis of endocarditis as recommended by the American Heart Association are listed in Table 3. The antibiotic regimens suggested for endocarditis prophylaxis are entirely different from

Table 3 Prevention of Bacterial Endocarditis in Patients Undergoing Dental, Oral, or Upper Respiratory Tract Procedures

Patient Category	*Agent*	*Route*	*Dosage*		*Time*
			Pediatric	*Adult*	
A. Low Risk, able to take oral medications					
Nonallergic to penicillin	Amoxicillin	Oral	50 mg/kg	3.0 g	1 hr before
			25 mg/kg	1.5 g	6 hr after
Allergic to penicillin	Erythromycin	Oral	20 mg/kg	800 mg	2 hr before
			10 mg/kg	400 mg	6 hr after
	Clindamycin	Oral	10 mg/kg	300 mg	1 hr before
			5.0 mg/kg	150 mg	6 hr after
B. Low Risk, unable to take oral medications					
Nonallergic to penicillin	Ampicillin	IV/IM	50 mg/kg	2.0 g	30 min before
			25 mg/kg	1.0 g	6 hr after
Allergic to penicillin	Clindamycin	IV	10 mg/kg	300 mg	30 min before
			5.0 mg/kg	150 mg	6 hr after
C. Very High Risk					
Nonallergic to penicillin	Ampicillin	IV/IM	50 mg/kg	2.0 g	30 min before
	Gentamycin	IV/IM	2.0 mg/kg	80 mg	30 min before
	Amoxicillin	Oral	25 mg/kg	1.5 g	6 hr after
Allergic to penicillin	Vancomycin	IV	20 mg/kg	1.0 g	Over 1 hr before only

those required for the prophylaxis of acute rheumatic fever. Antibiotics for prophylaxis of bacterial endocarditis should be administered in two doses, before and after the procedure. Moreover, they should be given to all patients with rheumatic valvular disease even if they are on current secondary prophylaxis.

REBOUNDS OF RHEUMATIC ACTIVITY

Clinical or laboratory evidence of rheumatic activity may reappear when antirheumatic therapy is discontinued. Such reactivation has been termed a "rebound" and should clearly be distinguished from a recurrence. Spontaneous rebounds do not occur more than 5 weeks after complete cessation of all antirheumatic therapy; the majority occur within 2 weeks, but most occur within a few days or while the dosage is being reduced. Mild rebound episodes can be characterized by fever, arthralgia, or mild arthritis. Some patients may have only laboratory evidence of relapse such as re-elevation of the C-reactive protein level and the erythrocyte sedimentation rate. Murmurs may reappear. In patients with carditis, rebounds may be severe, and a flare-up of pericarditis or congestive heart failure may occur and, eventually, may be more severe than during the initial period of treatment. Mild rebounds subside spontaneously within 1 or 2 weeks and do not require medication. If treatment is necessary, salicylates are preferred. Severe rebound episodes often can be prevented or minimized by giving salicylates as the corticosteroid dosage is tapered.

CONTINUING MANAGEMENT

The responsibility of the physician to the patient with acute rheumatic fever does not cease with treatment of the acute disease. The first responsibility is to insure that the patient is started and continues on antistreptococcal prophylaxis. Secondary prophylaxis offers the only hope for healing and recovery from cardiac disease. For the patient with residual cardiac involvement, monitoring of the cardiac disease and its management (both medical and, if necessary, surgical) should be continued. Patients should be seen at frequent intervals initially, later at monthly and bimonthly intervals, and then at biyearly or yearly intervals, to ensure that prophylaxis is being complied with. Education of the patient should continue through adolescence. Part of the continued care includes emphasis on dental hygiene and increasing the patient's awareness regarding the need for prophylaxis against bacterial endocarditis. The patient should be encouraged and informed that these efforts will result in good control of the cardiac disease and a return to a normal way of life.

ANTISTREPTOCOCCAL VACCINE

Despite the efficacy of antibiotics and chemotherapeutic drugs, infectious diseases have been eradicated only by vaccines and/or improved environmental sanitation. Attempts to develop a streptococcal vaccine are based on studies of M proteins, the only streptococcal components that elicit protective antibodies. These efforts have been hampered by the lack of highly antigenic and well-tolerated preparations. Preparations of M proteins that are highly immunogenic in man and relatively free of side effects are now available. However, even highly purified M proteins contain epitopes that cross-react with heart and brain antigens, and thus they may cause rheumatic fever instead of preventing it. Two possible solutions are now under investigation using selected fragments of M proteins. The first is to use fragments of the highly conserved C-terminus region, which is common among the different serotypes. This type of vaccine will offer the advantage of protection against all serotypes of rheumatogenic streptococci but it is likely to induce the formation of autoantibodies. The second approach is to produce a multivalent vaccine containing fragments from the highly variable N-terminus region. This preparation will immunize only against selected serotypes, but it will carry a reduced risk of autoimmune reactions. Studies are currently ongoing in humans to evaluate the safety and effectiveness of these vaccines. However, until sufficient data are available, antibiotic prophylaxis remains our mainstay for prevention of acute rheumatic fever.

SUGGESTED READING

Anonymous. Guidelines for the diagnosis of rheumatic fever. Jones Criteria, 1992 update. JAMA 1992; 268:2069–2073.

Ayoub EM. Resurgence of rheumatic fever in the United States. The changing picture of a preventable illness. Postgrad Med 1992; 92:139–142.

Berrios X, del Campo E, Guzman B, Bisno AL. Discontinuing rheumatic fever prophylaxis in selected adolescents and young adults. Ann Intern Med 1993; 118:401–406.

Lue HC, Wu MH, Wang JK, et al. Long-term outcome of patients with rheumatic fever receiving benzathine penicillin G prophylaxis every three weeks versus every four weeks. J Pediatr 1994; 125:812–816.

Taubert KA, Rowley AH, Shulman ST. Seven-year national survey of Kawasaki disease and acute rheumatic fever. Pediatr Infect Dis J 1994; 13:704–708.

POSTCARDIAC INJURY SYNDROME

CLIFFORD J. KAVINSKY, M.D., Ph.D.
JOSEPH E. PARRILLO, M.D.

The postcardiac injury syndrome (PCIS) encompasses a group of disorders characterized by a pericarditis syndrome occurring several days to several months following a myocardial or pericardial insult as a result of infarction (postmyocardial infarction syndrome; Dressler's syndrome), cardiac surgery (postcardiotomy syndrome), or trauma (postcardiac trauma syndrome). A similar syndrome has been reported following pulmonary embolism/infarction and after cardiac pacemaker placement. Whether the inciting event is myonecrosis, wide incision of the pericardium, or extravasation of blood into the pericardial space, the end result is a systemic inflammatory process consisting of constitutional symptoms, pleuropericarditis, and occasionally pneumonitis. This disorder generally occurs 1 to 4 weeks after the initial insult with a range of 1 week to several months.

Postcardiac injury syndrome is thought to complicate 1 to 4 percent of myocardial infarctions and up to 30 percent of cardiac surgeries. Although this disorder is considered to be self-limited, generally resolving over a period of weeks, recurrences are common and may occur as late as 2 years after the initial insult. As many as 50 percent of patients with PCIS experience recurrence, which usually occurs 2 to 4 months after the initial bout and often coincides with tapering of anti-inflammatory therapy. In addition, rare but potentially serious sequelae such as pericardial tamponade, severe incapacitating chest pain, pneumonitis, premature coronary bypass graft occlusion, unstable angina requiring surgical revascularization, and the late development of chronic constrictive pericarditis have all been reported in association with PCIS.

Predisposing factors for the development of this syndrome are poorly understood. Epidemiologic studies have identied recent viral infection, young age, history of pericarditis, prior treatment with prednisone, B-negative blood type, and halothane anesthesia as imparting increased risk for the development of PCIS after cardiac surgery. In patients following myocardial infarction, postmyocardial infarction syndrome was more common in those with anterior or recurrent infarcts and in diabetics.

The precise mechanisms responsible for the pathogenesis of PCIS are unclear. However, accumulated clinical and laboratory evidence supports immune-mediated tissue injury to be at least partially responsible for the clinical expression of this syndrome. An autoimmune process is suggested by the presence of a latent period between the initial myocardial insult and the onset of symptoms, polyserositis, the self-limited nature of the syndrome, the presence of heart reactive antibodies, the often dramatic response to anti-inflammatory therapy, and the tendency for recurrences. It is proposed that damage to the myocardium or pericardium or damage caused by the entry of blood into the pericardial space results in cellular injury that after a latent period triggers an autoimmune response involving both humoral and cell-mediated arms of the immune system directed against heart cell antigens and leading to release of cellular mediators of inflammation. This is supported by several studies demonstrating the occurrence of anti–heart antibodies in postinfarction and postcardiac surgery patients who developed PCIS. Engle has reported a close correlation between high titers of anti–heart antibodies and the clinical appearance of PCIS in postsurgical patients. Further studies have identified reactive antigenic determinants residing within a variety of myocyte cellular components, including the major contractile proteins, actin and myosin. In addition, some investigators have demonstrated rising antibody titers directed against viral antigens in patients with PCIS. This has led to the hypothesis that reactivation of latent viral or recurrent viral infection may provide an immune stimulus that serves to initiate the cascade of events leading to the brisk systemic inflammation seen in this disorder.

CLINICAL FEATURES

The postcardiac injury syndrome is characterized by the onset of constitutional symptoms, fever, chest pain, and shortness of breath most commonly occurring 2 to 3 weeks after the initial insult (Table 1). The chest pain is often pleuritic, worse in the supine position, precordial or substernal in location, and may radiate to the left shoulder or posteriorly to the interscapular area. Fatigue and malaise are common associated findings. Physical examination will often reveal pericardial and pleural friction rubs. In the postcardiac surgery setting where pericardial friction rubs are the rule, the presence of fever and persistent chest pain are suggestive of PCIS.

Table 1 Major Clinical Findings in Postcardiac Injury Syndrome

Signs and Symptoms	*Percentage*
Chest pain	91
Fever	66
Pericardial rub	63
Dyspnea	57
Pleural rub	46
Rales	51

Table 2 Diagnostic Findings in the Postcardiac Injury Syndrome

Test	*Percentage*
Elevated erythrocyte sedimentation rate	96
Leukocytosis	49
Chest radiograph abnormalities	94
Pleural effusion	83
Pulmonary infiltrates	74
Enlarged cardiac silhouette	49
Pericardial effusion (echocardiography)	60
ECG abnormalities	50

Pleural effusions, pulmonary infiltrates, and enlargement of the cardiac silhouette are often noted on chest radiograph (Table 2). Echocardiography will reveal pericardial effusions in approximately one-half of patients. The pericardial effusions are usually small and cardiac tamponade occurs rarely. Fluid drained from either the pleural or pericardial space may be either serosanguinous or hemorrhagic and is always exudative with high protein contents (4 to 5 g per deciliter) and leukocyte counts less than 1,000 per cubic millimeter. The electrocardiogram may show changes consistent with pericarditis such as PR segment depression, ST segment elevation, or T-wave inversion. Finally, elevation of acute phase reactants, particularly the erythrocyte sedimentation rate and total blood leukocyte count, are frequently observed.

There are no pathognomonic findings in the PCIS to aid in establishing the diagnosis; thus, the diagnosis of this disorder relies on clinical criteria. Laboratory and diagnostic test data may be used to provide supportive evidence. In cases of suspected PCIS other illnesses capable of causing similar symptomatology such as myocardial ischemia or infarction, other collagen vascular disorders, pneumonia, pulmonary embolism, heart failure, or infection must be effectively ruled out.

THERAPY

Salicylates

Postcardiac injury syndrome is usually a self-limited illness lasting from 4 to 6 weeks, although as previously mentioned recurrences are common, particularly when tapering anti-inflammatory therapy. The self-limited nature of this disorder makes assessment of the efficacy of anti-inflammatory therapy difficult. The various treatments for PCIS are summarized in Table 3. Patients with mild constitutional symptoms, chest pain, and shortness of breath without large pericardial effusions, tamponade, or pneumonitis on physical examination or diagnostic evaluation may be treated with salicylates (Table 4). Aspirin at a dose of 650 mg every 4 hours usually results in a symptomatic response after a few doses, with improvement in chest pain and fever and a general sense of well-being. Although symptoms improve, other indices of disease activity such as acute phase reactants and pleural and pericardial effusions are usually unaffected by aspirin. However, since PCIS is self-limited, providing symptomatic relief may be all that is necessary. In patients who achieve a therapeutic response to salicylates, mild lingering residual chest discomfort may be treated with small doses of analgesics such as codeine, oxycodone, or hydrocodone. In patients responding to aspirin, a 2- to 3-week course of therapy is usually recommended to prevent recurrence of symptoms.

Salicylates, as well as other nonsteroidal anti-inflammatory drugs (NSAIDs), exert their beneficial effects in the PCIS through their antipyretic, analgesic, and anti-inflammatory properties, which occur as a result of inhibition of cyclooxygenase-mediated prostaglandin synthesis. Aspirin, as well as other NSAIDs, may cause gastric irritation and ulceration with upper gastrointestinal bleeding. Adverse gastrointestinal side effects can be minimized by taking tablets after meals or with antacids. Alternatively, patients exhibiting gastrointestinal symptoms may be treated with sucralfate or misoprostol. Aspirin also results in inhibition of platelet function and prolongation of the bleeding time and should be generally avoided in patients taking warfarin or in those patients with a bleeding diathesis. Aspirin may cause reversible elevation of serum transaminases as well as depression of renal function and should be used cautiously in patients with underlying liver or kidney dysfunction.

Nonsteroidal Anti-inflammatory Drugs

Patients with mild to moderate PCIS who do not respond to several days of aspirin therapy should receive a nonsteroidal anti-inflammatory drug. Several NSAIDs have been used in this setting and are summarized in Table 4. A cautionary note should be invoked when using NSAIDs. Isolated studies have described an adverse affect of NSAIDs on left ventricular remodeling following myocardial infarction. NSAIDs, in particular ibuprofen and indomethacin, have been associated with scar thinning as well as infarct expansion, which may potentially lead to aneurysm formation and myocardial rupture. In addition, these agents can adversely effect coronary vascular resistance. However, these effects are largely experimental and theoretical and there is little published clinical data which suggests that patients treated with NSAIDs after myocardial infarction have an adverse short- or long-term outcome. Conversely, large published clinical trials have shown NSAIDs to be both effective and safe when used in the setting of PCIS. However, because of the aforementioned considerations, aspirin is the preferred initial therapy for PCIS, with NSAIDs reserved for those who fail to respond.

Table 3 Treatment Modalities in Postcardiac Injury Syndrome

Salicylates
Nonsteroidal anti-inflammatory drugs
Corticosteroids
Cytotoxic immunosuppressive agents
Analgesics
Pericardiocentesis
Pericardiectomy

Table 4 Salicylates and NSAIDs in Postcardiac Injury Syndrome

Agent	*Dose and Interval*
Aspirin	325-650 mg every 4 hours
Ibuprofen	400-800 mg every 8 hours
Naproxin	375-500 mg every 12 hours
Indomethacin	25-50 mg every 8 hours

In those patients who do require an NSAID, ibuprofen or naproxin are initially recommended rather than indomethacin since they are generally better tolerated and have less impact on infarct healing after myocardial infarction. As with aspirin, NSAIDs are useful in relieving fever and symptoms but do not affect other indices of systemic inflammation such as acute phase reactants or effusions. Besides the adverse gastrointestinal side effects described earlier, NSAIDs can cause reversible elevation in serum transaminases and inhibition of platelet aggregation. In addition, NSAIDs can adversely affect kidney function and cause acute renal failure, nephrotic syndrome, acute interstitial nephritis, and glomerulonephritis. Therefore, these agents should be used with caution in patients with underlying liver or kidney disease and periodic monitoring of renal and hepatic function should be carried out. Furthermore, NSAIDs can also cause sodium and fluid retention, peripheral edema, and exacerbation of heart failure in susceptible individuals. Patients with impaired heart function should be watched closely for signs and symptoms suggestive of heart failure and treated with diuretics when such evidence appears.

In patients who fail to respond to aspirin, ibuprofen, or naproxin and in those with more severe symptoms of chest pain, dyspnea, fever, and malaise, a trial of indomethacin is warranted. Therapy is generally begun at 25 mg three times per day and titrated upwards to a maximum of 75 mg three times daily. Many patients will achieve prompt relief of even severe symptoms of PCIS even if a suboptimal clinical response was previously noted with aspirin or other NSAIDs. Patients will usually note symptomatic improvement after several doses, but it may take 2 to 3 days to achieve maximum therapeutic benefit. If indomethacin therapy is effective, it should be continued for 2 to 3 weeks to prevent relapses. Recrudescent symptoms occurring after cessation of therapy can be treated with reinstitution of indomethacin at the dose previously known to be effective. Indomethacin therapy may be tapered to provide longer term anti-inflammatory benefit while minimizing adverse side effects.

Corticosteroids

Corticosteroids are extremely effective in treating the signs and symptoms of PCIS. Corticosteroids also suppress the systemic inflammatory state associated with this syndrome. However, because of the potentially serious long-term adverse effects associated with steroid use and the potential for recurrence during tapering of therapy, these drugs should be reserved for patients with severe symptoms, symptoms that are unresponsive to more conservative therapy, or for those patients with the more serious sequelae of PCIS (Table 5).

Patients with severe incapacitating chest pain and shortness of breath, as well as those patients who do not achieve an adequate clinical response to salicylates or

Table 5 Indications for Corticosteroids in Postcardiac Injury Syndrome

Severe symptoms
Symptoms unresponsive to aspirin or NSAIDs
Multiple recurrences
Pneumonitis
Cardiac tamponade
Large pericardial effusions without tamponade

NSAIDs, should be treated with systemic corticosteroids. In addition, patients with multiple recurrences of PCIS may become increasingly refractory to aspirin and NSAIDs and will often require corticosteroids for control of symptoms.

Corticosteroids can be given orally or intravenously. Steroid therapy can usually be initiated with oral prednisone at a dose of 60 mg per day. Most patients will have dramatic clinical response with resolution of chest pain, shortness of breath and fever, as well as an increased sense of well-being. Unlike aspirin or NSAIDs, which improve symptoms without altering the systemic inflammatory state, patients treated with corticosteroids will exhibit normalization of acute phase reactants as well as resolution of pleural and pericardial effusions. If patients achieve a complete clinical response with resolution of symptoms and signs of systemic inflammation, steroids may be tapered over a 10-day period, avoiding suppression of the pituitary-adrenal axis and the requirement for "stress-dose" steroids.

Patients who exhibit flaring of symptoms during tapering or after discontinuation of corticosteroid therapy can be treated with aspirin or NSAIDs. Alternatively, such patients can have reinstitution of full-dose steroid therapy followed by a more prolonged, graded tapering of therapy. Alternate-day tapering is recommended by many using 5 mg decrements in the alternate-day dose such that after several weeks the patient is taking 60 mg per day of prednisone with no steroid dose on alternate days. During this tapering regimen one should watch closely for exacerbation of symptoms. The adverse side effects of long-term corticosteroid administration such as glucose intolerance, osteoporosis, muscle weakness, hypertension, fluid retention and edema, and cataract formation are markedly diminished with alternate-day prednisone therapy.

Once alternate-day prednisone therapy is successfully achieved without recurrence of symptoms, the remaining prednisone may then be slowly tapered over a period of 2 to 6 weeks. Patients seldom exhibit recurrences with this type of prednisone dosing regimen. Those patients who demonstrate recrudescent symptoms should have the alternate-day prednisone dose increased, followed by a more gradual tapering course. Alternatively, flares occurring during steroid tapering can be treated with small doses of NSAIDs. Patients who require corticosteroid therapy for more than 4 to 6 weeks should be tapered to a dose of 5 mg prednisone every other day for several weeks before totally discontinuing therapy to avoid suppression of the pituitary-adrenal axis.

Pericardiocentesis

Patients presenting with any of the severe complications of PCIS such as large pleural or pericardial effusion, cardiac tamponade, or severe pneumonitis should be immediately hospitalized and undergo careful clinical assessment. For patients presenting in a shock-like state with impaired organ perfusion, hypotension, distant heart sounds, elevated jugular venous pressure, and pulsus paradoxicus, cardiac tamponade should be considered and immediately evaluated with two-dimensional and doppler echocardiography. Echocardiography may reveal a pericardial effusion of variable size with signs of tamponade physiology, which include right atrial and ventricular diastolic wall collapse and respirophasic variation in the doppler signal across the atrioventricular valves. Patients with findings of cardiac tamponade should undergo emergent percutaneous needle pericardiocentesis. The echocardiogram should verify the presence of significant fluid in the anterior pericardial space so that coronary artery laceration and myocardial perforation are avoided during the procedure. Pericardiocentesis is most safely performed using the subxiphoid approach with the needle attached to a V lead of an electrocardiogram to avoid myocardial perforation. A pressure transducer may also be attached to the needle to monitor intrapericardial pressure and to signal entry into the right ventricular cavity. Entry into the pericardial space will result in return of serous or hemorrhagic fluid. Removal of even small amounts of pericardial fluid (10 to 20 cc) will usually result in significant hemodynamic improvement. To ensure complete drainage of pericardial fluid it is recommended that a soft catheter be advanced into the pericardial space over a guide wire and left in place for several hours or days.

Patients with PCIS complicated by cardiac tamponade should be immediately treated with corticosteroids. In this setting therapy is best initiated with intravenous methylprednisolone 60 mg followed by 20 mg IV every 8 hours for 1 to 2 weeks to prevent recurrence of tamponade. Following completion of intravenous therapy the patients should be given a course of oral prednisone, which is slowly tapered using the alternate-day approach previously described. Most patients treated in this manner do not experience recurrent tamponade and alternate-day prednisone therapy should be tapered after 2 to 3 months.

Patients who have PCIS complicated by pneumonitis or significant pleural or pericardial effusions without tamponade physiology are also best treated with corticosteroids. Again, initially intravenous therapy is preferred with methylprednisolone 60 mg followed by 20 mg every 8 hours. In many instances the pericardial effusion will rapidly resolve on steroid therapy. Likewise, pneumonitis almost always resolves with corticosteroid administration. Parenteral therapy should be continued for

1 to 2 weeks, followed by a course of oral prednisone as previously described.

Pericardiectomy

Patients with recurrent pericardial effusion and cardiac tamponade despite full courses of corticosteroid therapy should be considered for surgical pericardiectomy. This procedure has a low major complication rate and virtually eliminates the chance of recurrent tamponade. In addition, pericardiectomy reduces chest pain in most patients. An occasional patient may suffer from some chest pain even after pericardiectomy and will require a prolonged course of alternate-day prednisone therapy to control symptoms.

Rarely patients who have had PCIS will present late with refractory heart failure due to chronic constrictive pericarditis. The incidence of this complication is low. Echocardiography may suggest thickening of the pericardium with findings of pericardial constriction. Cardiac catheterization will demonstrate pulmonary hypertension with elevation and equalization of right and left sided diastolic filling pressures. Confirmation of pericardial thickening using computed tomography or magnetic resonance imaging aids in establishing the diagnosis. Patients who develop constrictive pericarditis with heart failure are best treated with a surgical pericardial stripping procedure, which is often curative.

Cytotoxic Immunosuppressive Agents

Occasionally, patients will have recurrent symptoms despite a prolonged course of steroid therapy. In order to minimize the adverse effects of long-term prednisone therapy, cytotoxic immunosuppressive agents have been successfully employed. Patients may be treated with azathioprine 2 mg per kilogram per day or cyclophosphamide 1 to 2 mg per kilogram per day along with alternate-day prednisone therapy. This therapeutic approach can also be employed to treat patients with recurrent pericardial effusion and tamponade. Patients should be closely monitored for adverse effects of cytotoxic therapy such as bone marrow suppression. Cytotoxic therapy can be continued for 1 to 2 years, after which all anti-inflammatory therapy can be tapered and discontinued without recurrence of symptoms.

SUGGESTED READING

Engle MA, Gay WA, Zabriskie JB, Senterfit LB. The postpericardiotomy syndrome: 25 years' experience. J Cardiovasc Med 1984; 9:321–332.

Gregoratos G. Pericardial involvement in acute myocardial infarction. Cardiol Clin 1990; 8(4):601–608.

Horneffer PJ, Miller RH, Pearson TA, et al. The effective treatment of postpericardiotomy syndrome after cardiac operations. J Thorac Cardiovasc Surg 1990; 100:292–296.

Khan AH. The Postcardiac Injury Syndrome. Clin Cardiol 1992; 15:67–72.

Stelzner TJ, King TE Jr, Antony VB, Sahn SA. The pleuropulmonary manifestations of the postcardiac injury syndrome. Chest 1983; 84(4):383–387.

INFLAMMATORY MYOCARDITIS

PETER J. RICHARDSON, M.D., F.R.C.P.

Inflammatory myocarditis is one of the most common diseases to affect the myocardium and when longstanding may lead to a dilated cardiomyopathy. Although molecular techniques for the detection of enterovirus in the myocardium, both by in situ hybridization and polymerase chain reaction (PCR), have demonstrated virus in up to 30 percent of patients, it should not be forgotten that there are many other infectious agents such as bacteria, rickettsiae, fungi, and parasites that may be responsible for causing inflammation in heart muscle. Myocarditis is twice as frequent in males as in females with the exception of secondary myocarditis due to the collagen diseases. The definition of different types of myocarditis is not possible on the basis of the cardiovascular signs and symptoms, although inflammatory heart muscle disease "myocarditis" may be an accompanying feature of a systemic illness. In the absence of clear signs of the latter, careful investigation may be required to establish the pathogenetic origin of the inflammatory heart muscle disease.

The presentation of inflammatory heart muscle disease may include all degrees of cardiac failure or an arrhythmia, but it may even be asymptomatic.

DEFINITION AND DIAGNOSIS OF INFLAMMATORY MYOCARDITIS

The advent of endomyocardial biopsy has made it possible to obtain myocardial biopsy tissue from patients with suspected inflammatory heart muscle disease. This has enabled not only the confirmation of the suspected clinical diagnosis of myocarditis by histopathologic evaluation, but also the demonstration of enterovirus in the myocardium. Other pathogens have included such infectious agents such as *Borrelia,* coccidioidomycosis, and tuberculosis.

Table 1 Systemic Connective Tissue Disorders or Autoimmune Diseases

Acute rheumatic fever	Scleroderma
Still's disease	Mixed connective tissue disorder
Rheumatoid arthritis	Polyarteritis nodosa
Systemic lupus erythematosus	Wegener's granulomatosis
Ankylosing spondylitis	Sarcoidosis

Myocarditis may be defined as a "process characterized by an inflammatory infiltrate of the myocardium with necrosis and/or degeneration of the adjacent myocytes not typical of the ischemic damage associated with coronary arterial disease." In the clinical context biopsy-proven myocarditis may be further classified into active, healing, or healed phases, the healed phase being indistinguishable histologically from dilated cardiomyopathy. These histologic classifications of myocarditis enabled a more acute description of the response of the myocardium to treatment with immunosuppressive therapy (Table 1).

In some patients with inflammatory myocarditis there may be concomitant myopericarditis. This is particularly common with a viral infection. There are almost always underlying epicardial-myocardial lesions. Myopericarditis has been defined as a clinical syndrome of pericardial effusion associated with cardiomegaly with or without segmental wall motion abnormalities, with the latter occurring as the result of a focal myocarditic process. Pericarditis, defined as an inflammation of the pericardium, is usually associated with pericardial fluid. The pericarditis may be recurrent or persistent and constriction may occur as a late sequel. The pathogen most frequently encountered in constrictive pericarditis is tuberculosis, although in many patients no specific cause can be identified.

TREATMENT

In considering the treatment of inflammatory myocarditis it is important to determine whether there is a specific connective tissue disorder or a specific pathogen responsible for the myocardial inflammatory disease. In both the latter groups specific treatment may be available. Table 1 lists the systemic connective tissue disorders or autoimmune diseases. With the exception of acute rheumatic fever, which is treated with aspirin with or without prednisolone, the treatment for the other conditions is immunosuppression using steroids, azathioprine, or cyclophosphamide. The most commonly encountered is sarcoid heart disease. Sarcoid involvement of the conducting system and arrhythmias are not infrequent and complete heart block will require a pacemaker. The treatment of this multisystem disease is monitored in the usual way (see the chapter *Sarcoidosis*). Serum angiotensin-converting enzyme (ACE) levels may be useful in assessing activity of the disease.

Specific infections that may affect the myocardium are classified as bacterial, fungobacterial, fungal, and parasitic. The common pathogens are listed in Table 2. In those with bacterial infection the appropriate antibiotics should be employed. In tuberculous infection, antituberculous therapy is indicated. However, it may be found that there is pericardial involvement. The concomitant pericardial fluid can produce tamponade, requiring pericardiocentesis. Pericardial biopsy may be required if aspiration of the pericardial fluid has not identified the pathogen. In those patients in whom there is recurrent tamponade or in whom constriction has developed, a pericardial window or pericardiectomy may be indicated. In rickettsial infection, tetracycline may be required for 3 to 6 months and similarly in *Borrelia* infection (Lyme disease) antibiotics for 3 to 6 months may also be indicated. In the fungal group the appropriate antimycotic treatment should be given. In parasitic infections, for example, amoebiasis should be treated with metronidazole or dihydroemetine. Echinococcal cysts should be excised if possible. Toxoplasmosis may be treated with pyrimethamine and sulfadiazine or spiromycin. In some of the latter cases pericardiectomy may be required.

Table 2 Specific Pathogens

Bacterial	*Fungobacterial*
Mycobacterium tuberculosis	*Actinomyces*
Pneumococcus	*Nocardia*
Staphylococcus	
Streptococcus	*Fungal*
Rickettsiae	*Candida*
Borrelia	*Histoplasma*
	Coccidioides
Parasitic	
Amoebae	
Toxoplasma	
Echinococcus	

VIRAL HEART DISEASE

At the present time although viral heart disease may be diagnosed by in situ hybridization or PCR of biopsy tissue, no specific antiviral therapy is available. Ribavirin has been used in animal models with some success, and preliminary studies with interferon alpha have shown that it inhibits virus replication and reduces the inflammatory response in the myocardium. There are some preliminary clinical data that suggest that interferon may be of some value. The results of more detailed and controlled clinical trials, however, are required before this treatment should be employed more generally.

IMMUNOSUPPRESSIVE THERAPY

While viruses may be responsible for inflammatory myocarditis it should be recognised that the majority of patients in whom viral infection occurs will recover spontaneously without any specific treatment. It is only in those patients who have important sequelae such as focal or diffuse myocardial involvement that more specific treatment may be indicated. Although the viral origin has been substantiated it is recognised that the virus does not persist in its normal replicating form but rather as a defective mutant virus. This has been thought to produce further heart muscle damage by immune mediated mechanisms. Various forms of immunosuppression have been tried in experimental murine Coxsacke B3 myocarditis. Prednisone, cyclosporine and monoclonal antibodies, T helper and cytolytic suppressor T lymphocytes have been employed. Similarly the effects of tumor necrosis factor, interleukin II and anti-interleukin II receptor antibodies have been studied. In the majority, however, it has been difficult to demonstrate any consistent benefit using these forms of treatment.

Considerable interest has focused on the possibility of using immunosuppressive therapy for the treatment of inflammatory myocarditis where no specific pathogen has been isolated. The use of immunosuppression was suggested following the recognition that this could be successfully used to treat cardiac transplant rejection. The initial observations were made by Mason and colleagues at Stanford who treated 10 patients with biopsy-proven myocarditis, five of whom showed improvement. Relapse followed withdrawal of treatment. A similar observation was made by Daly and colleagues who investigated 18 patients; nine had acute inflammatory myocarditis on biopsy and in seven there was substantial clinical improvement with treatment. These early studies, however, were uncontrolled. A review of the papers published up to 1993 showed a total of 112 patients who were identified as suffering from acute myocarditis, and in 59 percent improvement was observed primarily using prednisolone and azathioprine.

The Myocarditis Treatment Trial was designed to evaluate the efficacy of immunosuppression in patients with myocarditis and at the same time to identify immunologic markers of the severity of the disease and their relationship to the response to therapy. The trial was specifically designed to determine whether improvement of left ventricular function occurred in response to immunosuppressive treatment. One hundred and eleven patients with a histopathologic diagnosis of acute myocarditis and an ejection fraction (EF) of less than 45 percent were randomly allocated to receive conventional therapy alone or a 24-week regimen of immunosuppressive therapy in combination with conventional therapy. The immunosuppressive therapy consisted of prednisolone with either cyclosporin or azathioprine. The primary outcome measurement was the change in the left ventricular ejection fraction after 28 weeks of treatment. In the group as a whole, the mean left ventricular ejection fraction improved from 25 percent at baseline to 34 percent at 28 weeks ($p < 0.001$). The mean change of the left ventricular ejection fraction at 28 weeks did not differ significantly between the two groups of patients. It was found that certain factors predicted a better outcome, namely a higher left ventricular ejection fraction at the baseline, the need for less conventional treatment, and disease of short duration. There was no significant difference in survival between the two treatment groups. The mortality rate for the entire group was 20 percent at 1 year and 56 percent at 4.3 years. It was concluded as a result of this study that ventricular function improved regardless of whether or not the patients received immunosuppressive therapy. The mechanism of improvement is unclear. An important observation was that there was a high long-term mortality.

In light of the Myocarditis Trial finding, it is difficult to recommend immunosuppression in patients with acute biopsy-proven myocarditis. However, certain observations are pertinent, namely that in the study of Quigley and co-workers (1984) it was clear that approximately 50 percent of patients may improve on follow-up within a period of 6 months and recovery was not confined to those with poor EFs. Late improvement of ejection fraction at 6 months is unusual but has been reported. The persistence of an inflammatory infiltrate in the myocardium appears to predict the possibility of subsequent improvement in these patients. The finding on serial biopsy of a pattern consistent with a dilated cardiomyopathy indicates that there is little likelihood of significant improvement in ventricular function if the patients have already been treated conventionally for heart failure. The detection of enterovirus RNA in the myocardium of patients with suspected heart muscle disease with or without inflammatory changes on biopsy is associated with a poorer prognosis and a reduced survival rate. The influence of virus could not be assessed in the Myocarditis Treatment Trial, although an increased natural killer cell activity and a higher white cell count were found to be consistent with a more effective inflammatory response. It was suggested that in patients with myocarditis a prominent immunologic response may be a benefit rather than a cause of the disease.

CONVENTIONAL TREATMENT

Although the benefit of immunosuppression has been carefully investigated in inflammatory myocarditis, the mainstay of treatment must be conventional for the majority of patients. This includes treatment of cardiac failure, treatment of arrhythmias, and the prevention of embolic complications. When the standard treatment of heart failure fails, hemodynamic support must be considered with aortic balloon pumping and finally cardiac transplantation.

Arrhythmias

In inflammatory heart disease both supraventricular and atrial dysrhythmias, particularly atrial fibrillation, are frequent. Treating patients with digoxin is of benefit in controlling the heart rate and improving the inotropic response. Digoxin is given initially as a loading dose of

250 to 750 μg, with 250 μg three times a day for the first 24 hours, which thereafter is reduced usually to between 125 and 250 μg daily. Digoxin is usually given in addition to a diuretic and against this background it is important to monitor the level of the serum potassium since hypokalemia is more likely to result in digitalis provoked arrhythmia.

Supraventricular arrhythmias may be treated in the usual way, but it should be remembered that the majority of agents may exert negative inotropism and should not be used when there is significant depression of left ventricular function. Amiodarone can be used in this context and can also be given for ventricular arrhythmias. Other antiarrhythmic agents such as disopyramide or mexiletine are negatively inotropic and drugs such as flecainide may have a proarrhythmic effect. Drug resistant ventricular tachycardia, which is inducible, may benefit from an automatic implantable defibrillator system.

Cardiac Failure

One of the most common manifestations of inflammatory myocarditis is impairment of ventricular function, which may affect both ventricles, although in some patients either ventricle may be affected in isolation. The major management options for treatment (Table 3) are shown in Figure 1.

It has long been recognized that prolonged bedrest may be of value in patients with active myocarditis. Experimental data suggest that myocyte injury can be promoted by continued physical activity when the inflammatory process is still active. As a general measure restriction of salt intake is of value, certainly in patients with New York Heart Association (NYHA) grades III and IV heart failure.

Diuretics

The use of diuretics is necessary in the majority of cases and the most frequently used are the loop diuretics, furosemide, or bumetanide. When a mild diuresis is required a thiazide diuretic may be sufficient. In more severe failure the use of the thiazide-like diuretic, metolazone, may be of benefit. Enhancement of the diuretic response and conservation of the potassium, thus obviating hypokalemia, may be achieved either by the use of amiloride, which largely has a potassium-sparing effect and little diuretic effect, or spironolactone, which has both a significant diuretic and

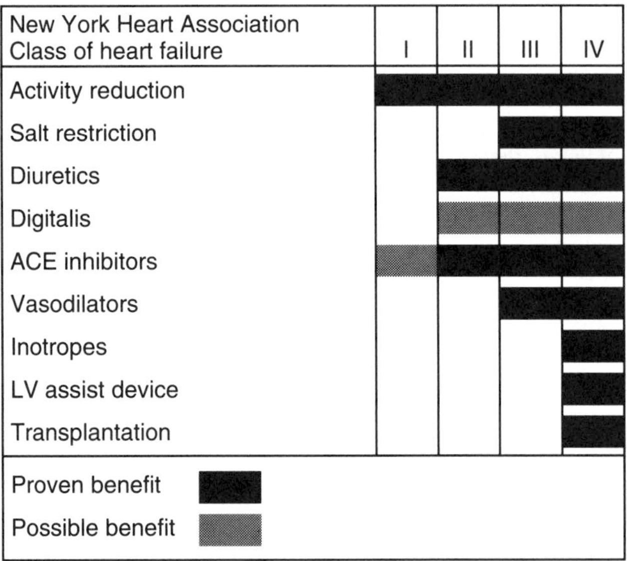

Figure 1 Management options in the treatment of myocarditis and dilated cardiomyopathy.

Table 3 Treatment of Cardiac Failure

Class	*Drug*	*Dosage* *Initial*	*Dosage* *Maintenance*
Glycosides	Digoxin	250-750 μg	125-250 μg daily
Diuretics			
Loop	Furosemide	20-40 mg IV 40-80 mg oral	40-250 mg daily
	Bumetanide	2-5 mg oral	1-5 mg daily
Thiazide	Bendrofluazide	5-10 mg	5-10 mg daily
Thiazide-like	Metolazone	5-10 mg	5-10 mg daily
Potassium-sparing diuretic	Spironolactone	50-100 mg	25-50 mg daily
	Amiloride	5-10 mg	5-20 mg daily
Vasodilators			
	Hydralazine	25 mg t.i.d.	Up to 50-75 mg t.i.d.
Nitrates	Isosorbide dinitrate	10-20 mg t.i.d.	10-30 mg t.i.d.
	Isosorbide mononitrate	10 mg b.i.d.	10-20 mg b.i.d.
ACE inhibitors	Captopril	6.25 mg t.i.d.	25-50 mg t.i.d.
	Enalapril	2.5 mg daily	5-20 mg daily
	Lisinopril	2.5 mg daily	5-20 mg daily
Beta-blockade			
	Metoprolol	6.25-10 mg daily	10-150 mg daily

b.i.d., twice daily; *t.i.d.*, three times daily.

potassium-sparing effect. The latter drug may be particularly useful when secondary hyperaldosteronism has developed with development of persistent edema. In the latter situation we have found that a number of patients may respond to the combination of the two loop diuretics furosemide and bumetanide. Very careful monitoring of renal function and the potassium level is required. The diuretic response in these patients, however, can be extremely positive.

Vasodilators

The benefit of vasodilatation in patients with cardiac failure is well recognized and indeed should be considered in all patients with a dilated heart and impaired systolic ventricular function. Initially benefit was achieved either by using the vasodilator hydralazine or combined with the venodilators of the nitrate group. More recently, however, the ACE inhibitor group has been shown to be extremely beneficial in this type of patient. With respect to the use of the ACE inhibitors it is important to recognize that there may be a hypotensive response related to the initiation of treatment, particularly when the patients are either salt or volume depleted. In view of this, the initial dose of all ACE inhibitors should be low when treatment is commenced. The advantage of enalapril and lisinopril over captopril is that the former may be given as a single daily dose. The use of ACE inhibitors has been associated with improved survival and also a reduction of arrhythmias. In V-HEFT II both enalapril and the combination of hydralazine and isosorbide dinitrate or 4 years produced a small sustained improvement in ejection fraction. SOLV-D data provide evidence that ACE inhibitors favorably influence the long-term prognosis process in cardiac failure. In none of these studies has the effect been specifically studied with respect to inflammatory heart muscle disease.

Beta-blockade

It has long been recognized that there is a group of patients with postmyocarditic dilated cardiomyopathy who may respond to beta-blockade. It has been known for some time that patients with cardiac failure have increased myocardial adrenergic neurotransmission and high circulating catecholamines. The result of this has been the down regulation of the beta-adrenergic receptors. It has further been recognized that in acute inflammatory myocarditis antibodies to the beta-receptors can develop, and this further decreases the inotropic response of the ventricle to catecholamines. Against this background the use of beta-adrenergic blockade in patients with dilated cardiomyopathy has been shown to be of benefit.

The benefit of beta-blockade has been further confirmed by the results of the Metoprolol Treatment Trial. This large multicenter study aimed to find out whether metoprolol improved overall survival and morbidity in 383 patients with heart failure from idiopathic dilated cardiomyopathy (ejection fraction <0.40). They were randomly assigned placebo or metoprolol; 94 percent were in NYHA functional classes II and III, and 80 percent were receiving background treatment. A test dose of metoprolol (5 mg twice daily) was given for 2 to 7 days; those tolerating this dose (96 percent) entered randomization. Study medication was increased slowly from 10 mg to 100 to 150 mg daily. There were 34 percent fewer primary endpoints in the metoprolol than the placebo group. Two and 19 patients respectively deteriorated to the point of needing transplantation and 23 and 19 died. The change in ejection fraction from baseline to 12 months was significantly greater with metoprolol than with placebo (0.13 vs 0.06, $p > 0.0001$). Exercise time at 12 months was significantly greater ($p = 0.046$) in metoprolol-treated than in placebo-treated patients. In patients with idiopathic dilated cardiomyopathy, treatment with metoprolol prevented clinical deterioration and improved symptoms and cardiac function.

Although the study just described relates to dilated cardiomyopathy, there is no contraindication to the use of beta-blockade in patients with myocarditis. Metoprolol can be used beginning with a low dose of 6.25 mg daily. With improvement of the ejection fraction the dose of beta-blockers can be increased to a maximum of 150 mg of metoprolol daily. As with ACE inhibitors, it is important that the systolic pressure is maintained at 90 mm Hg or above and that renal function is also monitored.

Anticoagulants

Thromboembolic events are commonly encountered in patients with biopsy-proven inflammatory myocarditis. The mural thrombus on the inflamed endomyocardial surface is frequently seen on histologic examination. In our own experience, we have found that approximately 25 percent of our patients, some without dilated left ventricles, had an embolic event either from the right or left heart. It is therefore important to consider anticoagulation. In those patients where thrombus has been demonstrated either by echocardiography or angiography or, alternatively, on endomyocardial biopsy examination, it is mandatory. In the majority of patients, embolic phenomena occur when the ejection fraction is less than 30 percent. Anticoagulation is achieved with warfarin and controlled on the prothrombin time with an International Normalized Ratio (INR) between 2 and 3.5.

Intractable Cardiac Failure

Inotropic support with dopamine given by intravenous infusion may improve cardiac function. This may allow a window of opportunity to enable the patient to be stabilized while a donor heart is found. In many others, inotropic support may be sufficient to bring about improved renal function and thereby increased effectiveness of conventional therapy. In the event of the cardiac failure being resistant, intra-aortic balloon pulsation must be considered. This may also be used in the patient who presents in acute cardiogenic shock. For many of these patients the only treatment option is cardiac transplantation.

Cardiac Transplantation

When intensive medical therapy has failed and the patient remains in intractable cardiac failure despite inotropic support, transplantation is the only available treatment. It is important to recognize, however, that patients with active myocarditis have an increased likelihood of cardiac transplant rejection. In one study of cardiac transplantation a multicenter retrospective analysis of patients revealed that the frequency of rejection and of mortality was more than two-fold greater for those with myocarditis than those without myocarditis. When transplantation is considered, the presence of active myocarditis, the age of the patient, and the presence of multisystem disease should all be taken into account.

SUGGESTED READING

Al-Nakib W. Prospects for treatment and prevention of virally induced heart disease. In: Banatvala JE, ed. Viral infections of the heart. London: E. Arnold, 1993:231.

Aretz HT, Billingham ME, Edwards WD, et al. Myocarditis: A histologic definition and classification. Am J Cardiovasc Pathol 1986; 1:3–14.

Daly K, Richardson PJ, Olsen EGJ, et al. Acute myocarditis: Role of histological and virological examination in diagnosis and assessment of immunosuppressive treatment. Br Heart J 1984; 51:30–35.

Mason JW, Billingham ME, Ricci DR. Treatment of acute inflammatory myocarditis assisted by endomyocardial biopsy. Am J Cardiol 1980; 45:1037–1044.

Mason JW, O'Connell JB, Herskowitz A, et al. A clinical trial of immunosuppressive therapy for myocarditis. New Engl J Med 1995; 333:269–275.

Richardson PJ, Why HWF, Maisch B. Myocarditis, myopericarditis and dilated cardiomyopathy. In: Julian DG, Camm AJ, Fox K, et al, eds. Diseases of the Heart. 2nd ed. London: Baillière Tindall, 1995 (in press).

Waagstein F, Bristow MR, Swedberg K, et al. Beneficial effects of metoprolol in idiopathic dilated cardiomyopathy. Lancet 1993; 342:1441–1446.

Why HJF, Meany BT, Richardson PJ, et al. Clinical and prognostic significance of detection of enteroviral RNA in the myocardium of patients with myocarditis or dilated cardiomyopathy. Circulation 1994; 89:2582–2589.

GASTROINTESTINAL DISEASE

ULCERATIVE COLITIS

STEPHEN B. HANAUER, M.D.

Ulcerative colitis and Crohn's disease comprise the idiopathic inflammatory bowel diseases. Ulcerative colitis is distinguished from Crohn's disease by a pattern of diffuse, continuous, superficial ulcerations beginning in the rectum at the anorectal verge and involving a proximal portion of the colon that varies among individuals. Once the upper margin has been delineated it usually remains constant in the patient, but occasionally moves more proximal in up to 40 percent of patients, usually early in the course. Approximately one-third of patients have disease confined to the rectum and sigmoid (proctitis or proctosigmoiditis), one-third have disease up to the splenic flexure (left-sided colitis), and in the remaining third the entire colon (pan-extensive or pancolitis) is inflamed. The course of ulcerative colitis is also variable. Most patients will have chronic, continuous activity that can be suppressed by acute and then maintenance therapy. Approximately 15 percent of patients may have chronic, refractory activity despite ongoing medical therapy. The course of colitis may be modified by acute infections, cigarette smoking, pregnancy, or concurrent therapy with nonsteroidal anti-inflammatory drugs (NSAIDs). NSAIDs should be avoided because of their potential to exacerbate inflammatory bowel disease. The approach to therapy will depend upon the mucosal extent and severity of inflammation, as well as the patient's response to prior interventions.

DRUG THERAPY

Aminosalicylates

Therapy with mesalamine and its various delivery systems is the first-line approach to patients with mild to moderate ulcerative colitis and to maintain remissions (prevent relapse). Sulfasalazine was originally conceived to deliver both a sulfa antibiotic (sulfapyridine) in conjunction with an anti-inflammatory compound (5-aminosalicylic acid) into the connective tissue of patients with ulcerative colitis and rheumatoid arthritis. Sulfasalazine subsequently was demonstrated to be effective in a dose-dependent manner for maintaining remissions in ulcerative colitis and for treating mild to moderate active disease. Thirty years after its introduction, the concept of delivering the compound into connective tissues was found to be erroneous. Instead, sulfasalazine remains intact through the stomach and small intestine until it reaches the colon. Within the colon, sulfasalazine is broken down by azo-reductase activity of normal colonic flora into sulfapyridine and 5-aminosalicylic acid (mesalamine). The sulfapyridine component is absorbed, acetylated by the liver, and eliminated in the urine. The 5-aminosalicylic acid (ASA) moiety remains within the colon, is acetylated by colonic epithelium, and is excreted primarily as N-acetyl 5-aminosalicylic acid within the feces.

Clinical trials have demonstrated that the 5-ASA component contains the active therapeutic properties of sulfasalazine. The sulfapyridine acts primarily as a "carrier" to deliver mesalamine into the colon. This observation has opened the door for alternative mesalamine-delivering formulations that can be divided into oral versus topical (rectal) applications. In the United States, rectal mesalamine may be administered as suppositories or enemas. Oral formulations include delayed- or continuous-release preparations, or alternative carrier systems for mesalamine (Table 1).

In clinical trials, no formulation has been superior to sulfasalazine when equimolar concentrations of 5-ASA are compared. However, these newer formulations without sulfapyridine no longer carry the risk of sulfa-related side effects such as intolerance (nausea, headache, myalgias), hypersensitivity reactions (fever, rash, hepatitis, or hemolytic effects), or sperm abnormalities. In addition, these formulations offer site-specific delivery of mesalamine "targeted" to locations of inflammation along the digestive tract. In addition, the newer aminosalicylates can be utilized in higher doses than possible for sulfasalazine without inducing intolerant side effects. Nevertheless, they should not be considered "superior" to sulfasalazine, which remains the first-line standard of treatment because of its low cost and long track record.

The mechanism of action of the aminosalicylates is unknown. Virtually all mediators of inflammation attrib-

Table 1 Aminosalicylate Preparations

Preparation	Size	Formulation	Delivery	Dose
Topical/Rectal				
Mesalamine enema	1, 4 g	60-100 ml	Left colon	1-4 g hs acute 1 g hs maintenance
Mesalamine suppository	500 mg-1 g	–	Rectum	500 mg b.i.d.-t.i.d. acute 500 mg hs maintenance
Oral				
Azo-bond				
Sulfasalazine	500 mg	Sulfapyridine-carrier	Colon	4-6 g divided dose acute 2-4 g divided dose maintenance
Olsalazine	250 mg	5-ASA dimer	Colon	1.5-3 g divided dose maintenance
Delayed-release				
Asacol	400 mg	Eudragit S (pH 7)	Distal ileum, colon	2.4-4.8 g divided dose acute* 800 mg-4.8 g divided dose maintenance*
Sustained-release				
Pentasa	250, 500 mg	Ethylcellulose-micro-granules	Stomach to colon	2-4 g divided dose acute* 1.5-3 g divided dose maintenance*

*Comparative studies are inadequate to fully assess dose-response in active vs. maintenance ulcerative colitis.

uted to ulcerative colitis are influenced by these agents. Sulfasalazine has a modest antibacterial effect related to the sulfa moiety, but it also inhibits Fimetolearphe (FMLP) binding and activation of neutrophils. The aminosalicylates have multiple effects on arachidonic acid metabolism by increasing prostaglandin production in the mucosa, but diminishing some prostanoid metabolites, including thromboxane synthetase. These agents also inhibit the lipoxygenase pathway and reduce mucosal production of leukotriene B_4. Production of interleukin-1, platelet activating factor, and immunoglobulins by plasma cells are inhibited, and both 5-ASA and sulfasalazine scavenge and prevent release of reactive oxygen species.

The aminosalicylates are utilized as a first-line agent for the induction of remission for mild to moderate ulcerative colitis and to maintain remissions in quiescent disease. Both properties are dose related (see Table 1) and once remission has been induced, it should be maintained, essentially indefinitely, on a long-term basis.

Glucocorticoids

The primary role of glucocorticoid therapy in ulcerative colitis is to induce remission in moderate to severe disease. Steroid preparations are useful when administered topically, orally, parenterally, or via adrenocorticotropic hormone (ACTH). The short-term effects of corticosteroids are not translated into long-term benefits. These agents should not be used to "maintain" remissions in ulcerative colitis because they have not been effective in maintenance studies and the well-established side effects preclude long-term use. Adverse effects associated with glucocorticoids are related to dose and duration of therapy. In addition, ACTH carries a risk of adrenal hemorrhage. Thus, glucocorticoids are usually reserved for moderate to severe ulcerative colitis with varied formulations, dose, and applicability (Table 2).

Table 2 Corticosteroids for Ulcerative Colitis in the United States*

Parenteral	
Hydrocortisone	300-400 mg
Methylprednisolone	40-60 mg
ACTH	80-120 U
Oral	
Prednisone	40-60 mg
Rectal	
Hydrocortisone enema (Cortenema)	100 mg
Hydrocortisone foam (Cortifoam)	80 mg
Budesonide enema	2 mg†

*Daily dose.
†Pending FDA approval.

Similar to the aminosalicylates, the mechanism of action is complex. Corticosteroids affect arachidonic acid liberation from membranes, are lymphocytotoxic, and inhibit the generation of multiple cytokines.

Newer formulations with enhanced potency, yet increased first-pass hepatic metabolism, are currently under development. Agents such as budesonide have already reached clinical utility in distal ulcerative colitis, and oral, controlled-release formulations are under evaluation for ileocecal and colonic disease. Because of their enhanced potency the small proportion that reaches the systemic circulation has increased binding to the glucocorticoid receptors. It remains to be determined whether the mucosal effects can be divorced from systemic activity.

Immunosuppressants

Immunosuppressants such as azathioprine and 6-mercaptopurine have been used for several decades as "steroid-sparing" agents in ulcerative colitis and Crohn's disease. Until recently, their role in ulcerative colitis has been limited by the potential curability of the disease via colectomy, thus avoiding long-term exposure to potential immune suppression. However, over the past decade, clinical trials have supported the efficacy of azathioprine and 6-mercaptopurine to maintain remissions in ulcerative colitis in previously steroid-dependent patients and they have accumulated an extended safety profile. The primary difficulty in employing these agents has been a delayed onset of action, up to 6 to 12 months. This time frame has required some patients to continue low to moderate dose steroids in addition to aminosalicylates while awaiting the impact of the immune modifiers. Most recently, cyclosporine has been utilized in severe or fulminant ulcerative colitis. Cyclosporine has dramatic short-term efficacy and improves symptoms in steroid-unresponsive patients within a matter of days. Unfortunately, the short-term effects of cyclosporine have not translated into long-term benefits unless patients are transferred to alternative immunosuppressants. Here, the risk-benefit ratio must be weighed on an individual basis to determine whether curative colectomy or long-term medical management is warranted.

The mechanisms of action of azathioprine and 6-mercaptopurine in ulcerative colitis are unknown. There has been a correlation of effect with reduction of circulating lymphocyte populations (natural killer cells) in observational studies of Crohn's disease, but no data are available regarding ulcerative colitis. On the other hand, cyclosporine has well-documented effects on interleukin-2 and T-lymphocyte signaling.

The two primary precautions regarding the use of azathioprine or 6-mercaptopurine are bone marrow toxicity and leukopenia or hypersensitivity reactions, including pancreatitis, seen in up to 15 percent of patients with inflammatory bowel disease. The former is managed by frequent monitoring of the complete blood count (CBC). Patients should be warned about the possibility of developing new abdominal symptoms related to pancreatitis and to discontinue the medication if abdominal pain or nausea arise.

The side effects of cyclosporine are much more extensive. Patients' blood levels of cyclosporine should be monitored to maintain steady state or trough levels between 200 to 400 ng per milliliter by high-performance liquid chromatography (HPLC). Kidney function and blood pressure also need to be monitored. Hypocholesterolemia is a relative contraindication to cyclosporine use because of the risk of grand mal seizures. In addition, use of these agents should be restricted to practitioners experienced in managing immune compromised patients because there is a risk of opportunistic infections, including pneumocystis pneumonia.

DIETARY AND SYMPTOMATIC TREATMENT

Diet does not play a primary role in ulcerative colitis. No specific factor has been identified that increases colonic inflammation. Furthermore, neither elemental diets nor hyperalimentation and bowel rest have been found to affect the course of ulcerative colitis. On the other hand, diet is used to minimize symptoms in patients already disposed to diarrhea and abdominal cramping. Low-residue and lactose-free diets are employed for patients with frequent loose bowel movements or lactose intolerance.

In patients with mild disease, antispasmodics and antidiarrheals can be utilized. It should be recognized that patients with distal ulcerative colitis generally have delayed transit in the right colon (essentially constipation), and antidiarrheals may be of limited value in this population. These agents should be proscribed in patients with severe disease because of the potential of initiating or exacerbating toxic megacolon related to impaired colonic muscular action. Nutritional supplements, especially iron, may be necessary in patients with chronic blood loss and calcium supplementation may be necessary in those on long-term steroid therapy.

SPECIFIC CLINICAL SITUATIONS

The therapeutic approach and options for patients with ulcerative colitis depend upon the extent and severity of colonic ulceration and response to prior interventions. Before initiating therapy some assessment of the overall severity and mucosal extent is necessary. In patients with mild to moderate symptoms (Table 3), a colonoscopic examination defines the mucosal extent and severity. Patients with evidence of systemic toxicity (fever, tachycardia, or abdominal tenderness) should not undergo instrumentation. In this setting an abdominal radiograph will usually define the upper margin of disease and exclude the presence of colonic dilatation or free air. Occasionally, indium-labeled leukocyte scans may be useful in defining the extent of colonic inflammation.

Ulcerative Proctitis

Approximately one-third of patients presenting with ulcerative colitis have disease limited to the rectum. This affords the potential of either oral or topical therapy. In the setting of mild disease, sulfasalazine or an alternative aminosalicylate can be used orally, although topical application of mesalamine suppositories or enemas will provide faster relief of symptoms. Alternatively, rectal administration of hydrocortisone, prednisolone, or budesonide is effective. Patients should be treated continuously until symptoms are completely relieved, after which the frequency of topical treatment with mesalamine is reduced to alternate nights or several times weekly, or use of an oral preparation may be substituted for maintenance therapy. The clinician should anticipate a dose-response in maintaining remissions, and patients who have repeated flares should be treated with higher dose maintenance therapy.

Patients with ulcerative proctitis are often constipated and may benefit from the additional use of a bulk laxative such as psyllium. Antispasmodics may be useful,

Table 3 Modified Truelove Witts Criteria for Ulcerative Colitis Severity

Variables	*Mild/Moderate**	*Severe*	*Fulminant*
Bowel frequency	< 4/day	> 6/day	> 10/day
Blood in stool	+/−	++	Continuous
Fever	Normal	> 37.5° C	> 37.5° C
Pulse	Normal	> 90/min	< 90/min
Hemoglobin	Normal	< 75%	Transfusion required
Erythrocyte sedimentation rate	< 30 mm/hr	> 30 mm/hr	> 30 mm/hr
Colon radiography		Colonic air, edematous wall, thumbprinting	Dilated colon
Clinical sign		Abdominal tenderness	Abdominal distention and tenderness

*Moderate has features between mild and severe.

but antidiarrheals should be avoided, because these patients already have proximal constipation.

Patients refractory to initial interventions with oral aminosalicylates or topical steroids should be treated with high-dose rectal mesalamine, either with suppositories 500 mg three times daily or a nightly 4 g enema. Occasionally, patients will benefit from co-administration of topical hydrocortisone foam (Cortifoam) and mesalamine suppositories administered twice daily. Oral steroids are *rarely* indicated for distal ulcerative colitis. Once administered, they should be rapidly tapered. Immune modifiers such as azathioprine or 6-mercaptopurine are occasionally indicated for patients with resistant ulcerative proctitis used in conjunction with both oral and topical aminosalicylates.

Left-Sided Disease

More than one-half of the patients presenting with ulcerative colitis have disease limited distal to the splenic flexure. Usually these patients will present with mild to moderate symptoms, but occasionally may manifest severe or fulminant colitis and rarely toxic megacolon. Mild to moderate disease is treated with either oral or topical aminosalicylates similar to treatment for ulcerative proctitis. These patients' disease may be more difficult to manage and often requires a combination of oral therapy for long-term treatment, as well as topical, short-term administration of either mesalamine or steroid enemas. Patients should be treated until complete symptomatic recovery after which a maintenance regimen of oral therapy, with or without rectal mesalamine, should be continued on a long-term basis. Up to 4.8 g of oral mesalamine may be necessary to maintain patients with left-sided disease. Patients unable to taper the dosage regimen of topical mesalamine are maintained utilizing interval dosing on an alternate or every-third-night basis to continue symptomatic remission.

Patients with more moderate to severe disease require short-term administration of prednisone to induce remission, after which maintenance therapy with an oral and/or topical aminosalicylate should be maintained.

Patients who fail oral steroid administration should be hospitalized for intensive intravenous steroid treatment (see following discussion). Individuals who respond to steroids but cannot taper despite combinations of oral and topical aminosalicylates can benefit from the addition of azathioprine or 6-mercaptopurine in selective situations if surgery (colectomy) is refused.

Symptomatic therapy for mild to moderate disease includes dietary adjustments to avoid diarrhea and the use of antispasmodics and antidiarrheals. The latter should be avoided in more severe disease. Long-term management of patients with left-sided ulcerative colitis should include surveillance colonoscopies after 10 years of disease, monitoring for dysplasia (see following discussion).

Extensive Colitis

Ulcerative colitis extending proximal to the splenic flexure necessitates oral administration of an aminosalicylate for mild to moderate disease or oral steroids for moderate to severe symptoms. The principles of acute and maintenance therapy continue to apply. Once patients have responded, they should be maintained on an oral aminosalicylate to prevent relapse. Patients treated acutely with steroids should be weaned and maintained on an oral aminosalicylate. Patients who flare despite optimal dosing of an aminosalicylate (up to 4.8 g of mesalamine) require azathioprine or 6-mercaptopurine as steroid-sparing agents. Optimal dosing for the latter has not been established, although commonly employed doses include up to 2.5 mg per kilogram of azathioprine or 1.5 mg per kilogram of 6-mercaptopurine. Monitoring of the CBC should prevent leukopenia. Dietary interventions depend upon symptoms, but maintenance of iron status should be confirmed.

Fulminant Colitis and Toxic Megacolon

Fulminant ulcerative colitis is a medical emergency necessitating management by medical and surgical teams. Patients should be hospitalized, and fluid and electrolyte resuscitation along with blood transfusions to maintain the hematocrit above 30 percent instituted. In addition, an intensive regimen of intravenous steroids, either hydrocortisone 300 to 400 mg daily or methylprednisolone 40 to 60 mg daily, should be initiated. We favor continuous infusion over intermittent administration. Patients with severe abdominal pain, nausea, or vomiting should have nothing by mouth temporarily. However, bowel rest is not necessary for patients who wish to continue eating. Either an elemental or low residue diet is prescribed according to the patient's desire and tolerance. Individuals presenting with abdominal distention or rebound tenderness with evidence of a small bowel ileus require a nasogastric tube decompression. Broad-spectrum antibiotics have not been proven to be of benefit in clinical trials, but most experienced clinicians add a broad-spectrum regimen such as an aminoglycoside and metronidazole or a second-generation cephalosporin for patients with evidence of transmural ulcerative colitis (manifest by abdominal tenderness, rebound or colonic dilatation). Antibiotics are only required short-term, although patients should be monitored for *Clostridium difficile* co-infection.

Patients who fail to respond to the aforementioned intravenous regimen within 5 to 10 days should be considered for either cyclosporine therapy or colectomy. Intravenous cyclosporine therapy has "salvaged" patients unresponsive to steroids, but the long-term benefits remain to be established.

Once patients have responded to the intensive intravenous regimen and are able to resume a low-residue diet they are transferred to an oral steroid regimen (prednisone 40 to 60 mg daily or in divided doses) and an aminosalicylate for maintenance therapy. Steroids are then gradually tapered according to the time course of response, generally 5 to 10 mg weekly to a maximum dose of 20 mg and then 2.5 to 5 mg weekly thereafter. Patients requiring cyclosporine should probably be considered for long-term maintenance therapy with azathioprine or 6-mercaptopurine in conjunction with an aminosalicylate.

Surgical Indications

Ulcerative colitis is a curable disease. Either proctocolectomy or colectomy with mucosal proctectomy and ileoanal anastomosis removes the mucosa at risk. Most patients favor the latter, sphincter-saving operations, to maintain continuity of their digestive tract and allow evacuations per anorectum. Indications for colectomy in ulcerative colitis include perforation, unresponsive toxic megacolon, refractory disease, persistent growth retardation in children, complications of medical therapy (e.g., osteonecrosis or steroid dependency), dysplasia, or cancer. Although proctocolectomy and ileostomy afford a long-term "cure" the ileoanal procedures are potentially complicated by recurring inflammation in the "neorectum" referred to as pouchitis. The pathogenesis of pouchitis is uncertain, but the majority of patients affected respond to antibiotic therapy with either metronidazole or ciprofloxacin. Occasionally, chronic therapy with antibiotics is necessary to prevent recurrent episodes of pouchitis manifested by abdominal cramps, increased frequency of defecation, rectal bleeding, and occasionally, fevers or extraintestinal manifestations.

Long-Term Management

Ulcerative colitis is a chronic, medically incurable disease. However, quality of life in a symptom-free state of remission is the goal for the majority of patients. The long-term management of patients with ulcerative colitis requires a surveillance program to monitor the risk of colonic neoplasia that is increased in patients with extensive colitis, long duration of disease, or those with hepatobiliary complications (sclerosing cholangitis). At present, colonoscopy with mucosal biopsies throughout the colon is recommended after 10 years of ulcerative colitis and the interval schedule of screening is inversely proportional to the duration of disease. Biyearly examinations are indicated in patients who have had ulcerative colitis for 10 to 20 years, after which yearly colonoscopic surveillance is advised.

The peak incidence of ulcerative colitis occurs in childbearing years. Fertility is not affected (except in men on sulfasalazine where reversible sperm abnormalities may transiently impair fertility) by ulcerative colitis and neither is its therapy. Pregnant women with ulcerative colitis are treated similar to nonpregnant females. Sulfasalazine or aminosalicylates should be continued as acute or maintenance therapies. Corticosteroids may be required for pregnancy-related flare-ups. Immunosuppressives have been employed successfully without recognized consequences on fetal development.

SUGGESTED READING

Hanauer SB. Medical therapy of ulcerative colitis. Lancet 1993; 342:412–417.

Hanauer SB. Medical therapy in ulcerative colitis. In: Kirsner JB, Shorter RG, eds. Inflammatory Bowel Disease: 4th ed. Baltimore, Md: Williams and Wilkins, 1995:664.

Hanauer SB, Stathopoulos G. Risk-benefit assessment of drugs used in the treatment of inflammatory bowel disease. Drug Safety 1991; 6:192–219.

Hodgson HFJ, Mazlam MZ. Review article: Assessment of drug therapy in inflammatory bowel disease. Aliment Pharmacol Therap 1991; 5:555–584.

Kornbluth AA, Salomon P, Sacks HS, et al. Meta-analysis of the effectiveness of current drug therapy of ulcerative colitis. J Clin Gastroenterol 1993; 16:215–218.

Sutherland LR, May GR, Shaffer EA. Sulfasalazine revisited: A meta-analysis of 5-aminosalicylic acid in the treatment of ulcerative colitis. Ann Intern Med 1993; 118:540–549.

CROHN'S DISEASE

JOSEPH M. POLITO II, M.D.
THEODORE M. BAYLESS, M.D.

Crohn's disease is a form of idiopathic inflammatory bowel disease characterized by transmural inflammation that can involve any part of the gastrointestinal tract. The etiology of Crohn's disease remains unknown, but it is generally believed to result from immunologic dysregulation that is influenced to varying degrees by genetic predisposition and/or environmental exposure.

It is important to recognize the existence of well-characterized clinical patterns for Crohn's disease that influence management and prognosis. These subtypes can be separated by anatomic location, either ileocecal, jejunoileitis, or colonic disease only, and type of disease, (inflammatory, stricturing, or fistulizing). Fistulizing disease, which often declares itself early with spontaneous fistula or free perforation, is the most aggressive form and often requires recurrent surgeries. Patients with the stricturing subtype of ileitis tend to declare themselves after approximately 8 to 9 years of inflammatory disease and will often have a relatively indolent postoperative course after resection. The inflammatory subtype is the most common form seen in Crohn's colitis and comprises about one-third of patients with ileitis. It is characterized by episodes of active inflammation that may require resection for intractability or bleeding.

The course of Crohn's disease may vary from patient to patient; 10 to 20 percent of patients will experience a prolonged remission after the first episode, while others will have chronic relapsing disease, and still others are steroid dependent or have refractory disease.

Each of the drug types available for use in Crohn's disease have different anti-inflammatory effects; thus, multiagent combination therapy should be used when treating active disease. There are currently few controlled trials of multiple-drug regimens. Medications should usually be started at high doses in order to achieve a remission and then tapered down once a response is seen. Patients receiving corticosteroids should also receive other less toxic medications at a maximum dose to achieve maximal steroid sparing. For symptoms of rectosigmoid involvement, topical therapy in the form of enemas, foams, or suppositories is useful in Crohn's proctocolitis, as it is in other forms of proctocolitis. Because of the wide spectrum of clinical presentations, complications, and individual drug responses (Table 1), medical and surgical therapy needs to be carefully tailored for each patient with Crohn's disease.

5-ASA DERIVATIVES

Sulfasalazine is a sulfapyridine moiety linked to 5-aminosalicylic acid (5-ASA) through an azo bond; it has been used successfully at doses of 3 g per day in the management of ulcerative colitis for several decades. In the distal ileum and colon, small intestinal bacteria that possess an intracellular azo reductase cleave the active 5-ASA from the sulfa moiety. It is not surprising therefore that sulfasalazine is most efficacious in the management of mild to moderate ileocolitis and colitis, but not in isolated small bowel Crohn's disease. Sulfasalazine is useful in both attaining and maintaining remission, especially in the colon. Sulfasalazine use is sometimes limited by a 10 to 20 percent incidence of side effects, including headache, nausea, and anorexia, which appear to correlate with high blood levels of sulfapyridine. Some of these adverse effects can be avoided at lower doses or with enteric-coated forms. Allergic reactions, manifested by rash and fever, are usually due to sulfa sensitivity rather than the active 5-ASA component. More serious side effects include hypersensitivity-related pancreatitis, hepatitis, and pneumonitis, as well as neutropenia and hemolytic anemia. Such reactions mandate discontinuation of the drug. Male patients interested in starting a family should be warned that sulfasalazine reversibly decreases spermatogenesis and can result in infertility. Its use in women who are pregnant or lactating, however, appears to be safe. Since sulfasalazine competitively inhibits folic acid absorption, theoretically patients on chronic therapy should receive folate supplementation if red cell folate levels are not being monitored.

Recognition of 5-ASA as the active moiety in sulfasalazine has led to the development of other 5-ASA derivatives that can be delivered to various disease sites. Delayed-release forms of mesalamine (Asacol) dissolve at a pH over 7 and are released in the distal ileum and colon. Pentasa is a sustained-release form that is released throughout the small bowel and colon and therefore is useful in extensive jejunoileitis or duodenitis, as well as colonic disease. Olsalazine (Dipentum) is a 5-ASA dimer released in the colon.

In general, these products are as efficacious as sulfasalazine in the management of Crohn's disease, while avoiding the side effects associated with the sulfa moiety (although at much greater expense). For some patients the use of Dipentum for Crohn's colitis is limited by the occurrence of a watery diarrhea caused by enhanced small bowel secretion. Although not yet approved by the FDA for Crohn's disease, Pentasa can be used at a dose of 4 g per day. Asacol at 2.4 g per day is effective in active mild to moderate small bowel Crohn's disease, and based on the work with ulcerative colitis, additional benefit may be obtained by increasing the dose to 4.8 g per day.

Crohn's proctitis is a real syndrome and 5-ASA enemas are ideal agents as topical therapy either alone or in combination with topical steroids.

GLUCOCORTICOIDS

Patients with active Crohn's disease unresponsive to 5-ASA or sulfasalazine therapy clearly benefit from steroids. The addition of steroids to a 5-ASA regimen

Table 1 Medical Therapy for Crohn's Disease

Drug	*Indications*	*Advantages*	*Disadvantages*
Sulfasalazine	Mild, moderate inflammation of colon or terminal ileum, maintenance of remission (unproven)	Inexpensive, effective and safe in pregnancy	High frequency of toxic, allergic side effects; limited effect in small bowel disease; male infertility
Asacol	Mild, moderate inflammation of colon, terminal ileum; maintenance of remission in selected patients	Delivery to distal ileum, colon; maintenance of remission, including postsurgical	More expensive than sulfasalazine; delivery erratic with rapid transit
Pentasa	Mild, moderate inflammation of small bowel and colon; maintenance of remission in selected patients	50% delivered to small bowel	More expensive than sulfasalazine; large daily number of pills required
Dipentum	Mild, moderate inflammation of colon; maintenance of remission	Delivery to colon	Secretory diarrhea
Glucocorticoids	Moderate, severe inflammation	Rapid onset of antiinflammatory action; effective	Steroid side effects; enhanced formation of fistula if obstructed; may mask infectious complications
Azathioprine/6-MP	Moderate, severe refractory inflammation, steroid sparing, improving fistula; consistent maintenance of remission proven	Most effective treatment for refractory disease; steroid sparing	Slow onset of action (3 mo); myelosuppression; allergic and toxic reactions; theoretical cancer risk; expensive
Cyclosporine	Severe refractory inflammation; rapid onset of action desired	Very rapid onset of immunosupressive effect with IV use (days)	Significant toxicity; erratic oral absorption; requires close monitoring; long-term efficacy variable
Methotrexate	Severe refractory inflammation	Intermediate onset of immunosuppressive effect (6-8 weeks)	Myelosuppression; allergic pneumonitis; hepatotoxicity; requires close monitoring; long-term efficacy unknown; average duration <2 years
Metronidazole	Mild, moderate inflammation of colon and ileum; perianal disease with fistula	Lower potential toxicity for treatment of perianal disease than azathioprine/6-MP; inexpensive	Nausea; disulfiram-like effects; severe paresthesias if >1 g/day used
Ciprofloxin	Mild, moderate inflammation of colon, perianal disease	Low toxicity in treatment of perianal disease in metronidazole intolerant or contraindicated patients	Efficacy unknown (investigational); expense

Modified from James S, Strober W. Crohn's disease. In: Lichtenstein LM, Fauci AS, eds. Current therapy in allergy, immunology, and rheumatology, 4th ed. St Louis: Mosby, 1992.

leads to an accelerated improvement in symptoms as compared to using 5-ASA alone. To minimize steroid side effects, we always use another anti-inflammatory agent, and often, an antibiotic as well when prednisone is needed to suppress inflammation. It should be noted that because of the potential side effects of glucocorticoids some physicians reserve these agents for more refractory or serious disease. As stated, we feel that there are methods of minimizing steroid side effects, including rapid tapering, use of combination therapy, switching to a single morning dose after 2 to 3 weeks of divided dose therapy, and use of alternate-day therapy to maintain remission. Newer topically active and rapidly metabolized steroids such as budesonide (9 mg seemingly equivalent to 40 mg prednisone) will probably also prove useful in avoiding steroid side effects and perhaps for maintenance of remission. Daily and alternate-day prednisone seem to reduce the frequency of relapses in patients in clinical remission. Extraintestinal manifestations of Crohn's disease (seen in up to 20 percent of patients) such as pyoderma gangrenosum, arthritis, erythema nodosum, and uveitis also appear to benefit from steroid therapy.

When used systemically, steroids should be begun at high enough doses to induce remission and then tapered on an outpatient basis. Forty to sixty milligrams of prednisone per day given as a divided dose for 2 weeks and then as a single morning dose can be used. Patients requiring hospitalization receive 60 mg Solu Medrol intravenously per day. Once response to therapy has been achieved, steroids should be gradually tapered. Flares during this period result from too rapid tapering. Prednisone can usually be reduced by 10 mg every 2 weeks initially until a dose of 30 mg per day is achieved. At this level a less rapid tapering schedule is needed and an attempt should be made to switch over to alternate-day therapy because this may reduce the incidence of side effects. We do this by slowly reducing the alternate, even-day dose, while maintaining the odd-day dose. Once the even day dose is zero, one can begin adjusting the odd-day dose downward to 20 mg every other day. Adverse effects diminish with prolonged low-dose alternate-day steroid use.

Topical steroids in the form of enemas can be useful in the management of distal disease. Although systemic absorption from cortisone enemas is not totally avoided via this route, budesonide, a potent glucocorticoid with extensive first-pass hepatic metabolism, results in fewer side effects and less adrenal-axis suppression (2 mg of budesonide is equivalent to 100 mg of hydrocortisone). Budesonide is currently undergoing trials in an ileal-release form and may make steroid toxicity far less problematic in the future (9 mg is seemingly equivalent to 40 mg prednisone).

The side effects of steroid use are well known to physicians, and patients should be informed of these before starting therapy. Adverse effects include the symptoms of diabetes, peptic ulcer, and hypertension; the common symptoms of iatrogenic Cushing syndrome, including weight gain, redistribution of fat, and facial, mood and sleep changes; and aseptic necrosis of the femoral head, shoulders, and knees, which can be devastating, especially in younger patients. Risk factors include very active inflammatory bowel disease (IBD); long-term high-dose steroids; high-impact, weight-bearing activities; alcoholism; and smoking.

Osteoporosis is a more common and insidious problem that can be minimized and even partially corrected with the use of calcitonin. Long-term steroid dosages should be minimized as previously discussed, and patients receiving steroids should be maintained on calcium and vitamin D supplements. The degree of osteoporosis can be followed with periodic dual photon absorptiometry measurements. Serum osteocalcin and 2-hour urine pyridinium cross-linked collagen levels are useful measures of excessive bone turnover.

Most textbooks advise against long-term steroid use, but we have found alternate-day prednisone in doses of 20 to 30 mg every other day in combination with sulfasalazine or an appropriate 5-ASA agent, and if necessary, azathioprine or 6-mercaptopurine, to be both useful and safe in preventing relapses over a 4-year period.

IMMUNOMODULATORY AGENTS

Immunomodulatory agents are effective in 70 percent of patients with chronic Crohn's disease. These drugs are not used as initial therapy and are reserved for patients with more severe or refractory situations. Nonetheless, there are specific circumstances in which their use can have substantial benefits. The most common scenario in which they should be considered is in the patient with chronic active Crohn's disease who is steroid dependent or steroid resistant and in whom there is concern about complications of long-term steroid use such as cataracts, osteoporosis, and physical appearance, or mood changes. Typically these patients will have a flare of symptoms whenever their oral prednisone dose is tapered below a certain level, usually around 20 mg per day, and there is a need to provide some "steroid sparing." Seventy percent of such patients would be expected to respond. Patients with Crohn's disease who have had recurrent, relapsing disease and in whom surgery has resulted in a "short gut," or in whom disease is so extensive that repeated resections are not advisable, may benefit from immunomodulatory agents in an attempt to prolong remission between relapses, but this is as yet unproven. Finally, a subset of patients with severe perianal fistulous disease unresponsive to local surgical procedures or metronidazole may benefit with decreased drainage from the fistulas and, hopefully, less progression of fistula formation.

Azathioprine and 6-Mercaptopurine

Azathioprine and its active metabolite, 6-mercaptopurine (6-MP), have had the most proven success of the immunomodulatory agents in Crohn's disease. Overall, approximately 70 percent of patients with refractory or steroid-dependent Crohn's disease can be expected to respond with either induction of clinical remission or successful steroid tapering. In addition, approximately two-thirds of patients with fistulous disease (i.e., enteroenteric, enterocolonic, or perianal) will demonstrate improvement, and up to 30 percent will heal entirely, especially those with a single perianal fistula. Patients with enterocutaneous fistulas in old surgical tracts or patients with enterovesicular or enterovaginal fistulas may not do as well and often require surgery. Long-term efficacy of azathioprine and 6-MP in the maintenance of remission of disease has been shown in controlled trials and the probability of relapse following withdrawal of azathioprine is seemingly inversely correlated with duration of therapy.

Therapy with azathioprine is generally started at 50 mg per day orally while maximizing multiagent therapy with prednisone 5-ASA drugs and metronidazole or ciprofloxacin. If patients tolerate this dose for 3 weeks without allergic side effects, it can usually be increased to 1.5 mg per kilogram per day. We will gradually increase the dose to 125 or 150 mg in particular patients, usually those with Crohn's colitis, to achieve a response. Some clinicians believe maximal benefit can only be achieved if the dose is pushed to the point of myelosuppression; however, this is not usually necessary. The median duration to response is 3 months after initiating therapy; however, some patients will respond within 2 months, while others may take as long as 6 to 9 months. In our experience 80 percent of those who were going to respond had done so by 4 months of therapy, and in our published series of 78 patients all nine of the nonresponders had colonic disease. Intravenous administration of azathioprine seemingly speeds up the onset of action to one or two weeks in some patients.

Azathioprine and 6-MP have significant toxicities of which the patient should be made fully aware. There is a 5 percent incidence of allergy usually seen in the first 3 weeks of treatment. This may manifest itself as fever, rash, arthralgias, or myalgias. Some patients who had arthralgias on azathioprine did not on 6-MP. Pancreatitis is seen in less than 2 percent, and myelosuppression can occur, so patients should be alerted to an increased risk of infection. Patients starting therapy should have a complete blood count (CBC), liver function tests, and amylase checked every 2 weeks for 6 weeks and then a CBC every 6 weeks thereafter. The risk of malignancy, specifically non-Hodgkins lymphoma, has been raised primarily as a reflection of the organ transplant literature; however, recent reports regarding azathioprine and 6-MP use in IBD patients suggest that this risk is, to date, not enhanced. The risk of colon cancer was not increased over that expected in IBD in a 20-year British study. Finally, there is no evidence that azathioprine taken during pregnancy is associated with an adverse outcome; however, most physicians believe that it is prudent to avoid this exposure if at all possible. A recent abstract describing 8 patients on 6-MP and 100 others who had 6-MP prior to pregnancy was seemingly well-tolerated.

Cyclosporine

Cyclosporine (CYA) has not had as clear a benefit in Crohn's disease as compared to azathioprine and 6-MP; however, it is useful in certain situations. The most significant benefit of CYA is its rapid onset of effect, often within 5 to 10 days when given intravenously, even in steroid-resistant patients. This is particularly useful in hospitalized patients with severe Crohn's disease who might otherwise require emergent surgery for refractory disease and therefore cannot wait 3 months for azathioprine to be effective. Unfortunately, there is a high relapse rate when CYA is tapered. Long-term therapy with oral CYA (perhaps 6 months) or azathioprine may be needed to maintain a remission. A recent controlled trial of orally administered CYA found it to be more effective than placebo in patients who absorbed enough to have therapeutic blood levels, who were also on prednisone at the same time, and who were not already candidates for surgery for obstruction.

CYA is best started with continuous IV infusion at 4 mg per kilogram per day, and after a response is achieved, it can be converted to an oral dose of 6 to 8 mg per kilogram per day. Serum trough levels need to be followed closely, and patients are monitored for renal toxicity, tremors, hypertension, and other side effects that are common with CYA in the transplant setting. CYA is contraindicated in patients with a cholesterol of less than 120 because this is associated with severe neurotoxicity. Topical CYA as an enema has been reported, anecdotally, but not in a controlled trial, to be of help in some patients with refractory proctosigmoiditis unresponsive to topical steroids and 5-ASA products. In addition, CYA has been shown to be helpful in closing chronic perianal fistulas, but long-term immunomodulatory therapy seems to be necessary to maintain this beneficial effect. Pyoderma gangrenosum has also been treated successfully according to several case reports.

Methotrexate

Methotrexate (MTX) has been effective in over 50 percent of patients with Crohn's disease unresponsive to azathioprine. A controlled trial has confirmed the early open trial by Kozarek. Colonic disease responded best and did so in 6 to 8 weeks. Remissions do not usually last over 9 months. MTX can be started as 25 mg intramuscularly every week for 12 weeks, and once a response is seen, converted to 12.5 mg or 15 mg orally or intramuscularly once per week.

MTX is contraindicated during pregnancy because of its teratogenic effects. In addition, it is myelosuppressive and is reported to be hepatotoxic; therefore patients should have CBCs and liver function tests monitored periodically. Hepatotoxicity is related to cumulative dose, and liver biopsy is appropriate at greater than 2 g of exposure. Because of adverse synergistic effects of alcohol exposure, patients on MTX should be advised of this risk. Although uncommon, allergic pneumonitis is a potentially fatal complication, if unrecognized.

Experimental

Anti-TNF (tumor necrosis factor) has shown anti-inflammatory effects when given once to a small number of patients with active Crohn's disease. Whether this medication will be effective when given repeatedly remains to be determined.

ALTERING LUMINAL CONTENTS

There is some experimental evidence that luminal contents, including colonic type bacteria, play a role in mediating and maintaining ileal and colonic disease activity in Crohn's disease. Defunctioning ileostomies result in improvement in both colonic and perianal disease. Total parenteral nutrition, bowel rest, and elemental diets, which are absorbed in the upper gastrointestinal tract, may presumably have their beneficial effect by lessening antigenic exposure and altering luminal bacterial concentration. Antibiotics, as discussed in the next section, can be effective "anti-inflammatory" therapy in some situations, perhaps by altering luminal contents as well.

Antibiotics

An intra-abdominal abscess should be ruled out by CAT scan with oral and intravenous contrast in patients presenting with an abdominal mass. Broad-spectrum antibiotics such as ampicillin, gentamicin, and metronidazole are given intravenously whenever there is concern about potential perforation or abscess. Even if a frank abscess cavity is not seen, prophylactic broad-spectrum coverage is usually initiated.

Metronidazole has been shown in controlled trials to be effective in the treatment of chronic active Crohn's disease. Its benefit is most clear in the treatment of perianal disease, including fistulas; however, it is also often useful in ileocolonic Crohn's disease in combination with other medications. Metronidazole is not as consistently effective in isolated small bowel disease, where colonic flora are probably not an important factor. Therapy is usually begun with an oral form administered at 250 mg three or four times a day. Additional benefit in perianal disease may be seen by increasing to over 1 g per day; however, peripheral neuropathy is almost universal at this dosage. Frequent side effects include a metallic taste and nausea, which may be unacceptable for some patients. Alcohol consumption in large amounts may result in a disulfram-like reaction when taken concomitantly with this medication. Women should be warned about potential mutagenic effects if taken in the first trimester of pregnancy.

Ciprofloxacin has also been used in perianal Crohn's disease when metronidazole therapy is not tolerated or has failed. Although there are no controlled trials of this agent, a dose of 500 mg twice per day can be used.

Nutrition

Poor nutrition in Crohn's disease can result from anorexia, food avoidance due to abdominal pain, malabsorption, or short-gut syndrome due to surgical resection. Often these patients also have increased nutritional requirements due to chronic disease and steroid use. Specific trace elements and vitamin deficiencies such as zinc, iron, vitamins B_{12} and D, can be supplemented as needed. Evidence of more significant protein calorie malnutrition should be approached initially by encouraging increased quantity and frequency of meals, as well as the addition of antimotility agents in patients with diarrhea, to aid fluid and electrolyte absorption in nondiseased intestine. Some patients with severe disease or partial obstruction will require liquid formula diets.

Elemental diets are more easily absorbed and theoretically deliver a lower antigenic load to the gut and probably lessen the bacterial population of the colon. Sedimentation rates can fall in 1 week on elemental diets and intestinal permeability improves. They have been found to be helpful in achieving remission in 60 to 75 percent of patients with small bowel disease but are less effective in patients with colonic or perianal disease. Unfortunately, the use of elemental diets is limited by a lack of palatability and expense.

Total parenteral nutrition (TPN), presumably by altering luminal contents, is helpful in achieving remission in more severely active Crohn's disease. TPN can also be of benefit by allowing patients with fistulous disease some degree of bowel rest. Most importantly, TPN has a well-proven beneficial role in malnourished patients with stricturing or fistulous disease awaiting elective surgery, and nutritional status can usually be adequately corrected before surgery in all but the most emergent situations.

SURGERY

Surgical intervention is eventually needed in over two-thirds of patients with small bowel Crohn's disease. The predominant site of disease location in Crohn's disease is a good predictor of the likelihood of bowel resection. The need for resection in isolated colonic disease has decreased with adequate medical intervention. Nonetheless, refractory bleeding, perforation, and obstruction can still occur and require surgery. Stricturoplasties are useful as a bowel-preserving procedure in patients with jejunoileitis.

Because of the multifocal nature of Crohn's disease, surgery does not represent a cure; however, it is clearly beneficial as a "fresh start" in certain situations. Patients with disease confined only to a short segment of distal ileum will benefit from surgical resection. Often these patients will present after 7 to 9 years of active inflammatory disease with fixed fibrostenosis. These are proving to be ideal candidates for laparoscopically assisted ileocolonic resections. Patients with ileocolonic fistulizing disease tend to require surgery for abscess or free perforation much earlier in the course of their disease. Frank abscess formation, often defined by CAT scan, generally requires some form of drainage, either percutaneously or with laparotomy. Patients with ileojejunitis usually come to surgery for obstruction somewhat later than those with terminal ileitis, often after 12 to 15 years. Short strictures of the ileum and jejunum are well suited for stricturoplasties.

Recurrence after bowel resection is a concern as well. Patients with isolated colonic disease appear to have low rates of recurrence, while ileocolonic disease frequently recurs in the neoterminal ileum. There is evidence that maintenance therapy with oral controlled-release 5-ASA may lower the incidence of this after ileal resection. Severe perianal disease, especially rectovaginal fistulas, may require surgical intervention, including diversion of the fecal stream. Reanastomosis is occasionally successful in the patient with a grossly normal rectum.

SUGGESTED READING

Greenberg G, Feagan B, Martin F, et al. Oral budesonide for active Crohn's disease. N Engl J Med 1994; 331:836–841.

Linn FV, Peppercorn MA: Drug therapy for inflammatory bowel disease: Part I. Am J Surg 1992; 164:85–89.

O'Brien J, Bayless T, Bayless J. Use of azathioprine or 6-mercaptopurine in the treatment of crohn's disease. Gastroenterol 1991; 101:39–46.

Prantera C, Pallone F, Brunetti G, et al. Oral 5-aminosalicylic acid (Asacol) in the maintenance treatment of Crohn's disease. Gastroenterology 1992; 103:363–368.

Present DH, Meltzer S, Krumholz MP, et al. 6-Mercaptopurine in the management of inflammatory bowel disease. Short- and long-term toxicity. Ann Intern Med 1989; 111:641–649.

Sandborn WJ, Tremaine WJ. Cyclosporine treatment of inflammatory bowel disease. Mayo Clin Proc 1992; 67:981–990.

CHRONIC HEPATITIS

MICHAEL P. MANNS, M.D.
CHRISTIAN P. STRASSBURG, M.D.

DEFINITION AND PRESENTATION

Chronic hepatitis is a syndrome characterized by an inflammatory process affecting the liver without improvement for a period of at least 6 months. Inflammatory diseases of the liver can be classified as acute and chronic hepatitis. Histologic evidence of hepatitis is surprisingly uniformly characterized by hepatocellular inflammation usually involving periportal inflammation with piecemeal necrosis. Regardless of the underlying pathophysiologic process, chronic hepatitis ultimately leads to liver cirrhosis and liver failure. Nevertheless, sound knowledge of the presenting clinical picture and the classification of chronic hepatitis is essential for precise risk assessment of the involved patient, consequently leading to a specific, effective, and safe treatment strategy. This includes knowledge about etiologic agents, immunologic processes, and interpretation of biochemical, clinical, and immunologic laboratory parameters. Additionally, knowledge about the pharmacologic and biologic functions of commonly used medications ranging from interferons to immunosuppressive agents is warranted.

The presenting clinical picture of chronic hepatitis is nonspecific. It is generally characterized by fatigue and often by incapacitating exhaustion. Right upper quadrant abdominal pain, jaundice, palmar erythema, and spider nevi may be present. In later stages of chronic hepatitis the effects of portal hypertension—ascites, encephalopathy, and esophageal variceal bleeding are noted. In addition, chronic viral hepatitis C and autoimmune hepatitis can be characterized by extrahepatic autoimmune syndromes that may precede the diagnosis and manifestations of hepatic disease. Among these are thyroiditis, vitiligo, alopecia, nail dystrophy, ulcerative colitis, rheumatoid arthritis, and even conditions such as glomerulonephritis and diabetes mellitus. Although a thorough history will usually reveal the aforementioned symptoms of chronic hepatitis, most patients will present with abnormal liver function tests and usually elevated aspartate aminotransferase (AST) and alanine aminotransferase (ALT) values.

Classification of Chronic Hepatitis

Classification of the different entities of chronic hepatitis strongly relies on biochemical and immunologic laboratory investigations. Patients with suspected chronic hepatitis are classified to allow for the association of a specific, well-defined condition with an effective therapy. Not all forms of chronic hepatitis, however, have established and scientifically verified treatment protocols, and some do not require treatment at all. The current international consensus view of chronic hepatitis subclassifies chronic hepatitis into four principal categories: (1) chronic viral hepatitis, (2) autoimmune hepatitis, (3) drug-induced hepatitis, and (4) cryptogenetic hepatitis (Table 1).

Chronic viral hepatitis is caused by the hepatitis C (HCV), hepatitis B (HBV), or hepatitis D virus (HDV) (superinfection of ongoing hepatitis B or simultaneous infection of hepatitis B and D virus). *Chronic hepatitis B* requires the presence of serum hepatitis B surface antigen (HBsAg) and the detection of HBV-DNA. *Chronic hepatitis C* is diagnosed by anti–HCV antibodies and more accurately by HCV-RNA. In *hepatitis D* anti-HDV antibodies or HDV-RNA are detected in addition to markers of chronic HBV infection.

In *autoimmune hepatitis* markers of viral hepatitis (hepatitis A-E) and other markers of hepatotropic viral or other infection (herpes simplex virus, Epstein-Barr

Table 1 Classification of Chronic Hepatitis

Hepatitis Type	*HBsAg*	*HBV-DNA*	*Anti-HDV (HDV-RNA)*	*Anti-HCV (HCV-RNA)*	*Autoantibodies*
B	+	+/−	−	−	−
D	+	−	+	−	~10% anti–LKM-3
C	−	−	−	+	~2% anti–LKM-1
Autoimmune hepatitis					
Type 1	−	−	−	−	ANA
Type 2	−	−	−	−	LKM-1
Type 3	−	−	−	−	SLA/LP
Drug-induced	−	−	−	−	Some ANA, LKM, LM
Cryptogenic	−	−	−	−	−

Modified from Desmet VJ, Gerber M, Hoofnagle JH, et al. Classification of chronic hepatitis: Diagnosis, grading and staging. Hepatology 1994; 19(6):1513–1520.

ANA, Antinuclear antibodies; *LKM,* anti–liver-kidney microsomal antibodies; *LM,* anti-liver microsomal antibodies; *LP,* anti–liver pancreas antibodies; *SLA,* antibodies against soluble liver antigen.

virus, varicella zoster virus, cytomegalo virus, toxoplasma gondii) are absent. Additionally, no signs of genetic (Wilson's disease, hemochromatosis, alpha-1-antitrypsin deficiency), metabolic (galactosemia, storage diseases), or toxic (drugs, alcohol) liver disease are found. A number of tissue and non–tissue specific autoantibodies are detectable that are currently the basis of further subclassification. The oldest recognized form of autoimmune hepatitis is classical *autoimmune hepatitis type 1* (earlier named lupoid hepatitis). It is characterized by antinuclear (ANA) and anti–smooth muscle antibodies (SMA). *Autoimmune hepatitis type 2* is characterized by liver-kidney microsomal antibodies (LKM-1) that are directed against cytochrome P450 2D6. A third group *(autoimmune hepatitis type 3)* displays antibodies against soluble liver antigen (SLA) and in some patients also against liver pancreas antigen (LP).

Autoimmune hepatitis affects predominantly (75 percent) young female patients with 50 percent of patients being between 10 and 20 years of age. A second peak of incidence is around age 50 (mainly type 1 autoimmune hepatitis and hepatitis C associated autoimmune hepatitis). Otherwise the classification according to prevalent autoantibodies has not led to an impact on the therapeutic management of these patients. Antibodies against microsomal antigens, however, have recently claimed a role beyond the immunopathologic search for pathophysiologic models of autoimmune hepatitis. Autoantibodies against microsomal antigens have been implicated in differentiating between virus-associated autoimmunity and autoimmune hepatitis, thereby attempting a rational basis for the decision of whether to employ interferon treatment versus immunosuppression.

Drug-induced chronic hepatitis implies the absence of markers and factors mentioned for chronic viral and chronic autoimmune hepatitis. The exclusion of these criteria leads to the suspicion of drug-related hepatitis. Drugs typically implicated are propylthiouracil, alpha-methyl dopa, estrogens, anabolic drugs, isoniazid, and nitrofurantoin. A second aspect in drug-mediated chronic hepatitis is a drug-induced immunologic *hypersensitivity* reaction. This entity has similarity with autoimmune hepatitis but is, in contrast, self-limiting upon discontinuation of the inducing drug in most instances. Interestingly, this reaction is accompanied by the appearance of antimicrosomal antibodies that are directed against cytochrome P450 2C9 (LKM-2, drug: ticrynafen) and P450 1A2 (LM, drug: dihydralazine).

Cryptogenic chronic hepatitis is a collecting pool of patients with the clinical, biochemical, and histologic signs of chronic hepatitis in absence of a detectable cause. Many aspects of cryptogenic chronic hepatitis resemble autoimmune hepatitis and further research will help to constantly decrease this group of patients.

These considerations regarding the classification of chronic hepatitis illustrate that the search for adequate treatment strategies and for correct prognosis assessment has been the driving force of the definition of disease entities.

Table 2 Index of Hepatic Inflammation

Inflammatory Activity	*Serum ALT Activity*	*Serum ALT (times upper normal value)*
Mild	<100 U/L	<3×
Moderate	100-400 U/L	3-10×
Severe	>400	>10×

NATURAL HISTORY, SEVERITY OF DISEASE, AND PROGNOSIS

The single most reliable predictor of the severity and prognosis of chronic hepatitis is the degree of inflammation. Together with the histologic evaluation of liver needle biopsy specimens, ALT values are used to determine the grade of disease activity (Table 2). Mild inflammatory activity can be considered with a three-fold ALT increase or values up to 100 U per liter, moderate with up to ten-fold ALT increases or 100 to 400 U per liter, and severe disease with ALT values exceeding 10 times the upper normal or amounting to more than 400 units per liter.

The major risk of chronic inflammatory liver disease that ultimately determines mortality is the development of cirrhosis. Cirrhosis may be present well before clinical signs of portal hypertension are apparent. Unfortunately clinical experience shows that the levels of aminotransferases do not always correlate with the rate and grade of liver cirrhosis. This fact stresses the importance of liver biopsy evaluation in every patient who is suspected of having chronic hepatitis. Additionally, scoring systems resulting in indices that allow for prognostic assessment of cirrhosis are employed. Among the most widely used to date is the Child-Pugh classification that utilizes bilirubin values, albumin values, prothrombin time, ascites, and encephalopathy to determine a score of severity (Table 3). A clinical evaluation system aimed at determining both the grade of inflammation and the grade of cirrhosis is particularly useful in chronic viral hepatitis B, C, and D. Here specialized tests for viral markers rapidly lead to the establishment of the diagnosis, and the mentioned indices determine the assessment of risk and, most importantly, the beginning of treatment. The Child-Pugh score has been found to correlate with the outcome of interferon therapy of patients with chronic hepatitis B.

Although roughly 300 million humans are infected with the hepatitis B virus, exact data on the natural course are difficult to obtain. The rate of chronicity appears to be 10 percent in adults and up to 90 percent in neonates with perinatal infection. The course of disease is extremely variable and also appears to depend on geographic factors. In general, a high grade of inflammation, older age, persistence of hepatitis B-DNA, and bridging necrosis indicate a poorer prognosis. When hepatitis D superinfection occurs prognosis is again much poorer with chronicity rates of 80 percent.

Table 3 Child-Pugh Classification for the Assessment of Liver Cirrhosis

Score	*Bilirubin (mg/dl)*	*Albumin (g/dl)*	*Prothrombin Time (sec)*	*Hepatic Encephalopathy (grade)*	*Ascites*
1	<2	>3.5	1-4	None	None
2	2-3	2.8-3.5	4-6	1-2	Mild
3	>3	<2.8	>6	3-4	Severe

Child classification: A: 5 to 6; B: 7 to 9; C: >9.

Hepatitis C will progress to chronic hepatitis in 60 percent of affected patients, and since the identification of the HCV virus in 1989 has been recognized as one of the major causes of chronic hepatitis. The course of disease is similarly variable as in hepatitis B. The markers of inflammation, however, tend to increase and decrease more than in HBV infection, thereby leading to apparent intermediate remissions. Hepatitis C is additionally interesting with regard to the discrimination of autoimmune liver disease and viral infection. Rates of virus-induced autoimmune diseases and immunologic autoimmune phenomena are higher in hepatitis C than in other viral infections. This requires precise diagnostic discrimination and initiation of correct therapeutic strategies.

Autoimmune hepatitis has received considerable attention and has been the focus of intense investigation. The diagnosis is difficult and is reached through the exclusion of other causes of chronic hepatitis. Therefore a scoring system is employed and guarantees the highest possible reliability (Table 4). This system reflects the current international consensus view and incorporates hypergammaglobulinemia, autoantibody titers, sex, immunogenetic predisposition, and status of markers of viral hepatitis. Interestingly, the effect of immunosuppression (corticosteroids and azathioprine) has also been incorporated and is seen as a diagnostic criterium of autoimmune hepatitis. This fact stresses the significance of the connection between immunologic laboratory findings and treatment response in establishing the diagnosis of autoimmune hepatitis. Therefore, when discussing the therapy of autoimmune hepatitis, broad emphasis and awareness of the immunopathologic background is imperative.

Overall, the natural course of chronic hepatitis has been well documented in autoimmune hepatitis. Patients with moderate to severe inflammatory activity of chronic hepatitis have a 5-year mortality of 80 to 90 percent. Eighty-two percent of patients presenting with bridging necrosis develop cirrhosis in 5 years and have a mortality of 50 percent. Patients initially presenting with cirrhosis have a 5-year mortality of over 50 percent. In mild chronic hepatitis survival can be normal and associated with a probability of cirrhosis as low as 20 percent. It appears, however, that patients with chronic autoimmune hepatitis suffer from a more severe course of their disease when compared to patients with chronic viral hepatitis.

Hepatocellular carcinoma (HCC) has to be appreciated as an additional and serious complication of chronic hepatitis. It does not appear to correlate with the type of disease leading to cirrhosis but rather with presence of cirrhosis itself. Risks for HCC are estimated as being between 30 to 300 times higher in patients with cirrhosis compared to those who do not have cirrhosis.

Table 4 Diagnostic Criteria of Autoimmune Hepatitis

	Score
Hypergammaglobulinemia	+3
Autoantibodies:	
ANA, SMA, LKM-1	+3
SLA, ASGPR, LP,	+2
AMA	−2
Female sex	+2
AST/ALT <3.0	+2
Complete response to immunosuppression	+2
Anti-HAV IgM, HBsAg, anti–HBc IgM	−3
HCV-RNA (PCR)	−3
Anti-HCV	−2
Other virus infections	−3
Ethanol intake	
Males <35 g/day females <25 g/day	+2
Immunogenetics: HLA-B8-DR3 or DR4	+1
Value of score >15 before and >17 after therapy: AIH certain	
Value of score 10-15 before and 12-17 after therapy: AIH probable	

Modified from Johnson PJ, McFarlane IG. Hepatology 1993; 18:998-1005.
PCR, polymerase chain reaction; *ANA,* antinuclear antibodies; *SMA,* smooth muscle antibodies; *LKM-1,* liver-kidney microsomal antibodies; *SLA,* antibodies against soluble liver antigen; *ASGPR,* antibodies against asialoglycoprotein receptor; *LP,* liver pancreas antibodies; *AMA,* antimitochondrial antibodies.

Drug-related hepatitis and drug-related hypersensitivity reactions are usually self-limiting once the cause has been identified and is discontinued. Elevation of aminotransferases (alanine aminotransferase, aspartate aminotransferase) and markers of cholestasis (alkaline phosphatase, gamma glutamyl transferase, bilirubin) sometimes take extended periods (up to 12 months and longer) until they are completely normalized.

WHEN TO BEGIN TREATMENT

Not all forms of chronic hepatitis require treatment. As discussed previously, drug-induced hepatitis or drug-related hypersensitivity reactions usually reach remission upon discontinuation of the inducing agent. The main problem lies in rapidly identifying this form of hepatitis. Here, autoantibody testing may be of additional diagnostic help (i.e., LM autoantibodies in dihydralazine-induced hepatitis). In viral and autoimmune chronic hepatitis, however, treatment is warranted when biochemical parameters indicate active or aggressive hepatic disease (Table 5). Importantly, the precise diagnosis must be immunologically established.

Since chronic hepatitis C is associated with multiple immunopathologic phenomena the indication for treatment of both chronic hepatitis C virus infection and autoimmune hepatitis will be discussed in this section.

Multiple international trials have confirmed the beneficial effect of interferon-alpha in the treatment of chronic hepatitis C in which interferon-alpha is currently recognized as the standard treatment regimen. The indication for treatment is present once a second generation ELISA test for anti-HCV antibodies and HCV-RNA *(polymerase chain reaction)* are positive, liver biopsy reveals signs of chronic hepatitis, and aminotransferase levels are increased 1.5 times the upper normal limit. Since chronic hepatitis C leads to liver cirrhosis and this is regarded to be the major risk factor of hepatocellular carcinoma, the indication for interferon treatment may be considered in young patients despite possible low elevations of aminotransferase levels. This issue is, however, not yet decided because of a lack of long-term scientific study data.

A number of prognostic factors influence the response to interferon treatment. Patients younger than 40 to 45 years of age with a short history of chronic hepatitis show a favorable outcome. Also, mild elevation of aminotransferases is associated with better treatment results. Factors that are viewed as indicators of poor treatment response include the presence of liver cirrhosis, a high elevation of the gamma glutamyl transferase, iron overload (high ferritin), and the presence of HCV genotype II according to Okamoto's classification or genotype Ib according to Simmonds. Because interferon is a powerful therapeutic agent, there are several absolute and relative contraindications to its use (Table 6). If autoimmune disease is present interferon therapy must be conducted cautiously with a higher frequency of physical examinations and meticulous monitoring of organ function tests (thyroid) and immunologic serum parameters such as autoantibodies.

The indications for treatment of autoimmune hepatitis are similar (see Table 5). Signs of viral, toxic, metabolic, or genetic liver disease are excluded and a score indicative of autoimmune hepatitis is documented. In contrast to viral hepatitis C (and B and D) the standard therapy in autoimmune hepatitis regardless of the type (types 1–3) consists of immunosuppression. Aminotransferase levels exceeding 1.5 times the upper normal limit, elevation of gamma globulin levels of 2 times the upper normal limit, and liver biopsies showing hepatocellular inflammation and necrosis constitute absolute indications. A relative indication is the presence of extrahepatic incapacitating symptoms.

A number of prognostic factors influence the treatment response in autoimmune hepatitis. Autoimmune hepatitis shows a dual age peak incidence. The younger patient group with a high inflammatory activity and high aminotransferases shows a poorer treatment response than the older patient group with lower markers of inflammatory activity. Interestingly, the younger group is characterized by the immunogenetic association with *human leukocyte antigen* (HLA) DR3, the older patient group is associated with HLA-DR4, both of which are viewed as independent risk factors and are also incorporated into the diagnostic scoring system of autoimmune hepatitis (see Table 4).

As previously mentioned, the indication for treatment should also be influenced by the risk of hepatocellular carcinoma in the cirrhotic liver. More so than in chronic viral hepatitis, patients with untreated autoimmune hepatitis have the tendency to rapidly progress to liver cirrhosis. Since these patients are generally much younger than patients with chronic viral hepatitis, their lifetime risk of liver cancer will be appreciably higher.

VIRUS-INDUCED AUTOIMMUNITY

Chronic hepatitis C virus infection and, as suggested by recent data, chronic hepatitis D virus infection are associated with multiple signs and symptoms of autoimmunity. This includes hepatic and extrahepatic manifestations (Table 7). Earlier studies showed that patients with autoimmune hepatitis type 2 (LKM-1 positive) had markers of HCV infection in up to 90 percent depending

Table 5 Treatment Indications in Chronic Viral Hepatitis C and Autoimmune Hepatitis

Indications for Treatment of Chronic Viral Hepatitis C
Aminotransferases 1.5 × upper normal limit
Anti–HCV-ELISA (2nd generation) positive
HCV-RNA (PCR) positive
Liver biopsy: chronic hepatitis, moderate to severe activity
Indications for Treatment of Autoimmune Hepatitis
No signs of viral, toxic, metabolic, genetic liver disease
Presence of serum autoantibodies
Gamma globulin 2 times upper normal limit
Aminotransferases 1.5 times upper normal limit
Liver biopsy: chronic hepatitis, moderate to severe activity

Table 6 Contraindications for Interferon Treatment

Autoimmune hepatitis
Liver failure (decompensated cirrhosis)
Immunosuppression
Pregnancy
Mental disorders (i.e., depression)
Thrombocytopenia $<50{,}000/\mu l$
Leukopenia $<2{,}000/\mu l$
Bilirubin >2.5 mg/dl
Relative contraindication: autoimmune diseases

on the geographic origin of patients. In untreated chronic hepatitis C, cryoglobulins are found in 36 percent, rheumatoid factor in 70 percent, salivary gland lesions in 49 percent, lichen planus in 5 percent, and anti–tissue antibodies (antinuclear antibodies, smooth muscle antibodies, liver kidney microsomal antibodies, and antithyroid antibodies) in 41 percent. Disease manifestations include membranoproliferative glomerulonephritis, Sjögren's disease, porphyria cutanea tarda, vasculitis, autoimmune thyroid disease, and autoimmune hepatitis. A direct etiologic role of the HCV virus is suspected and evidence has been provided in HCV-induced autoimmunity (LKM autoantibodies), cryoglobulinemia, and membranoproliferative glomerulonephritis. Chronic hepatitis C–associated and clinically apparent autoimmune disease are rare. LKM autoantibodies occur in about 2 to 3 percent of patients with chronic hepatitis. While LKM autoantibodies in autoimmune hepatitis are predominantly directed against an eight aminoacid core peptide of cytochrome P450 2D6, targets of LKM autoantibodies in HCV-associated autoimmunity are heterogenous. In HCV-associated autoimmunity LKM autoantibodies are regularly detectable upon immunofluorescence, but further molecular evaluation provides evidence for epitope diversity, conformational epitopes, and recognition to date of unidentified microsomal antigens. More frequently autoimmune thyroid disease such as Hashimoto's thyroiditis is encountered in chronic hepatitis C. Up to 30 percent of patients with chronic hepatitis C have antithyroid antibodies (antithyroglobulin antibodies, antimicrosomal antibodies).

Interferon not only has antiviral and antiproliferative effects but is also a powerful immunomodulator through which it has a well-documented capability of inducing autoimmunity. In viral hepatitis interferon's antiviral and immunodulatory effects are the basis of treatment. When accidently used in autoimmune hepatitis, interferon leads to disease exacerbation with ALT levels increasing to up to 50 to 100 times the upper normal limit, a dramatic rise in inflammatory activity, and the progression to liver failure. Similarly, quiescent autoimmune thyroid disease can be exacerbated, sometimes leading to persistent hypo- or hyperthyroidism. These considerations illustrate the triangular relationship of the hepatitis C (and other) virus, which is an inducer of autoimmunity, interferon, which is also an inducer of autoimmunity and the standard therapeutic agent of chronic hepatitis C, and autoimmunity itself, which is treated by immunosuppression (Fig. 1). Chronic hepatitis C must therefore be considered within the scope of immunologic diseases. This raises two important points—the diagnosis of viral hepatitis and autoimmune hepatitis must be precise and performed according to the molecularly defined and accepted methods (autoantibodies, PCR) in order to initiate the correct therapeutic strategy; and treatment protocols must take the possibility of inducing autoimmunity into account and must include screening for autoimmunity in order to assure safe and effective interferon treatment.

Table 7 HCV-Associated Autoimmunity and Extrahepatic Diseases

Tissue-specific autoantibodies (ANA, LKM, SMA, antithyroid)
Cryoglobulinemia
Lymphocytic sialadenitis
Membranoproliferative glomerulonephritis
Autoimmune thyroid disease
Porphyria cutanea tarda
Lichen planus
Vasculitis

ANA, Antinuclear antibodies; *LKM,* liver-kidney microsomal antibodies; *SMA,* anti–smooth muscle antibodies.

Beyond the above-mentioned distinctions hepatitis C–associated autoimmunity and genuine idiopathic autoimmune hepatitis represent two clinically distinct syndromes (Table 8). When viral replication is detectable in the absense of markers of autoimmunity the standard treatment is interferon alpha. In autoimmune hepatitis without markers of replicative viral infection the standard treatment is immunosuppression. In the overlap of both—chronic replicative viral hepatitis with markers of autoimmunity—interferon may be administered cautiously requiring consequent clinical, immunologic, and biochemical monitoring for adverse effects. Data of large trials evaluating this treatment group, however, are not yet available.

TREATMENT OF VIRAL HEPATITIS C

Interferon is currently regarded as the standard therapeutic agent of chronic hepatitis B, C, and D. In hepatitis B the rate of hepatocellular damage is deter-

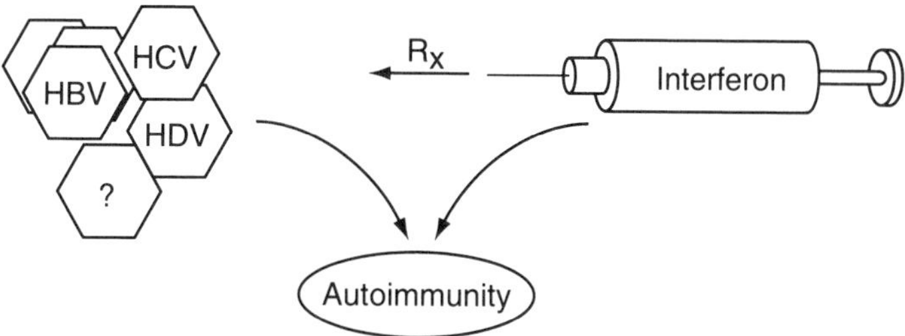

Figure 1 Viruses, interferon, and autoimmunity. From Strassburg CP, Manns MP. Autoimmune hepatitis versus viral hepatitis C. Liver 1995;15:225–232.

mined by the immunologic T-cell response of the infected organism. In contrast to hepatitis C the associated autoimmunity in hepatitis B and its clinical implications are extremely rare. Chronic hepatitis C, however, displays an array of immune and autoimmune phenomena. Therefore therapy of chronic hepatitis C is discussed here.

Once the diagnosis of hepatitis C has been confirmed and a liver biopsy has been evaluated, patients will be screened for autoimmune disease and markers of autoimmunity. If no contraindications are present, patients receive 5 million units of interferon alpha subcutaneously three times per week for 6 to 12 months. A normalization of aminotransferases is usually achieved within 3 to 4 months. The therapeutic response can be monitored in 4-week intervals at which a physical examination, a complete blood count, aminotransferase and gamma-glutamyl transferase levels, bilirubin, ferritin, and prothrombin time are determined. In patients with signs of autoimmune disease or with serum autoantibodies the monthly tests will include ANA, LKM, SMA, SLA, and antithyroid antibody determinations. Thyroxine, triiodothyronine, and thyroid stimulating hormone are also monitored to allow for an early detection of thyroid dysfunction. With a history of thyroid disease and the pretreatment presence of antithyroid antibodies the initiation of interferon treatment should be carefully monitored weekly during the first month. Upon exacerbation of autoimmune disease, interferon treatment is discontinued. Exacerbated thyroid disease is treated immediately since this appears to be beneficial for the prevention of persistent hypo- or hyperthyroidism (Table 9).

A needle liver biopsy is performed at the end of treatment to provide reliable documentation of the inflammatory hepatocellular status. Approximately 50 percent reach a complete remission (complete normalization of aminotransferases, negative HCV-RNA) at the end of therapy. About 14 percent reach a partial response (50 percent reduction of initial aminotransferase levels). The remaining patients are nonresponders with no changes. If there is no measurable treatment response within 4 months, interferon therapy should be discontinued. In 50 percent of the initial responders a reactivation of the HCV virus occurs requiring reinitiation of therapy. The retreatment regimen is identical except for an increased dose of 5 to 10 million units of interferon alpha given subcutaneously 3 times per week. Overall, 15 to 20 percent will remain complete responders. The therapeutic problem of patients with complete response and the recurrence of minimally active chronic hepatitis C after cessation of

Table 8 Clinical Features of Autoimmune Hepatitis Type 2 and HCV-Associated Autoimmunity (LKM)

	Autoimmune Hepatitis Type 2	*Chronic Hepatitis C Associated with LKM-1 Autoantibodies*
Age	Young	Older
Sex	90% female	No prevalence
ALT	↑ ↑ ↑	↑
LKM-1 titer	↑ ↑ ↑	↑
Immunosuppression effective	+ + +	−
Interferon effective	−	(+)?
HLA-DR3	+ +	+
C4A-Q0	+	+
Anti–HCV/HCV RNA	−	+

ALT, Alanine aminotransferase; *C4A-Q0,* null allele of the complement factor C4A haplotype; *HCV,* hepatitis C virus; *HLA-DR3,* human leukocyte antigen DR 3; *LKM-1,* anti–liver-kidney microsomal antibodies.

Table 9 Treatment of Chronic Hepatitis C

	First Treatment	*Retreatment*
Interferon-α:	5 million U SC 3 times per week	5-10 million U SC 3 times per week
Duration:	6-12 months	6 months

Follow-up

Test	*Before Therapy*	*During Therapy (q4wk)*	*Remission*	*After Therapy (q3mo)*
Physical examination	+		+	+
Liver biopsy	+		+	
Blood count	+	+	+	
Aminotransferases	+	+	+	+
Gamma-glutamyl transferase	+	+	+	
Bilirubin	+	+	+	
Coagulation	+	+	+	
Ferritin	+	+	+	+
Autoantibodies*	+	+/−		
Thyroid function*	+	+/−		

*If autoantibodies or abnormal thyroid function tests are found before initiation of therapy, screening every 4 weeks during therapy is required.

interferon therapy is not yet satisfactorily resolved. Response rates of patients with detectable autoantibodies during therapy do not appear to differ from those without signs of autoimmunity.

MECHANISMS OF ACTION AND SIDE EFFECTS OF INTERFERON

Interferon is a potent cytokine that exerts antiproliferative, antiviral, and immunomodulatory effects. Treatment of viral hepatitis B, C, and D profits from interferon's antiviral properties and to some extent possibly also from the immunomodulatory effects. The immunomodulatory effects are the basis of the observed tendency of interferons to newly induce or exacerbate pre-existing autoimmunity. A number of effects account for this observation. Interferon leads to an upregulation of HLA class I and HLA class II antigens that play an important role in antigen presentation and activation of immunologically competent cells. The activity of cytotoxic T cells is increased and the activity of suppressor T cells is decreased. A decrease of suppressor T cells is also found in autoimmune hepatitis. These observations are implicated in the induction of autoimmunity.

On the other hand a number of adverse side effects are frequently associated with interferon treatment, including a flulike syndrome, nausea, diarrhea, abdominal discomforts, thrombocytopenia, and leukocytopenia. Rare side effects include depression, neurologic symptoms such as paresthesias and dysgeusia, and toxic reactions with elevation of the gamma glutamyl transferase and bilirubin values (Table 10).

Table 10 Adverse Effects of Interferon

Flu-like syndrome
Gastrointestinal symptoms
Thrombopenia
Leukopenia
Depression
Paresthesia, dysgeusia
Induction or exacerbation of autoimmune disease
Induction of autoantibodies
Toxic reaction (elevation of bilirubin and gamma glutamyl transferase)

TREATMENT OF AUTOIMMUNE HEPATITIS

After biochemical and immunologic confirmation of the diagnosis and evaluation of the liver biopsy two principal treatment strategies can be employed. One is a single drug regimen using prednisolone and the other is a combination regimen of prednisolone and azathioprine (Table 11). Both regimens are equally suited to induce biochemical and histologic remission in patients with autoimmune hepatitis. There are, however, a number of considerations that may lead to the preference of one regimen.

Prolonged therapy with corticosteroids leads to a number of cosmetic and metabolic side effects. Unfortunately the majority of patients treated for longer than 12 months develop side effects such as obesity, moon-shaped face, hirsutism, abdominal and chest striae, acne, and dorsal hump formation. Especially the cosmetic changes can severily impair patient compliance (Table 12). Additional side effects that also lead to serious

Table 11 Treatment of Autoimmune Hepatitis

	Single-Drug Regimen	*Combination Regimen*
Prednisolone	50 mg for 10 days; taper 5 mg every 10 days; maintenance 20 mg or lower as required	50 mg for 10 days; taper 5 mg every 10 days; maintenance 10 mg or lower as required
Azathioprine	None	100 mg for 3 weeks; 50 mg
Upon remission (treatment 24 months)		
Prednisolone	Taper 2.5 mg every week	Taper 2.5 mg every week
Azathioprine	None	Taper 25 mg every 3 weeks
Follow-up		

Test	*Before Therapy*	*During Therapy (q4wk)*	*Remission*	*After Therapy (q3wk × 4)*	*(q3 mo)*
Physical examination	+		+	+	+
Liver biopsy	+		+		
Blood count	+	+	+	+	+
Aminotransferases	+	+	+	+	+
Gamma-glutamyl transferase	+	+	+		
Gamma globulin	+	+	+	+	+
Bilirubin	+	+	+	+	+
Coagulation	+	+	+	+	+
Autoantibodies	+	+/−			
Thyroid function	+	+/−			

Table 12 Adverse Effects of Corticosteroids

Acne
Moon-shaped face
Striae rubrae
Dorsal hump formation
Hirsutism
Obesity
Osteoporosis
Aseptic bone necrosis
Mental disorders (euphoria, psychosis, depression)
Diabetes mellitus
Cataract
Hypertension

long-term complications are osteopenia, aseptic bone necrosis (head of the hip, vertebrae), euphoria, depression, steroid diabetes mellitus, hypertension, and cataract formation.

The combination of azathioprine with prednisolone can result in a substantial reduction of required corticosteroid dose during the course of treatment. Several international trials and our own experience find this regimen to be as effective as the single-drug regimen. The rate of appreciable side effects is much lower than that of steroid treatment. Patients complain of abdominal discomfort, diarrhea, nausea, and exanthemas. The blood profile reveals thrombocytopenia and leukopenia in a minority of patients. Azathioprine, however, has other potential risks. The main point of concern is the hypothetical teratogenic and oncogenic potential of the drug. Azathioprine is a false metabolite whose target is to block purin synthesis (adenine, guanine). As a result this leads to an interference with normal DNA synthesis, which raises the possibility of somatic and germline mutations, potentially leading to neoplastic transformation. In the mouse model azathioprine was capable of inducing skeletal deformation, cleft palate, hypoplasia of the thymus, and hematologic abnormalities. In humans only a few effects have been conclusively demonstrated so far. The risk of tumor formation appears to be increased to 3 percent after 10 years of treatment. Other data fail to show a correlation of the duration of azathioprine therapy and cancer risk. The risk of malignancy is estimated to be 1.4 times greater than in a reference population (Table 13).

The consideration of side effects leads to the necessity of patient selection. This can be illustrated in two examples. A postmenopausal patient with osteoporosis, hypertension, elevated serum glucose, and a Cushing phenotype after prednisolone therapy will be a candidate for combination therapy. Young and fertile women, pregnant women, or patients with hematologic disorders will be candidates for prednisolone monotherapy.

Prednisolone monotherapy will typically be initiated at a dose of 50 mg daily. The dose is tapered by 5 mg every 10 days up to a maintenance dose of around 20 mg initially. Under close supervision of the aminotransferase values the prednisolone dose is tapered to the minimally required dose that still leads to aminotransferase normalization. In patients that respond well the maintenance dose can be as low as between 2.5 and 10 mg per day.

Table 13 Adverse Effects of Azathioprine

Nausea
Vomiting
Abdominal discomforts
Hepatotoxicity
Exanthema
Leukocytopenia
Teratogenicity ?
Oncogenicity ?

Combination therapy is begun with 100 mg azathioprine and 50 mg prednisolone. Prednisolone is tapered as described above to a minimally effective dose and then azathioprine can be reduced to 50 mg per day. The maintenance dose will typically be 2.5 to 10 mg prednisolone and 50 mg azathioprine.

Patients that do not respond to the single-drug regimen are transferred to the combination regimen that, in our experience, is beneficial in some patients with an incomplete response to prednisolone alone. Therapy is continued beyond the achievement of complete remission for a period of 24 months. During this time a program of regular follow-up tests is implemented. The single most reliable test is the determination of ALT and AST values (every 2 to 4 weeks). Additionally, gamma immunoglobulin levels, bilirubin (every 2 to 4 weeks), full blood count, complete liver function tests, and coagulation studies (every 6 to 8 weeks) are performed. Upon remission a needle liver biopsy is obtained to assess the grade of hepatocellular inflammation and necrosis. Biochemical normalization usually precedes histologic normalization. After this period of time withdrawal of therapy can be tried. After a prolonged period of corticosteroid treatment prednisolone must be tapered to prevent withdrawal symptoms. Usually, the dose is reduced in 5 to 2.5 mg decrements at weekly intervals until discontinuation. In the combination regimen the daily azathioprine dose is reduced by 25 mg every 3 weeks and then discontinued (Table 11).

Histologic findings have the greatest predictive value of treatment response. Patients that show a normal liver biopsy upon remission have a risk of relapse within the next 6 months of only 20 percent. Patients with mild hepatitis have a 50 percent risk and those with disease progression to cirrhosis during therapy have a 100 percent risk of relapse. The risk of relapse decreases with the duration of remission. After discontinuation of therapy patients should be monitored and ALT and AST levels assayed every 3 to 4 weeks for 6 months and then at 3-month intervals. With this regimen a complete response can be achieved in about two-thirds of patients. Although prednisone is converted to prednisolone in the liver there has to date been no conclusive evidence that there is a therapeutic benefit of prednisolone versus prednisone in the therapy of autoimmune hepatitis.

UNSATISFACTORY RESPONSE

There are four principal situations in which unsatisfactory responses are encountered:

1. Treatment failure (disease progression and deterioration in spite of immunosuppression),
2. Severe side effects that require discontinuation of therapy,
3. Failure to reach complete remission, and
4. Relapse or multiple relapses after discontinuation of therapy.

Disease progression and deterioration is the most serious complication that is seen in about 10 percent of patients and is associated with a high mortality rate. In this case higher doses of prednisolone (i.e., 100 mg) and azathioprine (i.e., 150 mg) than suggested in the aforementioned regimens are administered. If despite these efforts biochemical parameters do not improve, patients have to be evaluated for liver transplantation. Liver transplantation represents the ultimate treatment strategy and has survival rates exceeding 80 percent in 5 years. A number of experimental drug regimens are currently being evaluated for this group of patients. A promising approach appears to be the administration of cyclosporine A. At this point, however, cyclosporine should only be given in the context of controlled studies in the hands of an experienced hepatologist.

Side effects account for termination or alteration of treatment protocols in about 13 percent of patients. If treatment is impossible and disease progresses the possibility of experimental protocols or the evaluation of liver transplantation remains.

Failure to reach complete remission usually requires a change from the single-drug to the combination regimen. If this is not effective, again higher-than-normal doses of immunosuppression are administered. This way, many patients can be maintained in a stable situation for longer periods of time. They should, however, also be evaluated for liver transplantation.

Finally, a number of patients reach complete remission but relapse after tapering and discontinuation of therapy. In these patients a long-term, possibly indefinite administration of corticosteroid treatment is effective. Doses can typically be maintained well below 10 mg thereby minimizing and in most instances eliminating Cushingoid side effects. At regular intervals (12 to 24 months) disease progression should be monitored by needle liver biopsy. Most patients' disease can be kept stabilized with significantly reduced mortality. From general considerations it is advisable to favor prednisolone for permanent treatment since the effects of long-term administration of azathioprine cannot be calculated.

In summary, immunosuppressive therapy offers an effective treatment strategy in the well-characterized and precisely diagnosed patient that substantially reduces the considerable mortality of the natural history of autoimmune hepatitis. Care must be taken to identify virus-associated autoimmunity and autoimmune disease before administering interferon for chronic viral hepatitis.

SUGGESTED READING

Arroyo V, Bosch J, Rodés J. Treatments in hepatology. Barcelona, Spain: Masson SA, 1995.

Desmet VJ, Gerber M, Hoofnagle JH, et al. Classification of chronic hepatitis: Diagnosis, grading and staging. Hepatology 1994; 19(6): 1513–1520.

Durazzo M, Philipp T, Van Pelt FNAM, et al. Heterogeneity of microsomal autoantibodies (LKM) in chronic hepatitis C and D virus infection. Gastroenterology 1995; 108:455–462.

Johnson PJ, McFarlane IG. Meeting report: International autoimmune hepatitis group. Hepatology 1993; 18:998–1005.

Manns MP, Griffin KJ, Sullivan KF, Johnson EF. LKM-1 autoantibodies recognize a short linear sequence in P45011D6, a cytochrome P-450 monoxygenase. J Clin Invest 1991; 88:1370–1378.

Manns MP, Krüger M. Immunogenetics of chronic liver diseases. Gastroenterology 1994; 106:1676–1697.

Strassburg CP, Manns MP. Autoimmune hepatitis versus viral hepatitis C. Liver 1995; 15:225–232.

PRIMARY BILIARY CIRRHOSIS

MARSHALL M. KAPLAN, M.D.

Primary biliary cirrhosis (PBC), a chronic, progressive, liver disease that occurs predominantly in middle-aged women, is characterized by the destruction and subsequent disappearance of small intralobular bile ducts. The etiology is unknown but appears to be related to some abnormality of immunoregulation. The destruction of small bile ducts causes a chronic, progressive impairment of bile flow with a resultant retention of potentially toxic substances such as bile acids within the liver. Ultimately, there is destruction of liver cells, progressive portal fibrosis, the development of cirrhosis, and, finally, liver failure. Although not common, PBC is of major economic importance because it is one of the leading reasons for liver transplantation. Its prevalence has been reported to range from 3.7 to 14.4 per 100,000 population, but recent experience in the United States suggests that this figure is low, perhaps by as much as 50 percent.

CLINICAL FEATURES

Clinically, PBC mimics extrahepatic bile ducts obstruction. The most common initial symptoms are fatigue and itching. Many patients note darkening of the skin due to the increased deposition of melanin in skin. Jaundice is usually a later manifestation. Other manifestations of PBC include osteoporosis with bone pain and spontaneous fractures of vertebrae and ribs; hypercholesterolemia with xanthoma and xanthelasmas; and an increased incidence of other autoimmune disorders such as sicca syndrome, hypothyroidism, calcinosis, Raynaud's phenomenon, esophageal hypomotility sclerodactyly, telangiectasias (CREST) syndrome, and arthritis. It is important that the diagnosis of PBC be considered in all patients with unexplained cholestatic liver disease so that appropriate diagnostic tests can be done and unnecessary invasive tests or surgery is avoided.

The diagnosis of PBC is based on characteristic liver function tests (i.e., greatly elevated serum alkaline phosphatase and gamma-glutamyl transpeptidase and only moderately elevated serum aminotransferase levels, usually less than 300 IU). Ninety-five percent of patients with PBC will have a positive antimitochondrial antibody test. Most will have elevations of serum IgM. It is essential that mechanical bile duct obstruction be excluded. Techniques such as ultrasonography and computed tomography imaging are adequate except in patients with negative antimitochondrial antibody test results. Endoscopic cholangiography should be done in this group of patients to rule out primary sclerosing cholangitis. Diagnosis should be confirmed by percutaneous liver biopsy, which will also allow histologic staging and aid in prognosis.

Histologically, PBC has been divided into four stages. In stage I, there are so-called florid bile duct lesions, characterized by the infiltration and destruction of small bile ducts by mononuclear cells, predominantly T lymphocytes. Inflammation is confined to portal triads. Stage II is characterized by ongoing bile duct destruction and the absence of bile ducts in some portal triads and atypical bile duct proliferation in others. Inflammation extends from the portal triads into the surrounding parenchyma, a process termed "piecemeal necrosis." In stage III, there is more extensive fibrosis and linkage of adjacent portal triads by bands of scar tissue. Stage IV is characterized by cirrhosis. It is often distinguishable from other types of cirrhosis by a striking diminution in the number of small bile ducts seen in the liver biopsy specimen. Granulomas are often seen in patients with early PBC and suggest a more benign course than in patients without them.

PROGNOSIS

The course of PBC is variable but usually slowly progressive. The typical patient with recently discovered PBC is an anxious, minimally symptomatic 40-year-old woman who has been told (or has read) that her disease is untreatable and that she will die of her disease or require a liver transplantation within 5 to 8 years. This is incorrect. Survival is better than stated in most textbooks, even without treatment, now that the disease is recognized more commonly and at earlier stages. In addition, there appears to be effective treatment for patients with precirrhotic disease. I now care for many patients with precirrhotic PBC whose disease appears to have gone into remission in response to treatment with colchicine, ursodiol, methotrexate, or combinations of the three. Because so many patients with PBC are depressed and discouraged by what they have read and heard about PBC, I find it helpful to reassure such patients that it may be possible for their disease to respond to treatment and go into remission. Survival in asymptomatic patients with PBC is longer than in symptomatic patients. Median survival (referral for liver transplantation) in untreated symptomatic patients is approximately 9 years. Most asymptomatic patients develop typical symptoms within 3 to 5 years of diagnosis. Hence, a better term for this phase may be presymptomatic PBC.

THERAPY

The management of PBC has two goals: (1) management of the symptoms and complications that result from chronic cholestasis, and (2) an attempt to suppress or reverse the underlying pathogenic process, destruction of small intralobular hepatic bile ducts.

Management of Symptoms and Complications

Pruritus

The earliest and most disconcerting symptom in PBC is pruritus. The itching is worse at bedtime and may cause insomnia and extensive excoriations because of the overwhelming urge to scratch. The pruritus is caused by the inability of the liver to excrete certain substances into bile, which presumably accumulate in the skin and produce the itching. The pruritogenic substance is not known but binds to cholestyramine, a nonabsorbed quaternary ammonium resin. Cholestyramine taken orally will relieve the itching associated with PBC in 95 percent of patients as long as there is adequate bile flow (i.e., stools are not acholic [clay colored]). The usual dosage of cholestyramine is 4 g three times a day, taken just before or with meals. Cholestyramine takes 2 to 4 days to relieve itching from the time it is started. If itching fails to respond to the usual dose of cholestyramine within 4 days, the dose should be increased in 4 g increments up to 24 g per day. Doses above 24 g per day are rarely more effective, although doses as high as 36 g per day have been tolerated by some patients. Some patients have difficulty taking cholestyramine because of its taste and consistency. Its palatability can be improved by mixing it with fruit juice, applesauce, or pureeing it with fruits in a food processor.

Cholestyramine may cause severe constipation. This

can be treated with laxatives or bulking agents. Many drugs will bind to cholestyramine and be poorly absorbed. Hence, medications should be taken as far apart from the cholestyramine as possible, at least 2 hours before or after cholestyramine is taken. Blood levels of fat-soluble vitamins A, D, E, and K should be periodically monitored or replacement therapy given, since patients requiring cholestyramine may malabsorb fat-soluble vitamins. Cholestyramine usage has also been associated with folic acid deficiency. Concomitant treatment with folic acid, 1 mg per day, is recommended, or serum folate should be monitored. For patients who cannot tolerate cholestyramine, colestipol hydrochloride, another nonabsorbed anion exchange resin, may be used. It is as effective as cholestyramine and has the same side effects. The starting dose is 5 mg three times a day orally.

Rarely, the pruritus in PBC will not respond to cholestyramine. In such instances, large-volume plasmapheresis may be effective. Unfortunately, plasmapheresis is expensive and impractical if used chronically. Its beneficial effects usually last 2 to 4 weeks, at which time the plasmapheresis must be repeated. Antihistamines and other related anti-itch medicines are rarely, if ever, effective as treatment for severe pruritus, but they may be helpful in mild pruritus if given before bedtime.

A number of patients with pruritus note that their itching worsens if they eat rich, fatty meals. Conversely, some have reported that their itching improves if they eat a low-fat diet. Diet treatment has not been critically evaluated but is innocuous. If these measures fail to relieve the itching, rifampin may be tried. The dose is 150 mg orally twice a day if the serum bilirubin is greater than 3 mg per deciliter and 150 mg three times a day if the serum bilirubin level is lower. If all of these fail, there are anecdotal reports of patients whose itching has responded to phototherapy with UVB light, phenobarbital, methyltestosterone, glucocorticoids, and cimetidine. In addition, the itching may respond to the opiate inhibitor, naloxone. It has to be given intravenously, but there are effective antiopiates that can be taken orally that are available in England and Europe.

Malabsorption

Many patients with PBC who are clinically jaundiced have steatorrhea. In some, the steatorrhea causes obvious diarrhea, including troublesome nocturnal diarrhea. The steatorrhea is due primarily to inadequate concentrations of bile acids within the small intestinal lumen, below the critical micellar concentration. Patients with concomitant sicca syndrome may also have pancreatic insufficiency. This may be detected with the bentiromide test and treated with replacement pancreatic extract. Symptomatic steatorrhea can be partially corrected by restricting dietary fat. Medium-chain triglyceride may be added if caloric supplementation is required to maintain body weight. Each milliliter of medium-chain triglyceride oil contains 7.5 calories. Most patients can tolerate 60 mg per day without difficulty. The medium-chain triglyceride oil may either be taken directly by the teaspoon or be used in cooking as a substitute for shortening and oil.

Patients with PBC may malabsorb the fat-soluble vitamins A, D, and K. Deficiencies of vitamin E are uncommon except in patients with advanced disease awaiting liver transplantation. Vitamin A deficiency occurs in approximately 30 percent of patients but is rarely symptomatic. It is as practical to prevent vitamin A deficiency with dietary supplements of vitamin A, 15,000 units per day (three times the recommended daily allowance), as it is to measure serum levels on a regular basis. Vitamin K deficiency rarely occurs in PBC unless the patient takes cholestyramine on a regular basis and is deeply jaundiced. The prothrombin time is normal in most patients until late in the course of disease when there are signs of liver failure. Vitamin K rarely has to be given except to these patients.

Bone Disease

Osteopenia with spontaneous bone fractures is a serious problem that occurs in approximately 20 percent of patients with PBC. The metabolic bone disease most commonly associated with PBC is osteoporosis, not osteomalacia. Osteomalacia occurs rarely and only in patients with advanced disease. The osteoporosis is manifested by bone pain and spontaneous fractures, usually of the vertebral bodies and ribs. Neither the cause nor the treatment of the osteoporosis is known. Patients with PBC may have low serum levels of 25-hydroxy vitamin D, but serum levels of the most active vitamin D metabolite, 1, $25(OH)_2$ vitamin D, are normal. The following treatment regimen is suggested, more in the belief that it will not hurt and may have placebo effect than the conviction that it will stabilize or reverse the bone loss. Oral calcium supplements are given, 1.0 to 1.5 g of calcium per day. The use of TUMS is a good, well tolerated, inexpensive way to give calcium supplements; its safety can be easily monitored by measuring serum calcium levels and 24-hour urinary calcium excretion. Twenty-four-hour urinary calcium excretion should be less than 200 mg per day. If serum levels of 25-hydroxy vitamin D are low, supplementation with 25-hydroxy vitamin D_3, 20 μg per day, may be given. The goal is the maintenance of the serum 25-hydroxy vitamin D level in the high-to-normal range. Treatment with 25-hydroxy vitamin D will correct or prevent the osteomalacia that occurs in patients with advanced disease. There is no information about the efficacy or safety of medications used to treat postmenopausal osteoporosis, such as calcitonin, etidronate, or sodium fluoride. They are best not used.

Xanthomas

Less than 10 percent of patients with PBC develop xanthomas. Planar xanthomas may occur on the palms of the hands, become painful, and interfere with manual dexterity. Xanthomas on the soles of the feet may also cause pain and make walking difficult. If xanthomas become truly symptomatic, they can be treated with large-volume plasmapheresis done at 1- to 2-week intervals. The goal is to remove cholesterol from the body. Each plasmapheresis will lower the serum cholesterol level by approximately 50 percent. Once the serum cholesterol level approaches normal, xanthomas will gradually resolve.

Anemia

Iron-deficiency anemia may occur in PBC, often in patients without obviously advanced disease. A thorough search for a site of gastrointestinal blood loss should be done, even in the absence of overt gastrointestinal blood loss. Some patients may have unexpectedly severe portal hypertension. Chronic intermittent blood loss from congestive gastropathy or esophageal varices is a possible cause. If treatment with oral iron is not adequate, the usual modalities to treat bleeding from portal hypertension should be considered: beta-blockers, variceal rubber band ligation, sclerotherapy, and transjugular intrahepatic portosystemic stent shunt, in that order. If the bilirubin and albumin are normal and bleeding cannot be controlled with beta-blockers or endoscopic therapy, a distal splenorenal shunt (Warren shunt) is preferable to the transjugular intrahepatic portosystemic stent shunt (TIPSS).

Autoimmune Disorders

Other autoimmune disorders, such as Sjögren's syndrome and the CREST syndrome, may occur in patients with PBC. Treatment is symptomatic. More importantly, as many as 25 percent of patients with PBC may have (or develop) hypothyroidism. Routine tests for thyroid function, such as the total T_4 or free T_4 index, may be misleading because these patients have increased serum concentrations of thyroid-binding globulin. Hypothyroidism is best evaluated by measuring the thyroid-stimulating hormone. Patients with hypothyroid biliary cirrhosis respond normally to replacement thyroid hormone.

Liver Failure

Patients with advanced PBC develop symptoms of liver failure, such as ascites and bleeding esophageal varices, similar to patients with other types of liver disease. Management is similar. Liver transplantation is recommended in patients with impending liver failure and those who have bled from portal hypertension and have cirrhosis or jaundice. The efficacy of liver transplantation in prolonging survival in PBC is proven. It is best not to delay transplantation until patients have advanced liver failure with recurrent hepatic encephalopathy, intractable ascites, or florid muscle wasting. If there is any doubt about the severity of the disease, patients should be referred to medical centers that perform liver transplantation for consultation.

Treatment of the Underlying Process

The management of patients with PBC is rapidly changing. There are two reasons for this. First, drugs such as colchicine, ursodeoxycholic acid, and methotrexate appear to combine efficacy and safety. Second, there is now agreement that PBC is a progressive disease in virtually all patients. It eventually becomes irreversible, usually at the time that cirrhosis develops. The risk-benefit ratio of drugs such as colchicine, ursodeoxycholic acid, and methotrexate is clearly better than that of no treatment and awaiting liver failure with the need for liver transplantation. In addition to the risk of major surgery, patients who survive liver transplantation face a lifetime of treatment with the combination of cyclosporine, tacrolimus (FK-506, i.e., Prograf), glucocorticoids, azathioprine, and antihypertensive agents, a treatment regimen that is more problematic than colchicine, ursodeoxycholic acid, and methotrexate, alone or in combination. Because specific therapy is a rapidly evolving and still controversial area, relevant clinical data are reviewed.

Drugs that are Ineffective, Toxic, or Both

Results with the drugs used to treat most autoimmune disease have been disappointing. A prospective, controlled trial of glucocorticoids confirmed the experience of most hepatologists, that glucocorticoids have little beneficial effect on the course of the disease and accelerate the progression of osteoporosis, an already serious problem in PBC. This predictable complication outweighs any short-term improvement in biochemical tests.

Seven prospective, controlled trials of D-penicillamine have been conducted in PBC. All show no efficacy and much toxicity. D-penicillamine was evaluated because it was known to be beneficial in patients with Wilson's disease. PBC, like Wilson's disease, is characterized by increased hepatic copper stores. The hope was that removal of hepatic copper would be as beneficial in PBC as it is in Wilson's disease. D-penicillamine also has anti-inflammatory effects and can impair the maturation of collagen, a process that might slow the development of cirrhosis. Unfortunately, none of the theoretical promise of D-penicillamine has been fulfilled. Of equal importance, D-penicillamine was associated with a high incidence of serious side effects, up to 30 percent in some studies, and there were several deaths attributed to its use. D-penicillamine should clearly not be used to treat PBC.

Azathioprine in doses ranging from 1 to 2 mg per kilogram body weight per day was initially shown to be of no therapeutic benefit in two prospective, controlled trials. However, one of these studies was continued for a longer period, and on reanalysis, survival in the azathioprine group was shown to be longer than that in the placebo group. Unfortunately, no biochemical or histologic data were given in this report, nor have they been published since. Based on personal experience, I do not recommend azathioprine in the treatment of PBC.

Chlorambucil, an alkylating drug with immunosuppressive properties, was evaluated in a small pilot study. Its beneficial effects in stabilizing or improving serum bilirubin, aminotransferase, albumin, and IgM levels were offset by its bone marrow toxicity. The study was discontinued because of chlorambucil's observed and potential toxicity.

Cyclosporine has been evaluated in several controlled trials. In the doses used, 3 to 4 mg per kilogram body weight per day, cyclosporine was only minimally effective and had predictable toxicity, hypertension and some worsening of renal function. Cyclosporine did not improve symptoms or liver histology and had no effect on survival unless survival was corrected with the Cox multiple hazards model because patients treated with cyclosporine were sicker at baseline. There is little enthusiasm for its use in PBC.

Drugs that are Promising and Being Evaluated

We and others have studied the effects of colchicine, 0.6 mg twice a day, versus placebo in PBC during the past 15 years. We found that colchicine-treated patients had significantly improved levels of serum albumin, bilirubin, alkaline phosphatase, aminotransferases, and cholesterol after 2 years compared with those on placebo. Of greater importance, colchicine appeared to decrease the risk of dying of liver failure. Four years after entry, the cumulative mortality from liver disease was 21 percent in colchicine-treated patients and 47 percent in patients taking placebo. However, there was no improvement noted in the histologic progression of the disease or in symptoms or physical findings. There was little toxicity. Several patients developed diarrhea, which disappeared when the dose was lowered to 0.6 mg once a day. Two other studies have results similar to ours. With meta-analysis, colchicine clearly decreases the risk of dying of liver failure. It also stabilizes sulfobromophthalein clearance, a sensitive indicator of bile secretion. These studies suggest that colchicine slows the progression of PBC but does not stop it. It is safe and well tolerated.

The results of studies employing ursodeoxycholate, 10 to 15 mg per kilogram body weight per day, are encouraging. Ursodeoxycholate produces striking reductions in serum alkaline phosphatase, gamma-glutamyl transpeptidase, alanine aminotransferase, and aspartate aminotransferase levels and some decrease or stabilization in serum bilirubin. Histologic improvement is less impressive. Inflammation may be decreased, but there is no improvement in fibrosis. These studies, now carried out for 4 years, indicate that ursodeoxycholic acid also decreases the risk of dying or being referred for liver transplantation. Ursodeoxycholic acid lessens the need for cholestyramine in some patients with pruritus and appears to lessen manifestations of autoimmunity. Little toxicity, other than diarrhea, has been reported. These results suggest that ursodeoxycholic acid is safe and may be effective. Of note, most of the beneficial biochemical effects of ursodeoxycholic acid occur within 2 to 3 months of initiating therapy. Its efficacy appears to be limited to patients with precirrhotic disease whose serum bilirubin is less than 2 mg per deciliter.

We have reported our experience with low-dose oral pulse methotrexate in 14 patients with precirrhotic PBC. We are currently engaged in a prospective, double-blind trial of methotrexate versus colchicine. There was a striking improvement in biochemical tests in response to methotrexate and the disappearance of debilitating fatigue and itching in symptomatic patients. There was an encouraging improvement in liver histology, much less inflammation after 1 and 2 years of methotrexate, and an apparent decrease in fibrosis in patients treated for 2 years or longer. Of note, most patients had a striking but transient increase in aminotransferase levels, up to five-fold elevations, 1 to 8 months after beginning methotrexate. Aminotransferase levels then improved in all of these patients and became normal in some. Paradoxically, worsening aminotransferase levels appear to be a marker for an ultimately good response to methotrexate. No hepatotoxicity has been seen. However, bone marrow suppression occurs rarely and allergic pneumonitis occurs in approximately 12 percent of PBC patients. In contrast to the ursodeoxycholic acid response that occurs within 2 to 3 months of initiating therapy, the response to methotrexate occurs slowly and is often not obvious until 6 to 10 months after starting methotrexate. There then appears to be sustained biochemical and histologic improvement. Patients with advanced PBC, those with cirrhosis and jaundice and/or portal hypertension, do not respond to methotrexate or to any drug studied so far. On the positive side, I follow more than 10 patients with PBC whose disease appears to have gone into remission on methotrexate, with some having now been followed for up to 12 years. This improvement includes improvement or normalization of liver histology. I do not hesitate to add ursodiol, colchicine, or both to patients whose biochemical tests of liver function have improved but not normalized on methotrexate. It is possible that the use of several agents together will be more effective as it is in patients on immunosuppression for liver transplantation or in patients with Hodgkin's disease.

RECOMMENDATIONS

Virtually all patients with PBC have a progressive and potentially serious disease. If one waits too long to treat, patients may develop cirrhosis and irreversible disease. Hence, all patients without advanced disease, i.e., those in need of liver transplantation, should be treated. Ideally, each patient should be enrolled in a prospective, randomized treatment trial. However, this is neither practical nor possible for most patients with PBC. For those patients who can not be enrolled in treatment trials, treatment should be initiated with ursodeoxycholic acid, 10 to 15 mg per kilogram of body weight per day. After 3 months of treatment, when the maximal effect of ursodeoxycholic acid is typically achieved, colchicine, 0.6 mg twice a day, should be added. Each acts differently, and their efficacy may be additive. Treatment should be continued indefinitely.

My own experience suggests that methotrexate is more effective treatment than either ursodeoxycholic acid or colchicine. However, it is potentially more toxic.

I have found methotrexate, 15 mg per week orally, encouragingly effective in symptomatic precirrhotic patients. If methotrexate were to be used outside of a treatment trial, a percutaneous liver biopsy should be done at baseline and after 1 and 2 years of treatment. A complete blood count and platelet count should be done monthly and biochemical tests of liver function done every 2 months. Patients should be seen every 3 months and should receive folic acid, 1 mg per day.

The next several years should see more results of treatment trials in PBC. Prospects are good that there will be effective treatment and that hepatologists will feel comfortable prescribing treatment early in the course of PBC.

SUGGESTED READING

Kaplan MM. Methotrexate treatment of chronic cholestatic liver diseases: Friend or foe? Q J Med, New Series 1989; 72:757–761.

Kaplan MM. Primary biliary cirrhosis. N Engl J Med 1987; 316: 521–528.

Kaplan MM, Alling DW, Zimmerman HJ, et al. A prospective trial of colchicine in primary biliary cirrhosis. N Engl J Med 1986; 315:1448–1454.

Lombard M, Portmann BP, Neuberger J, et al. Cyclosporine A treatment in primary biliary cirrhosis: Results of a long-term placebo controlled trial and effect on survival. Gastroenterology 1993; 104:519–526.

Poupon RE, Poupon R, Balkau B. UDCA-PBC Study Group. Ursodiol for the long term treatment of primary biliary cirrhosis. N Engl J Med 1994; 330:1342–1347.

HEMATOLOGIC DISEASE

IMMUNOLOGIC THROMBOCYTOPENIA

DIANE M. REID, M.D.
N. RAPHAEL SHULMAN, M.D.

Immunologically mediated thrombocytopenias are a leading cause of hemorrhagic diathesis. Sensitizing agents can be autoantigens, alloantigens, drugs, or infectious organisms. Autoimmune idiopathic thrombocytopenic purpura (ITP) is the most common of all acquired hemorrhagic disorders. Acute ITP occurs primarily in children before puberty, equally in both sexes, and completely subsides within 6 months to a year with or without therapy. Chronic ITP, the chief topic discussed, can occur at any age but most often affects adults, women 2 to 3 times more often than men, and permanent remissions are unusual. Thrombocytopenia may accompany various infections, particularly viral, most often at a time when antibodies against the infectious agent begin to form. The high frequency of thrombocytopenia in HIV infection is attributable usually to immunologic platelet destruction by antibodies, and sometimes to inhibition of platelet production. Thrombocytopenias caused by alloantibodies or drug-induced antibodies are uncommon but readily recognizable syndromes that respond promptly to treatment. Neonatal thrombocytopenias, due to transplacental transfer of maternal auto- or alloantibodies, raise special ante- and postnatal therapeutic considerations.

CHRONIC ITP

Diagnosis

ITP is a clinical diagnosis based on findings of thrombocytopenia, a normal bone marrow with normal or increased numbers of megakaryocytes, and exclusion of other disorders that could account for thrombocytopenia such as infection, splenic enlargement, or use of specific drugs. In rare instances when differentiation between increased platelet destruction and inadequate production is difficult, platelet survival studies can help. Autoantibodies against surface epitopes of platelet membrane glycoproteins appear to be specific for ITP and can be measured in a majority of patients. However, antibody tests are not necessary for diagnosis and have unknown significance in prognosis.

Symptomatology: A Guide to Therapy

Idiopathic thrombocytopenia occurring for the first time in patients older than 20 years of age is almost always chronic. There is no singular antecedent event related to its development. Onset is often insidious and initially detected by a routine platelet count, but may be fulminant with severe hemorrhagic symptomatology. Patients with milder forms of ITP may have no symptoms with a subnormal platelet level that does not vary significantly for years. However, temporary symptomatic exacerbations lasting weeks or months may occur, sometimes coincident with infection or stress. Severe-onset symptomatic ITP with a platelet count less than 10,000 per microliter may respond promptly to initial therapy and then become relatively mild, or may require continued, increasingly aggressive forms of treatment. Regardless of initial severity, spontaneous remissions of variable degree can occur that may last weeks, months, or even years.

Hemorrhagic manifestations in ITP may be surprisingly slight at platelet levels that are frequently associated with marked bleeding in patients with aplastic anemia, leukemia, or chemotherapy-induced marrow suppression. The short platelet life span in ITP results in circulation of younger, hemostatically more effective platelets. ITP patients characteristically have no spontaneous hemorrhage, including petechiae, when platelet counts are above 10,000 to 20,000 per microliter. There may be excessive bruising after trauma at these platelet levels, but the risk of serious hemorrhage is minimal. Intracranial hemorrhage, the one occurrence responsible for almost all of the 1 to 2 percent mortality associated with ITP, does not occur in the absence of trauma unless severe symptoms such as generalized petechiae, periodontal bleeding, hemorrhagic mucous membrane bullae, and retinal hemorrhages are present. These ominous symptoms characteristically occur when platelets are falling and reach levels below 5,000 per microliter. In contrast, a stable count of 5,000 per microliter or even lower is often not associated with significant bleeding.

Treatment

If the presenting platelet count is above 30,000 per microliter and increased bruising after trauma is the only symptom, treatment is not necessary unless a patient's activities involve increased risk of injury. The platelet count can be monitored at appropriate intervals to evaluate its stability with the understanding that the patient will report significant changes such as development of petechiae or other spontaneous hemorrhage that may herald the need for treatment. To prevent overtreatment, it is best to base therapy on symptomatology rather than on maintenance of some presumed "safe" platelet level.

When patients present with very low platelet counts and spontaneous hemorrhage, destruction of platelets exceeds compensatory production, which at most can be two to three times normal. Although symptomatically similar, these patients will vary in their individual responses to the same therapy. Platelets sensitized by ITP antibodies are destroyed by phagocytosis in the reticuloendothelial system (RES), the inhibition of which is the primary goal of most therapies. Since inhibition at best is only partial, varying degrees of platelet sensitization by different ITP antibodies most likely account for unequal responses to therapy. Currently there is no serologic test to accurately assess degree of platelet sensitization.

All patients with ITP should be cautioned against use of aspirin and nonsteroidal anti-inflammatory agents, such as ibuprofen, that inhibit platelet function and increase hemorrhagic symptoms at any given platelet level.

Glucocorticoids

Glucocorticoids act primarily by inhibiting the RES. This effect is immediate, very sensitive to in vivo drug levels, and dissipates at a rate paralleling pharmacologic decay of the drug. A treatment regimen in which the same total daily glucocorticoid dosage is given in divided doses may be more effective than a single dose, but twice the daily dose given every other day is usually less effective. In the long term, glucocorticoids may decrease antibody production. They do not increase platelet production, and there is no convincing evidence that they promote capillary integrity without a concomitant, albeit sometimes slight, rise in platelet level.

The initial dose should be sufficient to maximally inhibit platelet sequestration (e.g., prednisone, 1.0 to 1.5 mg per kilogram per day). All glucocorticoids appear to be equally effective provided equivalent dosages are given. A favorable clinical response (at least partial correction of the platelet count and subsidence of symptoms) is obtained in 70 to 80 percent of patients. Responses usually occur within 1 to 3 days, and reach a maximum within 5 to 10 days. If there is no response to glucocorticoids in 10 days, continued administration is unlikely to be beneficial. If platelets return to above 50,000 per microliter, the initial high glucocorticoid dosage should be tapered to determine the amount that will maintain the platelet count in the range of 25,000 per microliter to 50,000 per microliter. A reasonable incremental decrease for prednisone is 10 to 15 percent of the initial dose every third day until 60 to 70 percent of the dose is reached. After that, a decrease of 2.5 to 5.0 percent of the initial dose every third day is appropriate. This regimen permits rapid assessment of the minimal effective dosage, provided platelet counts are determined two to three times a week. If the platelet count falls below 25,000 per microliter, dosage is increased to the amount given prior to the fall, and this is usually a satisfactory maintenance dose. In the initial course of treatment, the maintenance dosage is continued for about 4 weeks before attempting another incremental decrease. Amelioration of the disease permitting lower maintenance dosages of glucocorticoids may occur over a period of 6 months to a year.

Slower tapering schedules than just described must be used to avoid symptoms of adrenocortical insufficiency in patients who have taken high doses of steroids for prolonged periods. Intercurrently, or within a year after discontinuing long-term steroid therapy, stressful situations such as operative procedures should be covered by intravenous hydrocortisone, 100 mg every 8 hours, which can be tapered rapidly the day after surgery.

Patients who know their response to glucocorticoids can increase their dosage or start treatment themselves if symptoms such as spontaneous mucosal hemorrhage develop and there is no immediate access to a physician.

Patients refractory to usual steroid dosage as well as to other forms of therapy may respond to intermittent intravenous infusion of megadoses of glucocorticoids (e.g., monthly courses of dexamethasone, 40 mg per day on 4 consecutive days or methylprednisolone, 1 g per day for 3 days). There are too few observations on this form of therapy to provide a response rate. These regimens may avoid some side effects of daily low dosages of steroids, but effects related to cumulative dose may be unchanged or greater since the total doses per month of suggested intermittent therapy are equivalent to 35 mg prednisone per day.

If glucocorticoids are required in high doses or for prolonged periods of time to prevent hemorrhage, splenectomy should be considered to avoid immediate and chronic deleterious side effects. These include adrenocortico-suppression, fluid retention, muscle weakness, osteoporosis, hyperglycemia, cataract development, impaired wound healing, thinning of the skin, mood swings, moon facies, centripetal obesity, and hair loss.

Splenectomy

Platelets weakly sensitized by ITP antibodies are more effectively removed by the spleen than by the liver, although both organs participate in platelet destruction at all degrees of sensitization. Amounts of radiolabeled platelets sequestered in spleen compared to liver during platelet survival studies, however, do not predict responsiveness to splenectomy or to any other form of treatment. In some studies, patients who responded well to glucocorticoids were likely to have favorable results from splenectomy. The overall favorable response rate to splenectomy is 70 to 90 percent with complete remission in 50 to 65 percent. Even if splenectomy does not prevent the recurrence of symptoms, it usually facilitates management by decreasing requirements for steroids or other therapeutic agents. There is also a perception that less bleeding may occur at a given platelet level after splenectomy.

Preoperative treatment with glucocorticoids and/or intravenous immunoglobulin G (see next section) is given to raise platelets to safe hemostatic levels (20,000 per microliter), but even if this level is not attainable, the amount of intraoperative and postoperative hemorrhage is usually surprisingly scant. Peritoneal drainage can lessen abdominal complications from hemorrhage if there is no response to splenectomy. Platelet transfusions (see following section) are not given preoperatively. When necessary intraoperatively, platelet transfusions are most effective if given after the splenic pedicle is clamped.

The rate of platelet rise after splenectomy in those who have a good response is at least 20,000 per microliter per day and may be several times that. A favorable long-term response is more likely if the peak platelet level, usually reached in 7 to 12 days, is greater than 500,000 per microliter. A peak of 1,000,000 per microliter is not uncommon and values of 2,000,000 per microliter are observed occasionally. If counts exceed 1,000,000 per microliter, aspirin, 300 mg per day, or low-dose heparin therapy is sometimes temporarily instituted as prophylaxis against thrombosis, but the value of this therapy has not been substantiated.

Symptoms suggestive of intracranial bleeding in patients not immediately responsive to other forms of therapy are an indication for emergency splenectomy, which may have to be performed when platelet counts are less than 2,000/μL. Under these circumstances, platelet transfusions are used immediately (see following discussion). The reported mortality from emergency splenectomy in ITP ranges from 1.4 to 4.9 percent. However, mortality from intracranial hemorrhage approaches 100 percent, and splenectomy reduces this to less than 50 percent.

There is a slight increase in susceptibility to infection following splenectomy, much less in adults than in children. All patients undergoing splenectomy should receive vaccines against *Streptococcus pneumoniae* and *Haemophilus influenza b* beforehand, if possible. Some recommend that children should, in addition, receive prophylactic penicillin until puberty.

Accessory spleens may cause failure to respond to splenectomy in the immediate postoperative period or several months to years later. Because accessory spleens are present in as many as 20 percent of patients, a preoperative radioisotopic scan is recommended to detect splenic tissue that may be distant from the splenic pedicle. Laparoscopic splenectomy would not be an optimal technique for identifying and removing accessory spleens. Removal of an accessory spleen for recurrent thrombocytopenia some time after splenectomy results in improvement in 50 percent or fewer cases.

Radiation of the spleen has been occasionally successful as alternate therapy in elderly patients with ITP who are poor risks for splenectomy.

Intravenous Immunoglobulin G

High-dose intravenous immunoglobulin G-(IVIgG) produces a significant rise in platelets in as many as 75 percent of ITP patients. It appears to block the RES and may contain anti-idiotypic antibodies. Standard dosages are 1 g per kilogram per day for 1 to 2 days or 0.4 g per kilogram per day for 5 days, given in an outpatient setting. The most common side effects are headache, nausea, myalgia, and minor allergic reactions such as hives. However, sensitized IgA-deficient individuals may have anaphylactoid reactions. Although made from human plasma, IVIgG is manufactured under strict FDA regulations to prevent transmission of hepatitis and HIV viruses. IVIgG acts synergistically with steroids and splenectomy. Platelets rise typically within 1 to 3 days after IVIgG, reach a maximum level within 1 week, and then fall to pretreatment levels within about 1 week. Because of its prohibitive cost, long-term IVIgG therapy is not practical in adults able to tolerate other options, but it has a place in management of emergency hemorrhagic events and in preparation for surgery.

Anti-D

Intravenous anti-D is thought to block the splenic RES with sensitized red cells in Rh-positive patients but, paradoxically, has been reported to benefit an Rh-negative patient. Reported successes have been primarily in children, many not previously treated, and most with acute ITP (see following discussion). Responses occur after 1 to 2 days and may last 2 to 3 weeks; splenectomized patients are less responsive. Anti-D treatment, while not toxic or expensive, is not as effective or reliable for chronic ITP as more established forms of therapy. The primary side effect is a mild reduction in hemoglobin level.

Platelet Transfusions

Platelet transfusions have only an emergency role in management of ITP patients, primarily for those who have signs of intracranial bleeding or require emergency surgery. Five to ten random units of platelets given every 4 to 6 hours along with high doses of IVIgG and glucocorticoids may help hemostasis even if platelet recovery or survival is not measurable. Continuous infusion of platelets may be more beneficial than intermittent administration.

Therapy for Refractory Patients

Patients who remain symptomatic after splenectomy, and do not respond to glucocorticoids in low to moderate dosages (5 to 30 mg per day) may respond to other therapies, but the choices are not well defined in terms of potential benefits weighed against toxic side effects and/or expense.

High-dose Glucocorticoids

Short-term, high-dose schedules as described earlier, combined with IVIgG if necessary, are the most reliable option for emergency or temporary treatment of refractory ITP.

Danazol

Danazol, an attenuated androgen that suppresses the pituitary-ovarian axis, may decrease Fcγ receptors on monocytes, causing impaired RES function. In different reports, dosages of 400 to 800 mg per day produced partial to complete remissions in as few as 10 percent to as many as 60 percent of patients with refractory ITP. Benefits occurred after 2 to 6 weeks of therapy with maximal effects at 6 to 10 weeks. Continued therapy was necessary for a sustained response, during which corticosteroids could be tapered or discontinued. In one study, danazol at 50 mg per day appeared to be as effective as higher doses, but responses were delayed. None of the studies were controlled with respect to ancillary treatment. Side effects include fluid retention, menstrual irregularity, acne, mild hirsuitism, and hepatic toxicity. There are reports of danazol-associated thrombocytopenia, which must be borne in mind if a precipitous decrease in platelets occurs during therapy.

Vinca Alkaloids

Vincristine inhibits phagocytes by binding to tubulin. It also appears to stimulate release of platelets without having an effect on long-term production. Given as an intravenous bolus of 1 to 1.5 mg per square meter, it can produce elevations of platelet counts beginning within 2 or 3 days, peaking in 4 to 10 days. Thereafter, platelets usually fall to pretreatment levels within 1 to 2 weeks. Occasionally, a sustained remission is obtained for several weeks to months. The best responses have occurred in splenectomized patients. Repeated doses can be given at 1- to 2-week intervals. If there is no response to three doses, further therapy is unlikely to produce benefit. Toxic effects, including leukopenia and neuropathies, can be cumulative and progressively severe, but usually reverse after discontinuation of the drug. Patients older than 50 years of age are particularly susceptible to severe neuropathies and should not be given more than 1.5 mg per square meter for three doses at 2-week intervals, with careful neurologic evaluation before each dose. Platelets preincubated with vincristine or vinblastine and given by slow infusion have essentially the same therapeutic and toxic effects as vincristine but can cause greater myelotoxicity. These drugs generally are too toxic for maintenance use.

Cytotoxic Agents

Oral immunosuppressive therapy with azathioprine (150 mg per day) or cyclophosphamide (50 to 150 mg per day) may produce responses in refractory cases of ITP if given daily for a minimum of 1 to 4 months. Results are difficult to interpret because the best responders in some series were those who had the disease less than 1 year, a time during which spontaneous amelioration of symptoms is frequent, and many were treated when their initial platelet counts were above 20,000 per microliter. These drugs should be used only for the most severe cases of ITP, realizing that suppression of thrombopoiesis is a possible side effect that can exacerbate an already threatening degree of thrombocytopenia. Other toxic effects include leukopenia, increased risk of malignancy, hypogonadism or sterility, and alopecia. Noteworthy is a high mortality rate (10 percent) from bleeding in a report on 53 patients with ITP treated with azathioprine. Both pulse intravenous cyclophosphamide and combination chemotherapy with cyclophosphamide, prednisone, vincristine, and procarbazine or etoposide have been used with success in the short term for small numbers of refractory patients, but it is unclear if these treatments will carry an unacceptable risk of marrow suppression and development of secondary malignancy.

Unproved Therapies

Because the natural course of ITP is variable, it is difficult to evaluate a new therapy. This is particularly true if the patients studied were recently diagnosed, responses occurred only after prolonged observation, conventional therapy was used along with experimental therapy, or trials were not designed to eliminate bias. Selected case reports of good responses to a new drug in patients with refractory ITP are not necessarily testimony to its benefits because many ITP patients (8 of 15 in one report) who don't respond to any form of treatment, including immunosuppression, will develop a spontaneous remission of variable length within a 3- to 12-year period without receiving any therapy.

Colchicine. Colchicine, which binds to tubulin, produced responses in 20 to 40 percent of a small series of patients refractory to splenectomy and glucocorticoids. Response occurred within 2 weeks. Diarrhea or constipation, maladsorption, myopathy, and peripheral neuritis were reversible side effects.

Apheresis. Apheresis procedures to remove antibody or antigen-antibody complexes, including use of *Staphylococcus* protein A columns or plasma exchange, produce transient beneficial results in relatively few patients. Use of expensive immunosorption columns in refractory ITP is particularly controversial since they remove very little of the total circulating IgG, and reported results are based primarily on studies sponsored by the manufacturer. Side effects may include fever, chills, pain, nausea, urticaria, and even anaphylaxis.

Interferon alpha-2b. Interferon alpha-2b, 3 to 5 million units every 2 to 3 days for 4 weeks to 3 months, has produced a complete response in a few reported cases, partial transient responses in about 25 percent of cases, and worsening of the platelet count in about 10 percent. This treatment does not seem promising in ITP but may be more effective in HIV-associated thrombocytopenia (see following discussion).

Cyclosporine. Cyclosporine, 5 to 12 mg per kilogram per day for 3 or more months, has produced transient corrections of platelet counts in only a few cases of refractory ITP by possible modulation of immune responses. Other forms of therapy were given concomitantly. Risks include hypertension, renal toxicity, and potential secondary malignancy.

Ascorbic acid. Improvement of platelet counts in ITP patients receiving ascorbic acid, 2 g per day, was reported several years ago, but has not been reproducible in more recent studies. Although relatively nontoxic, vitamin C is not a reliable treatment option.

Thrombopoietin. Endogenous levels of thrombopoietin, a newly characterized cytokine responsible for regulating platelet production, are low to normal in patients with ITP. Trials may be under way shortly to determine whether administration of recombinant thrombopoietin would be effective in elevating platelet counts in ITP patients.

ACUTE ITP

ITP occurring before puberty is acute in 65 to 95 percent of cases. It often develops 1 to 3 weeks after a viral illness. Over 80 percent of patients have mild or no hemorrhagic symptoms and recover spontaneously within a few weeks to months. The 10 percent who do not recover within 6 months to a year are considered to have chronic ITP. Treatment is reserved only for those with serious hemorrhagic manifestations and is aimed at tiding patients over the symptomatic period, anticipating complete recovery. Symptoms are usually most pronounced at onset and tend to ameliorate within several weeks, even if the platelet count remains below 20,000 per microliter. High-dose IVIgG (see Chronic ITP) is usually more effective than prednisone; either one or both can be given initially. After subsidence of symptoms and rise in platelets to greater than 15,000 per microliter, prednisone can be tapered rapidly (10 percent every other day). If further treatment is necessary, adequate responses are often obtained by single doses of IVIgG, 0.4 to 1.0 g per kilogram or by short courses of high-dose glucocorticoids (see Chronic ITP). Treatment for suspected CNS hemorrhage is as described for chronic ITP, which includes consideration of emergency splenectomy. Splenectomy for less threatening hemorrhage is not a therapeutic option. Neither cytotoxic drugs nor vinca alkaloids have application in acute ITP. When platelet counts are above 10,000 per microliter and there are no symptoms, children do not require special restriction at school or home other than avoidance of activities that might lead to excessive bruising or head trauma.

ITP AND PREGNANCY

Mothers with symptomatic ITP are treated similarly to other cases of ITP, but potentially teratogenic and oncogenic drugs are not used. IVIgG may be preferable to high-dosage glucocorticoids because it has fewer side effects. Splenectomy is avoided if possible because operative morbidity is high and the incidence of postoperative abortion is about 25 percent. There have been no reports of maternal mortality due to hemorrhage from ITP.

Antibodies responsible for ITP can be passively transferred to the fetus, but there is currently no serologic test to predict this occurrence. Generally, if the platelet count of a nonsplenectomized mother is greater than 100,000 per microliter, her infant is less likely to be affected than if the maternal count is less than 100,000 per microliter; but there is no close correlation between the maternal and fetal or neonatal platelet counts. Overall incidence of neonatal thrombocytopenia in infants of mothers with ITP is about 25 percent. Although the thrombocytopenia is usually asymptomatic, about 10 percent are severely affected, and 3 percent have, or may develop, intracranial hemorrhage. Fetal platelet level can be determined by cordocentesis, but this procedure, even if done by an experienced specialist, is associated with a risk (<1 percent) of fetal mortality. Some investigators recommend cesarean section if the fetal platelet count is less than 50,000 per microliter, but the mode of delivery does not appear to affect the incidence of neonatal central nervous system hemorrhage. There is no clear evidence that any medication administered to the mother increases the fetal platelet count, and risks attending cordocentesis without clear benefit appear to rule out this procedure.

Infants affected by ITP antibodies characteristically have a progressive fall in platelet count during the first few days after birth, and their thrombocytopenia, even if mild, may last for weeks to months. Treatment is only for symptomatic thrombocytopenia and is similar to that for children with acute ITP (see earlier discussion). In rare instances of poor response to other remedies, blood exchange along with platelet transfusions is effective. Splenectomy should not be done.

GESTATIONAL THROMBOCYTOPENIA

During pregnancy, approximately 8 percent of normally healthy women with no history of ITP develop mild to moderate asymptomatic thrombocytopenia (as low as 50,000 per microliter, but usually closer to 100,000 per microliter). The etiology is unknown. In different series,

0 to 4 percent of infants of these mothers had thrombocytopenia; none had a count less than 50,000 per microliter or was symptomatic. Mothers with this syndrome should not be treated and cordocentesis should not be done.

DRUG-INDUCED THROMBOOCYTOPENIA

Drugs, most commonly quinine and quinidine, can induce antibodies that bind to platelets in the presence of the drug and cause thrombocytopenia that can mimic ITP. Withdrawal of the offending drug results in return to normal platelet counts within 1 to at most 2 weeks. Drug purpura often requires urgent treatment in addition to withholding the suspected drug. Glucocorticoids, IVIgG, and platelet transfusions as used for ITP can be effective for serious hemorrhage before platelets return. However, in heparin-induced thrombocytopenia, platelet transfusions should not be used because they can exacerbate a predisposition to thrombosis that exists in this disorder. There is no role for splenectomy in acute drug purpura.

Gold-induced thrombocytopenia, in contrast to other drug purpuras, may persist for months to years, possibly because of the slow excretion of gold or the induction of autoantibodies. For treatment, gold chelation as well as other ITP therapies, including splenectomy, have been used successfully.

ITP-LIKE SYNDROMES ASSOCIATED WITH OTHER DISEASES

Systemic Lupus Erythematosus

Thrombocytopenia of apparent autoimmune etiology occurs in 7 to 26 percent of patients with systemic lupus erythematosus (SLE), and SLE may develop in approximately 2 percent of patients diagnosed months to years previously with ITP. Only about 5 to 10 percent of thrombocytopenic patients with SLE have hemorrhagic symptoms, and death from hemorrhage is very rare. Thrombocytopenia is often corrected when other manifestations of lupus regress. Therapy for symptomatic thrombocytopenia is the same as that for ITP. Cytotoxic drugs such as cyclophosphamide should be avoided unless needed for other complications of lupus such as nephritis. Splenectomy is rarely necessary.

Lymphoproliferative Disorders

Hodgkin's disease and non-Hodgkin's lymphoma are associated with ITP-like thrombocytopenia in 0.5 to 1 percent of cases, sometimes months or years before signs of lymphoma are apparent. When thrombocytopenia occurs in chronic lymphocytic leukemia, the underlying diagnosis is almost always apparent. Thrombocytopenia usually responds to therapy that controls the lymphoproliferative disorder, and is also responsive to general therapeutic approaches used for ITP. Thrombocytopenia occurring in patients with lymphoma in remission is more likely to be refractory.

HIV and Other Infections

Thrombocytopenia similar to that in chronic ITP occurs in up to 30 percent of HIV-infected individuals. It may be a presenting manifestation, but occurs more frequently as the infection progresses. Severe bleeding due to this complication is uncommon. Zidovudine and interferon-alpha have beneficial effects on HIV-related thrombocytopenia most likely because of their antiviral effects. Glucocorticoids elevate platelets as in ITP, but should be given only in short courses because of their immunosuppressive effect. IVIgG is preferred, but its effect, as in ITP, is short-lived. Splenectomy is effective in more than 65 percent of cases and does not have a deleterious effect on the course of HIV infection.

The acute and/or convalescent phase of many viral, bacterial, and protozoal infections is associated with thrombocytopenia that is usually mild and resolves spontaneously (see also Acute ITP).

NEONATAL ALLOIMMUNE THROMBOCYTOPENIA

Fetomaternal incompatibility with respect to a platelet alloantigen can result in production of maternal IgG alloantibodies that cross the placenta and attach to fetal platelets, causing their destruction. Neonatal alloimmune thrombocytopenia (NAT) occurs in approximately 1 in 2,000 live births, the first born can be severely affected, and there is significant morbidity and mortality due primarily to the 10 to 30 percent incidence of intracranial hemorrhage. Sensitization to the Pl^{A1} or Br^{a} platelet alloantigens account for most cases of serologically confirmed NAT in Caucasians. Those involving Pl^{A1} tend to be the most severe. However, there is no correlation between maternal antibody level and severity of NAT. If NAT has occurred previously in a family, the high risk of fetal morbidity in subsequent pregnancies justifies cordocentesis to monitor fetal platelet counts. If the fetal count is below 50,000 per microliter, antenatal treatment to the mother that appears to have a beneficial effect on the fetus includes corticosteroids that resist metabolism by the placenta, high-dose IVIgG, or both. Treatment to the fetus involves direct infusion of IVIgG or transfusion of irradiated compatible platelets via cordocentesis. If maternal nonantigenic platelets are used for transfusion, washing is necessary to remove antibody-containing plasma. Delivery by cesarean section is usually recommended for severely affected infants, in part to prepare for prompt postnatal treatment, which consists of glucocorticoids, IVIgG, and compatible platelet transfusions. Once platelets attain a safe level of 50,000 per microliter, usually no further treatment is necessary.

POST-TRANSFUSION PURPURA

Post-transfusion purpura (PTP) is characterized by a precipitous fall in platelets 5 to 8 days after receiving transfused blood or blood fractions from a donor whose platelets contain an alloantigen absent in the recipient. Antibody against the donor's alloantigen is present in the patient's serum at the time thrombocytopenia develops. The mechanism of autologous platelet destruction is unclear, but is believed to be secondary to binding of alloantigen-antibody complexes. PTP can be distinguished from ITP by the clinical circumstances and reliable serologic tests for alloantibody. Treatment often is required urgently because of platelet counts less than 5,000 per microliter and marked symptomatic hemorrhage. IVIgG as for chronic ITP is effective in most cases, but one or more plasma exchanges, each of approximately an 80 percent volume, is often effective in cases refractory to IVIgG. Transfusion of random or antibody-compatible platelets may not be effective in raising the platelet count during the initial stages. Glucocorticoids alone are ineffective.

SUGGESTED READING

Berchtold P, McMillan R. Therapy of chronic idiopathic thrombocytopenic purpura in adults. Blood 1989; 74:2309–2317.

Bussel J, Kaplan C, McFarland J, and the Working Party on Neonatal Immune Thrombocytopenia of the Neonatal Hemostasis Subcommittee of the Scientific Standardization Committee of the ISTH. Recommendations for the evaluation and treatment of neonatal autoimmune and alloimmune thrombocytopenia. Thromb Haemost 1991; 65:631–634.

George JN, El-Harake MA, Raskob GE. Chronic idiopathic thrombocytopenic purpura. New Eng J Med 1994; 331:1207–1211.

Marroni M, Gresele P, Landonio G, et al. Interferon-α is effective in the treatment of HIV-1-related, severe, zidovudine-resistant thrombocytopenia. A prospective, placebo-controlled, double-blind trial. Ann Int Med 1994; 121:423–429.

Picozzi VJ, Roeske WR, Creger WP. Fate of therapy failures in adult idiopathic thrombocytopenic purpura. 1980; Am J Med 69:690-694.

Reiner A, Gernsheimer T, Slichter SJ. Pulse cyclophosphamide therapy for refractory autoimmune thrombocytopenic purpura. Blood 1995; 85:351-358. See also letter to editor in Blood 1995; 86:414–415.

Shulman NR, Reid DM. Platelet immunology. In: Colman RW, Hirsh J, Marder VJ, Salzman EW, eds, Hemostasis and thrombosis: Basic principles and clinical practice. 3rd ed. Philadelphia: JB Lippincott, 1994: 414.

AUTOIMMUNE HEMOLYTIC ANEMIA

MICHAEL M. FRANK, M.D.

The autoimmune hemolytic anemias (AIHA) are a group of disorders characterized by the autoantibody-mediated destruction of erythrocytes. These disorders have an incidence of about 1 in 60,000 population per year. More than 70 percent of the new cases affect patients over 40 years of age, with peak incidence between 60 and 70 years of age. For diagnostic purposes, AIHA can be classified as primary or secondary to an accompanying disease or drug. In the secondary cases, treatment of the concurrent disease or suspension of the causative drug often improves the anemia. AIHA generally are classified with regard to the isotype of the autoantibody involved. In general, there are two major classes of antibody that produce AIHA IgG and IgM, although a limited number of cases due to IgA antibody have been reported. Antibodies of the IgG isotype in general are reactive with the red cell surface at 37° C, causing so-called "warm antibody" mediated hemolytic anemia. In contrast, antibodies of the IgM isotype usually react optimally with erythrocytes at 4° C, and react poorly at 37° C. These antibodies cause cold hemagglutinin disease. In rare cases IgG cold reactive antibody of the Donath-Landsteiner type reacts with cells at temperatures below 37° C, activates complement, and induces intravascular hemolysis. Intravascular hemolysis in general is an unusual consequence of autoantibody-mediated erythrocyte destruction. IgG antibody in AIHA almost always causes sequestration of antibody-sensitized erythrocytes in phagocytes of the reticuloendothelial system, with subsequent destruction. Intravascular hemolysis is more common with IgM antibody but, even so, extravascular sequestration and destruction is the most common event. The pattern of red cell clearance, site of organ sequestration, response to treatment, and prognosis all are determined by the class of antibody involved.

IgM-INDUCED HEMOLYTIC ANEMIA

AIHA caused by IgM antibody is most commonly seen in cold hemagglutinin disease, which usually affects the elderly; the cause of the disease is unknown (idiopathic). In some cases cold agglutinin disease follows infection, particularly that caused by mycoplasma pneumoniae, although it also may follow infectious mononucleosis, and less commonly, other viral infections. The antibody found in cold agglutinin disease and mycoplasma pneumonia recognizes an erythrocyte antigen designated I; that found in mononucleosis usually recognizes the i antigen, an allotypic variant. The production of cold agglutinin antibody may accompany immunoproliferative disease, as in chronic lymphocytic leukemia or non-Hodgkin's lymphoma.

In this disease, hemolysis depends on the capacity of the antibody to activate the complement system while remaining cell bound. The IgM antibody tends to dissociate from the erythrocyte surface at 37° C but may be associated at lower temperatures. Therefore, at core body temperature, the antibody is not erythrocyte bound. As blood circulates, it leaves the 37° C environment of core body temperature as it circulates to fingers, toes, ear lobes, and so forth, and is exposed to temperatures below 37° C. High titer or more importantly a wide thermal amplitude of the IgM antibody (indicating that the antibody remains cell bound and activates complement at a relatively high temperature) positively correlates with the extent of erythrocyte destruction. As the antibody-coated cells circulate, they become coated with complement proteins before they return to the core body temperature and the antibody dissociates. IgM and complement-coated erythrocytes are cleared from the circulation by hepatic macrophages. The mechanism of clearance involves binding of the C3-coated erythrocytes to the surface of hepatic macrophages, which have C3 receptors on their surface, with subsequent ingestion. C3 and IgM sensitization of erythrocytes are poor triggers for erythrocyte ingestion. A second signal such as IgG on the erythrocyte interacting with IgG Fc receptors, or cytokines released during inflammation activating the phagocytes, triggers the ingestion process. For this reason, marked red cell destruction in cold agglutinin disease is less common and patients may tolerate the disease for years. In about 5 percent of cases, disease may be caused by IgM autoagglutinin IgM antibody reactive at 37° C. As might be expected this finding is associated with a poorer prognosis than that of cold agglutinin.

IgG-INDUCED HEMOLYTIC ANEMIA

As is the case with IgM-mediated cold agglutinin disease, IgG-induced hemolytic anemias often will occur without an apparent underlying disease (idiopathic type). However, they may also accompany an immunoproliferative disorder, such as non-Hodgkin's lymphoma, chronic lymphocytic leukemia, Sézary syndrome, or T-cell lymphoma, or other autoimmune disease such as systemic lupus erythematosus or chronic inflammatory bowel disease. In general, the detection of IgG bound to the erythrocyte surface (Coombs' direct test) establishes the diagnosis. In most cases of autoimmune hemolytic anemia, the specificity of the IgG is difficult to characterize with precision, but the antibody appears to recognize the Rh family of antigens and does not bind to cells with the Rh null phenotype. Except in rare cases, the antibody does not activate the complement cascade. The titer of the antibody, its antigenic specificity, and its capacity to activate complement all play a role in determining the extent of intravascular hemolysis and the rate of erythrocyte destruction.

The macrophages of the reticuloendothelial system not only bear receptors for C3 but also have receptors for the Fc portion of IgG. These IgG Fc receptors detect IgG-coated erythrocytes and bind and ingest them even in the absence of complement. However, complement deposited on the red cell surface enhances the phagocytic process. Partial ingestion of erythrocyte surface membrane by phagocytes leads to the formation of spherocytes, characteristic of AIHA. Splenic macrophages primarily are responsible for clearance of IgG-coated erythrocytes from the circulation. This is in sharp contrast to the situation with IgM- and complement-coated cells in which hepatic macrophages are responsible for clearance. Hepatic macrophages are able to remove IgG-sensitized erythrocytes from the circulation, but only with high levels of sensitization.

THERAPEUTIC MEASURES

In patients with both IgG- or IgM-induced immune anemia the need for therapeutic intervention and the aggressiveness of the intervention are determined by the degree of hemolysis. In cases in which the hemolysis is mild no treatment may be necessary. In cases secondary to other diseases or drugs, treatment of the underlying disease or suspension of the associated drug often will bring the hemolytic anemia under control. However, if the patient has clinically severe anemia, therapeutic intervention is in order. It should be emphasized that the goal of therapy is not necessarily complete hematologic remission. Although remission is desirable, one balances the ability to achieve a compensated hemolytic anemia with ongoing hemolysis against the prospect of increased toxicity due to more aggressive therapeutic manipulation.

IgG-Induced Hemolytic Anemia

Glucocorticoids

Glucocorticoids are used in the initial treatment of patients with AIHA. This group of drugs is thought to act by influencing three separate processes. First, they decrease the production of the abnormal IgG. This effect is delayed in onset and may lead to a gradual decrease in hemolysis and increase in hemoglobin over the course of 2 to 6 weeks. Second, glucocorticoids are reported to induce a fall in the affinity of the antibody with the erythrocyte surface, thereby decreasing the extent of antibody sensitization of the cells improving the red cell survival. This is probably a relatively minor effect of this therapy. Third, glucocorticoids interfere, both in vitro and in vivo, with macrophage Fc (IgG) and C3b and iC3b (CR_1 and CR_3) receptor expression. These receptors are responsible for the binding of erythrocytes to the surface of phagocytes, leading to their ultimate destruction. This effect may be rapid and is thought responsible for the rise in hemoglobin that initially occurs within days in most patients.

Approximately 70 to 80 percent of patients treated with 1 to 1.5 mg per kilogram of prednisone per day respond to therapy. The onset of response is usually within days. Initial response may be noted in as little as 1 to 2 days. The median duration of therapy before discernible response in some series is 7 days, and relatively few responses occur after 3 weeks of therapy. Therefore, failure to respond within 3 weeks of therapy is considered a therapeutic failure. Once a therapeutic response is achieved (hematocrit greater than 30 percent), glucocorticoids should be tapered. Sudden cessation of therapy often results in prompt relapse; a progressive but slow tapering of the dosage is necessary. A useful schedule is as follows: weekly reduction of the daily dose of prednisone by 10 mg until a dose of 30 mg per day is reached. At this point we attempt to convert the patient to an every-other-day dosage schedule by tapering 5 mg every other day, reducing dosage once per week. We taper every other day until a dosage of 15 mg per day alternating with 30 mg per day is reached. Subsequently, we reduce dosage 2.5 mg every other day every 1 or 2 weeks until the patient receives 30 mg every other day. At this point the every other day dose is tapered slowly first by 5 mg per week till 15 mg every other day is reached, then 2.5 mg per week. If a relapse occurs, the dose is raised by two steps and slowly tapered. Occasionally when a patient relapses on a slowly tapering dose, the dose must be raised again to 60 mg per day and the slow taper restarted.

Using this approach, 10 to 20 percent of patients will remain in complete remission, 20 to 50 percent (in various series) will require permanent low doses of prednisone, and 20 to 50 percent will fail and require other forms of therapy.

Splenectomy

The spleen has unique circulatory pathways and acts as a fine filter for minimally abnormal cells. The splenic circulation results in intimate contact between macrophages with surface IgG Fc receptors and the IgG-coated red cells. This intimate contact leads to binding of the erythrocytes to the macrophage surface and phagocytosis. Since the spleen is the major site of red cell sequestration in IgG-induced hemolytic anemias, removal of the spleen is an effective therapeutic strategy. In the days before the availability of glucocorticoids, splenectomy represented the best available therapy for treatment of AIHA. The majority of patients responded to therapy but most of these patients relapsed as the level of erythrocyte IgG antibody built up on the circulating cells until they were sequestered and phagocytosed by Kupffer cells in the liver.

Patients who do not respond to glucocorticoids, who relapse when attempts are made to lower the dosage, or who have unacceptable side effects from glucocorticoid therapy are candidates for splenectomy. Overall response rate for treatment with splenectomy plus glucocorticoids is at least 70 percent. The patients often continue to require small doses of glucocorticoids to maintain adequate clinical remission. Those patients who initially do not respond to glucocorticoids are less likely to achieve complete remission with splenectomy plus glucocorticoids.

The complications of splenectomy vary greatly from institution to institution. We have generally attempted to identify one or two surgical colleagues who carry out most of the splenectomies on our patient population. The morbidity of the procedure (10 to 20 percent) includes postoperative thrombosis and infections both above and below the diaphragm. The mortality is approximately 2 to 10 percent in various series. The risk of mortality and morbidity is greater in older patients, in those with related underlying disease (benign or malignant immunoproliferative disorders), in those with complicating medical problems, and, to some extent, is influenced by the degree of glucocorticoid side effects. Thus, a thoughtful analysis of the benefit-versus-risk factors needs to be undertaken for each patient. A final consideration is that patients who undergo splenectomy have a statistically increased risk of life-threatening septicemia, particularly with high-grade encapsulated pathogens like pneumococcus. We generally immunize patients with pneumococcal vaccine some weeks before elective splenectomy in an effort to reduce this long-term complication. Those patients who do not respond to glucocorticoid therapy, with or without splenectomy, or who need an unacceptable dose of glucocorticoids must receive additional and often more aggressive therapy.

Alternative Therapies

Immunosuppression. Immunosuppressive drugs used to decrease the production of antibody have been used extensively in patients unresponsive to glucocorticoids or splenectomy. The agents most frequently used are the thiopurines (6-mercaptopurine, cyclophosphamide, and chlorambucil).We tend to use cyclophoshamide as the initial chemotherapeutic agent. We begin treatment at 1.5 to 2 mg per kilogram and adjust the dose downward to maintain a leukocyte count over 3,500, a granulocyte count over 1,500, and a platelet count over 50,000 per cubic millimeter. Following the onset of clinical benefit the dosage is maintained for an additional 6 months and then is tapered over several months. During therapy, patients are advised to maintain a high fluid intake to reduce the incidence of hemorrhagic cystitis. Also, they are instructed to have weekly blood counts to monitor bone marrow suppression. Gonadal suppression may help decrease the infertility associated with cytotoxic therapy.

In this moderate dosage range, the immunosuppressive agents are well tolerated. However, a variety of side effects may be noted including bone marrow suppression, hemorrhagic cystitis, nausea, partial alopecia, amenorrhea, impaired spermatogenesis, and the long-term potential for increasing the incidence of malignancy. These side effects require that the clinical indications for an immunosuppressive therapy be strong and that patient exposure to the drug be limited. Nevertheless, a glucocorticoid-sparing effect of the glucocorticoids is often observed, and some patients who respond to glucocorticoids poorly initially will respond well in the presence of cytotoxic therapy.

Intravenous Immunoglobulin. The clinical use of high doses of intravenous immunoglobulin G (IVIgG) was developed following the observation of resolution of autoimmune thrombocytopenic purpura in patients with congenital agammaglobulinemia by replacement therapy with IgG. Since then, the indication of IVIgG has expanded to patients with other immune cytopenias including AIHA. Several mechanisms of action of IVIgG are postulated. Competitive blockade of macrophage Fc receptors, anti-idiotypic downregulation of autoantibody synthesis, and inhibition of complement deposition on the sensitized cell are all postulated mechanisms of IVIgG action.

IVIgG is less effective in treatment of AIHA than of idiopathic thrombocytopenic purpura. A recent review suggested that about one-third of 73 patients responded to therapy. Interestingly patients with hepatomegaly with or without splenomegaly were more likely to respond.

The usual dose of IVIgG is 0.4 g per kilogram per day for three to five consecutive doses, although even higher doses have been used with success. In some patients with AIHA, IVIgG induces a rapid increase in hemoglobin concentration. Responses are often less dramatic than those seen in idiopathic thrombocytopenic purpura. Even so because this agent is extremely safe, it is used with increasing frequency. It should be noted that this is safe but extremely expensive therapy. In cases with ongoing severe hemolysis the use of IVIgG may allow the patient time to respond to glucocorticoid therapy. Responses to IVIgG are in general short lived and no permanent remissions are observed. In some patients, the initial response is maintained by periodic (every 3 weeks) infusions of IVIgG.

Miscellaneous Therapies. Plasmapheresis has been used in patients with severe AIHA, but has met with limited success. This reflects the fact that more than one-half of the total IgG is extravascular and that the plasma tends to contain low affinity antibodies (the high avidity antibodies being on the red cell surface). IgM antibodies are predominantly intravascular in distribution and more easily removed by plasmapheresis, but they less commonly cause disease. Reduction of antibody level by plasmapheresis is often followed by an increased rate of antibody synthesis. Success has been reported by using apheresis followed by cytotoxic therapy.

Rare reports of successful therapy of AIHA with heparin or thymectomy have not led to clear indications for these treatment modalities. Recently antithymocyte globulin has been used in combination with cytotoxic agents to treat refractory patients with AIHA and SLE. Other immunoregulatory agents like cyclosporin have been used in anecdotal reports. Other measures that have been used effectively in some patients are vincristine, vinblastine infusions, and hormonal therapy. The most exciting development in hormonal therapy is the recent success of danazol. Danazol is a synthetic androgen with limited masculinizing effect. It has been shown, in nonrandomized studies, to improve immune thrombocytopenia as well as AIHA. In our hands the effect has not been dramatic, but this agent is safe and may allow for decreased glucocorticoid dosage. There is some suggestion that it may function to downregulate IgG Fc and C3 receptors.

IgM-Induced Hemolytic Anemia

In contrast to IgG-induced hemolytic anemia, cold hemagglutinin disease usually has a milder course but also a poorer response to treatment. Acute management should include primarily increasing the peripheral body temperature by warming, and more chronically, avoidance of cold exposure. In some cases, patients severely affected consider moving to areas of temperate weather.

As discussed previously, in cold hemagglutinin disease, intravascular lysis of erythrocytes is unusual, the complement-coated cells are usually destroyed through interaction with complement receptors on liver macrophages. Glucocorticoids have not been found to alter complement-mediated intravascular hemolysis and have only a modest effect on the binding and ingestion of C3-coated cells by macrophages. Thus, in general, glucocorticoids are of limited usefulness in cold hemagglutinin disease. A few unusual patients have been noted to improve with glucocorticoid therapy; presumably these patients have IgG autoantibody as well as IgM cold agglutinin present in their illness. If a patient responds to glucocorticoid therapy the same guidelines are followed that are outlined for warm AIHA. Since the clearance of IgM-sensitized erythrocytes is always due to hepatic sequestration, splenectomy plays no role in the treatment of this disease.

A common scenario is that patients with compensated cold agglutinin disease have a sudden exacerbation at the time of an unrelated infection. Presumably cytokines released during the course of the infection increase phagocytosis of C-coated erythrocytes by hepatic macrophages. Often controlling the infection will lead to a marked slowing of the hemolytic process.

In the rare cases in which cold agglutinin diseases persist in a severe form, immunosuppressive drugs have been the major and most effective strategy. Alkylating agents (cyclophosphamide or chlorambucil) have been the drugs used most commonly and appear to have a beneficial effect in 50 to 60 percent of the cases.

There are now multiple case reports in the literature suggesting the usefulness of interferon alpha-2b in the treatment of IgM-mediated cold agglutinin disease, although there are no well-controlled clinical trials.

Transfusion Therapy

Many patients with AIHA do not require transfusion therapy because the anemia has developed gradually and physiologic compensation has occurred. However, some patients experience acute and/or severe anemia and require transfusion for support. Transfusion therapy is complicated by the fact that the blood bank may be unable to find any "compatible" blood. This usually is due to the presence of an autoantibody directed at a core component of Rh substance, which is present in the erythrocytes of virtually all donors, regardless of Rh subtype. The usual recommendation is for the blood bank to identify the most compatible units of blood of the patient's own major blood group and Rh type and to transfuse the patient with the most compatible units available. One never withholds blood in a life-threatening situation because of incompatibility but transfuses the most compatible units.

In cold hemagglutinin disease it is important to prewarm all intravenous infusion including whole blood to 37° C, since a decrease in blood temperature locally in a vein can enhance the binding of the IgM antibody to the infused red cells and accelerate the hemolytic process. Furthermore, agglutination of the chilled or even room temperature cells in small peripheral vessels during the transfusion can result in severe ischemic changes and vascular compromise.

SUGGESTED READING

Fest T, de Wazieres B, Lamy B, et al. Successful response to alpha-interferon 2b in a refractory IgM autoagglutinin-mediated hemolytic anemia. Ann Hematol 1994; 69:147–149.

Flores G, Cunningham-Rundles C, Newland AC, Bussel JB. Efficiency of intravenous immunoglobulin in the treatment of autoimmune hemolytic anemia: Results in 73 patients. Amer J Hematol 1993; 44:237–242.

Jefferies LC. Transfusion therapy in autoimmune hemolytic anemia. Hematol Oncol Clin North Am 1994; 8:1087–1104.

Schreiber AD, Rosse WF, Frank MM. Autoimmune hemolytic anemia. In: MM Frank, KF Austen, HN Claman, ER Unanue, eds. Samter's immunologic diseases. 5th ed. Vol II. Boston: Little, Brown, 1995: 903–918.

AUTOIMMUNE LEUKOPENIA

GORDON STARKEBAUM, M.D.
DAVID C. DALE, M.D.

The terms "autoimmune leukopenia," "autoimmune granulocytopenia," and "autoimmune neutropenia" are often used synonymously to describe conditions in which autoantibodies to mature neutrophils, or their precursors, lead to cell destruction and a reduced blood neutrophil count. Leukopenia is generally defined as a reduction in the total white blood cell count to less than 4,000 cells per deciliter; neutropenia is defined as a neutrophil count of less than 1,800 cells per deciliter. Neutropenia has numerous causes and mechanisms; the most frequent cause is reduced cell production by the bone marrow. Neutropenia also occurs because of abnormalities in the distribution of cells between the circulating and marginated pools of cells in the blood and accelerated cell destruction. Autoimmune leukopenia can be caused by any of these mechanisms.

Although the term "leukopenia" often implies "neutropenia," there are many pathologic conditions in which not only neutrophils but also lymphocytes, monocytes, eosinophils, and basophils are concomitantly or specifically reduced. Lymphocytopenia is a common feature of the stress response to many infections and acute inflammatory illnesses. It occurs in systemic lupus erythematosus (SLE) and other collagen vascular diseases. Lymphocytopenia, monocytopenia, and eosinopenia are regularly seen with corticosteroid therapy. Reductions in any of the white blood cell elements may reflect an important ongoing pathologic process. Severe neutropenia, that is, fewer than 500 blood neutrophils per microliter, predisposes to serious problems with recurrent and potentially life-threatening infections.

TESTING FOR ANTINEUTROPHIL ANTIBODIES

Multiple methods for detecting antineutrophil antibodies have been described. These can be roughly categorized as immunoassays for IgG or functional assays, detecting the effect of antineutrophil antibodies. The immunoassays include immunofluorescence tests, radioimmunoassays, and enzyme-linked immunoassays to detect neutrophil-bound or neutrophil-eluted IgG. Functional tests often measure opsonization or chemiluminescence. Other tests include assays for leukoagglutination, granulocytotoxicity, complement fixation, and the use of myeloid cell lines to detect antibodies against immature neutrophil precursors. No single method has been widely accepted as the best way to assay for neutrophil antibodies. With increasing availability of flow cytometry in clinical laboratories it is likely that indirect immunofluorescence with flow cytometry will become the general standard. The ability to gate specifically on the granulocyte population makes highly purified preparations of cells unnecessary. Also, the results are semiquantitative and can be readily performed without radioisotopes by technicians who use flow cytometry for other assays. It may also be possible to distinguish antineutrophil antibodies from neutrophil-binding immune complexes based on the histogram pattern of immunofluorescence, and both IgG and IgM antibodies can be detected if needed. Controversy exists regarding whether freshly purified polymorphonuclear leukocytes (PMNs) or paraformaldehyde-fixed PMNs are optimal.

Recent studies have examined the sensitivity and specificity of antineutrophil antibodies in various disorders. Maher and Hartman found that none of 37 patients with rheumatoid arthritis (RA) without neutropenia had PMN-reactive IgG using direct immunofluorescence and flow cytometry with freshly isolated PMNs. In contrast, 51/244 (21 percent) of non-neutropenic patients with SLE and other connective disorders had antineutrophil antibodies. Of patients with suspected immune neutropenia with collagen vascular disorders such as Felty's syndrome or SLE, 20/26 (77 percent) had elevated neutrophil-binding IgG. Of all neutropenic patients tested, 59/159 (37 percent) had evidence for antineutrophil antibodies. Logue and colleagues tested sera of patients with chronic idiopathic neutropenia using a radioimmunoassay for IgG and IgM and paraformaldehyde-fixed PMNs. Approximately one-third of the sera had antibodies to PMNs; such patients tended to be older, female, and to have other cytopenias, splenomegaly, and infections compared to the patients without antineutrophil antibodies.

Whether or not to test for antineutrophil antibodies may be questioned. The benefits of testing may include confirmation of an antibody-mediated process. In some cases, finding antineutrophil antibodies may support the use of corticosteroids or immunosuppressive agents in treating the autoimmune neutropenia in patients with recurrent infections (see following discussion). On the other hand, test results for antineutrophil antibodies should be interpreted with caution even those from well-established laboratories. The assays may be neither sensitive nor specific for antibodies to neutrophils. Testing for antibodies to mature neutrophils may not detect antibodies that are directed against immature neutrophil progenitors. Cell-mediated immune processes, such as T-cell suppression of granulocytopoiesis, also may cause neutropenia.

PATIENT EVALUATION

Evaluation begins with a careful history and physical examination. The family history is important; it may reveal other individuals with recurrent fevers, infections, and leukopenia, as well as previously diagnosed autoimmune diseases. The drug history and current medications are also extremely important. The physical examination should give special attention to the skin and mucous membranes, especially the gingiva, oropharynx, and perianal areas. Examination for arthritis, lymphadenopathy, splenomegaly, hepatomegaly, and bone tenderness are also very important.

Laboratory examination begins with a complete blood count. Measurement of the hematocrit and hemoglobin, reticulocytes, and platelets are helpful to recognize serious hematologic diseases such as aplastic anemia, myelodysplasia, or leukemia. A bone marrow aspirate and biopsy may also be necessary. It may also be helpful to obtain serologic tests for autoimmune diseases such as antinuclear antibodies, rheumatoid factor and other specialized tests; liver function tests; and tests for chronic viral infections, including hepatitis, infectious mononucleosis, and HIV. Results from these tests will direct further work-up and consultation, and assays for antineutrophil antibodies generally follow these preliminary assessments.

Measurements of neutrophil kinetics (i.e., glucocorticosteroid test of the bone marrow reserves), epinephrine infusion to measure the degree of neutrophil margination, and radioisotopic studies to measure neutrophil turnover are best performed by research laboratories. Measurement of the growth of bone marrow cells with in vitro culture systems is also a specialized procedure. Many clinical laboratories now examine the immunophenotype of blood leukocytes; this procedure may be useful in identifying clonal disorders of the immune system such as the large, granular lymphocyte syndrome that is associated with neutropenia.

ACUTE NEUTROPENIA

Patients presenting with fever and severe neutropenia (i.e., febrile neutropenia), require urgent attention with appropriate cultures and immediate broad-spectrum antibiotic therapy. Acute febrile neutropenia is usually due to drugs, either as a toxic response to treatment with chemotherapy or immunosuppressive agents or as an idiosyncratic reaction to other drugs. Drug-induced neutropenia or leukopenia may be immune-mediated or result from direct effects of drugs on the cell formation in the bone marrow. There are currently no reliable and specific ways to distinguish between these two possibilities, but the toxic effects of many agents are well recognized. With acute febrile neutropenia of uncertain cause, all suspicious medications should be discontinued immediately.

For many years, much research has focused on efforts to stimulate neutrophil production and to replace neutrophils by transfusions. Transfusions remain logistically complex and of uncertain value in most situations. The colony-stimulating factors (CSFs), granulocyte colony-stimulating factor (G-CSF), and granulocyte-macrophage colony-stimulating factor (GM-CSF), are now widely used to stimulate marrow recovery. These agents will hasten marrow recovery with chemotherapy-induced neutropenia and are probably efficacious in other conditions that cause acute neutropenia. The use of the CSFs in idiosyncratic drug-induced neutropenia has not been studied in randomized trials but has gained considerable acceptance in practice. G-CSF (3 to 5 μg per kilogram per day SC) is the most frequently used treatment.

CHRONIC IDIOPATHIC AND AUTOIMMUNE NEUTROPENIA

Patients with chronic neutropenia can be stratified by their neutrophil counts as mild (below normal but greater than 1.0×10^9 per liter), moderate (0.5 to 1.0×10^9 per liter), or severe (less than 0.5×10^9 per liter).

They may also be broadly divided into primarily hematologic conditions that may be due to autoantibodies and conditions associated with recognized autoimmune diseases. At birth, neonates may have immune neutropenia, but this is not an autoimmune disorder. It is caused by antibodies of maternal origin and predictably passes within a few weeks. Young children may develop neutropenia associated with viral syndromes, which may be on an autoimmune basis. This condition is likely to remit spontaneously and permanently within months to years. It generally requires no therapy because there is little in the way of serious problems with bacterial infections. Some children, however, with a similar presentation but lower neutrophil counts will have recurrent fevers and infections. They will respond to long-term G-CSF treatment (usually 1 to 5 μg per kilogram per day) with increased neutrophils and decreased symptoms. Treatment can be discontinued if the condition remits spontaneously. Treatment with glucocorticoids is generally no longer recommended. Gamma-globulin therapy, as is sometimes used for the treatment of idiopathic thrombocytopenic purpura (500 mg per kilogram per day for 3 to 4 days with maintenance therapy at approximately monthly intervals), is used in some centers. Plasmapheresis is generally not recommended.

Older children and adults may have idiopathic or autoimmune neutropenia. General laboratory testing and neutrophil antibody tests do not unequivocally distinguish between these diagnoses. Therapy is determined primarily on the basis of the pattern of recurrent fevers and infections, including the occurrence of mouth ulcers, gingivitis, sinusitis, and lower respiratory tract and skin infections. For patients with recurrent infections, long-term treatment with G-CSF is effective. Patients with and without autoantibodies appear to respond to treatment similarly.

TREATMENT OF NEUTROPENIA ASSOCIATED WITH OTHER AUTOIMMUNE DISEASES

In most cases of SLE or Sjögren's syndrome complicated by neutropenia, the underlying disease is active and treatment of the disease flare, usually with corticosteroids or immunosuppressive agents, improves the neutropenia. In contrast, patients with Felty's syndrome or with leukemia of large granular lymphocytes generally have chronic neutropenia in the absence of active arthritis. In this situation, treatment directed specifically at the neutropenia appears warranted.

Felty's Syndrome

The risk of infection in patients with Felty's syndrome is particularly increased in patients with neutrophil counts less than 0.2×10^9 per liter. In such patients, mortality is substantially increased compared to patients with uncomplicated rheumatoid arthritis (RA). The neutropenia of Felty's syndrome is the result of a complex immune-mediated process, which is a manifestation of the underlying rheumatoid arthritis in a genetically susceptible (HLA-DR4 positive) individual. Reflecting this mechanism, drugs that are effective for RA are often useful in treating Felty's syndrome. These include gold salts, D-penicillamine, cyclophosphamide, azathioprine, methotrexate (see following discussion), cyclosporine, and corticosteroids. Modalities that are not effective include intravenous gammaglobulin, plasmapheresis, and total nodal irradiation.

Patients with Felty's syndrome may respond to methotrexate, frequently with a prompt rise in neutrophils. Given the potential marrow suppressive effect of methotrexate, however, patients should be monitored closely and its use should be avoided in patients with impaired renal or hepatic function; hypoalbuminemia may also increase risk of toxicity from methotrexate.

Recently, recombinant hematopoietic growth factors have been used in Felty's syndrome. Improvement of neutropenia and a decrease in infections has been reported with both G-CSF (1 to 5 μg per kilogram per day) and GM-CSF (similar doses). Complications of CSF treatment have included flare of arthritis, anemia and thrombocytopenia, and vasculitis. In rare patients, combination treatment with either G-CSF and methotrexate or G-CSF with cyclophosphamide were needed to correct the neutropenia.

Splenectomy has been used for many years in the treatment of the neutropenia of Felty's syndrome. Although up to 50 percent of patients respond with a rise in neutrophil count after splenectomy, it is not possible to predict which patients will respond. Furthermore, patients are at risk of postsplenectomy sepsis, especially those patients with recurrent infections presplenectomy. Nevertheless, in patients not able to tolerate drug treatment or those who fail to respond, splenectomy should be considered an option. Of note, splenic embolization has been reported to be successful in Felty's syndrome.

Based on these considerations, we recommend treating patients with Felty's syndrome who have had infections, regardless of the neutrophil count. Generally, we begin with G-CSF in patients who are acutely ill. If the patient responds, we add low-dose pulse methotrexate to achieve a stable remission and eliminate the need for chronic G-CSF. In asymptomatic patients without infections, the decision when to treat may be more difficult. If the neutrophil count drops to 200 per microliter, however, we recommend treatment, given the high risk of serious infections. In such patients, we begin with 2.5 to 5 mg per week of methotrexate and slowly increase the dose, for example, by 2.5 mg per week each month. Thus, it may take 3 to 4 months for the patient to reach 10 to 12.5 mg per week of oral methotrexate. In patients with renal insufficiency or hepatic disease, in whom methotrexate is contraindicated, we recommend G-CSF or GM-CSF on a long-term basis. In such patients, splenectomy should be considered if no response is seen or if complications such as disease flare or vasculitis occur.

Treatment of LGL Leukemia

In patients with LGL leukemia, lymphocytosis itself is usually not progressive; morbidity results from neutropenia and resultant infections. Treatment has included splenectomy, GM-CSF, G-CSF, and prednisone. Recently, methotrexate was found to be helpful in 6 of 10 patients, resulting in a rise in neutrophil counts and a decrease in infections. In three patients achieving a complete clinical response on methotrexate, molecular analyses of T-cell receptor gene rearrangement could not detect the abnormal clone. Of note, two of the responding patients did not have RA.

SUGGESTED READING

Dale DC, Bonilla MA, Davis MW, et al. A randomized controlled phase III trial of recombinant human G-CSF for treatment of severe chronic neutropenia. Blood 1993; 81:2496–2502.

Fiechtner JJ, Miller DR, Starkebaum G. Reversal of neutropenia with methotrexate treatment in patients with Felty's syndrome. Correlation of response with neutrophil-reactive IgG. Arthritis Rheum 1989; 32:194–201.

Logue GL, Shastri KA, Laughlin M, et al. Idiopathic neutropenia: Antineutrophil antibodies and clinical correlations. Am J Med 1991; 90:211–216.

Loughran TP Jr, Kidd PG, Starkebaum G. Treatment of large granular lymphocyte leukemia with oral low-dose methotrexate. Blood 1994; 84:2164–2170.

Maher GM, Hartman KR. Detection of antineutrophil autoantibodies by flow cytometry: Use of unfixed neutrophils as antigenic targets. J Clin Lab Anal 1993; 7:334–340.

Shastri KA, Logue GL. Autoimmune neutropenia. Blood 1993; 81:1984–1995.

APLASTIC ANEMIA

EMMANUEL N. DESSYPRIS, M.D.

Aplastic anemia is a disorder characterized by severe bone marrow hypoplasia or aplasia with replacement of hematopoietic cells by fatty tissue resulting in pancytopenia. The diagnosis should be established by bone marrow biopsy. The severity of aplastic anemia can be assessed by the magnitude of pancytopenia. In severe aplastic anemia the absolute neutrophil count is lower than 500 cells per microliter, the platelet count is lower than 20,000 cells per microliter, and the reticulocyte count is lower than 20,000 cells per microliter. Such severe pancytopenia is usually associated with a marrow cellularity lower than 30 percent. Cases with less severe pancytopenia and/or higher marrow cellularity are classified as nonsevere aplastic anemia.

Acquired aplastic anemia results from an injury to pluripotent hematopoietic stem cells that reduces or abolishes the ability of these primitive cells to undergo proliferation and differentiation. In the majority of cases the bone marrow stroma seems to maintain normal function. Injury to stem cells that results in marrow aplasia may occur during the course of a variety of viral infections (hepatitis, Epstein-Barr virus, cytomegalo virus, parvovirus B19, herpes 6); autoimmune diseases (systemic lupus erythematosus, diffuse eosinophilic fascitis); certain neoplasms (thymoma); some hematologic disorders (paroxysmal nocturnal hemoglobinuria, preleukemia); or, more commonly, after exposure to certain drugs, chemicals, or radiation. In more than one-half of cases, however, no association can be established with any underlying disease or previous exposure to myelotoxic chemical or physical agents. Although the exact nature of the injury to stem cells is still unknown, indirect evidence has accumulated that indicates that the immune system may play an important role either in the initial events leading to, or in maintaining the dysregulated stem cell function. There has been recent demonstration of clonal hematopoiesis in a proportion of cases of idiopathic aplastic anemia; it is not known whether this is the result of the initiating bone marrow injury or if this represents a manifestation of abnormal residual hematopoiesis.

THERAPY

Once the diagnosis is established by bone marrow biopsy, any exposure to chemicals or drugs should be discontinued and the patient should receive supportive treatment and be observed for signs of marrow recovery, which is expected to occur within 2 to 3 weeks. After this period of time spontaneous remissions are very rare. Unfortunately, even in cases of well-documented exposure to myelotoxic agents, removal of the offending agent is only rarely followed by bone marrow recovery. Recovery can usually be documented by an increasing absolute neutrophil, platelet, or reticulocyte count.

Bone marrow transplantation and immunosuppression are the two major types of effective therapy for patients with aplastic anemia. The type of therapy that is indicated in an individual case depends on the severity of aplastic anemia, the age of the patient, and the availability of a histocompatible related bone marrow donor. Patients with severe aplastic anemia who are younger than 45 years of age and have a histocompatible related bone marrow donor should be treated with bone marrow transplantation. Young patients who do not have a histocompatible marrow donor, patients older than 45 years of age, as well as patients with less than severe aplastic anemia and non–life-threatening pancytopenia, should be considered for immunosuppressive therapy.

Bone Marrow Transplantation

After the diagnosis of severe aplastic anemia is made in a patient younger than 45 years of age, HLA typing of the patient and family members should be initiated as soon as possible in preparation for bone marrow transplantation. Female patients should be started on antivulatory medicines to prevent severe bleeding from menstruation. In candidates for bone marrow transplantation, administration of blood products (red blood cells and platelets) should be kept to a minimum, since they increase the risk for sensitization to minor histocompatibility antigens with subsequent higher rates of graft rejection. Blood products from family members that are potential marrow donors should be avoided for the same reasons. Severe anemia (Hemoglobin concentration as low as 5 to 6 g per 100 ml) can be tolerated quite well by young persons, particularly if their activities are limited. Transfusions of washed red cells should be given only if cardiorespiratory symptoms develop. Platelet transfusions should be avoided if the platelet count is above 10,000 per microliter and the patient is stable in the sense that no new petechiae or wet purpura develop and there is no bleeding. All blood products should be administered through leukocyte filters. Such a strict policy for transfusions can be relaxed once it is determined that the patient has no matched related donor. It has been estimated that a matched related donor can be identified in only 20 to 30 percent of cases. Transplantation of histocompatible bone marrow from an unrelated donor identified through a national or international bone marrow donor registry may be considered as a reasonable option for children but still remains an experimental procedure for patients older than 20 years of age.

Once a histocompatible related marrow donor is identified, the patient should be transferred to a bone marrow transplantation center. After conditioning the patient with fractionated total body radiation or cyclophosphamide for induction of sufficient immunosuppression to allow marrow grafting, bone marrow collected from the donor is infused intravenously. Collection of donor marrow is performed under general anesthesia by multiple aspirations from different sites of the pelvis. A total volume of 700 to 1,500 ml is harvested, which usually provides an adequate number of nucleated cells for successful grafting (3 to 9 $\times$ 10^8 nucleated marrow cells per kilogram.

Successful grafting of donor marrow occurs in 97 to 99 percent of cases. Engraftment is manifested by an increasing monocyte and granulocyte count within 2 to 4 weeks posttransplantation. Normalization of peripheral blood counts takes place within 40 to 60 days, although platelet counts may stay subnormal for a longer period of time. All patients routinely receive graft versus host disease (GVHD) prophylaxis with cyclosporin and prednisone.

The major complications seen in bone marrow recipients include graft rejection; acute and chronic GVHD; severe immunosuppression resulting in viral, bacterial, and fungal infections; idiopathic interstitial pneumonia; veno-occlusive disease of the liver, leukoencephalopathy; and cataracts. These complications are responsible for a 10 to 30 percent mortality within the first year post-transplantation. The overall 5-year survival of patients undergoing bone marrow transplantation for severe aplastic anemia is in the range of 60 to 65 percent. Patients with aplastic anemia treated successfully with bone marrow transplantation are cured from their disease and late relapses or hematologic complications are extremely rare.

Immunosuppression

Antilymphocyte globulin (ALG) or antilymphocyte serum (ALS) and cyclosporin-A are the two immunosuppressive agents that have been used successfully in aplastic anemia. Patients who for any reason are not candidates for bone marrow transplantation should receive immunosuppressive treatment. ALG and cyclosporin-A are equally effective as single agents in inducing remission of aplastic anemia.

Antilymphocyte Globulin

ALG is prepared by immunizing horses or rabbits with lymphocytes obtained by cannulating the thoracic duct. After absorption with human red cells, either the whole immune serum or purified immune IgG are used as therapeutic agents. The optimal dose and duration of treatment with ALG has not yet been studied. A commonly used regimen consists of administration of 15 mg of immune IgG per kilogram of body weight daily for 10 days in combination with 60 mg of oral prednisone daily for 10 days with rapid tapering over the following 3 weeks. High-dose corticosteroids do not add to the therapeutic efficacy and are associated with a higher rate of side effects, in particular infections. Androgenic steroids, frequently used in the past in combination with ALG, have not been found to increase the response rate and thus, should not be used routinely.

ALG is diluted in normal saline (1 mg per milliliter) and infused, preferably through a central venous line, over 6 to 12 hours. Before administering the first dose, a skin test is performed with a 1:1,000 dilution of the preparation. Patients with a positive skin test should receive ALG from another species. Both skin testing and intravenous infusion of ALG should be performed under close medical supervision, and the physician should be appropriately prepared to promptly treat possible anaphylaxis. Fever, chills, skin rash, arthralgias, anaphylactic reactions, serum sickness, exacerbation of thrombocytopenia, subclinical hemolysis, and transient hypotensive or hypertensive episodes are the complications associated with ALG therapy. Most of the allergic reactions can be managed successfully by temporarily increasing the dose of corticosteroids.

Response to ALG, as documented by an increase in the peripheral blood counts, is usually slow and occurs at the earliest in 2 to 3 months after initiation of therapy. About 40 to 60 percent of patients with severe aplastic anemia respond to ALG by increasing their peripheral blood counts to levels that allow cessation of transfusions. Almost one-half of the responders normalize their blood counts, with the remaining patients continuing to have mild cytopenia that does not require any treatment. In most cases the hematologic response to ALG is maintained without any further therapy. About 10 to 15 percent of responsive patients relapse within the first 6 to 36 months after ALG therapy. Late relapses may be seen as well. The overall relapse rate over a 14-year follow-up period is about 25 to 35 percent. Patients responding to ALG early after its administration have the highest risk for relapse. Relapsing patients have the same chance of responding to a second course of ALG. Nonresponders should receive cyclosporin A.

Patients responsive to ALG have a 60 to 70 percent survival at 15 years after the diagnosis. However, a significant proportion of these patients, as high as 40 percent, may develop a clonal hematologic disorder, such as myelodysplastic syndrome, paroxysmal nocturnal hemoglobinuria, or, less frequently, acute leukemia, during the 10-year period following the diagnosis of aplastic anemia. Because of the high incidence of relapses and late development of clonal hematologic disorders, treatment with ALG should be reserved only for those patients that are not candidates for bone marrow transplantation.

Cyclosporin A

Cyclosporin A has been shown to be equally effective with ALG in inducing remissions in patients with severe aplastic anemia. In addition, patients unresponsive to ALG may respond to cyclosporin and vice versa. Cyclosporin is given orally at a daily dose of 10 mg per kilogram of body weight in two divided doses. Patients receiving cyclosporin should be followed with serial measurements of serum creatinine and serum cyclosporin concentrations. The response to cyclosporin is as slow as that for ALG, and usually improvement in peripheral blood counts is not seen until 8 to 12 weeks of treatment. After improvement of peripheral blood counts, treatment with cyclosporin A continues until either normalization or maximum improvement of blood counts is seen. Then the dose of cyclosporin is slowly tapered over a 2- to 3-month period. The long-term results of treatment of aplastic anemia with cyclosporin are not yet well known.

It has not yet been determined whether ALG or cyclosporin should be used first for the treatment of severe aplastic anemia. A combination of both drugs does not seem to accelerate recovery, but evidence exists that such a combination results in a higher response rate. In patients with very severe aplastic anemia (absolute neutrophil count lower than 200 per microliter) the combination of these two drugs should be used initially. For the remaining patients, selection between cyclosporin and ALG depends on the experience of the treating physician.

Hematopoietic Growth Factors

Hematopoietic growth factors such as erythropoietin, G-CSF, GM-CSF, and IL-3, have been used in clinical trials for the treatment of aplastic anemia. These factors are capable of promoting proliferation and differentiation of hematopoietic progenitors both in vitro and in vivo. In aplastic anemia, the numbers of hematopoietic progenitors in the marrow, which are the cells on which these factors exert their action, are significantly reduced. Therefore, it is not surprising that growth factors do not have any effect in severe aplastic anemia. The role of these agents is limited to cases of less than severe aplastic anemia in which residual progenitors may be stimulated by growth factors and produce a higher number of mature cells. In such cases, improvement of cytopenias may occur, but the improvement is totally dependent upon continuous administration of growth factors. In only rare exceptions the beneficial effect of growth factors may continue after their discontinuation.

Supportive Care

Symptomatic anemia and thrombocytopenia should be managed by transfusions of appropriate blood products. A conservative approach to platelet transfusions is wise since sensitization occurs in all patients in a predictable fashion. Patients without bleeding and with a platelet count in excess of 10,000 per microliter may tolerate thrombocytopenia for a prolonged period of time. Infections should be treated aggressively with appropriate antibiotics. Minor infections can be managed on an outpatient basis, and hospitalization of asymptomatic neutropenic patients should be avoided if possible. Because of the short life span of granulocytes, granulocyte transfusions for all practical purposes cannot be recommended as routine treatment of patients with neutropenia.

SUGGESTED READING

Storb R. Bone marrow transplant for aplastic anemia. Cell Transplantation 1993: 2:365–379.

Young NS, Alter BP. Aplastic anemia, acquired and inherited. Philadelphia: WB Saunders, 1994.

Young NS, Barrett AJ. The treatment of severe acquired aplastic anemia. Blood 1995: 85:3367–3377.

PHAGOCYTE FUNCTION DISORDERS

MARK S. KLEMPNER, M.D.
MARK P. EPSTEIN, M.B., B.Ch.

Phagocytes, or "cells that eat," play a central role in the elimination of invasive, foreign particles such as bacteria and fungi. The success of these cells, principally neutrophils, but also monocytes and eosinophils, in eliminating pathogenic microorganisms requires a coordinated series of separate functions that are analogous to any successful feast: there must be a sufficient number of participants to ensure a sociable gathering, food that produces appetizing aromas to attract the assembled masses, and the participants need to be able to recognize and move in the direction of the delicacies and to possess the appropriate machinery for ingesting and digesting the spread. We have often used this banquet metaphor to simply explain the disorders in phagocyte function, which we routinely evaluate in a host defense evaluation laboratory, to referring physicians, patients, and their families. In more formal terms, an adequate number of neutrophils must express cell surface adhesion molecules to adhere to resting and stimulated endothelial cells, emigrate from the circulation by chemotaxis toward microbial or host-generated chemoattractants, and bind opsonized particles to cell surface receptors, which induce particle phagocytosis and digest (kill) these particles using both preformed lysosomal antimicrobial components and newly generated, labile oxygen derivatives. We will consider the specific neutrophil defects (Table 1) in leukocyte adhesion, chemotaxis, granule formation and function, and oxygen metabolism following a general description of the presentation of patients with these disorders.

Patients with clinically significant defects of neutrophil function most often come to medical attention because of one of three circumstances: (1) an unusually severe manifestation of infection with a common organism (e.g., pyogenic liver abscess due to *Staphylococcus aureus* or a severe, poorly healing skin or soft tissue infection), (2) recurrent infections with common bacterial pathogens (e.g., recurrent bacterial pneumonias or soft tissue infections), or (3) infection with a pathogen that is unusual in a normal host (e.g., *Aspergillus* or *Boldheria* [formerly *Pseudomonas*] *cepacia*). Recurrent viral upper respiratory tract infections do not signify a likely phagocyte defect and do not merit laboratory evaluation of neutrophil function. Similarly, recurrent *(S. aureus)* furunculosis in an adult is a common referral for neutrophil function testing but is unlikely to be associated with abnormal neutrophil function.

Since most of the major defects are congenital, clinical presentation is often in childhood. However, milder defects and even major functional abnormalities may not become apparent until adulthood. Lack of a history of recurrent childhood infections in no way excludes the diagnosis of abnormal phagocyte function. A family history of unusual, frequent, or particularly severe infections should be sought in all patients. Consanguinity of parents is a risk factor for some of the heritable disorders and should be specifically questioned in patients suspected of abnormal neutrophil function.

Physical examination may provide important clues to possible neutrophil dysfunction. Poor or very prolonged healing of soft tissue infections is common, sometimes resulting in multiple scars. Because the gingiva is a major site of confrontation between bacteria and phagocytes, poor oral hygiene, poor dentition, or severe gum recession is often found in patients with neutrophil dysfunction.

Management of cases usually involves classification and identification of the functional defect through specific laboratory tests, provision of treatment for acute infections, chemoprophylaxis against future infection, and genetic counseling. Following is a discussion of the major defects of neutrophil function as presented in Table 1.

LEUKOCYTE ADHESION DEFICIENCY TYPES 1 AND 2

Neutrophils localize to sites of infection first by adhering to endothelial cells, then by emigrating from the intravascular space through the basement membrane into the extravascular space. Adhesion is mediated by at least three major cell surface moieties: cell surface glycoproteins, which have selective carbohydrate binding domains (the selectins); integral membrane proteins either $beta_2$ or leukocyte integrins, which bind to extracellular matrix components (e.g., fibronectin and collagen) and to adhesion molecules on the endothelial cell (e.g., ICAM 1 and 2); and a homophilic glycoprotein (platelet-endothelial cell adhesion molecule-1 or PECAM-1), which is expressed on both neutrophils and at endothelial cell junctions where it facilitates neutrophil emigration.

Mutations in the gene for the common beta-subunit of the leukocyte integrins LFA-1, Mac-1, and gp 150, 95 are inherited in an autosomal recessive pattern and are termed leukocyte adhesion deficiency type 1 (LAD-1). Typically, patients with LAD-1 have recurrent, necrotic, and indolent bacterial infections involving the skin, oral mucosa, genital mucosa, respiratory tract, and intestinal tract. Infections begin in the neonatal period, and a hallmark of this disease is delayed separation of the umbilical cord. A broad range of bacteria and fungi, including *S. aureus,* enteric gram-negative bacteria, *Candida,* and *Aspergillus* cause infections in these patients. Rapidly spreading cellulitis may occur. Because of the inability to localize neutrophils to infected sites, pus formation is limited in infections of patients with LAD. A persistently high white count or an unusually

Table 1 Phagocyte Function Disorders

Disorder	*Inheritance*	*Clinical Features*	*Defect*	*Diagnosis*
Leukocyte adherence deficiency (LAD 1 and 2)	Autosomal recessive	Granulocytosis Delayed umbilical cord separation Recurrent skin, oral, and respiratory infections	Absent or abnormal β subunit CD-11/18 Absent Sialyl-Lewis X ligand of E-selectin in LAD-2	FACS analysis of peripheral blood leukocytes for CD-11/18 Measurement of Sialyl-Lewis X antigen
Hyperimmunoglobulin E recurrent infection syndrome (Job's syndrome)	Autosomal dominant (incomplete penetrance)	"Cold" skin abscesses Pulmonary fungal infection Chronic eczematous dermatitis Coarse facies Mucocutaneous candidiasis	Profoundly reduced chemotaxis Putative T-lymphocyte deficit	Serum IgE >2,500 IU/ml Mild eosinophilia
Specific granule deficiency	Autosomal recessive	Recurrent bacterial infections – cutaneous, sinopulmonary, and otic common Attenuated inflammatory response	Deficiency in specific granule formation	Deficiency of lactoferrin by ELISA/Western blot Absent or deficient granules on Wright's stain or by electron microscopy of peripheral blood neutrophils
Myeloperoxidase deficiency (MPO)	Autosomal recessive (variable expression)	Normal clinically Disseminated fungal disease in association with diabetes mellitus Acquired deficiency in AML/CML	Pre-and posttranslational precursor processing deficits	Delayed bacterial killing Deficiency of peroxidase positive cells as measured in automated white cell differential
Chédiak-Higashi syndrome (CHS)	Autosomal recessive	Partial occulocutaneous albinism Recurrent bacterial infections Prolonged bleeding time Nystagmus and peripheral sensorimotor neuropathy	Ineffective granule morphogenesis	Giant granules in peripheral blood neutrophils by Wright's stain
Chronic garnulomatous disease (CGD)	X linked: 65% Autosomal recessive: 36%	Multiple granulomas Liver abscess or pneumonia Recurrent infections – catalase positive bacteria and fungi	Respiratory burst NADPH oxidase	NBT test Superoxide quantitation Genetic analysis

high neutrophil count at times of acute infection are typical of patients with LAD.

Five classes of mutations have been described for the gene located on chromosome 21, which encodes the beta chain of the leukocyte integrins. Some mutations result in less complete deficiency of integrin expression, and these patients have a less severe phenotype. The magnitude of deficiency is directly related to the severity of disease. Functionally, neutrophils adhere poorly to endothelial cells or to protein-coated surfaces. Chemotaxis and cell aggregation are deficient in proportion to the deficiency of the membrane proteins.

As is the case for most phagocyte function disorders, treatment depends on the severity of infection and identification of the specific microbial pathogens. Broad-spectrum empiric therapy should be started early with a low threshold for adding an antifungal agent if clinical improvement is not seen. Prophylactic trimethoprim-sulfamethoxazole may be useful for preventing recurrent bacterial infections and is recommended. Bone marrow transplantation is the treatment of choice for patients with the severe phenotype and should be considered early in the course of the disease. In vitro correction of LAD lymphocytes using a retrovirus-mediated gene transfer has been successful and provides the basis for optimism in gene therapy for this disease.

Recently leukocyte adhesion deficiency type 2 was described in two unrelated boys. Both boys lacked the Sialyl-Lewis X ligand of E-selectin and had the Bombay (hh) blood phenotype. Clinically both had severe mental retardation, short stature, recurrent bacterial infections, periodontitis, recurrent otitis media, and cellulitis without pus formation. Infections were associated with a marked leukocytosis. Functional abnormalities in adhesion to endothelial surfaces and chemotaxis were found. These are the only two reported cases of this syndrome.

HYPERIMMUNOGLOBULIN E RECURRENT INFECTION SYNDROME

Hyperimmunoglobulin E (HIE) recurrent infection syndrome is a rare disorder that is also known as Job's syndrome. "Cold" staphylococcal skin abscesses, which lack the usual signs of acute inflammation, are the clinical hallmark of this disease. Sinusitis, otitis media, and recurrent pneumonia sometimes with pneumatoceles, occur frequently. *S. aureus* is the usual pathogen. Septic arthritis, cellulitis, osteomyelitis, and chronic mucocutaneous candidiasis are also seen in patients with this syndrome. Chronic eczematous dermatitis is an early feature of the disease and manifests in early childhood. While originally described in red-haired, fair-skinned females, this syndrome also occurs in males and in African-Americans. Coarse facial features with a broad, flattened nasal bridge are common.

Abnormal immune regulation is prominent in patients with the HIE recurrent infection syndrome. A marked elevation in serum IgE, which is usually greater than 2,500 IU per milliliter, is observed in all patients. Hyperimmunoglobulinemia E results from decreased catabolism of IgE. IgE antibodies against staphylococci and *Candida* species are also present in serum from these patients but not in serum from patients with hyperimmunoglobulin E due to atopy. Interferon (IFN-γ) gamma production by stimulated lymphocytes is also depressed. A neutrophil chemotactic defect is found during the course of the disease in most patients but varies from normal to severely depressed in serial determinations on any single patient. The magnitude of the defect in neutrophil migration correlates with the severity of eczema.

Treatment is directed against the acute infection. Early, aggressive drainage and prolonged antibiotic therapy are advocated. Trimethoprim-sulfamethoxazole may be used as prophylaxis against infections, particularly *S. aureus.* A controlled trial of levamisol did not decrease the rate of recurrent infections in these patients. Dermatitis usually responds to topical steroid application. No controlled studies have been completed to show efficacy of treatment with IFN-γ, although uncontrolled studies have shown clinical improvements with this treatment.

SPECIFIC GRANULE DEFICIENCIES

Secondary or specific granules of neutrophils contain lactoferrin, vitamin B_{12} binding protein, and lysozyme and function as a storage pool of receptors (e.g., C3bi) and respiratory burst oxidase components (e.g., cytochrome b $_{558}$), which are mobilized to the cell surface upon activation of the cells. Complete absence of specific granules is extremely rare, having been described in only five patients. Patients who lack specific granules experience recurrent bacterial infections beginning in early childhood. Both congenital and acquired forms of specific granule deficiency have been described, with the congenital form demonstrating autosomal recessive inheritance. The acquired form may be seen in neonates and in thermally injured patients, in which granules fuse prematurely with the plasma membrane, resulting in functional impairment of neutrophil function.

Clinically, patients present with recurrent bacterial infections. The inflammatory response to infection is usually diminished, which underestimates the severity of infection. Cutaneous, sinopulmonary, and otic infections are common. Diagnosis is based on examination of blood smears prepared with Wright's stain, in which neutrophil granules appear absent because the azurophil or primary granules do not stain with Wright's stain. However, azurophil granules are seen by peroxidase stain. Antibiotics are directed towards the specific offending pathogen and should be continued until several weeks after resolution of the infection.

MYELOPEROXIDASE DEFICIENCY

This is the most common of inherited neutrophil abnormalities, a partial deficiency of the enzyme myeloperoxidase (MPO) occurs in approximately 1 in 2,000 and a complete deficiency occurs in approximately 1 in 4,000 individuals. Inheritance is autosomal recessive with variable penetrance. Automated white cell differentials, which detect peroxidase negative granulocytes, allow for more accurate detection and prevalence figures. The gene that encodes for MPO is located on chromosome 17. Strong evidence exists that both pre- and post-translational abnormalities account for the decrease in myeloperoxidase. Acquired MPO deficiency is often associated with hematologic disorders, acute and chronic myelogenous leukemia, myelodysplastic syndrome, refractory megaloblastic anemia, and aplastic anemia. There have also been reports of MPO deficiency in pregnancy, the neonatal period, and in lead intoxication.

Laboratory studies usually reveal normal neutrophil chemotaxis, phagocytosis, and degranulation, with an enhanced respiratory burst. Microbicidal activity against bacteria is delayed but not absent. In contrast, killing of *C. albicans, C. tropiacalis, C. stellatoidea,* and *C. cruzi* is markedly depressed or absent. The majority of patients with MPO deficiency are clinically normal and do not require prophylactic antibiotics or evaluation of host defense mechanisms. Although this is the most common abnormality of neutrophils, only six patients have been described with significant infections. Three of four patients with MPO deficiency and systemic candidiasis also had diabetes mellitus, which was the more likely predisposition to infection.

CHÉDIAK-HIGASHI SYNDROME

Approximately 200 cases of Chédiak-Higashi syndrome (CHS), a rare autosomal recessive syndrome, have been described in which profound defects in intracellular granules occur. Intracellular granules fuse together to form giant granules within the cytoplasm of the cell. This phenomenon is seen in all granule-containing cells, affecting cellular function and resulting in neutrophil dysfunction, prolongation of bleeding time, partial oculocutaneous albinism, mixed sensorimotor peripheral neuropathy, and nystagmus. The inflammatory response is depressed due to slowed chemotaxis, despite normal or increased numbers of chemotactic receptors.

Patients develop recurrent bacterial infections most commonly involving the skin, soft tissues, and upper and lower respiratory tracts. Viral, fungal, and parasitic infections are uncommon in the early stages of CHS. *S. aureus* and *Haemophilus influenzae* are the most common pathogens isolated from pyogenic infections. *Staphylococcus epidermidis* and enteric gram-negative organisms may also be seen. Three to six major infections per year is not uncommon, with extensive scarring from drainage of subcutaneous infections being common in older children. Children surviving into their teens develop an accelerated phase of the disease characterized by lymphadenopathy, hepatosplenomegaly, and lymphocytic infiltration of many organs. This acceleration of the disease may be precipitated by infection due to Epstein-Barr virus.

Because the fundamental abnormality in CHS is unknown, treatment is based on treating the recurrent infections. Prophylaxis against infection has been successful with trimethoprim-sulfamethoxazole. Some patients have shown improved neutrophil function after administration of ascorbic acid. Treatment of the accelerated phase of the disease is difficult. Bone marrow transplantation has shown limited success. There has also been a case report of improvement in a 10-year-old patient following splenectomy. Using fetal blood sampling at 17 weeks, prenatal diagnosis for CHS has recently been reported.

CHRONIC GRANULOMATOUS DISEASES OF CHILDHOOD

Chronic granulomatous diseases (CGD) are a genetically heterogenous group of inherited disorders characterized by the failure of phagocytic cells to produce superoxide. The condition affects approximately 1 in 750,000 individuals. Neutrophils, eosinophils, and monocytes are affected. Patients are susceptible to recurrent infections that may be life threatening.

The clinical presentation of CGD is variable. Most patients will present in childhood, but a few patients will not be identified until adulthood, including a patient whose initial presentation was at 69 years of age. Infections in patients with CGD may be indolent and are usually not accompanied by a pronounced inflammatory response. Fever may or may not be present. Pneumonia occurs in 70 to 80 percent of patients with CGD, with *S. aureus* being isolated in almost one-half of all pneumonias. Lymphadenitis, cutaneous infections, and hepatic and perihepatic abscesses occur commonly. Less commonly, patients present with osteomyelitis, perirectal abscesses, and septicemia. Brain abscess, pericarditis, and meningitis are uncommon infections in CGD. *S. aureus,* enteric gram-negative bacteria, *Serratia marcesens, Burholderia cepacia* (formerly *Pseudomonas*), and *Aspergillus* spp. are frequently encountered pathogens.

Although overt clinical signs of infection are usually less dramatic in patients with CGD, there is an accumulation of inflammatory cells, which leads to the formulation of granulomas. Granulomas are commonly found in the lungs, liver, and spleen but may form in all tissues. Large granulomas may cause urinary and gastrointestinal obstruction.

When assessing a patient with CGD, a detailed history and physical examination are extremely important. New areas of inflammation may be sites of active infection. Commonly the erythrocyte sedimentation rate is raised and the white cell count may be elevated. An attempt should be made to identify the source and location of any infection with definitive culture of the offending organism through aspiration or biopsy. Blood cultures should be routine when assessing a suspected infection in a CGD patient. Lumbar puncture is generally not recommended in initial evaluation because meningitis is uncommon in these patients. Definitive diagnosis of CGD is made by a nitroblue tetrazolium (NBT) slide test or quantitation of superoxide production. The NBT slide test, which is available in many hospital laboratories, assesses the reduction by stimulated neutrophils of a yellow dye to blue/black formazan. Neutrophil superoxide production is only measured in a few university-based research laboratories.

A chest radiograph is helpful in diagnosing pneumonia, although infiltrates are usually subtle. Ultrasound is usually helpful in identifying intra-abdominal abscesses. Computerized tomography is sensitive in identifying pulmonary and abdominal infections.

THERAPY

Prevention of infection is important in the management of patients with CGD. Minor cuts and abrasions should be cleansed promptly, and a topical antibiotic should be applied. Careful attention to oral hygiene, including regular flossing and professional teeth cleaning, can control gingivitis and aphthous ulcers. Extremely dusty environments, smoking, and the use of humidifiers should be avoided. Administration of all childhood immunizations is recommended.

Prophylactic administration of trimethoprim-sulfamethoxazole has been shown to significantly decrease the incidence of bacterial infections and increase latency between infections. Studies addressing fungal prophylaxis are ongoing. A recent multicenter study has shown efficacy in reducing the frequency of severe infection by the administration of IFN-γ at 50 μg per square meter subcutaneously three times per week. This beneficial effect was not accompanied by an improvement in respiratory burst function.

Early recognition of infection, culture of the pathogen, adequate doses of antibiotic, and long courses of treatment ensure the most favorable result when treating CGD patients. Surgical intervention is required in cases where compression or obstruction of visceral organs occurs. Ureteral obstruction can cause pyelonephritis and hydronephrosis and may be treated with steroids when surgical access is poor.

Granulocyte transfusions may aid in the treatment of some infections, but their efficacy has not been proven in controlled trials. In a recent report intralesional granulocyte installation and concomitant IFN-γ were employed for the treatment of multiple hepatic abscesses, with clinical and radiographic improvement. Cyclosporine has also been used successfully in the treatment of CGD colitis in a 12-year-old boy, however, the risk-benefit ratio of this treatment must be carefully evaluated because infectious complications can be disastrous.

Prenatal diagnosis can be achieved by sequencing fetal DNA obtained from amniocentesis or chorionic villus sampling. In a recent publication, a p47 phox-deficient EBV-transformed B-cell line underwent successful transfer with a functional p47-phox cDNA, restoring its capacity to generate superoxide. This successful gene transfer in vitro is encouraging for future strategies in human gene therapy.

SUGGESTED READING

Curnette JT. Disorders of phagocyte function. In: Hoffman R, Benz EJ, Shattil SF, eds. Hematology: Basic principles and practice. 2nd ed. 1995. New York: Churchill Livingstone, 1995.

Etzioni A, Frydman M, Pollack S, Avidor I. Brief report: Recurrent severe infections caused by a novel leukocyte adhesion deficiency. N Engl J Med 1992; 327:1789–1792.

Gallin JI. Disorders of phagocytic cells. In: Gallin JI, Goldstein IM, Snyderman R, eds. Inflammation: Basic principles and clinical correlates. 2nd ed. New York: Raven Press, 1992.

Klempner MS, Malech HL. Phagocytes: Normal and abnormal neutrophil host defenses. In: Gorbach SL, Bartlett JG, Blacklow NR, eds. Infectious Diseases. 2nd ed. Philadelphia: WB Saunders, 1995.

Klempner MS, Styrt B. Prevention of recurrent staphylococcal skin infections with low-dose oral clindamycin therapy. JAMA 1988; 260:2682–2685.

EOSINOPHILIA-MYALGIA SYNDROME ASSOCIATED WITH L-TRYPTOPHAN INGESTION

LEE D. KAUFMAN, M.D., F.A.C.P.
LAUREN B. KRUPP, M.D.

GENERAL BACKGROUND OF CLINICAL DISEASE AND ETIOPATHOGENESIS

The eosinophilia-myalgia syndrome (EMS) is a unique multisystem disorder. It has been recognized since 1989 when an epidemic developed in association with the ingestion of L-tryptophan–containing products. Clinical and epidemiologic studies during the past 5 years have defined the natural history and outcome of EMS. The overlapping features of this recently described disease with systemic sclerosis, eosinophilic fasciitis, systemic lupus erythematous, and the Spanish toxic oil syndrome (1981) related to the ingestion of denatured rapeseed oil, highlight the critical role of environmental agents in the development of idiopathic connective tissue diseases.

EMS includes acute, intermediate, and chronic stages (Table 1). Significant morbidity (Table 2) and a mortality estimated to be 2.7 percent after the first year of disease have been reported. The acute illness is characterized by diffuse erythematous maculopapular skin rashes and striking peripheral edema in association with fever, fatigue, and weight loss. Over the course of days to weeks, proximal myopathy, peripheral neuropathy, scleroderma-like skin thickening (diffuse, limited, or localized), xerostomia, and alopecia are characteristic clinical manifestations.

The chronic sequelae of EMS continue to evolve with predominantly neuromuscular, articular, and constitutional symptoms. These consist of distinctive muscle cramping that has been related to myoclonus in some patients, arthralgia (and rarely polyarticular synovitis), myalgia, and peripheral neuropathy, which is occasionally progressive. Movement disorders, including a postural tremor and myokymia, have been identified in some patients. Marked sclerodermatous thickening persists among some patients, although a general trend has been softening with cosmetically disturbing hyperpigmentation over the trunk and extremities.

Chronic dyspnea is also a common and frequently difficult problem. In some cases, dyspnea can be ascribed to interstitial lung disease or pulmonary hypertension. In most patients, it is probably related to respiratory muscle fatigue. In these individuals, clinical impression can be substantiated by the demonstration of normal results on pulmonary functions tests (with and without exercise) and echocardiography, in association with abnormal mouth pressure measurements of inspiratory force.

A high prevalence of severe fatigue and chronic neuropsychiatric disorders are noted among EMS patients. These include primarily sleep disturbance, depressive symptoms, and cognitive deficits. Some of these problems are likely to be premorbid conditions exacerbated by the development of a systemic disease. Others appear to develop concurrently with EMS.

Insomnia is particularly common among EMS patients, since many of them originally took L-tryptophan for this complaint. In many cases sleep problems become more severe as a result of pain and mood changes. Self-reported sleep difficulties are correlated with self-reported depressive symptoms and fatigue.

Table 1 Clinical Stages of EMS

Acute (≤2 mo)	*Intermediate (2-6 mo)*	*Chronic (>6 mo)*
Myalgia	Myalgia	Myalgia
Arthralgia[a]	Arthralgia	Arthralgia[a]
Fever/fatigue	Fatigue	Fatigue
Diffuse erythematous rash	Scleroderma-like skin thickening[b]	Scleroderma-like skin thickening[b]
Hyperesthesia	Neuropathy[c]	Neuropathy[d]
Dyspnea/cough[e]	Dyspnea[f]	Dyspnea[g]
Diarrhea	Myopathy	Myopathy
Myocarditis	Muscle cramps	Muscle cramps[h]
	Alopecia	Cutaneous hyperpigmentation
	Xerostomia	Cognitive impairment
		Tremor[i]
		Myokymia

[a]Occasional synovitis.
[b]Peau d'orange (eosinophilic fasciitis) and/or induration resembling systemic sclerosis (diffuse, limited, or localized).
[c]Sensory or sensorimotor (occasionally with ascending Guillain-Barré–like paralysis).
[d]Sensory or sensorimotor > mononeuritis multiplex.
[e]Parenchymal or interstitial infiltrates > pulmonary hypertension.
[f]Interstitial lung disease; pulmonary hypertension.
[g]Respiratory muscle fatigue > interstitial lung disease; pulmonary hypertension.
[h]In some patients associated with myoclonus.
[i]Effort and posture related.

Fatigue is present in almost all patients. In some, it is less intense following recovery from the acute phase of EMS, but for a large proportion it lingers as a persistent problem. Fatigue severity correlates with pain intensity and depressive symptoms. Many EMS patients use a variety of medications for various problems (pain, insomnia, muscle spasm, and other concurrent medical disorders). Fatigue appears to be greater for patients on multiple medications compared to those on only one or two drugs, suggesting that medication side effects may also contribute to fatigue.

Cognitive complaints, consisting of problems with memory, concentration, and confusion, are reported by over two-thirds of patients to have followed EMS. Neuropsychologic testing reveals that most individuals with EMS have high levels of premorbid intellectual ability, scoring high on standard intelligence test measures and in reading skills. However, specific cognitive areas appear to be affected in EMS. These patients performed poorly on tests of verbal memory retrieval, visual memory, and motor speed compared to age- and education-matched healthy controls. Statistically adjusting for group differences in depressive symptoms does not change these findings. EMS patients score worse in these same cognitive areas when compared to controls matched for level of depressive symptoms. Therefore, depression does not fully explain the cognitive impairment. In prospective studies conducted over 2 years at our institution, cognitive function has remained the same in most patients. At the present time, neuropsychologic testing in EMS is most useful for assessing neurocognitive function over time in symptomatic patients and should not be considered for establishing a diagnosis.

Mood disturbance is a well-recognized feature of chronic illness. The majority of EMS patients report symptoms of depression. However, structured psychiatric interviews, which have greater specificity and accuracy than symptom surveys in diagnosing psychiatric conditions, reveal that only 5 to 25 percent of EMS patients have current psychiatric disorders of which depression and dysthymia occur the most frequently. Cognitive deficits are as common in EMS patients with concurrent psychiatric disorders as they are in those without.

Epidemiologic data have demonstrated discordant results regarding the potential role of age and amount of L-tryptophan consumed as potential risk factors of disease. No study has demonstrated an association with EMS and gender. In one survey, a reduced severity of disease was reported in those patients who had consumed a daily multivitamin during the 3 months before EMS onset.

The etiology of EMS remains unknown. Nevertheless, analysis of implicated L-tryptophan from the 1989 epidemic has demonstrated a link with at least two contaminants that have been identified by high performance liquid chromatography as 1, 1′-ethylidenebis (tryptophan) (EBT), known as peak E or peak 97, and 3-(phenylamino)alanine (PAA) referred to as peak UV-5. Of note, PAA is chemically similar to an aniline derivative identified in samples of implicated oil from the toxic oil syndrome, suggesting potential pathogenic overlap between the two epidemics. However, these agents have not yet been demonstrated to be causative in animal models and may simply be surrogate markers for an unidentified agent(s).

Accumulated clinical, pathologic, and serologic evidence suggests important roles for cellular and humoral immune-mediated injury and fibrosis in the pathogenesis of EMS. This includes the presence of inflammatory cell infiltrates in skin, muscle, and nerve, of activated T lymphocytes, macrophages, eosinophils, fibroblasts, and mast cells, and the detection of antinuclear antibodies in the sera of approximately 50 percent of patients from clinical case series during acute disease. At least two potentially specific autoantibodies have been identified by immunoprecipitation: one recognizing an antigen with an approximate molecular weight of 63 kD and a second pattern consisting of a strong 110 kD band coupled with a weak 95 kD band. These antigenic proteins have not been further characterized. In addition, immunohistochemical studies have demonstrated a role for transforming growth factor beta and platelet-derived growth factor in the fibrosis accompanying the inflammatory lesions of skin, muscle, and nerve.

Table 2 Prevalence of Selected Chronic Features in EMS*

Manifestation	*Percentage*
Fatigue	35-95
Myalgia	50-91
Neuropathy	30-91
Muscle cramps	43-90
Subjective cognitive impairment	33-86
Sclerodermatous skin change	44-82
Arthralgia	41-77
Myopathy	40-75
Dyspnea	8-50
Hyperpigmentation	25-42

*Summary of follow-up data ranging from 12 to 36 months.

DIAGNOSIS OF EMS

Formal clinical and/or laboratory criteria for the diagnosis of EMS have not been established. The initial diagnostic guidelines formulated in 1989 by the Centers for Disease Control (CDC) for national surveillance (Table 3) are thought by some to have underestimated the total number of individuals effected with EMS by approximately twofold to threefold. Observations among case series have indicated that peripheral blood eosinophilia may be absent in patients who otherwise demonstrate many representative clinical and/or pathologic features of EMS. This may be important in helping to identify sporadic cases of EMS, and in differentiating them from related disorders. During acute or subacute disease, the constellation of myalgia, scleroderma-like skin changes (most often resembling eosinophilic fascii-

Table 3 Initial CDC Surveillance Criteria for the Diagnosis of EMS

Peripheral blood eosinophilia of $\geq 1{,}000$ cells/mm^3
Generalized myalgia (at some point during the course of illness) of sufficient severity to affect a patient's ability to pursue his or her usual daily activities
Absence of an infection or neoplasm that could account for the eosinophilia or myalgia

tis), paresthesias, alopecia, and typical muscle cramping (frequently with trismus and subcostal involvement) are highly suggestive of EMS, and can be confirmed by the relatively specific neuropathologic findings (in that clinical setting) of perimyositis and epineuritis on muscle and nerve biopsies, respectively.

Unfortunately, there is no single diagnostic test currently available for EMS. The unique finding of an elevated serum aldolase (usually with a normal or low creatine kinase), in association with the clinical and biopsy findings, will distinguish EMS from myopathic or eosinophilic diseases such as polymyositis, the idiopathic hypereosinophilic syndrome, eosinophilic fasciitis (unrelated to EMS), and the Churg-Strauss subset of systemic necrotizing vasculitis. Serologic markers such as the autoantibodies previously referred to might prove to be suggestive; however, they have thus far been found in only a minority (15 percent) of patients.

In patients with chronic disease, symptoms at initial physician contact may be nonspecific and a suspected diagnosis is dependent upon data collected retrospectively. The muscle biopsy findings of late stage EMS are not well delineated and have not been as helpful as during acute disease. Moreover, the late manifestations of EMS must be carefully differentiated from the protean features of idiopathic connective diseases, chronic fatigue syndrome, soft tissue rheumatic syndromes (i.e., fibromyalgia), and unrelated neuromuscular disorders.

Careful categorization of isolated cases of EMS and related syndromes should assist in identifying additional environmental agents as triggers of rheumatic diseases. In that regard, L-tryptophan (or the etiologic contaminant of EMS) is the first agent to be clearly associated with eosinophilic fasciitis, a scleroderma spectrum disorder previously postulated to be drug- or toxin-induced.

THERAPY

Reports on therapy consist of anecdotal observations only. This is due to the highly epidemic nature with which EMS occurs, the distribution of a relatively small number of cases over many states, and the lack of previous experience with this disease. No specific therapy has been demonstrated to alter the natural history of EMS. In spite of these limitations, cumulative experience with EMS has led to some degree of consensus regarding management. Recommendations should be individualized depending upon the needs and clinical findings of each patient.

Cumulative Experience in Acute EMS

The abrupt onset of multisystem disease and inflammatory infiltrative lesions of skin, muscle, and nerve initially led most clinicians to extrapolate therapy from experience with idiopathic connective tissue diseases. Multiple immunomodulating agents were subsequently employed with disappointing results. Contrary to previous experience with corticosteroids, which have been quite effective for most acute diseases associated with peripheral blood and tissue eosinophilia, these appeared to be of very little use for the early or late clinical manifestations of EMS. The most impressive impact of these agents appeared to be on resolution of acute pulmonary infiltrates. In some physician-patient evaluations, modest global improvement and a decrease in myalgia and peripheral edema were noted. Nevertheless, retrospective epidemiologic surveys and 5 years of prospective clinical observations indicate that corticosteroids do not appear to influence the development of cutaneous, neuropathic, or chronic cardiopulmonary disease and cannot be advocated for these purposes. A short course of moderate to high-dose prednisone therapy (40 to 60 mg per day for 2 to 4 weeks with subsequent tapering over an additional 1 to 2 months) would be appropriate to assess individual response during acute disease. Chronic therapy with these agents in doses larger than 5 mg of prednisone per day is not indicated in EMS.

There also appears to have been little objective improvement in disease progression with the use of more aggressive immunosuppressive or cytotoxic therapy such as cyclophosphamide, azathioprine, hydroxyurea, or cyclosporine. In one study, methotrexate (7.5 to 10 mg per week) was evaluated prospectively in seven EMS patients over a mean of 4.5 months. A significant ($p < 0.05$) increase in functional class and reductions in skin thickening (assessed by total skin score) and edema were reported. These findings are encouraging; however, in the absence of a control group or data confirming these results from other centers, it is difficult to assess the measured improvement as related to therapy or secondary to natural history. Plasmapheresis and intravenous gammaglobulin have also been utilized with reports of subjective improvement in some individuals. Unfortunately, these potentially toxic and/or expensive interventions cannot be recommended because of a paucity of data demonstrating efficacy.

Anti-inflammatory or antirheumatic agents, including plaquenil, D-penicillamine, colchicine, isotretenoin, and flavinoids, have been advocated in small numbers of patients. As with other isolated reports of benefit, there is a lack of definition as to how improvement or resolution was determined in these subjects.

A tryptophanase adsorption column approved for the therapy of certain neoplastic diseases was reported to be helpful in at least one individual; however, this was not subsequently confirmed in other patients. Because it is unlikely that native tryptophan itself induced EMS, this does not appear to be an optimal form of treatment.

Oral administration of biologically "pure" (nonimplicated) tryptophan (500 to 3,000 mg per day) was

Table 4 Recommended Pharmacologic Therapy for Common Symptoms of Chronic EMS

	Agent	*Dosage*
Muscle Cramping	Amitriptyline (Elavil)	10-50 mg/day
	Baclofen (Lioresal)	10-80 mg/day
	Dantrolene (Dantrium)*	25-150 mg/day
	Cyclobenzaprine (Flexeril)	10-40 mg/day
	Benzodiazepines†	
Depression	Amitriptyline (Elavil)	10-200 mg/day
	Fluoxetine (Prozac)	20-60 mg/day
	Sertraline (Zoloft)	50-200 mg/day
Insomnia	Amitripytline (Elavil)	10-100 mg/day
	Trazodone (Desyrel)	25-100 mg/day
	Benzodiazepines†	
Fatigue	Pemoline (Cylert)	18.75-112.5 mg/day
	Amantadine (Symmetrel)	200 mg/day
	Methylphenidate (Ritalin)†	2.5-20 mg/day
	Fluoxetine (Prozac)	20 mg/day
Neuropathy	Amitripytline (Elavil)	10-100 mg/day
	Nortriptyline (Pamelor)	10-75 mg/day

*Potential for significant hepatotoxicity.
†In selected patients.

reported to produce improvement in all 20 patients treated in an open-label regimen. Outcome measurements were not specified, and this preliminary study has not been confirmed by a placebo-controlled trial. This unconventional approach should be viewed with caution and at present cannot be recommended.

Based upon the available information just summarized, no clear therapeutic efficacy has been demonstrated with any form of immunomodulatory treatment implemented to date. In view of these findings, most clinicians experienced in the care of EMS patients have concluded that immunosuppressive agents are not recommended for the cutaneous, neuromuscular, or constitutional manifestations of the disease.

Recommended Approach to Chronic EMS

The management of late EMS should be predicated upon the severity of symptoms. At our institution a multidisciplinary approach is utilized based upon neurologic, rheumatologic, neuropsychologic, psychiatric, and rehabilitative evaluations. Recommended agents of some benefit for the common features of chronic EMS are summarized in Table 4.

Myalgia, Neuropathy, and Muscle Cramping

Chronic myalgia does not respond to corticosteroid therapy, which should be avoided in view of the potential for long-term toxicity. Nonsteroidal anti-inflammatory agents, tricyclic antidepressants, cyclobenzaprine, benzodiazepines, dantrolene, and baclofen have all been employed for pain of neuromuscular origin with highly variable results. Although many patients demonstrate little benefit from these agents, careful titration either alone or in combination can result in a gratifying and long-lasting response. Preliminary studies have demonstrated abnormally low levels of tissue magnesium in patients with EMS, suggesting that replacement may be of clinical benefit. This is currently being evaluated in a multicenter study. Muscle pain in some patients has been so severe as to provoke suicide. For this reason, carefully supervised therapy with narcotic analgesics may be necessary (albeit they are often of only partial benefit). Intensive physical therapy has been reported to be very effective for some patients with severe neuropathy.

Dyspnea

In a minority of patients with EMS whose chronic dyspnea is demonstrated to be secondary to pulmonary hypertension, the therapeutic modalities currently available for treatment of primary pulmonary hypertension should be utilized. In some patients pulmonary hypertension resulting from EMS appears to improve with time and may be reversible. For those patients with established disease, therapy could include high-dose calcium channel blocking agents and consideration of continuous prostacyclin infusion (by ambulatory pump). Heart-lung transplantation may be appropriate for selected individuals with progressive disease.

Insomnia

In patients with sleep disturbance, certain symptoms may require further evaluation. Individuals with excessive snoring, apneic episodes, daytime sleepiness, and sleep attacks may benefit from polysomnography. Sleep disturbance in many cases can be managed by improved sleep hygiene. Avoiding daytime naps and sleeping only in designated areas are useful suggestions. Occasionally insomnia requires medication. Some patients are helped by antihistamines, others require trazodone, tricyclic antidepressants, or benzodiazepines.

Fatigue

Fatigue can be treated by first reviewing possible contributing factors. Improved management of pain can often ameliorate fatigue. Identifying sleep disorders is important. Patients with concurrent depression may not improve with respect to fatigue unless the depression is also treated. However, in our experience the correlation coefficient between fatigue and depression is only 0.4, indicating that fatigue can only partially be explained by depressive symptoms.

A behavioral approach administered by a psychologist knowledgeable in the methods applied for chronic pain can be helpful by allowing patients to better cope with fatigue, dwell on it less, and perform at a higher level of activity. For some individuals, rest periods are essential; others benefit from escalating exercise programs.

In some cases medication is appropriate. Medications widely used to treat fatigue in other disorders (such as multiple sclerosis) can also be used with good results in EMS. These include energizing antidepressants (fluoxetine, sertraline), dopaminergic agents (amantadine), and mild CNS stimulants (pemoline). In selected patients stronger stimulants such as methylphenidate may be appropriate.

Cognitive Deficits

Cognitive impairment is difficult to remediate. The role of cognitive rehabilitation is controversial. However, formal evaluation with a neuropsychologist will often include educating a patient regarding their cognitive strengths and weaknesses. By learning effective compensatory mechanisms, this approach can be therapeutic. Other patients require psychotherapy. In this way, individuals that are counseled will avoid exacerbating their current deficits. Pharmacologic treatment for cognitive loss has yielded conflicting results.

Mood Disturbance

Mood disturbances are very responsive to treatment in most patients. Both psychotherapy and medication have a role. Many EMS patients are extremely angry about their condition and require special counseling. Medications that may be helpful include tricyclic antidepressants (such as amitriptyline), serotoninergic agents, including fluoxetine, sertraline, and paroxetine, and trazodone. Combination treatment is often necessary.

DISCUSSION

In the absence of significant numbers of new cases, it is not likely that meaningful conclusions will become available regarding optimal therapy of acute EMS. This is of particular concern given a lack of effective therapy for two previous toxic epidemic syndromes accompanied by substantial morbidity and mortality. Although many uncertainties continue to exist regarding the prevalence, duration, and relationship to the disease process of continuing complaints in EMS, a supportive and thoughtful approach is an effective means of improving the quality of life for these patients.

Increasing interest in environmental agents will hopefully sustain a vigilant search for potential toxins that could trigger similar future epidemics. To that end, it is essential that cooperative efforts be in place prospectively to coordinate data collection and formulate appropriate therapeutic plans.

SUGGESTED READING

Clauw DJ, Ward K, Wilson B, et al. Magnesium deficiency in the eosinophilia-myalgia syndrome: Report of clinical and biochemical improvement with repletion. Arthritis Rheum 1994; 37:1331–1334.

Gaudino EA, Masur DM, Kaufman LD, et al. The effects of depression on cognitive functioning in the eosinophilia-myalgia syndrome. Neuropsychiatry, Neuropsychology, and Behavioral Neurology 1995; 8:118–126.

Kaufman LD. Eosinophilia-myalgia syndrome: Morbidity and mortality (editorial). J Rheumatol 1993; 20:1644–1646.

Kaufman LD. Evolving spectrum of eosinophilia myalgia syndrome. Rheum Dis Clin North Am 1994; 20:973–994.

Kaufman LD, Gomez-Reino JJ, Gruber BL, Miller F. Fibrogenic growth factors in the eosinophilia myalgia syndrome and the toxic oil syndrome. Arch Dermatol 1994; 130:41–47.

Krupp LB, Masur DM, Kaufman LD. Neurocognitive dysfunction in the eosinophilia-myalgia syndrome. Neurology 1993; 43:931–936.

Hertzman PA, Kaufman LD, Love LA, et al. The eosinophilia myalgia syndrome—guidelines for patient care. J Rheumatol 1995; 22: 161–163.

Varga J, Uitto J, Jimenez SA. The cause and pathogenesis of the eosinophilia-myalgia syndrome. Ann Intern Med 1992; 116:140–147.

IMMUNODEFICIENCY

COMMON VARIABLE IMMUNODEFICIENCY

MARTHA M. EIBL, M.D.

Common variable immunodeficiency (CVID) comprises a group of heterogeneous disorders characterized by hypogammaglobulinemia and the inability to produce specific antibodies after contact with a number of different antigens. Serum concentrations of one, several, or all immunoglobulin classes and subclasses may be decreased, and defects in cell-mediated immunity are variable. Previously referred to as acquired agammaglobulinemia, the term "acquired" is no longer used because "acquired immunodeficiency" is reserved to refer to patients with HIV infection.

The spectrum of the disease ranges from deficiency of a single Ig class such as IgA deficiency to agammaglobulinemia. The incidence of CVID is estimated to be 1 in 50,000 individuals, and it affects males and females equally. The usual age at presentation is the second or third decade of life, but patients with this predominantly antibody deficiency may become symptomatic at virtually any age.

CLINICAL SYMPTOMATOLOGY

The most common symptoms observed in patients with CVID, as in patients with other forms of antibody deficiency, are recurrent pyogenic infections of the upper and lower respiratory tract. These infections are often caused by encapsulated bacteria such as *Haemophilus influenzae, Streptococcus pneumoniae, Staphylococcus aureus,* and *Pseudomonas aeruginosa.* In addition, patients are susceptible to viral and fungal infections. Chronic sinusitis is often the first and leading clinical sign and the symptom that takes longest to disappear after initiation of treatment. Recurrent otitis media can lead to hearing loss, and recurrent infections of the lower respiratory tract may cause chronic progressive bronchiectasis and pulmonary failure. Infections with opportunistic pathogens such as *Pneumocystis carinii* and increased susceptibility to tuberculosis may occur and are likely due to the T-cell abnormalities often present in this disease.

Because these patients do not produce antibodies, serologic diagnosis of infections based on antibody detection is not applicable and results can only be expected on the basis of the detection of the respective microorganisms.

Hematologic disorders are fairly frequent in this patient population; between 20 and 50 percent are anemic and more than 5 percent have pernicious anemia associated with atrophic gastritis, achlorhydria, and an absence of intrinsic factor. Leukopenia and thrombocytopenia are common and may be due to autoimmune mechanisms or hypersplenism.

Gastrointestinal abnormalities are common as well. A spruelike syndrome, characterized by steatorrhea, malabsorption, folate and vitamin B_{12} deficiency, lactose intolerance, generalized disaccharidase deficiency, and protein-losing enteropathy are often seen and abnormalities of villus architecture detected. Infection with *Giardia lamblia* is frequent, and small bowel biopsy may be needed for proper diagnosis. Most patients with malabsorption syndromes and common variable immunodeficiency do not respond to a gluten-free diet. By contrast, celiac sprue associated with selective IgA deficiency often responds to gluten elimination. *Giardia* is rarely found in selective IgA deficiency.

CVID patients often develop autoimmune disease, such as thyroiditis and inflammatory joint disease resembling rheumatoid arthritis, dermatomyositis, and scleroderma. Chronic active hepatitis, parotitis, and Guillain-Barré syndrome have also been reported. Autoantibodies are often undetectable, but organ biopsies (e.g., gastric atrophy on biopsy of the stomach or lymphoid infiltration in other organs involved) are informative. Hepatosplenomegaly often present in CVID patients is usually due to lymphoid hyperplasia, which must be carefully differentiated from lymphoid malignancy. Lymphoreticular malignancies and gastrointestinal malignancies occur in this patient population with increased frequency.

IMMUNOLOGIC CHARACTERIZATION AND DIAGNOSIS

Primary diagnosis of CVID is based on the detection of hypogammaglobulinemia. Serum IgG levels are below 500 mg per deciliter and individual IgG subclasses may be decreased to different degrees. IgA and IgM concentrations are usually below the normal range, but these findings are not obligatory. However, all patients are deficient in producing IgG antibodies against ubiquitous, clinically relevant (i.e., bacterial) antigens. In the patients' blood, B cells and T cells are usually present and close to normal numbers. In rare instances B cells may be reduced. CD4-positive helper T cells may be reduced and CD8-positive effector T cells may be found in increased numbers. Lymphocyte responses to mitogens are normal in the majority of patients, but about 60 percent of patients have diminished proliferative responses to T cell–receptor stimulation and decreased induction of gene expression for IL-2, IL-4, and interferon-γ. There is no evident abnormality of the T-cell receptor. Gene analysis indicates normal heterogeneity of gene rearrangement. Decreased IL-2 production appears to result from an abnormality in CD4 cells, which could be a defect in signal transduction and correlates with diminished CD40 ligand expression.

Circulating B lymphocytes are present in CVID patients, but fail to mature and/or differentiate to secrete different classes of immunoglobulins. In a large subset of patients the defect is not intrinsic to the B cell but likely to be due to a defect in regulatory function of T lymphocytes. Patients, especially young males, with low numbers of B cells and with agammaglobulinemia have to be differentiated from patients with X-linked agammaglobulinemia (XLA). Clinical symptoms in XLA usually appear earlier. Patients with XLA do not have B lymphocytes in their circulation, and the defect, a mutation in a cytoplasmic tyrosine kinase (btk) leading to the arrest in B-cell differentiation, has been identified and localized in the long arm of the X chromosome (Xq21.3–22). Other patients with CVID who have normal or elevated levels of serum IgM with IgG and IgA lacking should be evaluated to exclude the hyper-IgM syndrome; 70 percent of patients with this disease show X-linked inheritance. The gene has been localized on the X chromosome (Xq26), and these patients have mutations in a glycoprotein gp39 expressed on the surface of helper T cells. This glycoprotein constitutes the ligand for CD40 on B cells and is needed for immunoglobulin class switching in B cells.

CVID must be distinguished from secondary immunodeficiency disease due to protein loss. Because the gastrointestinal (GI) tract is more commonly involved in CVID than in other forms of antibody deficiency syndromes, malabsorption and weight loss as well as diarrhea may be present at first clinical presentation, and sometimes proper diagnosis will have to await successful treatment of these conditions. The inheritance of CVID is autosomal recessive, and individual cases often appear to be sporadic. Individuals with IgA deficiency and with autoimmune disease are often found in first-degree relatives, suggesting a genetic basis of immunologic dysregulation. An association between CVID and a selected group of the major histocompatibility (MHC) genes (MHC class I, class II, and class III genes) on the short arm of chromosome arm 6 has been established. The MHC gene complex is essential and contains elements involved in antigen presentation and cognate T- or B-cell interaction as well as genes of unknown function. The association between the extended MHC haplotype and CVID is not obligatory, that is, histoidentical siblings of patients may be healthy, and CVID patients may be identified who do not express the extended haplotype.

TREATMENT

Immunoglobulin Replacement

Immunoglobulin replacement is the treatment of choice in patients with CVID. All patients with significantly diminished IgG levels and/or demonstrated severe impairment of antibody production should receive IgG replacement. Patients with less pronounced hypogammaglobulinemia (IgG serum levels 300 to 500 mg per deciliter) will need immunoglobulin therapy if they present with chronic sinusitis, recurrent otitis media, and especially with chronic obstructive lung disease.

Previously, antibody-deficient patients were treated with human serum immunoglobulin (HSIG) for intramuscular use. These products contained 16 percent immunoglobulin, mainly IgG. The initial loading dose was approximately 250 mg per kilogram given as 50 mg per kilogram IM injections on 5 consecutive days at different sites, followed by 100 mg per kilogram per month, usually divided into weekly or biweekly doses. The disadvantages of the intramuscular application of IgG are obvious. The injections are painful, the amounts that can be given are limited, absorption of the IgG from the local deposit is slow and incomplete, proteolytic degradation occurs at the injection site, and peak IgG serum levels representing 25 to 50 percent of the injected dose are not reached until several days after administration. Adverse reactions, both immediate and delayed, have been described in 15 to 55 percent of the recipients, and the transmission of viral agents such as hepatitis, even though rare, has been reported.

More recently HSIG preparations for intramuscular use have been given subcutaneously. This mode of application is now being tested in clinical trials. It is, however, important to realize that products for IM use are formulated with mercury-containing preservatives, and high-dose treatment carries the risk of chronic mercury poisoning. Thus, HSIG products to be applied in large amounts subcutaneously will have to be free of these preservatives.

During the last decade several gammaglobulin preparations for IV use (IVIG) have become available. Because of differences in the methods of production and purification, there are differences in chemical structure, electrophoretic profile, subclass composition, and aggregate content between the individual preparations. The early generation preparations produced by intensive enzyme treatment or chemical modification have been found to lack complete Fc function and cannot be considered satisfactory for the treatment of antibody-deficient patients. The products currently available have been mildly treated with proteolytic enzymes such as pepsin, by immobilized hydrolases, or treated during fractionation by adsorption to DEAE-Sephadex or PEG precipitation. These preparations have been shown to meet the requirements for safety, antibody content, in vivo half-life, and clinical efficacy. The convenience, ease of administration, and relative freedom from major side effects make this mode of application highly preferable. As much higher doses could be delivered by the IV route, it became evident that for the majority of patients the dose of gammaglobulin given intramuscularly was inadequate. Immediately after intravenous administration 100 percent of the infused dose can be found in the intravascular space. Over the next 3 to 4 days the infused material equilibrates with the extravascular pool and 70 to 80 percent of the dose remains in the circulation. Several studies indicate that half-life in normal controls and in immunodeficient patients varies from 17 to 30 days for total IgG. To maintain "trough" serum IgG levels 200 to 400 mg per deciliter above those produced by the patient, 300 to 500 mg IgG per kilogram per month (150 to 250 mg per kilogram every 2 weeks) will be required. If IV replacement is started early and if sufficient amounts are given with sufficient frequency, recurrent infections can be prevented and progressive lung damage can be arrested. It has been documented that high-dose treatment (500 to 600 mg per kilogram per month) may improve abnormal pulmonary function even in patients who had developed bronchiectasis.

Table 1 lists IVIG products that are licensed to be used in the treatment of primary immunodeficiency diseases. Most of these products are lyophylized and have to be reconstituted with diluent. Single dose vials or packages are available containing 500 mg to 12.5 g. Gamimune is formulated to a 5 percent solution. As these preparations are produced from large donor pools, they contain comparable amounts of antibodies with a broad spectrum of specificity, and IgG Fc-mediated functions (e.g., reactivity with FcγR-expressing cells and complement activation) are preserved.

Table 1 IVIG Products

IVIG Products	*Manufacturer*
Venoglobulin I, Venoglobulin S	Alpha Therapeutic Corp.
Polygam	American Red Cross, (prepared using Hyland's facilities)
Gammar IV	Armour Pharmaceutical
Gamimune	Cutter Biological Miles P.D.
Gammagard	Hyland Division of Baxter
Iveegam	Immuno U.S.
Sandoglobulin	Sandoz Pharmaceuticals Corp.

Adverse Reactions

Systemic reactions to IVIG have been described and occur in about 4 percent of patients repeatedly, but occur more often after the first and second application. Anxiety, back pain, chills, headache, pruritis, nausea, flushing, tightness of the chest, dizziness, hypotension, and pallor have been reported. Immediate anaphylactic and hypersensitivity reactions have been observed in exceptional cases. Reactions to IVIG are usually mild and transient and can be controlled by slowing the rate of infusion. Some of the infusion-related side effects may be due to reaction between free antigen in the circulation of the recipient and the antibodies administered, and this might be the reason why reactions are more likely to occur at the initiation of treatment and when the interval between infusions has been prolonged to 2 months or longer. Profoundly hypogammaglobulinemic patients are reaction prone, and so are patients with fever or an acute infection. Dividing the dose at initiation of treatment (e.g., 20 mg per kilogram and 30 mg per kilogram on the first day and 50 mg per kilogram twice on the second day) may be helpful. It is advisable to start infusion slowly at a rate of 0.01 ml per kilogram per minute, increasing it to 0.02 ml per kilogram per minute after 15 to 30 minutes. Most patients tolerate a gradual increase to 0.03 to 0.08 ml per kilogram per minute (1.8 to 4.8 ml per kilogram per hour). One to two tablets of aspirin or an antihistamine (e.g., 50 mg diphenhydramine-hydrochloride-benadryl IV before the infusion) can be given to prevent reaction. Hydrocortisone has also been applied, but it is usually unnecessary if the previously mentioned precautions are taken.

Only very rarely can reactions be attributed to antibodies against IgA. Antibodies to IgA have been detected in 17 to 40 percent of IgA-deficient individuals; however, in most instances individuals with detectable IgA antibodies in their circulation tolerate IVIG infusions well. IVIG infusions may be given to most of these patients with due caution. In very few patients IgE antibodies to IgA or to an IgG subclass were documented and reported to be the basis for severe immediate hypersensitivity reactions. In most instances, however, the true reason for reactogenicity is the presence of aggregates in the gammaglobulin preparations leading to reactions by releasing vasoactive mediators via the Fcγ-receptor. The reactions are anaphylactoid in nature and are most likely to occur in those who are agammaglobulinemic, thus in patients who are unable to produce antibodies to IgA.

Infusions of large amounts of IVIG may also lead to late complications. Such complications have been observed in patients treated for autoimmune diseases when high doses of IVIG, 1 to 2 g per kilogram, were given. The mechanism of action has not yet been identified but may be due to increased protein levels. These complications include rise in plasma viscosity, transient rise in serum creatinine, and aseptic meningitis.

Transmission of viral agents by IVIG is of steady concern because IVIG is usually prepared from the plasma of 5,000 to 10,000 or more blood and/or plasma donations. The experience gained with intramuscular preparations with respect to hepatitis B (HB) transmission has indicated that if the single donations of plasma were free of detectable HB surface antigen and if appropriate fractionation methodology were used, the end product could be considered safe with regard to the transmission of viral hepatitis. On the other hand, hepatitis B has been transmitted by intramuscular immunoglobulin in a number of instances when inadequate starting material and/or fractionation methodology was used. Plasma donations have to be nonreactive with licensed tests for HB surface antigen. The requirement for the presence of hepatitis B antibodies in IVIG preparations is an additional safety measure against transmission of this viral disease.

There is no documented case of transmission of HIV by an immunoglobulin product, not even in the early 1980s, when HIV transmission did occur with other preparations made of human plasma such as coagulation factors. The reason is that partition and inactivation of HIV during cold ethanol fractionation, and additional manufacturing steps have been effective in removing HIV from the plasma pool. More recently additional inactivation steps for IVIG products have been included to guarantee viral safety.

Since the 1980s small outbreaks of non-A, non B-hepatitis, probably hepatitis C, occurred in England, Scotland, Sweden, and the United States and were associated with the use of particular batches of IVIG, suggesting that transmission depended on the extent of viral load of the starting material and/or was connected with pilot production and thus not completely validated manufacturing practices. In the absence of a screening test for hepatitis C (HCV) antigen and antibody, most manufacturers used liver enzyme determinations as surrogate markers. More recently, HCV antibody testing and exclusion of HCV antibody-positive plasma from plasma pools was introduced and believed to improve hepatitis C viral safety. The opposite view has also been expressed, that is, that hepatitis C antibodies may be important, in analogy to hepatitis B, in preventing the transmission of hepatitis C. However, the view that HCV antibodies are a marker of infectivity prevailed, and since early 1993 all anti-HCV antibody positive donations have been excluded from plasma pools before fractionation. Still, between October 1993 and June 1994 a major outbreak of hepatitis C connected with the application of two products, produced by the same manufacturer using the same methodology, did occur. The HCV-contaminated lots have been recalled by the manufacturer. Currently available evidence on the extensive use of other licensed products provides no indication of viral transmission. Still, manufacturers are making continuous efforts to increase safety with respect to viral transmission by additional steps of viral inactivation and/or applying new technology in testing the products for freedom from viral constituents.

Antimicrobial Chemotherapy and Other Considerations

Chronic sinusitis is a frequent medical problem in CVID patients. Symptoms include nasal congestion and discharge; pain may be intermittent and a low-grade fever may be present. Patients may have a chronic cough due to postnasal drip. The most common organisms are *H. influenzae, S. pneumoniae* and other streptococci, and *Moraxella.* If purulent discharge is present, antibiotic treatment with amoxicillin-clavulanic acid, trimethoprim-sulfamethoxazole, or a second-generation cefalosporin for 2 to 4 weeks may be advisable. Patients with sinusitis that has not resolved following this antimicrobial therapy may be evaluated by endoscopy to obtain adequate specimens for culture, and endoscopic sinosurgery may be required to obtain histologic diagnosis, remove polyps, and establish proper ventilation of infected sinuses.

If chronic otitis media or chronic draining ear is present, the local bacterial flora often includes, in addition to the common pyogenic organism, *P. aeruginosa, S. aureus,* and anaerobic pathogens. Treatment is directed at eradicating infection with a combination of local care, antibacterial ear drops, and systemic antibiotics which, if possible, are selected according to antibiotic sensitivities defined by culture.

Chronic or recurrent lower respiratory tract infections in CVID may facilitate the development of bronchiectases. For patients with bronchiectasis and infrequent exacerbations, antibiotics are commonly used only during acute episodes. In patients with chronic purulent sputum despite short courses of antibiotics, more prolonged courses (e.g., with oral amoxicillin or trimethoprim-sulfamethoxazole) or intermittent but regular courses of rotating antibiotics may be used. If *Pseudomonas aeruginosa* is present, oral therapy with a quinolone or parenteral therapy with an aminoglycoside or third-generation cefalosporin may be appropriate. When bronchiectasis is localized and the morbidity is substantial, surgical resection of the involved region of the lung should be considered.

In chronic upper and lower respiratory tract infection combining intensive antibiotic treatment with a higher dose of IVIG therapy, 250 to 300 mg per kilogram biweekly over a period of 2 to 3 months may prove efficient. A similar regimen may also be carried out before and after operations.

In the treatment of *Giardia lamblia* infection, metronidazole (200 mg three times daily for 5 days) and quinacrine (100 mg twice daily for 5 days) are effective. Patients who fail to respond to initial treatment can be retreated with another drug or a longer course of the same drug. In cases refractory to multiple treatment courses, combined therapy with metronidazole (750 mg three times daily for 21 days) and quinacrine (100 mg twice daily for 21 days) has been successful.

SUGGESTED READING

Buckley RH, Schiff RI. The use of intravenous immune globulin in immunodeficiency diseases. N Engl J Med 1991; 325:110–117.

From the Centers for Disease Control and Prevention. Outbreak of hepatitis C associated with intravenous immunoglobulin admin-

istration—United States, October 1993-June 1994. JAMA 1994; 272:424–425.
Chapel HM for the Consensus Panel for the Diagnosis and Management of Primary Antibody Deficiencies. Consensus on diagnosis and management of primary antibody deficiencies. BMJ 1994; 308: 581–585.
Cunningham-Rundles C. Clinical and immunological analyses of 103 patients with common variable immunodeficiency. J Clin Immunol 1989; 9:22–33.
Eibl MM, Wedgwood RJ. Intravenous immunoglobulin: A review. Immunodefic Rev 1989; 1 (suppl):1–92.
Fischer GW. Uses of intravenous globulin to prevent or treat infections. Adv Pediat Infect Dis 1992; 7:85–108.
Fischer MB, Hauber I, Eggenbauer H, et al. A defect in the early phase of T-cell receptor-mediated T-cell activation in patients with common variable immunodeficiency. Blood 1994; 84: 4234–4244.
Genetic basis of primary immunodeficiencies. Immunol Rev 1994; entire volume 138. Ed. Göran Möller, Stockholm.
NIH Consensus Conference. Intravenous immunoglobulin: Prevention and treatment of disease. JAMA 1990; 264:3189–3193.
NIH Consensus Staement. Moderator: Sneller MC. New insights into common variable immunodeficiency. Ann Intern Med 1993; 118: 720–730.
Rosen FS, Cooper MD, Wedgwood RJP. The primary immunodeficiencies. N Engl J Med 1995; 333:431–440.

SEVERE COMBINED IMMUNODEFICIENCY DISEASE

ZEINA E. BAZ, M.D.
RAIF S. GEHA, M.D.

Severe combined immunodeficiency disease (SCID) is a term used to describe a heterogeneous group of genetic disorders of lymphoid development that result in a profound state of immunodeficiency characterized by the inability of T lymphocytes to respond to mitogens, antigens, or allogeneic cells and of B cells to generate an antibody in response to an antigen stimulus.

Clinically, three major phenotypic forms of SCID have been identified: (1) classic SCID, characterized by both T and B lymphocytopenia and agammaglobulinemia; (2) the more common SCID with B lymphocytes, in which normal to high numbers of B cells and variable quantities of serum immunoglobulins without demonstrable antibody activity are detected; and (3) SCID associated with adenosine deaminase (ADA) deficiency, which may present with either of the above lymphoid phenotypes.

The syndrome is present in infants with no circulating lymphocytes as well as those with normal numbers of T and B lymphocytes. Transplacental engraftment of maternal lymphocytes can occasionally result in the presence of adequate numbers of circulating T cells; however, T-cell function is always poor.

Affected children initially appear healthy, but within the first 6 months of life they become ill with recurrent infections caused by a variety of bacteria, viruses, and opportunistic pathogens. The overall pattern is one of failure to thrive. Oral candidiasis (thrush), pneumonia, especially that caused by *Pneumocystis carinii,* and protracted diarrhea are the most common manifestations, and infants fail to thrive as early as 2 to 3 months of age.

In SCID patients, live vaccines can cause overwhelming infection as with the smallpox vaccination in the past and more recently, Calmette-Guéin bacillus. Orally administered attenuated poliovirus rarely gives rise to poliomyelitis, probably because of neutralization by immunoglobulin G of maternal origin or by the slow onset of the infection.

The disease exists in both X-linked and autosomal recessive forms. The male to female ratio is 3:1 or 4:1. If untreated, most infants die before 12 months of age.

A number of different molecular causes of SCID phenotypes have been found, ranging from the absence of the appropriate lymphoid precursors (reticular dysgenesis, Swiss type SCID), to defects in the expression of surface molecules that are critical for immune responses (SCID with MHC class II deficiency, TCR/CD3 deficiency, CD7 deficiency), to specific enzyme deficiencies involved in the purine salvage pathway, mainly adenosine deaminase deficiency and purine nucleoside phosphorylase deficiency. All of these defects are usually inherited as autosomal recessive.

Recently, the molecular defect in X-linked severe combined immunodeficiency disease, which constitutes the majority of patients with SCID, has been assigned to the gene encoding the chain of the interleukin-2 receptor, IL-2 receptor gamma. There is now compelling evidence that IL-2 receptor gamma is a common gamma chain that is part of other cytokine receptors, namely IL-4, IL-7, and IL-9, IL-13, and IL-15 receptors in addition to IL-2 receptor. This would explain why T-cell development is absent in X-linked SCID but not in isolated IL-2 deficiency. Also, given the role of IL-2, IL-4, and IL-7 in B-cell activation and differentiation, gamma chain deficiency may explain why B cells from X-linked SCIDs fail to function after successful T-cell engraftment.

Very recently, a deficiency in the IL-2 receptor gamma chain-associated Janus Kinase 3 (JAK 3) was found to result in SCID with a phenotype similar to that of X-linked SCID (i.e., no T cells, normal number of B cells).

GENERAL THERAPEUTIC CONSIDERATIONS

Adequate caloric and fluid intake, reverse isolation, and appropriate antibiotic and fungal therapy are the mainstays of the supportive therapeutic program.

Patients with SCID are highly susceptible to the development of acute graft-versus-host disease (GVHD) after the administration of blood or blood products. Administration of as little as 5 cc of blood to these children has resulted in death from acute GVHD. To avoid this problem, fully oxygen saturated blood should be irradiated to eliminate viable white blood cells that may inappropriately engraft the patient. Blood transfusion is also safe when processed by freezing and centrifugation. However, lymphocytes are still viable in outdated blood, washed red blood cells, unprocessed plasma, and platelet preparations.

BONE MARROW TRANSPLANTATION

HLA-Identical Bone Marrow

The treatment of choice for X-SCID is bone marrow transplantation (BMT) because it provides stem cells that are able to differentiate into T lymphocytes. HLA-identical BMT does not necessitate myeloablation to achieve development of allogeneic T cells, and in about 50 percent of cases, B cells. Exceptions do exist, however. For example, some patients with ADA-SCID have residual immune function and have required multiple HLA-matched transplants to achieve engraftment; for such patients, administration of immunosuppressive drugs may be indicated to facilitate engraftment of lymphoid progenitors in a secondary transplant. For those variants involving more than the lymphoid lineage such as reticular dysgenesis preparative regimens incorporating both myeloablative and immunosuppressive agents have also been required to insure rapid and full hematopoietic and lymphoid chimerism and correction of observed lymphoid and myeloid abnormalities.

Engraftment is usually observed in 14 to 21 days. The establishment of immune competence may be indicated by improved clinical status (e.g., weight gain); T and B cells in the circulating blood; and/or genetic markers of donors, including enzyme activity in previously deficient patients. Of these the establishment of chimerism is the most reliable evidence of engraftment. Appropriate tests for mosaicism include sex and other chromosomal studies, restriction fragment length polymorphism (RFLP) analysis, HLA and red cell antigens, plasma protein, or enzyme allotypes.

For successful transplants, a single intravenous infusion of 5×10^7 nucleated marrow cells per kilogram of body weight is often sufficient, although as few as 5×10^6 (five million) cells have been used.

After receipt of HLA – identical marrow, the recipients may experience return of T and B cell function, including the presence of T-cell proliferation to phytohemagglutinin (PHA), as early as 2 to 3 weeks. Full immune reconstitution is usually present within 6 months, with the return of B-cell function, which is much more variable than T-cell function.

Although acute GVHD in the post-transplant period is not unusual, it is most often self-limited and rarely fatal in this group. When used, treatment consists of either methotrexate given at the earliest signs of GVHD or in vivo administration of pan T-cell monoclonal antibodies.

Results of HLA-identical bone marrow transplantation are now excellent, with a cure being obtained in about 90 percent of patients. The deaths following this type of BMT are mostly due to infections acquired before transplantation.

For patients who have failure to engraft post–HLA-identical BMT, further options include a second BMT versus alternative therapy, possibly enzyme replacement administration in ADA-deficient SCID.

Matched Unrelated Bone Marrow Transplantation

Two-thirds of patients who need bone marrow transplantation do not have a compatible donor. A number of successful bone marrow transplants from matched unrelated donors have been performed; such donors may be found in the registries of HLA testing. An increased incidence of GVHD has been noted almost universally in clinical trials of matched unrelated donor transplantation, presumably because of micro variations in HLA molecules that cannot be detected by serologic typing. Recent studies using molecular typing techniques have shown an association of class II HLA-DR mismatching with severe GVHD, and molecular DR matching of unrelated donors was associated with a markedly reduced incidence of severe GVHD, despite the presence of MHC class I disparities. Management of patients who receive matched unrelated bone marrow is identical to patients who receive haploidentical bone marrow transplantation (see next section).

Haploidentical Bone Marrow Transplantation

Severe and often fatal GVHD has regularly followed transplantation from a histocompatible donor, usually a haploidentical parent. Two new approaches have resulted in successful reconstitution of haploidentical marrow. The first approach is based on selective removal of T lymphocytes on lectin (soybean agglutination) columns. The second approach is to use specific monoclonal antibodies directed against T-cell antigens in the treatment of the bone marrow inoculum before transplant and GVHD in the post-transplant period. The monoclonal antibodies are used in conjunction with rabbit complement to kill the T cells. Alternatively the bone marrow is treated with (Fab')2 fragments of monoclonal antibodies conjugated to ricin. The later procedure has the advantage of not requiring repeated washes of the bone marrow cell suspension. The recipient is treated with lymphocytotoxic drugs (e.g., antilymphocytic serum and cyclophosphamide, 50 mg per kilogram per day for 4 days) before transplant.

Success with T-cell engraftment has been encouraging, but it has been difficult to establish B-cell engraftment with haploidentical bone marrow. Full reconstitution has been obtained with a longer delay than in HLA-identical donors. After haploidentical transplantation, the average time for T-cell recovery with restoration of antigen specific T-cell proliferation is 90 to 120 days. Return of appropriate B-cell function may occur anywhere from 18 months to 3 years.

The delay of B-cell maturation may be due to a less than optimal interaction of half-matched donor T cells with host antigen presenting cells and B cells, knowing that the B cells postrecovery are usually recipient in origin. Antibody function in particular may be inadequate in patients receiving haploidentical bone marrow. Supplemental use of intravenous immune globulin during this time may be necessary to provide humoral function.

The major disadvantages of haploidentical BMT are the delay that patients have in immunologic reconstitution and the additional delays and complications when cytoablation is used.

Fischer and associates reviewed the European experience with unfractionated HLA-identical and T-cell depleted haploidentical (or non–T depleted) bone marrow transplants in SCID and other forms of immunodeficiency disease. The survival rates in Europe for HLA-identical bone marrow transplants was around 60 percent between 1969 to 1983 and around 90 percent after 1983. The results of HLA nonidentical transplants ranged between 70 and 80 percent after 1989. There is currently no similar published summary for experience in the United States.

Patients who experience engraftment failure after haploidentical BMT without preconditioning may have a repeat BMT or receive ADA enzyme replacement in ADA-deficient SCIDs. Patients who do receive pretransplant conditioning who experience graft failure are less responsive to enzyme replacement because of the suppressive effects of the cytotoxic agents used during the preconditioning.

COMPLICATIONS

Graft-Versus-Host Disease

Success of bone marrow transplantation depends on the ability of the graft to "take." If the recipient recognizes foreign MHC and/or minor antigens, the graft is rejected. Similarly, the graft's immunocompetent cells can recognize foreign antigens present in the host and trigger GVHD.

When GVHD occurs, it generally appears 8 to 20 days after a transplant and is usually manifested by a maculopapular skin rash that initially involves the palms and soles and later progresses centrally, liver injury that is characterized by elevation of bilirubin and transaminases, and secretory diarrhea that is initially watery but as the disease progresses may become bloody. GVHD is graded from I to IV depending on the degree of organ system involvement.

The incidence of acute GVHD in HLA-identical or HLA phenotypically matched family members is 20 to 50 percent. In HLA-matched unrelated, or genotypically identical to one haplotype and differing in one, two, or three loci (either class I or class II), the incidence increases to 60 to 80 percent. In addition to histocompatibility, other factors associated with GVHD include increasing age of the host, donor-recipient sex mismatch, infection, increased number of T cells in the graft, and absence of prophylactic regimen.

Prevention of GVHD includes pretreatment of bone marrow donor, in vitro manipulation of bone marrow, and treatment of recipient after transplantation, the latter being the most conventional. The combination of methotrexate 15 mg per square meter IV on the first day, 10 mg post-transplant per square meter 3.6, and 11 days post-transplant and cyclosporin 1.5 mg per kilogram IV every 12 hours from the day before surgery until 50 days post-transplant has been shown to be the most effective chemotherapy prevention method.

Mild acute GVHD (grade I) does not warrant therapy, but extensive disease (grades II-IV) requires treatment to avoid morbidity and mortality from infection. The three therapies most extensively studied are corticosteroids, antithymocyte globulin (ATG), and cyclosporin. Intravenous corticosteroid, usually methylprednisolone given every 6 hours at doses ranging from 2 to 20 mg per kilogram per day, is a first choice treatment for acute GVHD. Severe acute GVHD warrants initiation of therapy at doses at the high end of this range to rapidly gain control of fulminant disease. Responses are typically apparent by 3 to 5 days after instituting therapy. Once disease control is achieved, the methylprednisolone dose can be cautiously tapered by 25 percent each week while continuously watching for relapse of the GVHD. Cyclosporin has been used at a dose of 1.5 mg per kilogram slowly infused intravenously over 2 hours every 12 hours or 6 mg per kilogram taken orally twice daily. Close monitoring of renal function and dosage adjustment based on plasma cyclosporin levels are essential. ATG at a dose of 15 mg per kilogram given every other day for six doses has been used; however, the drug is frequently in short supply and sometimes produces an unpleasant serum-sickness reaction.

Chronic GVHD usually develops 100 days or more after a bone marrow transplantation either following acute GVHD or as a de novo syndrome without acute GVHD. The manifestations include scleroderma-like skin lesions, dry eyes and mouth (sicca syndrome), chronic hepatitis with cholestasis, and occasionally, esophageal and bowel strictures. Treatment involves symptomatic treatment with emollient skin lotions, sun screen, artificial tears and saliva, as well as the immunosuppressive agents previously described.

Patients with chronic GVHD are immunocompromised and at a high risk of infection for pneumococcal and *Haemophilus influenza* sepsis, disseminated varicella zoster, cytomegalovirus and herpesvirus pneumonia, and disseminated candidiasis or aspergillosis. These infections should be expected and treated aggressively as soon as the diagnosis is made. The most common cause of death in patients with chronic GVHD is infection.

Infectious Complications

Tests of immunologic competence should be repeated periodically in successful cases, since subsequently gradual decline has been observed in some instances.

Cytomegalovirus (CMV) infection in patients who are neutropenic, especially after grafting, causes considerable morbidity, with viremia, gastroenteritis, and hepatitis. If CMV pneumonia develops, the outcome is usually fatal and doesn't respond to treatment with acyclovir. Several controlled studies have been carried out to determine the efficacy of IVIG in the prevention of infections in bone marrow recipients. Results have not been consistent. However, interstitial pneumonia is uniformly less frequent in IVIG-treated patients than in controls.

Children who are dramatically restored immunologically have also occasionally died of pre-existing pulmonary infections with *Pneumocystis carinii* or other organisms just after immunologic capacity has been restored. Prophylactic treatment with sulfamethoxazole-trimethoprim has proven useful in the treatment of these complications. General deaths from varicella have occurred in successfully transplanted immunodeficient patients; such patients should be passively protected with varicella-zoster immune globulin (VZIG) and acyclovir following exposure, if no circulating antibody can be demonstrated.

The risk of developing EBV-induced B cell lymphoma in transplant recipients, particularly of haploidentical bone marrow donations, has been a difficult problem that is yet unsolved. Polyclonal B-cell proliferation is the initial event, ultimately followed by monoclonal dominance and a lymphoma syndrome.

ENZYME THERAPY

The aim of enzyme replacement is to provide circulating adenosine deaminase (ADA) in sufficient concentration to deplete affected cells of their toxic metabolites, which are in equivalence between affected cells and the surrounding plasma.

The first "enzyme replacement" approach in the treatment of ADA deficiency utilized transfusion of irradiated red blood cells. This treatment was effective in reducing plasma levels of adenosine and deoxyadenosine, along with the urinary excretion of deoxyadenosine, but the beneficial effects were transient and often inadequate probably because of the low level of ADA in red blood cells.

Purified bovine ADA bound to polyethylene glycol (PEG-ADA) was developed as an alternative treatment for patients with ADA deficiency SCID who do not have an HLA-identical bone marrow donor.

Newly diagnosed patients need to be initiated on a dosage of 30 μg per kilogram intramuscularly administered twice weekly. The twice-weekly schedule is continued until metabolic abnormalities are corrected, the child is clinically stable, and immune function has improved. At that time, often 1 to 3 months after initiation of therapy, treatment may be reduced to 30 μg per kilogram weekly. Recovery of the immune system can begin within a few weeks to several months after metabolic correction. Lymphocyte counts increase during the first 6 to 12 months sometimes into normal range, followed by improvement in specific immune function. In some patients there is a return of thymic shadow on the chest roentgenogram. Lymphocyte counts may decrease during the second year of treatment, producing a lymphopenia that is maintained despite appropriate circulating ADA levels and normal metabolic function. Lymphocyte blastogenic response to mitogens begin to improve by 2 months of therapy and may continue to improve over the next 6 to 8 months. Serum immunoglobulins will rise during enzyme therapy with 50 percent of patients being able to discontinue IVIG within 3 to 6 months of initiation of therapy. These patients have demonstrated normal antibody titers both after immunization and after natural infection.

GENE THERAPY

The goal of gene therapy for ADA deficiency was that the delivery of the ADA gene into bone marrow stem cells would provide "one short cure" for this disorder. Unfortunately, bone marrow stem cells usually exist in a nonproliferative state (Go stage) of the cell cycle. The use of a disabled retrovirus vector, which requires cells that are actively dividing in order to insert the corrected ADA gene, is not possible unless manipulations to induce stem cell proliferation are applied.

The other rational choice for gene therapy is the use of circulating T lymphocytes. These T lymphocytes are stimulated to proliferate through culture with recombinant IL-2 and OKT3. After 24 hours in culture, as the cells begin to proliferate and begin to synthesize DNA the retroviral vector is introduced. After 9 to 12 days in culture, these T cells have expanded fiftyfold to 600-fold and are reinfused intravenously into the patient.

Currently it is not known whether cells now expressing the ADA gene will be able to expand sufficiently to maintain immunity and whether these cells will be able to provide sufficient ADA enzyme activity to prevent the accumulation of toxic metabolites. Therefore, the success of gene therapy cannot be determined until it is established that enzyme therapy can safely be discontinued in these patients.

Choice of Therapy in ADA Deficient SCIDs

Of the currently available options for the treatment of ADA deficiency, the treatment of choice remains transplantation of bone marrow from an HLA-identical donor. When an HLA identical-donor is not available, haploidentical bone marrow transplantation or enzyme replacement needs to be considered and evaluated on an individual basis. The major problem with PEG-ADA replacement is the expense of this mode of therapy, especially in the current era of managed care and health care reforms. Gene therapy, on the other hand, holds the promise of a new era of medical therapy for the inherited immunodeficiency disorders but is still under evaluation at this point.

INTERLEUKIN-2 REPLACEMENT

Recently a patient with severe combined immunodeficiency was found to have interleukin-2 deficiency. Initially, this patient was thought to have isolated IL-2 deficiency but later on it was discovered that he had multiple cytokine deficiency. Two other patients with IL-2 deficiency have been described. The first of three patients was treated with IL-2. Treatment with IL-2 has resulted in the improvement of the clinical condition, improvement of the in vitro T-cell function, and improvement in B-cell function in vivo and in vitro. The other two patients died before the institution of IL-2 replacement therapy. Based on the experience with this single patient, it will be important to establish whether IL-2 deficiency is the basis of severe combined immunodeficiency in patients who have normal numbers of T cells that fail to proliferate to mitogens. If the proliferative response of these cells is corrected by recombinant IL-2 in vitro, such an observation warrants the trial of IL-2 replacement.

SUGGESTED READING

Buckley RH, Schiff SE, Roberts JL, et al. Haploidentical bone marrow stem cell transplantation in human severe combined immunodeficiency. Semin Hematol, 1993; 30(suppl 4):92–104.

Cassano WF, Graft-versus-host disease. J Fl Med Assoc 1991; 78(1): 23–25.

Dror Y, Gallagher R, Wara DW, et al. Immune reconstitution in severe combined immunodeficiency disease after lectin-treated, T-cell-depleted haplocompatible bone marrow transplantation. Blood 1993; 81(8):2021–2030.

Hilman BC, Sorensen RV. Management options: SCIDS with adenosine deaminase deficiency. Ann Allergy 1994; 72:395–403.

O'Reilly RJ, Keever CA, Small TN, Brochstein J. The use of HLA-non-identical T-cell-depleted marrow transplants for correction of severe combined immunodeficiency disease. In: Rosen FS, Seligmann M, eds. Immunodeficiencies. Chur, Switzerland: Harwood Academic Publishers, 1993:689.

WHO Scientific Group Report. Primary immunodeficiency diseases. Immunodefic Rev 1992; 3:195–236.

CONGENITAL IMMUNODEFICIENCY DISEASES

REBECCA H. BUCKLEY, M.D.

Congenital, or primary, immunodeficiency diseases may affect one or more of the four major components of the immune system, including T and B lymphocytes, phagocytic cells, and the complement system. Although these conditions are rare, more than 50 have been described. Over the past 15 years, there has been an explosion of knowledge about the molecular causes of such diseases. The identification and cloning of the genes for several of the primary immunodeficiency diseases have obvious implications for potential future somatic cell gene therapy for these patients. During the same time period, there have also been tremendous advances in other therapy for these diseases. The rapid occurrence of these advances suggests that there will soon be many more to come.

Most patients with antibody deficiency syndromes have recurrent infections with extracellular encapsulated bacteria, which can eventually be eliminated with adequate antibiotic treatment; some with selective IgA deficiency or with transient hypogammaglobulinemia may have few or no infections. Patients with antibody deficiency have few problems with fungal or viral (except enterovirus) infections. On the other hand, patients with partial or absolute defects in T-cell function often have infections with low-grade or opportunistic bacterial, fungal, protozoal, and viral agents for which there is no effective treatment and/or infections that are of a more severe nature than those in patients with antibody deficiency disorders. It is also rare that patients with primary T-cell defects survive beyond infancy or childhood unless immunologic reconstitution can be achieved. Patients with phagocytic cell defects have recurrent and/or serious infections with bacterial (primarily staphylococcal and gram-negative organisms, but also mycobacteria) or fungal (*Aspergillus* species predominantly) agents. Patients with complement component deficiencies have recurrent bacterial infections, often resembling patients with antibody deficiency.

THERAPEUTIC APPROACHES

The principal modes of therapy for congenital immunodeficiency disorders include antibiotics, protective isolation, and immunologic reconstitution by transplantation of immunocompetent tissue (e.g., normal bone marrow). The complexities of both the immunodeficiency diseases and their treatment emphasize the need for such patients to be evaluated in centers where detailed studies of immune function can be carried out and where appropriate therapy can be initiated.

Antibody Deficiency Disorders

Until 1981, therapy of these disorders was primarily with antimicrobial agents and intramuscular (IM) immune serum globulin (ISG). Since then, the most common form of antibody replacement therapy has been with intravenous immune serum globulin (IVIG). This is primarily because of the well-known disadvantages of IM ISG (i.e., the requirement of large volume, painful injections to achieve even low-level replacement therapy, and the potential for nerve damage and abscess formation). The development of safe and effective IVIG has represented a major advance in the treatment of patients with severe antibody deficiencies, although such therapy is expensive.

Indications and Contraindictions for Immunoglobulin Replacement Therapy

The rationale for the use of immunoglobulin replacement therapy is to provide missing antibodies, not to raise the serum IgG concentration. Therefore, broad antibody deficiency should always be carefully documented before IVIG therapy is initiated. Specifically, IVIG should not be administered solely on the basis of a certain serum level of an immunoglobulin class or subclass. Examples of defects with severe impairment in antibody formation include X-linked agammaglobulinemia, common variable immunodeficiency, and the syndromes of severe combined immunodeficiency (SCID). In addition, antibody therapy is indicated for patients with immunodeficiency with hyper-IgM (regardless of cause) and even for patients with normal immunoglobulin levels who have a demonstrated marked and broad impairment in their ability to produce specific antibodies following immunization. The latter includes boys with the Wiskott-Aldrich syndrome, who have an inability to produce antibodies to polysaccharide antigens and blunted anamnestic responses to protein antigens. Profound impairment in antibody-forming capacity is also occasionally seen in ataxia telangiectasia and in other patients who have normal or near-normal serum immunoglobulin concentrations.

Deficits in humoral immunity in which gamma globulin replacement is not indicated include transient hypogammaglobulinemia of infancy and selective IgA deficiency. In the former situation, infants usually have a normal capacity to make specific antibodies in response to immunization, despite low serum concentrations of all or some of the immunoglobulins during the first few months or years of life. Administration of passive antibody could suppress this ability and do more harm than good. The same problem potentially exists in patients demonstrated to have selective IgG subclass deficiencies. Since there are no pure preparations of the individual IgG subclasses available for therapy, if IVIG is used to treat a deficiency of one subclass, there is a risk that antibody production in the other classes or subclasses will be suppressed.

In the case of selective IgA deficiency, the lack of appropriate replacement therapy is unfortunate, since this is the most common primary immunodeficiency, and a high percentage of individuals with IgA deficiency have recurrent mucous membrane infections. Fortunately, patients with selective IgA deficiency usually have the ability to normally produce antibodies of the other isotypes. Indeed, a significant proportion (33 percent) of such individuals produce antibodies to IgA, and these antibodies have been implicated as the cause of anaphylactic transfusion reactions in some IgA-deficient patients. For this reason and because all commercially available ISG and IVIG preparations do contain some IgA, gamma globulin replacement therapy is contraindicated in this form of immunodeficiency. Moreover, even if products containing IgA could be given safely to patients with selective IgA deficiency, they still could not effect replacement of IgA at mucous membrane surfaces because secretory IgA in normal individuals is derived from paragut and pararespiratory lymphoid tissue and is not transported from the intravascular compartment to external secretions.

Intravenous Immune Globulin Preparations

Seven IVIG preparations have now been approved by the Food and Drug Administration and are available in the United States; nearly three dozen more are under investigation or marketed abroad. Both ISG and IVIG preparations are isolated initially from normal plasma by the Cohn alcohol fractionation method or a modification of it. Although IgG constitutes 95 to 99 percent of the protein in Cohn fraction II, varying but small quantities of IgA, IgM, IgD, IgE and other proteins are also present. Cohn Fraction II is then further modified by treatment at low pH or by adding polyethylene glycol, DEAE-Sephadex, or ethanol at low ionic strength to remove aggregated IgG. Additional stabilizing agents, such as sugars, glycine, and albumin, are added to prevent reaggregation and to protect the IgG molecule during lyophilization. HIV is inactivated by the ethanol used in preparation of IVIG; such preparations have also recently been modified by the addition of a detergent to ensure that they are free of hepatitis viruses.

In 1982 a committee of the World Health Organization established the following criteria for the production of intravenous immune globulin: each lot should be derived from plasma pooled from at least 1,000 donors; it should be free of prekallikrein activator, kinins, plasmin, and preservatives; it should contain at least 90 percent intact IgG, with the subclasses present in normal ratios, and be as free as possible of aggregates; its IgG molecules should maintain all of their biologic activity, such as the ability to fix complement; and the preparations should be free of infectious agents and "other potentially harmful contaminants."

In practice, all plasma is screened for hepatitis B

surface and core antigens, as well as for antibodies to hepatitis A, B, and (more recently) C and to human immunodeficiency virus (HIV), and elevated levels of alanine aminotransferase. All commercial lots are produced from plasma pooled from 3,000 to 6,000 donors and, therefore, contain a broad spectrum of antibodies. Each pool must contain adequate levels of antibody to antigens in various vaccines, such as tetanus and measles. However, there is no standardization based on titers of antibodies to more clinically relevant organisms, such as *Streptococcus pneumoniae* or *Haemophilus influenzae.* Although there is some variation in antibody titers between preparations from the various manufacturers, as well as from lot to lot with each preparation, there is no evidence that there are consistent differences in antibody titers between the preparations. In general, the IVIG preparations currently available in the United States have similar efficacy and safety. The one exception is that Gammagard has very low levels of IgA, and carefully screened lots of it can be used safely in patients who have antibodies to IgA. There has been no documented transmission of HIV infection by any of these preparations; however, within the past 2 years hepatitis C virus infections were transmitted by some lots from two of them. The latter problem appears to have been resolved by the addition of a detergent.

Dosage of IVIG. It is important to emphasize that the ideal dose of IVIG is unknown. Recent experience suggests that 400 mg per kilogram per month of IVIG permits achievement of trough IgG levels 4 weeks later close to the normal range. However, there will be considerable variability in dosage requirements from individual to individual. This is due in part to the variability in half-life of IgG in different immunodeficient patients. The half-life of IgG ranges from 17.5 to 22.1 days in normal subjects, with a mean of 19.8 days. It is usually longer in agammaglobulinemic subjects, although the presence of active infection of any type, diarrhea with consequent protein-losing enteropathy, or intestinal infestation with *Giardia lamblia* may result in a shortening of the half-life in such patients and dosage requirements may escalate precipitously. In addition, antibodies specific for the infecting agent or agents will be rapidly consumed. Therefore, no matter what the serum level of total IgG is, the level of antibodies to the offending organisms will be rapidly depleted. Additional infusions will thus be needed when the patient is sick, since he or she has no capacity for an anamnestic response, as in patients with persistent echovirus infections of the central nervous system, which develop most commonly in those with Bruton's agammaglobulinemia. Several patients with this ultimately fatal complication have shown marked clinical improvement and negative CSF viral cultures following high-dose IVIG therapy; there is currently no other effective therapy.

Adverse Effects of IVIG. Nonanaphylactic reactions are the most common type of reaction to IVIG. They are typified by back or abdominal pain, nausea, and often vomiting within the first 30 minutes of the infusion. Usually there is no dyspnea, hypotension, or other change in vital signs. Chills, fever, headache, myalgia, and fatigue may begin at the end of the infusion and continue for several hours. Most of these reactions can be prevented by slowing the initial rate of infusion or by pretreatment with aspirin. More severe reactions may require pretreatment with corticosteroids. These reactions may be caused by the binding of the infused antibodies to the antigens of infectious agents in the patient. The frequency and severity of this type of reaction diminish after acute or chronic bacterial infections, particularly of the lungs, have been controlled with antibiotic therapy and regular administration of adequate doses of IVIG. True anaphylactic reactions to IVIG are rare. However, anaphylactic reactions caused by IgE antibodies (in the patient) to IgA (in the IVIG preparation) may occur in patients with common variable immunodeficiency (CVID) or IgA deficiency. All newly diagnosed patients with CVID should be screened for anti-IgA antibodies through the American Red Cross before undergoing IVIG therapy. If such antibodies are detected, IVIG therapy may still be possible by use of the one available IVIG preparation containing almost no IgA; carefully screened lots of it can be used safely in patients who have antibodies to IgA.

Antimicrobial Therapy. Probably because it is impossible to replace secretory IgA, a majority of patients with severe antibody deficiency experience chronic or recurrent infections of mucous membrane surfaces (ears, sinuses, lungs, gastrointestinal tract) despite IVIG therapy. Complications of chronic upper and lower respiratory tract infections, such as sinusitis and bronchiectasis, account for most of the morbidity seen in these conditions. Thus, antibiotic therapy is frequently required for control of such infections. Because of a predominance of *H. influenzae* organisms in sputum and other external secretions of such patients, antimicrobials effective against these organisms are preferred. I find ampicillin (or amoxicillin) or trimethoprim-sulfamethoxazole to be effective in most patients. These antibiotics are used either for specific infections at full therapeutic dosage or chronically at lower doses in patients with bronchiectasis or persistent pyogenic infections. If used chronically, I find it helpful to rotate the types of antibiotics, usually on a monthly or bimonthly basis. It is important to emphasize that the antibiotics be given *in addition to* IVIG replacement in those patients for whom the latter is indicated. For patients who become infected with beta-lactamase-positive *H. Influenzae,* cefaclor (Ceclor) or amoxicillin and potassium clavulanate (Augmentin) may be given; I have also found chloromycetin to be effective in that situation. Ampicillin or amoxicillin are preferable to trimethoprim-sulfamethoxazole if concurrent infection with *S. pneumoniae* or Group A beta-hemolytic streptococcal organisms is present. Staphylococcal and *Pseudomonas* infections are less common; cultures are helpful in alerting one to a need for antistaphylococcal agents or aminoglycosides. Chronic antistaphylococcal antibiotics are the treatment of choice for patients with the hyper-IgE syndrome. Percussion and postural drainage on a twice daily basis are also helpful adjuncts to therapy in patients with bronchiectasis. Pneumococcal vaccine is advocated for patients with selective IgA deficiency and for those with ataxia telangiectasia.

Cellular and Combined Immunodeficiency Disorders

Therapy for cellular and combined immunodeficiency disorders has, in general, been far less successful than for the antibody deficiency syndromes. Since these patients are highly susceptible to all infectious agents, it is imperative that the diagnosis be made as soon as possible after birth so that protective isolation can be instituted for those infants with SCID, complete DiGeorge syndrome, or combined immunodeficiency (CID). If there is a family history of such defects, the diagnosis can be made by enumeration of T cells and subsets in lymphocytes from fresh heparinized cord blood and assessment of T-cell function.

Ordinary reverse isolation is usually adequate if the diagnosis is made early and bone marrow transplantation can be done soon. The urgency in initiating such isolation is due to these patients' marked susceptibility to viral infections for which there is no available treatment and which could lead to their demise before immunologic reconstitution can be accomplished. Neither the patient nor his or her siblings should be given live virus vaccines. Protective isolation is not necessary for patients with partial cellular immunodeficiency, such as those with ataxia telangiectasia or Wiskott-Aldrich syndrome. However, the latter are at risk for fatal sequelae from varicella infections.

Antimicrobial Therapy. The same general principals as outlined for the antibody deficiency syndromes apply to antimicrobial therapy. The differences are that patients with severe T-cell defects are also susceptible to gram-negative, fungal, and viral infections, and to *Pneumocystis carinii* pneumonia. As soon as a diagnosis of SCID, complete DiGeorge's syndrome, or Nezelof's syndrome is made, the patient should be placed on prophylaxis for *P. carinii* with oral trimethoprim-sulfamethoxazole at a dose of 10 mg per kilogram per day of trimethoprim chronically or for 3 days out of each week. If *P. carinii* pneumonia is present, the dose should be 20 mg per kilogram per day of trimethoprim. Leukocyte counts should be monitored weekly and, if neutropenia develops, oral folinic acid (Leukovorin) therapy should be initiated at a dose of 1 mg per day chronically until the neutrophil count returns to normal. If oral or cutaneous moniliasis is present, therapy with ketoconazole (Nizoral) or fluconazole (Diflucan) should be instituted immediately at a dose of 50 to 100 mg per day. Liver function studies should be obtained before beginning either of these agents, followed by weekly or biweekly assessments thereafter. If varicella or herpes infections develop in patients with cellular or combined immunodeficiency, acyclovir (Zovirax) should be administered intravenously at a dose of 250 mg per square meter at a constant rate over 1 hour, every 8 hours for 5 to 7 days, as early in the course of the infection as possible.

Precautions in Use of Blood Products. Since all patients with severe T-cell deficiency are highly susceptible to graft-versus-host disease (GVHD) from donor T lymphocytes in whole blood, packed red cells, platelet units, and/or plasma, all blood and blood products (except IVIG) should be irradiated with 5,000 cGy from a cobalt source prior to administration. Because such patients are also highly susceptible to blood-borne viral agents, such as hepatitis, HIV, Epstein-Barr virus (EBV) and cytomegalovirus (CMV), plasma, whole blood, and platelet units should be avoided if at all possible. Glycerol-frozen red cells are the safest, since such cells are multiply washed when thawed; the final product contains no plasma and very few or no leukocytes. Omission of leukocytes is important for prevention of CMV transmission. The red cell preparation should still be irradiated, however.

Immunoglobulin Replacement. Since it is impossible to have normal B-cell function if there is severe T-cell deficiency, most patients with cellular or combined immunodeficiency have varying degrees of antibody deficiency as well. IVIG should be administered to any such patient on a regular basis unless bone marrow transplantation can be accomplished soon after diagnosis. If exposure to varicella is known sufficiently early, it can be prevented by IM zoster immune globulin (VZIG) or 400 mg per kilogram IVIG.

Management of Diarrhea and Nutrition. One of the earliest manifestations of severe T-cell deficiency is intractable diarrhea. This is usually due to one or more viral agents, including enteroviruses (such as polioviruses from oral vaccine), rotovirus, or enteroadenovirus, or to *Clostridium difficile* toxin. Diagnostic studies for these agents should be carried out as soon as possible. Oral vancomycin (Vancocin HCl) at a dose of 44 mg per kilogram in three divided doses is the treatment of choice for *C. difficile.* Although there is no completely effective therapy for enteric viral infections, high-dose IVIG (i.e., 400 to 500 mg per kilogram) may provide some amelioration. Whatever the cause of the diarrhea, it is important that the patient be given nothing by mouth, oral electrolyte solutions, or a predigested formula such as Pregestimil. Maintenance of adequate nutrition is the key to management of such infants, and often is best accomplished by early institution of total parenteral nutrition (TPN). I have only rarely had to use gut sterilization regimens; these are not helpful unless the patient is also maintained in laminar-flow sterile isolation and is given sterile or no feedings.

Definitive Therapy. Currently, transplantation of MHC-compatible or haploidentical parental bone marrow is still the treatment of choice for patients with fatal T-cell or combined T- and B-cell defects. Shortly after the discovery of HLA in 1967, immune function was conferred in two patients with invariably fatal primary immunodeficiency diseases by transplanting into them HLA-identical allogeneic bone marrow cells. That early success was followed by many disappointments over the next 15 years because of the rare availability of HLA-matched sibling donors for patients with lethal primary T-cell defects. Efforts to get around the lack of a match by using HLA-nonidentical bone marrow or transplants of fetal tissues were thwarted either by the recipient developing lethal GVHD from the former or by failure of immune reconstitution from the latter.

In the first report of the outcomes of bone marrow transplants for severe combined immunodeficiency (SCID) in 1977, only 18 of 80 SCID patients worldwide who were given marrow or fetal tissue transplants were surviving with functional grafts. Possibly because of both earlier diagnosis before untreatable opportunistic infections develop and the availability of better antimicrobials to treat infections, the results of bone marrow transplantation have improved considerably over the last 15 years. More importantly, the development of techniques to deplete all post-thymic T cells from donor marrow in the early 1980s now permits the safe and successful use of haploidentical (half-matched) bone marrow cells for the correction of SCID and other fatal immunodeficiency syndromes. These techniques have employed (1) soybean lectin incubation followed by sheep erythrocyte rosette-depletion or (2) incubation with monoclonal antibodies to T cells plus complement. Both methods enrich the final cell suspension for stem cells, but there is better T-cell depletion with the soybean lectin/sheep erythrocyte-rosetting method. However, the kinetics of immune reconstitution is vastly different when one uses lymphocyte-depleted bone marrow stem cells, as opposed to unfractionated marrow cells. With unfractionated marrow, immune reconstitution can occur in fewer than 3 weeks because of adoptive transfer and engraftment of fully mature immunocompetent donor T and B cells present in the marrow. After transplantation of T cell–depleted marrow, however, genetically donor immune cells cannot usually be detected until 3 to 4 months post-transplantation.

A recent worldwide survey that I conducted revealed that 210 of 265 (79 percent) of patients with primary immunodeficiency transplanted with HLA-identical marrow over the past 27 years survive. Most encouraging, however, are the results of T cell–depleted haploidentical (half-matched) marrow transplants in patients with primary immunodeficiency. From the same survey, it was ascertained that 554 such transplants have been performed in patients with a wide variety of congenital immunodeficiency disorders over the past 13 years and of these, 297 (54 percent) survive. The significance is even more impressive when it is realized that most of the 535 recipients would have died had not the new T-cell depletion techniques been developed.

T cell–depleted haploidentical stem cell transplantation is highly effective, lifesaving therapy for infants with SCID. Over the past 14 years, my associates and I have performed bone marrow transplants in 72 patients with SCID without pretransplant chemotherapy, and currently 56 survive. Only 12 of these infants had HLA-identical donors. The deaths occurred from viral infections for which there was no effective antiviral agent. All 52 of our patients who are more than 4 months post-transplantation have good T-cell function and all but two have 100 percent donor T cells. B-cell function is much more variable. Four of twelve recipients of HLA-identical marrow and 10 of 58 recipients of haploidentical marrow have some donor B cells. The children who received these transplants have also seemed to do very well in many other respects. Most grow very well and generally seem to be normal children.

Patients with less severe forms of cellular immunodeficiency than present in SCID patients (such as Nezelof syndrome, Wiskott-Aldrich syndrome, cytokine deficiency, or MHC antigen deficiency) reject even HLA-identical marrow grafts unless they are conditioned with sublethal doses of myeloablative and immunosuppressive agents before transplantation. Several patients with Wiskott-Aldrich syndrome, leukocyte adhesion deficiency type I (LAD-I), and other forms of partial cellular immunodeficiency have been treated successfully with HLA-identical bone marrow transplantation after immunosuppression. T cell–depleted stem cell transplants have not been as effective for immunodeficiency diseases requiring pretransplant chemotherapy to prevent graft rejection. The long time-course to development of immune function after T cell–depleted stem cell transplants leaves the ablated recipient at more risk for death from opportunistic infection. Nevertheless, even in those conditions, haploidentical stem cell transplants offer some hope, whereas there was none previously unless the patient had an HLA-identical donor. Overall, more than 900 bone marrow transplants have been done in immunodeficiency patients worldwide, with approximately 61 percent surviving. Thus, until somatic cell gene therapy is more fully developed, bone marrow transplantation remains the most important and effective therapy for these inborn errors of the immune system.

Enzyme Replacement. Enzyme replacement therapy with polyethylene glycol-modified bovine ADA (PEG-ADA) administered subcutaneously once weekly has resulted in both clinical and immunologic improvement in more than 30 ADA-deficient SCID patients. However, bone marrow transplantation remains the treatment of choice, so PEG-ADA therapy should not be initiated first, as it will confer graft-rejection capability.

SUGGESTED READING

Buckley RH. Breakthroughs in the understanding and therapy of primary immunodeficiency. Pediatr Clin North Am 1994; 41: 665–690.

Buckley RH, Schiff RI. The use of intravenous immunoglobulin in immunodeficiency diseases. N Engl J Med 1991; 325:110–117.

Buckley RH, Schiff SE, Schiff RI, et al. Haploidentical bone marrow stem cell transplantation in human severe combined immunodeficiency. Semin Hematol 1993; 30:92–104.

WHO Scientific Group. Primary immunodeficiency diseases: Report of a WHO scientific group. Clin Exp Immunol 1995; 99:1–24.

HYPERIMMUNOGLOBULIN E SYNDROME (JOB'S SYNDROME)

ROBERT L. ROBERTS, M.D., Ph.D.
E. RICHARD STIEHM, M.D.

The medical eponym, "Job's syndrome," was originally applied to two fair-skinned, red-haired girls with severe eczema, recurrent infections, and markedly elevated levels of immunoglobulin E (IgE). This clinical complex, which has now been described in both sexes and in most ethnic groups, is usually referred to as the hyperimmunoglobulin E syndrome (HIE).

CLINICAL AND LABORATORY FEATURES

Clinical Features

The clinical features of HIE include eczematoid rashes, which are present in all patients and usually begin in infancy (Table 1). The rash is often papular and pruritic, but may also be pustular and lichenified. The face, neck, and ears are often affected but may also be present on the flexural and extensor surfaces on the limbs. The eczematous skin is particularly susceptible to bacterial invasion resulting in impetigo as well as superficial fungal and herpetic infections. Recurrent pneumonias are the most serious infections in HIE, and they often result in pneumatocele formation and empyema. *Staphylococcus aureus, Haemophilus influenzae,* and *Candida albicans* are the most common lung pathogens, but other organisms may also be recovered including pneumococci and group A streptococci.

"Cold abscesses," those lacking external signs of inflammation, are often described in HIE patients. The patient may be afebrile and not appear acutely ill, although the abscess may contain large volumes of pus and extend over large areas. Chronic otitis media, otitis externa, and sinusitis occur frequently, and mastoiditis may be found in severe cases. Coarse facial features, present in the majority of patients with HIE, include a broad nasal bridge, prominent nose, and irregularly proportioned cheeks and jaw; these features become more distinctive in adolescence and adulthood. Osteoporosis, diagnosed by photon absorptiometry, has also been reported in some patients and may be associated with a greater tendency for bone fractures. Osteomyelitis is not frequent but may occur in bone underlying an abscess or cellulitis. Gingivitis and oral ulcerations may occur in HIE, and polyarticular arthritis responsive to nonsteroidal anti-inflammatory medications has been reported in adult patients. Recurrent keratoconjunctivitis complicated by corneal scarring has developed in some patients.

Table 1 Clinical Features of HIE

Present in Majority of Patients
Eczematous dermatitis with onset in infancy
Recurrent skin and soft tissue infections
Recurrent sinopulmonary infections
Pneumatocele formation and lung scarring
Coarse facies
Less Frequently Reported
Keratoconjunctivitis with corneal scarring
Osteomyelitis from adjacent abscess
Gingivitis and oral candidiasis
Polyarticular arthritis

Laboratory Studies

Laboratory studies may aid in diagnosis and monitoring of HIE. An extremely high serum level of IgE, often 20,000 IU per milliliter or greater, is typical of this disease, and such elevations may occur early in infancy. A high percentage of the IgE is directed to *S. aureus,* which distinguishes HIE from atopic dermatitis patients with very elevated IgE, although assaying for anti-staph IgE is only available on a research basis. Most patients with HIE have a mild to moderate eosinophilia, and the total white blood cell count may become markedly elevated during acute infections. The erythrocyte sedimentation rate is usually elevated, particularly during exacerbation of disease. Histamine levels may be increased in blood or in urine but are usually not of practical significance.

Immunologic Abnormalities

Several studies have shown that neutrophils from HIE patients are defective in chemotaxis, but this has not been a consistent abnormality in all patients. The impairment in chemotaxis appears to be due to a humoral factor in the serum such as an inhibitory cytokine or IgG anti-IgE immune complexes. Defects in specific antibody production to both protein and polysaccharide antigens have also been described in HIE, and various abnormalities in T-cell function have also been reported, including anergy in delayed hypersensitivity testing and poor in vitro proliferative responses to soluble antigens. There have been case reports of HIE syndrome developing in HIV-infected patients, suggesting that T cell immunoregulator defects may be operative in the etiology of HIE. See Table 2 for a summary of immunologic abnormalities in HIE syndrome.

THERAPY

The most important therapeutic measure for patients with HIE is recognition of complicating infections and institution of prompt and adequate treatment. The patients' lack of an inflammatory response may mask the seriousness of the infection, and delay of treatment may result in further complications such as pneumatocoele formation following pneumonia or osteomyelitis secondary to an overlying abscess.

Eczema and Superficial Infections

The dermatitis in HIE is often severe and may be the source of much physical discomfort as well as psychological distress. Emollients containing lanolin or petroleum jelly may be used to moisturize the skin after an antibacterial soap is used. Topical steroids are used to control the inflammatory dermatitis, using a potency appropriate for the skin involved (Table 3). Oral steroids are sometimes employed for short periods of time for severe exacerbations. Impetiginous lesions that occur around the ears and nostrils often respond to topical mupirocin (Bactroban). The addition of a topical antifungal medication such as clotrimazole or ketaconazole is also helpful for superficial fungal infections. Antihistamines such as hydroxyzine or diphenhydramine are helpful in reducing the pruritis, particularly if given at bedtime. A nonsedating antihistamine such as astemizole or loratidine may be used during the day. Oral candidiasis (thrush) may be treated with nystatin suspension in young children or clotrimazole troches in older patients. Herpes simplex or H. zoster infections should be treated with oral or parenteral acyclovir.

Table 2 Immunologic Abnormalities in HIE

Extremely elevated IgE (>2,000 IU/ml)
Eosinophilia of blood and secretions
Defective neutrophil chemotaxis—variable
Impaired specific antibody responses to both protein and polysaccharide antigens
IgG subclass abnormalities (low IgG2, high IgG4)
High amounts of IgE to *S. aureus* (>10% of total IgE)
Anergy in delayed hypersensitivity testing
Poor T-lymphocyte proliferative response to soluble antigens
Decreased suppressor T-cell function

Sinopulmonary and Other Infections

Prophylactic oral antibiotics benefit most patients with HIE, and dicloxacillin or trimethaprim-sulfamethoxazole has been used for this treatment (see Table 3). Deep-seated or extensive abscesses or pneumonias often require intravenous antibiotics, and cultures should be obtained when possible because patients with HIE are susceptible to infections caused by many other bacteria, including *Haemophilus influenzae, Group A Streptococcus, Pseudomonas aeruginosa,* and *Escherichia coli,* in addition to *S. aureus.*

Table 3 Routine Management of HIE

A. Topical Skin Care for Dermatitis
   1. Emollients: lanolin, petrolatum
   2. Topical steroids (potency dependent on severity)
      a. Lowest Potency: Hydrocortisone base, 1.0%-2.5% cream, ointment
      b. Low Potency: Triamcinolone, 0.025% cream, ointment
      c. Intermediate Potency: Triamcinolone, 0.1% cream, ointment
      d. High Potency: Fluocinomide, 0.05% cream, ointment
      e. Highest potency: Betamethasone dipropionate, 0.05% ointment
   3. Topical antifungal agents for candidiasis, tinea
      a. Clotrimazole: 1% cream
      b. Ketoconazole: 2% cream
   4. Antibacterial agents for impetigo
      a. Neomycin, Bacitracin, Polymyxin (Neosporin) ointment
      b. Mupirocin (Bactroban), 2% ointment

B. Prophylactic Oral Antibiotics*
   1. Co-trimoxazole: 40 mg TMP/200 mg SMX, b.i.d.
   2. Dicloxacillin: 500 mg, b.i.d.
   3. Erythromycin (Enteric-coated preferred): 500 mg, b.i.d.

C. Antihistamines (Rotate to increase efficacy)*
   1. Hydroxyzine (Atarax): 25-50 mg, q8h
   2. Diphenhydramine (Benadryl): 25-50 mg, q8h
   3. Cyproheptadine (Periactin): 4-8 mg, q8h
   4. Astemizole (Hismanal): 10 mg, q.d.
   5. Loratidine (Claritin): 10 mg, q.d.

D. Immunizations
   1. Routine childhood immunizations: DPT, Polio, MMR, *Haemophilus influenzae,* Hepatitis B
   2. Pneumococcal multivalent vaccine
   3. Yearly influenza A vaccine
   4. Varicella vaccine (delay immunization if patient is on systemic steroids)

E. Pulmonary Care
   1. Bronchodilators for bronchospasm: Albuterol: 90 μg/dose by metered dose inhaler, q6h, PRN, or 2.5 mg/dose by nebulizer, q6h, prn
   2. Chest percussion and drainage in selected cases

*Adult dosages for oral medications. Please consult Johnson KB. *Harriet Lane handbook,* 13th ed. St Louis: Mosby, 1993, for pediatric dosages.

Table 4 Complications of Therapy for HIE

A. Topical Steroids
   1. Local cutaneous side effects: Rosacea, hypopigmentation, telangiectasia, acne, striae, skin thinning
   2. Systemic side effects (prolonged or excessive use): Adrenal suppression, Cushing's syndrome, growth failure, cataracts
   3. Inappropriate use of steroids
      a. High-potency steroid to face, axilla, groin: Local side effects more likely
      b. Skin infection without appropriate antibiotics: Prolongs infection
B. Antihistamines
   1. Nonprescription antihistamines: Sedation but tolerance may occur
   2. Nonsedating antihistamines
      a. Terfenadine (Seldane): Cardiac arrhythmia with ketaconazole or erythromycin
      b. Astemizole (Hismanal): Caution in hepatic disease
      c. Loratidine (Claritin): Caution in hepatic disease
C. Topical Antibiotics
   1. Neomycin based: Allergic sensitization
   2. Mupirocin: Local irritation of skin
D. Oral and Parenteral Antibiotics
   1. General antibiotic complications
      a. Gastrointestinal disturbances: Usually mild
      b. Skin rashes: Usually mild
      c. Pancytopenia, neutropenia: Rare
      d. Pseudomembranous enterocolitis: Due to *Clostridium difficile*
      e. Coagulation abnormalities: Due to vitamin K depletion
      f. Development of resistant bacteria
   2. Specific antibiotic complications
      a. Trimethoprim-sulfamethazole: Neutropenia, Stevens-Johnson syndrome (rare)
      b. Aminoglycosides: Nephrotoxicity, ototoxicity
      c. Ketaconazole: Gastrointestinal disturbances, hepatotoxicity
      d. Amphotericin B: Chills, fever, headache, nephrotoxicity
      e. Acyclovir: Nephrotoxicity
E. Surgical Complications
   1. Delayed surgical intervention due to lack of inflammatory responses
   2. Secondary infection due to lack of adequate antibiotic coverage postoperatively
   3. Recurrence of pulmonary cysts after removal
   4. Loss of lung volume
   5. Scoliosis secondary to lobectomy, pneumonectomy

Fungal infections are also common in patients with HIE, particularly involving the nails, and appropriate cultures and potassium hydroxide preparations should be taken. Oral ketaconazole is useful for treatment of paronychia due to *Candida* and intraconazole may be a good alternative. Fungal infections of the lungs or the meninges require prolonged intravenous therapy with amphotericin B or other antifungal medication depending on the sensitivities of the organism. Patients exposed to varicella and with no detectable antibodies to varicella should be considered for treatment with varicella-zoster immune globulin depending on the severity of their disease, and oral or parenteral acyclovir should be administered if they begin to develop vesicles. Surgical treatment may be required for debridement or drainage of deep-seated abscesses. Chest tube placement and lobectomy or pneumonectomy may be necessary for loculated pneumonias and pneumatoceles. Keratoconjunctivitis usually responds to topical steroids, although referral to an opthalmologist is recommended to rule out infectious causes. Table 4 lists some of the significant complications of therapy.

Experimental Treatments

Plasmapheresis has been used in patients with HIE who do not adequately respond to conventional therapy. The treatment is reported to decrease the severity of their eczematoid rash, and restore normal neutrophil chemotactic responses and lymphocyte proliferative responses. Leung and Geha (1988) initially recommend five treatments in a 10-day period, followed by weekly plasmapheresis to maintain the beneficial effects. They also recommend following the plasmapheresis with intravenous gammaglobulin (IVIG) to reduce the frequency of serious infections. Clinical trials using IVIG alone to treat HIE are now under way at UCLA and other medical centers. We have observed marked improvement in anecdotal cases of severe atopic dermatitis (not HIE) treated with IVIG. Initially a 2 g per kilogram dose of IVIG is given over 2 days, followed by a 1 g per kilogram dose given every 3 to 4 weeks depending on the patient's response. The patient's IgE levels have greatly decreased as their skin has improved. IVIG therapy has an added advantage in the treatment of patients with HIE because it provides protective antibodies as well as playing an immunoregulatory role.

Other therapies such as ascorbic acid, cimetidine, and transfer factor have been used in the treatment of HIE patients based on in vitro studies, but these treatments have not been subjected to adequate clinical trials (Table 5). Levamisole was tested in a double-blind, placebo-controlled study, and patients on the drug were

Table 5 Experimental Therapies for HIE

Intravenous Gammaglobulin: Clinical trials in progress
Plasmapheresis: Case reports of improvement in HIE patients
Interferon Gamma: Improves neutrophil chemotaxis in vitro
Ascorbic Acid: Improves neutrophil function in vitro
Cimetidine and other H_2 histamine blockers
Transfer Factor: Stimulates T lymphocytes
Isotretinoin: Single case report of improvement
Levamisole: Found to be ineffective in clinical trials

found to have more infections than those on placebo. Interferon gamma will improve the chemotaxis of neutrophils from patients with HIE in vitro as well as decrease IgE serum levels in some patients, but its clinical effectiveness has not yet been proven.

PROGNOSIS

The prognosis of the patient with HIE for a near-normal life span is good for those who are diagnosed early and followed carefully. The patient who is not diagnosed until later in life after bronchiectasis or pneumatoceles have developed has a poor prognosis for prolonged life.

There have been at least four cases of lymphomas diagnosed in patients with HIE who were under 20 years of age. The association between the development of a lymphoid neoplasm and other forms of immunodeficiency is well established and thought to be due to defective tumor surveillance by the patient's immune system. The development of malignancies in patients with HIE as they are followed over a longer period of time may emerge as another example of abnormalities in the immune response of HIE syndrome.

SUGGESTED READING

Buckley RH, Sampson HA. The hyperimmunoglobulinemia E syndrome. In: Franklin EC, ed. Clinical immunology update. New York: Elsevier, 1981:148.

Donabedian H, Gallin JI. The hyperimmunoglobulin E recurrent-infection (Job's) syndrome: A review of the NIH experience and the literature. Medicine 1983; 62:195–208.

King CL, Gallin JI, Malech HL, et al. Regulation of immunoglobulin production in hyperimmunoglobulin E recurrent-infection syndrome by interferon γ. Proc Natl Acad Sci USA 1989; 86: 10085–10089.

Leung DYM, Geha RS. Clinical and immunologic aspects of the hyperimmunoglobulin E syndrome. Hematol Oncol Clin North Am 1988; 2:81–100.

Stiehm ER, ed. Immunologic disorders in infants and children, 4th ed. Philadelphia: WB Saunders, 1996.

HUMAN IMMUNODEFICIENCY VIRUS INFECTION

JOHN G. BARTLETT, M.D.

Acquired immunodeficiency syndrome (AIDS) was initially described in 1981 as a disease characterized by defective cell-mediated immunity expressed as *P. carinii* pneumonia in gay men. This has subsequently mushroomed into what many believe is the most important epidemic of the 20th century with an estimated prevalence of approximately 17 million cases in 1995 and a projection of 40 million by the year 2000. Despite its relatively brief history, this disease is probably the most studied and the best understood of all infectious diseases. The database is continuously evolving so that statements regarding natural history and therapeutic strategies are subject to constant change.

NATURAL HISTORY

HIV is transmitted by "exchange of body fluids." Sexual intercourse, needle sharing by injection drug users, and vertical transmission from pregnant women account for 99.8 percent of transmissions subsequent to 1985 when the blood supply underwent routine serologic testing.

The sequence of events following viral transmission across a mucocutaneous barrier is extension to regional lymph nodes, followed by massive viremia with extensive involvement of lymph tissue, followed by immune response with partial control of viral replication ascribed to a complex interplay of cytotoxic T-cell response, humoral response, and cytokines. These events usually take place over 8 to 12 weeks and are followed by persistent HIV replication with low-level plasma viremia and CD4 cell depletion over a period that averages 8 to 10 years. The eventual consequence is massive destruction of the immune system with susceptibility to opportunistic pathogens and opportunistic tumors.

Studies on the dynamics of HIV replication indicate

the rate at mid- and late-stage disease to be 10^8 to 10^9 per day indicating approximately one billion new virions produced daily. The major target of HIV is $CD4^+$ cells, and cell destruction appears to reflect viral clearance by cytotoxic T lymphocytes. It is estimated that 10 to 25 percent of $CD4^+$ cells are infected relatively early in the course of HIV, and the rate of $CD4^+$ cell destruction is approximately 10^9 per day. The viral mutation rate is 10^{-4} or about 1 per 10,000 cells. Thus, by late-stage disease there are over 10^8 genetic variants.

The course of HIV infection from the time of viral transmission to the time of an AIDS-defining diagnosis averages 10 years. Nevertheless, there is a great deal of variation so that some patients have a rapid course with rapid $CD4^+$ cell depletion; at the opposite extreme are "non-progressors," who are sometimes defined as patients with HIV infection for over 8 years, $CD4^+$ cell counts that persist in the normal range (over 500 per cubic millimeter), and no antiviral therapy. These variations in course are poorly understood, but contributing factors are presumably the virulence factors of HIV and its mutants and the immune response, especially the cytotoxic T lymphocytes (CTL) response.

Staging of HIV infection is largely based on $CD4^+$ cell counts, the cell that is the primary target of HIV. The mean count in healthy persons is approximately 1,000 per cubic millimeter with a range for most laboratories of about 500 to 1,500 per cubic millimeter. The average loss during the course of HIV infection is 30 to 50 per cubic millimeter per year. When patients reach a threshold of 200 per cubic millimeter they become vulnerable to opportunistic infections that reflect defective cell-mediated immunity. The following conditions are the standard AIDS-defining diagnoses, the most common being (in rank order as initial AIDS-defining conditions) *P. carinii* pneumonia, *Candida* esophagitis, disseminated cytomegalovirus (CMV) infection, toxoplasma encephalitis, disseminated *M. avium* infection, chronic mucocutaneous herpes simplex infection, cryptococcal meningitis, and cryptosporidiosis. Other common complications of late-stage disease include tuberculosis, HIV wasting syndrome, Kaposi's sarcoma, and lymphoma.

ANTIRETROVIRAL THERAPY

The main components of HIV care are therapy directed against HIV and antibiotics for the treatment and prevention of opportunistic infections.

Guidelines for the treatment of HIV infection were provided by the expert panel of the U.S. Public Health Service, which convened in June 1993. These recommendations serve as the standard, but are somewhat antiquated by more recent studies. In general, there are four issues that apply to antiretroviral therapy: when to start, what to start with, when to change, and what to change to.

The Expert Panel recommended initiating therapy when patients were symptomatic and had a $CD4^+$ T cell count less than 500 per cubic millimeter or were asymptomatic with a $CD4^+$ cell count less than 200 per cubic millimeter. The controversial group was the relatively large pool of patients who are asymptomatic and have a $CD4^+$ cell count of 200 to 500 per cubic millimeter; the conclusion of the panel was that antiretroviral therapy for patients in this category was arbitrary. The decision about the agent for initial therapy was considered noncontroversial and was AZT (zidovudine) in a dose of 600 mg per day based on studies demonstrating superiority of AZT as initial therapy compared to zalcitibine (ddC) or didanosine (ddI). Changing agents was considered appropriate if the patient developed toxicity to AZT or had progression of disease while receiving that drug. Progression is defined as complications in the form of new opportunistic infections or tumors, wasting, thrush, or an accelerated decline in the $CD4^+$ T cell count. As substitute therapy, the options available at the time of the Expert Panel meeting were ddI and ddC; these drugs are considered therapeutically equivalent, although somewhat different in terms of their toxicity profile. An additional possible indication for changing therapy is extensive exposure to AZT since a therapeutic trial indicated that the shift to ddI conferred a benefit in this setting. In practice, most clinicians change treatment when there is toxicity to AZT; when the rationale for changing treatment is progression, a common ploy is to simply add ddI or ddC.

After the Expert Panel recommendations were published in 1993, there have been several developments that impact the prior conclusions: two new nucleoside analogs have been added (d4T and 3TC); there is increasing enthusiasm for protease inhibitors that represent a new class; and the utility of AZT in preventing vertical transmission has been convincingly demonstrated. These and other relevant issues in antiretroviral therapy are addressed in the following discussion (Table 1).

AZT

Control trials have demonstrated the efficacy of AZT for the following indications: prolongation of short-term survival; prevention of opportunistic infections; improvement or stabilization of HIV-associated dementia; stabilization or increase in weight; improvement in Karnofsky score; increased platelet count in HIV-associated ITP; prevention of vertical transmission; increase in $CD4^+$ cell count; and reduction in quantitative HIV virology. The usual dosage is 200 mg three times daily except with dementia in which the dosage is 1 to 1.2 g per day. Side effects are dose related. Subjective side effects include nausea, headache, flulike illness, and fatigue. Marrow suppression (anemia or neutropenia) is reversible, dose related, and stage dependent, meaning it is more frequent in late-stage disease than in asymptomatic patients. Administration of AZT in early-stage disease results in a delay in the $CD4^+$ cell decline and a 0.5 log decrease in HIV concentrations in serum, but it has not been possible to

Table 1 Nucleoside Analogs

	Zidovudine (AZT, ZDV) (Retrovir)	*Didanosine (ddl) (Videx)*	*Zalcitabine (ddC) (HIVID)*	*Stavudine (d4T) (Zerit)*	*Lamivudine (3TC)*
Indications: FDA labeling	FDA: $CD4^+$ cell $<500/mm^3$ Expert panel: $CD4^+$ cell $<500/mm^3$ with symptoms or $CD4^+$ cell count $<200/mm^3$. Asymptomatic patients with $CD4^+$ cell counts $200\text{-}500/mm^3$: optional	FDA: Advanced HIV infection plus prolonged prior therapy with AZT *or* advanced infection plus AZT intolerance or significant clinical or immunologic deterioration during AZT treatment	FDA: Monotherapy for advanced HIV infection plus intolerance or progression with AZT *or* combined with AZT in selected patients with $CD4^+$ cell $<300/mm^3$	FDA: Advanced HIV infection plus tolerance to approved therapies with proven benefit or significant clinical or immunologic deterioration with these therapies	Treatment IND: $CD4^+$ cell <300 plus intolerance or refractoriness to other FDA approved agents (AZT, ddl, ddC, d4T)
Cost (standard dose—AWP)	$3,150/yr	$2,090/yr	$2,330/yr	$2,060/yr	$2,200
Usual dose (oral)	200 mg t.i.d.	(Tablet form) >60 kg: 200 mg b.i.d. <60 kg: 125 mg b.i.d. 250 mg/b.i.d (powder)	0.75 mg t.i.d.	>60 kg 40 mg b.i.d. <60 kg 30 mg b.i.d.	150 mg b.i.d.
Minimum effective dose	300 mg/day		Not studied	Not studied	Not studied
Oral bioavailability	60%	Tablet: 40% Powder: 30%	85%	86%	86%
Serum half-life	1.1 hr	1.6 hr	1.2 hr	1.0 hr	3-6 hr
Intracellular half-life	3 hr	12 hr	3 hr	3.5 hr	12 hr
CNS penetration (% serum levels)	60%	20%	20%	30%	10%
Elimination	Metabolized to AZT glucuronide (GAZT); renal excretion GAZT	Renal excretion: 50%	Renal excretion: 70%	Renal excretion: 50% unchanged	Renal
Major toxicity	Bone marrow suppression: anemia and/or neutropenia; subjective complaints	Pancreatitis; peripheral neuropathy	Peripheral neuropathy; stomatitis	Peripheral neuropathy; pancreatitis	(Minimal toxicity)

demonstrate that early therapy compared to late therapy is associated with prolongation of survival. In vitro resistance is noted after prolonged therapy with AZT; this correlates with clinical deterioration, but does not appear to be the entire explanation for the failure of continued response.

Other Nucleoside Analogues

ddI and ddC are other nucleoside analogs that may be given as alternatives to AZT or may be given in combination with AZT. HIV strains that are resistant to AZT retain sensitivity to ddI and ddC, although their use will usually result in the evolution of resistance to them as well. ddI must be given with adequate buffering to improve absorption. The usual dose is two 100 mg tablets twice daily. Prior studies have shown this drug increases the $CD4^+$ cell count, decreases viral load, and confers a clinical benefit in terms of reduced opportunistic infections in patients switched from AZT to ddI after at least 8 weeks of AZT therapy. The major side effects of ddI are pancreatitis and peripheral neuropathy.

ddC is given in a dose of 0.75 mg three times daily. It has demonstrated benefit in increasing the $CD4^+$ cell count and reducing viral load and is considered therapeutically equivalent to ddI for late-stage disease. Initial studies showed that ddC in combination with AZT had a beneficial effect on the $CD4^+$ cell count compared to AZT alone, but two large clinical trials could not substantiate the benefit of this change in patients who had received AZT previously. The major side effect of ddC is peripheral neuropathy.

d4T is advocated for patients with advanced HIV infection who are intolerant of alternative, approved therapy, or who have significant clinical or immunologic deterioration while receiving the alternative drugs. The usual dose is 40 mg twice daily, it is generally well tolerated, and the most common side effect is peripheral neuropathy. d4T has demonstrated benefit in increasing the $CD4^+$ cell count and reducing viral load. It is generally not given in combination with AZT because of possible in vitro antagonism.

3TC is a relatively new drug that, in combination with AZT, shows promise in providing a sustained benefit in terms of increased $CD4^+$ cell count and reduction in viral load of about 1 log. The usual dose is 150 mg twice daily. The drug is well tolerated and has little in the way of side effects. In vitro resistance develops quickly, but there appears to be a sustained benefit based on reversal in resistance to AZT.

Protease inhibitors inhibit HIV protease that is responsible for cleaving polyproteins into functional products in late stage replication. These are designer drugs in the sense that they are chemically designed based on a three dimensional structure. Major problems in development have been poor absorption, rapid excretion, and toxicity. These problems have been surmounted and several products have shown extraordinary activity in clinical trials: ritonavir (Norvir), indinavir (Crixivan), saquinavir (Invirase), and viracept. These drugs are the most potent anti-HIV drugs developed to date; in combination with nucleoside analogs, there is a decrease in viral burden exceeding 2 logs (99% decrease), often to the point that HIV can no longer be detected. The major concerns about these drugs are the durability of the response and resistance.

Resistance

In vitro resistance appears to be a universal feature of antiviral therapy in HIV infection with nucleoside analogs (AZT, ddI, ddC, d4T, 3TC). The biologic basis of resistance is amino acid substitutions on the *pol* gene that inscribes for reverse transcriptase, which is the target of these drugs. The development of in vitro resistance correlates with clinical deterioration, but is not the total explanation of the clinical course during treatment. Determination of resistance is not done in the context of clinical care, but is considered a research tool of possible clinical merit in the future.

Combination Treatment

The studies of the dynamics of HIV replication in vivo previously summarized indicated very rapid replication and high rates of mutation throughout the course of HIV infection. This work also showed nearly complete replacement of wild-type virus in plasma by drug-resistant variants within weeks of initiating treatment. An arbitrary conclusion from these observations is that therapy should be much more aggressive using multiple drugs based on the rationale of multiple drug therapy in tuberculosis. As a consequence, most authorities now recommend the use of combinations of two or three antiviral agents. The rationale increased in vitro activity (synergy or additive) and reduced resistance. These concepts are supported by clinical trials showing combination treatment is superior to monotherapy based on quantitative virology, increase in $CD4^+$ cell count, delay in the time to an AIDS-defining diagnosis, and survival.

Vertical Transmission

A large clinical trial (ACTG 076) demonstrated a reduction in the rate of vertical transmission of HIV in pregnant women from approximately 25 percent in the placebo group to 8 percent in those who received AZT. The clinical application of this study mandates that all pregnant women should be offered HIV serologic testing; those who are positive should be offered an abortion, and those who elect to carry the child should be offered AZT. Treatment is advocated during the second and third trimesters, it is given intravenously during delivery, and it is given to the infant for the first 6 weeks of life.

HIV Exposure in the Workplace

Numerous studies have shown the risk of HIV transmission to healthcare workers with a needlestick injury from an HIV-infected source is approximately 0.3 percent. Factors that correlate with increased efficiency of transmission are hollow bore needles (versus suture needles), a large needle, deep injury, visible blood on the device, vascular access procedure, lack of gloves, and a source with terminal HIV illness. The latter presumably relates to the high level plasma viremia in late-stage disease. A case control study by the CDC suggests that AZT prophylaxis to the healthcare worker with HIV exposure due to a needlestick injury appears to confer a benefit.

PREVENTION OF OPPORTUNISTIC INFECTIONS

The second major component of HIV management concerns the prevention of the opportunistic infections that characterize late-stage disease. Suggested guidelines are in Table 2. In terms of priorities, prophylaxis for *P. carinii* pneumonia is considered most important because it is the most common AIDS-defining diagnosis, the most common identifiable cause of death, and it is readily preventable. Multiple strategies are available, including treatment with trimethoprim-sulfamethoxazole (TMP-SMX), dapsone, or aerosolized pentamidine. The preferred drug is TMP-SMX. Additional salutory benefits include efficacy in preventing toxoplasmosis and bacterial infections. The rate of reactions to TMP-SMX in AIDS patients is 25 to 50 percent, and reactions are primarily rash, fever, leukopenia, and hepatitis. The cause of these reactions is not known, but it does not appear to be related to IgE, and many patients do well with rechallenge at a lower dose.

Tuberculosis is another high priority for prophylaxis. The current recommendations are for purified protein derivative (PPD) skin testing annually and administration of isoniazid (INH) prophylaxis for 1 year in those with a reaction of up to 5 mm induration, a history of a positive PPD without prior prophylaxis, or exposure to active disease. Anergy testing was previously recommended, but now is considered unreliable.

The third condition with a high priority for prophy-

Table 2 Prevention of Opportunistic Infections: Antimicrobial Prophylaxis

Disease and Priority	*Indications*	*Preferred Regimen*	*Comment*
Tuberculosis *High priority*	PPD plus ($\geq$5 mm induration); prior positive PPD; high-risk exposure	INH 300 mg/day plus pyridoxine 50 mg/day	Efficacy established; alternative is rifampin 600 mg/day × 12 mo
P. carinii pneumonia *High priority*	Prior PCP; $CD4^+$ cell <200/mm^3; Thrush or FUO	TMP-SMX 1 double strength tab/day	Efficacy established; cost effective; reduced morbidity and mortality; alternatives: dapsone 100 mg/day; regimens for toxoplasmosis (see below); or aerosolized pentamidine 300 mg/mo
Toxoplasmosis *High priority*	$CD4^+$ cell <100/mm^3 *plus* positive serology (IgG)	TMP-SMX 1 double strength tab/day	Efficacy established; main issue is use of alternative regimens in patients with TMP-SMX intolerance: dapsone 50 mg/day plus pyrimethamine 50 mg/wk plus leucovorin 25 mg/wk *or* dapsone 200 mg/wk plus pyrimethamine 75 mg/wk plus leucovorin 25 mg/wk
M. avium *Moderate priority*	$CD4^+$ cell <50-75/mm^3	Rifabutin 300 mg/day	Efficacy established; most breakthrough cases involve rafabutin-sensitive strains of *M. avium* Concerns are resistance of TB to rifampin (not established), cost and drug interactions; clarithromycin is more effective, but "breakthrough disease" usually involves clarithromycin-resistant strains
CMV *Not recommended*	CD4+ cell <50/mm^3	Oral ganciclovir 1,000 mg PO t.i.d.	Efficacy established; concerns are cost, promotion of ganciclovir resistance, and preliminary state of data
Deep fungal infection *Not recommended*	$CD4^+$ cell <100/mm^3	Fluconazole 200 mg/day	Efficacy established for prevention of cryptococcosis, *Candida* esophagitis and thrush; concerns are cost, ease of treating these complications, evidence for prolongation of survival, and promotion of infection with azole-resistant *Candida* species

CMV, Cytomegalovirus; *FUO,* fever of undetermined origin; *INH,* isoniazid; *PPD,* purified-protein derivative (tuberculin); *TB,* tuberculosis; *TMP-SMX,* trimethoprim-sulfamethoxazole.

laxis is toxoplasmosis. Patients with positive serology and a CD4$^+$ cell count of less than 100 per cubic millimeter should receive TMP-SMX; for those who cannot receive this agent, the alternative regimen is dapsone plus pyrimethamine.

Prophylaxis has also been shown to be effective for prevention of *M. avium* using rifabutin or clarithromycin. Although endorsed, it does not have a high priority because of the expense of these drugs, the frequency of side effects, and concern for resistance. Fluconazole has demonstrated efficacy in preventing cryptococcal meningitis and *Candida* esophagitis. However, its use is not recommended because of the high cost of treatment, the fact that these are readily treated complications, and the concern for promoting azole-resistant *Candida.*

FUTURE THERAPIES

As noted, therapy of HIV infection is in constant evolution with rapidly changing guidelines and introduction of multiple new drugs, drug combinations, and new concepts. The strategies noted here are largely limited to nucleoside analogues for anti-HIV treatment since these have dominated the first 10 years of anti-HIV therapy. There is increasing enthusiasm for a more aggressive attack on HIV, and combination treatment is now routinely recommended. In general, therapeutic trials in HIV infection have evolved into two very stereotyped patterns of study: the initial studies are designed to show changes in CD4$^+$ cell counts and viral burden as indicated by quantitative PCR or bDNA. Drug regimens that survive this initial trial are then subjected to large clinical trials in which the end points are a new AIDS-defining diagnosis or death. To date, AZT, ddI, d4T, AZT + ddI, AZT + ddC, delaviridine + AZT, and several combinations of protease inhibitors + nucleoside analogues have documented benefit in both trial models; other drugs and drug combinations have documented benefit only in the surrogate marker studies.

Immune-based therapy is also gaining popularity, and the initial studies with IL-2 appear promising. Despite the rapid evolution of new drugs and new concepts, most authorities believe that the current state-of-the-art has provided only a 1- to 2-year survival advantage. Much of this must be ascribed to the prevention of *P. carinii* pneumonia, which some believe is the most important therapeutic development to date.

Major changes in the future will be extensive use of combination therapy directed against HIV with quantitative virology as a major mechanism of therapeutic monitoring. Concerns are the evolution of resistance and the durability of the response.

SUGGESTED READING

Ho DD, Neumann AU, Perelson AS, et al. Rapid turnover of plasma virions and CD4 lymphocytes in HIV-1 infection. Nature 1995; 373:123–126.

Pantaleo G, Graziosi C, Fauci AS. The immunopathogenesis of human immunodeficiency virus infection. N Engl J Med 1993; 328:327.

Markowitz M, Saag M, Powderly WG, et al. A preliminary study of ritonavir, an inhibitor of HIV-1 protease, to treat HIV-1 infection. N Engl J Med 1995; 333:1534–1539.

Eron JJ, Benoit SL, Jemsek J, et al. Treatment with lamivudine, zidovudine, or both in HIV-positive patients with 200 to 300 CD4$^+$ cells per cubic millimeter. N Engl J Med 1995; 333:1662–1669.

Dolin R. Human studies in the development of human immunodeficiency virus vaccines. J Infect Dis 1995; 172:1175–1183.

Bridges SH, Sarver N. Gene therapy and immune restoration for HIV disease. Lancet 1995; 345:427–432.

ACQUIRED IMMMUNODEFICIENCY SYNDROME: TREATMENT OF OPPORTUNISTIC INFECTIONS

KATHERINE M. SPOONER, M.D.
MICHAEL A. POLIS, M.D., M.P.H.

As human immunodeficiency virus (HIV) infection progresses to the acquired immunodeficiency syndrome (AIDS), infected individuals are at increasing risk for various opportunistic infections. In the early years of the epidemic, the primary goal of managing these patients was to treat established opportunistic infections. More recently the emphasis has been placed on modalities to prevent the occurrence of such infections. In addition, the importance of maintenance therapy to prevent relapses of opportunistic infections has been recognized. A general approach to managing HIV-infected individuals includes the use of appropriate antiretroviral therapy, ongoing monitoring of the immune system, and the initiation of appropriate prophylactic agents to prevent opportunistic infections when the level of immunocompromise warrants.

As experience accumulates with the management of opportunistic infections, the following principles are increasingly appreciated:

1. The manifestations of opportunistic infections are varied, and a high degree of suspicion should be maintained with regard to new symptoms in an HIV-infected patient.
2. Many infections, such as toxoplasmosis and cytomegalovirus, represent reactivation of latent disease.

3. The CD4 cell count is a good, though imprecise, marker of progressive immunologic decline.
4. Opportunistic infections such as histoplasmosis, coccidioidomycosis, leishmaniasis, and tuberculosis are often geographically or socioeconomically clustered.
5. Newly described entities such as bartonellosis, microsporidiosis, disseminated penicillium infections, and rhodococcal disease are increasingly recognized as we become more familiar with the presentations, prophylaxis, and treatment of common opportunistic infections.
6. Often, several different opportunistic infections may be present simultaneously.
7. Although bacterial opportunistic infections may be cured, most opportunistic infections due to fungal or parasitic pathogens, such as *C. neoformans* and *T. gondii* are rarely cured; thus lifelong maintenance therapy is required.
8. Prophylactic regimens are improving and may lead to a better quality of life; however, there are significant concerns regarding the increasing use of prophylaxis. These include cost, drug interactions, and most importantly, the emergence of microbial resistance.

PNEUMOCYSTIS CARINII

Before the routine use of *Pneumocystis carinii* pneumonia (PCP) prophylaxis, PCP occurred in up to 75 percent of patients with AIDS, and was by far the most common and serious opportunistic infection in these individuals. Although PCP is still a commonly recognized life-threatening opportunistic infection, coincident with the widespread use of prophylaxis, the incidence has decreased since 1988. A recent estimate maintains that PCP is the AIDS-defining illness in 14.5 percent of persons receiving prophylactic treatment, and up to 28 percent of HIV-infected patients will ultimately develop PCP. Fortunately, the morbidity and mortality associated with acute PCP has decreased in the last few years because of advances in early diagnosis and treatment.

It is generally recommended that prophylaxis for PCP should be initiated when the CD4 cell count falls below 200 cells per cubic millimeter, since it rarely occurs in patients with higher CD4 cell counts. Because the rate of secondary infection approaches 66 percent in the 12 months following an initial episode, prophylaxis is also indicated after such an episode. The most commonly used regimens for PCP prophylaxis are summarized in Table 1.

Trimethoprim-sulfamethoxazole (TMP-SMX) is the most efficacious treatment for PCP, decreasing the rate of primary (and secondary) infection to less than 5 percent compared to an 11 percent rate of primary infection with aerosolized pentamidine. Unfortunately, 30 to 40 percent of HIV infected individuals will have adverse reactions to TMP-SMX, with fever, rash and pruritis, leukopenia, and nausea being the most common. Unless a severe toxicity is observed such as Stevens-Johnson syndrome or an immediate hypersensitivity reaction or severe hematologic compromise, most experts recommend reinstitution of TMP-SMX. This approach is justified not only by the significantly better efficacy for PCP prophylaxis, but TMP-SMX also provides excellent prophylaxis against toxoplasmosis, and may provide protection against various bacteria, including *Salmonella, Listeria, Nocardia, Streptococcus pneumonia, Haemophilus influenzae, Staphylococcus aureus,* and many gram-negative bacteria.

Although less efficacious than TMP-SMX, aerosolized pentamidine has been shown to be an effective alternative prophylactic treatment. It is generally well tolerated, with the predominant side effect of coughing

Table 1 Management of PCP in HIV Infected-Persons

Indication	*Drug/Dosage*	*Alternative*	*Duration*	*Comments*
Prophylaxis	TMP-SMX DS (double strength: 160 mg TMP, 800 mg SMX), 1 tablet PO q.d.	Dapsone 100 mg PO q.d. Aerosolized pentamidine 300 mg monthly	Lifelong	Initiate when CD4 <200 cells/mm^3 or after initial episode of PCP TMP-SMX 3 times weekly may be as effective for prophylaxis
Therapy: mild disease	TMP-SMX 2 DS tablets PO t.i.d. Dapsone 100 mg PO q.d. with trimethoprim 20 mg/kg/day PO in 3 divided doses	Atovaquone 750 mg PO t.i.d. with food Pentamidine 4 mg/kg IV q.d.	21 days	
Therapy: moderate to severe disease	TMP-SMX: 15-20 mg TMP IV daily in 3 divided doses	Pentamidine 4 mg/kg IV q.d. Trimetrexate 30 mg/m^2 IV with leukovorin 20 mg/m^2 IV q6h Primaquine 15 mg PO q.d. with clindamycin 600 mg IV q6h	21 days	If arterial $Po_2 \leq 70$ add oral prednisone taper: 40 mg b.i.d. × 5 days 40 mg q.d. × 5 days 20 mg q.d. × 11 days

or wheezing in 30 to 40 percent of patients. Since it is not systemically absorbed, disseminated pneumocystosis has been reported in association with its use. Dapsone has been shown to be as effective as aerosolized pentamidine for primary prophylaxis, although it is also less effective than TMP-SMX. Dapsone plus pyrimethamine has been shown to be as effective as pentamidine and additionally provides protection against toxoplasmosis. Dose-limiting adverse reactions to dapsone, including fever, rash, bone marrow suppression, and hemolytic anemia occur in up to 41 percent of patients.

Early diagnosis and intervention for acute infections before pulmonary dysfunction generally leads to uneventful recovery and good prognosis. Several agents are available for the treatment of PCP (Table 1), although TMP-SMX remains the preferred agent. For mild to moderate disease, an oral regimen is effective and well tolerated. Oral dapsone-TMP has been shown to be as effective as TMP-SMX in this situation, and one small study suggests that dapsone-TMP may have fewer adverse reactions. The combination of clindamycin and primaquine has been evaluated and may have similar efficacy to TMP-SMX, with fewer adverse reactions. Other oral treatment agents include atovaquone, a hydroxynapthoquinone, which is better tolerated, but less effective, than TMP-SMX.

Moderate to severe disease is manifested by significant pulmonary compromise, usually with increased arterial-alveolar oxygen gradient (>35 mm Hg and/or arterial Po_2 of <70 mm Hg). The preferred treatment in this setting is intravenous TMP-SMX with the addition of glucocorticoids. Early use of adjunctive corticosteroid therapy has been shown to improve survival and decrease the occurrence of respiratory failure in patients with severe disease. If TMP-SMX cannot be tolerated, other options include intravenous pentamidine, with close attention to the potential development of hypoglycemia, hypotension, renal impairment, and pancreatitis. Trimetrexate with leucovorin is effective in the treatment of moderately severe PCP and may be better tolerated than TMP-SMX, but it is only available in parenteral formulation. Other second-line choices include clindamycin plus primaquine and dapsone-TMP.

Treatment for PCP should be continued for 21 days, although patients responding well to therapy have been treated for only 14 days. Patients not responding after 5 to 10 days of therapy should be re-evaluated for the presence of other pathogens, and alternative PCP treatment should be considered. However, decreased oxygenation, or desaturation with exercise, is commonly seen between day 3 and 7 of successful treatment.

PROTOZOAL INFECTIONS

Reactivation of latent *Toxoplasma gondii* produces a common, treatable central nervous system encephalitis in AIDS patients. The incidence varies geographically, with higher rates seen in endemic areas such as Europe, Latin America, and Africa where latent infection is present in 75 to 90 percent of the population, compared with the prevalence in the United States of 10 to 40 percent. Between 30 and 50 percent of AIDS patients with serologic evidence of latent disease will develop active infection. Toxoplasmosis rarely develops in HIV-infected individuals with a CD4 count greater than 100 cells per cubic millimeter, thus prophylaxis should be considered at this point, with either TMP-SMX or dapsone-pyrimethamine.

Since toxoplasmosis is the most common treatable cause of multiple, ring-enhancing mass lesions, often with surrounding edema, patients with computed tomography or magnetic resonance imaging scans consistent with toxoplasmosis should receive empiric treatment. A brain biopsy should be strongly considered if clear radiologic and clinical improvement is not seen after 2 weeks. Other common brain space-occupying lesions in HIV-infected persons include lymphoma, tuberculoma, progressive multifocal leukoencephalopathy, and cryptococcoma. Recommended therapy for toxoplasmosis (Table 2) is with pyrimethamine plus sulfadiazine or clindamycin, with the addition of leucovorin to diminish the bone marrow toxicity of pyrimethamine. Anecdotally useful alternative agents include atovaquone and azithromycin.

Protozoal causes of diarrheal disease in persons with advanced HIV infection are often associated with marked debility. Cryptosporidiosis, caused by *Cryptosporidium parvum*, has become increasingly common as patients receive better prophylaxis and treatment for common opportunistic infections. Although cryptosporidiosis may be a self-limited disease in immunocompetent hosts, HIV-infected individuals develop a persistent enteritis that is most often refractory to treatment. In one study, patients with a CD4 count greater than 180 cells per cubic millimeter had self-limited infections, whereas of those with a CD4 count of fewer than 140 cells per cubic millimeter, 87 percent developed persistent disease. In addition to voluminous, watery diarrhea, cryptosporidial infection can involve the biliary tract. Anecdotally, paromomycin has led to improvement in some patients, but there is no consistently effective treatment, and most patients suffer chronic diarrhea, weight loss, and abdominal pain. Isosporiasis, a chronic watery diarrheal illness caused by *Isospora belli*, is endemic in AIDS patients from Haiti, and can be treated with TMP-SMX. Microsporidiosis caused by *Enterocytozoon bienusi* and other *Microspora*, is another chronic enteritis seen in HIV-infected persons with advanced immunosuppression. There is currently no adequate treatment for this entity. Most patients with chronic diarrhea require aggressive antimotility agents, and severe cases associated with wasting may require parenteral nutrition.

FUNGAL INFECTIONS

Oral candidiasis caused by *Candida albicans* is the most commonly encountered fungal infection in persons

Table 2 Management of Protozoal Infections in HIV-Infected Persons

Disease	*Prophylaxis*	*Treatment*	*Maintenance*	*Comments*
Toxoplasmosis	TMP-SMX 1 DS tablet PO q.d. *or* dapsone 100 mg PO q.d. with pyrimethamine 50 mg PO weekly	Pyrimethamine 50-100 mg PO q.d. plus sulfadiazine 1 gm PO q.d. *or* clindamycin 1,200 mg IV or 600 mg PO q6-8h 3 to 6 weeks acute treatment	Pyrimethamine 50-100 mg PO q.d. plus sulfadiazine 500-1,000 mg PO q.d. *or* clindamycin 300 mg PO q.i.d.	Folinic acid 10 mg PO daily with pyrimethamine
Cryptosporidiosis	None effective	Anecdotal success with paromomycin 25 mg/kg daily in 3 divided doses × 10 days	Antimotility agents routinely administered for persistent diarrhea	Somatostatin may offer symptomatic relief; may require parenteral nutrition
Microsporidiosis	None effective	None effective	Antimotility agents routinely administered for persistent diarrhea	Somatostatin may offer symptomatic relief; may require parenteral nutrition
Isosporiasis		TMP-SMX 1 DS tablet PO q.i.d. × 10 days, then b.i.d. × 21 days	TMP-SMX 1 DS tablet PO 3 × weekly	
		Pyrimethamine 75 mg PO q.d. × 14 days	Pyrimethamine 25 mg PO q.d.	Folinic acid 10 mg PO daily with pyrimethamine

with HIV infection and is seen in up to 45 percent of patients at the time of AIDS diagnosis. Topical treatment is adequate for mild thrush; however, more extensive disease, including esophageal candidiasis (which occurs in up to 11 percent of patients), requires systemic therapy (Table 3). The triazole antifungal agent fluconazole has proved to be well tolerated and effective. Although there is currently no established role for prophylaxis in patients without prior thrush, persons with recurrent episodes may benefit from suppressive therapy since the relapse rate may be as high as 50 percent in the first month following treatment. Ketoconazole is less commonly used for treatment since absorption is erratic due to the gastric hypochlorhydria common in HIV-infected individuals. For unknown reasons, although HIV-infected persons commonly develop fungemia due to cryptococcosis and histoplasmosis, candidemia is rare in this population in the absence of a chronic catheter.

Cryptococcus neoformans meningitis in patients with AIDS is the most common life-threatening fungal infection in most areas of the United States and accounts for up to 10 percent of opportunistic infections. CD4 counts are almost always less than 50 cells per cubic millimeter at the time of presentation. Fever, headache, and malaise are common presenting symptoms, with meningismus present in only one-fifth of patients. Diagnosis is confirmed by the presence of cryptococcal antigen in the serum and cerebrospinal fluid (CSF), as well as by CSF cultures. Cryptococcal disease may also present with pulmonary or skin involvement and rarely with urinary tract or bone marrow involvement.

Preliminary data suggest that the prophylactic use of fluconazole may prevent cryptococcal infections. However, most experts do not recommend the widespread use of primary prophylaxis against fungal infections because of the low morbidity associated with early diagnosis and treatment of candida and cryptococcal infections, the risk of developing fluconazole-resistant fungi, and the prohibitive cost of fluconazole. Therapy for cryptococcal meningitis should be initiated with intravenous amphotericin B, with close monitoring of its associated toxicities, particularly nephrotoxicity, fever, and anemia. Concomitant flucytosine does not appear to offer a significant benefit and may increase drug toxicities. In patients responding to treatment within 2 weeks, oral fluconazole may be substituted to complete acute treatment, followed by lifelong maintenance treatment (see Table 3). Initial therapy with fluconazole may be effective in selected individuals with mild disease, but determining which patients may respond is difficult.

Other fungal diseases of significance to patients with HIV infection include histoplasmosis, caused by *Histoplasma capsulatum,* and coccidioidomycosis, caused by *Coccidioides immitis,* both of which present as disseminated infections. These tend to be more restricted geographically in the United States: histoplasmosis is seen throughout the central river valleys, and coccidioidomycosis in the southwest. In some areas, coccidioidomycosis and histoplasmosis may be more prevalent than PCP in persons with AIDS. Another geographically restricted fungal infection recently described in HIV-infected patients is disseminated *Penicillium marnefii,* seen in patients from Thailand.

VIRAL INFECTIONS

Forty-five percent of persons with AIDS may ultimately develop disease due to cytomegalovirus (CMV), most commonly manifested by retinitis or colitis, which frequently leads to significant morbidity. Disease rarely develops before the CD4 count falls below 50 cells

Table 3 Management of Fungal Disease in HIV-Infected Persons

Disease	*Prophylaxis*	*Treatment*	*Maintenance*	*Comments*
Oral and eosphageal candidiasis	None recommended	Mild thrush only: clotrimazole 10 mg troche 5 × daily Systemic treatment: fluconazole 200 mg PO day 1, then 100 mg q.d. × 10 days For resistant candidal disease, amphotericin B .25 mg/kg IV q.d. up to 100-200 mg total dose	For persistent disease, fluconazole 100 mg PO q.d. (may be effective less frequently)	Consider fluconazole 100 mg PO q.d. as prophylaxis for patients with frequent recurrences
Cryptococcal meningitis	None recommended	Amphotericin B, .7 mg/kg IV q.d. × 2 weeks, then fluconazole 400 mg PO q.d.	Fluconazole 200-400 mg PO q.d. or amphotericin B 1 mg/kg IV weekly	Oral fluconazol as initial treatment for mild disease has been used Fluconazole is effective for prophylaxis, but not routinely recommended because of low incidence of disease and rapid response to treatment
Histoplasmosis	None recommended	Initially amphotericin B 1 mg/kg IV q.d. × 2 weeks, then itraconazole 200 mg PO b.i.d. for 12 weeks acute treatment Mild disease: itraconazole 200 mg PO t.i.d. × 3 days, then 200 mg b.i.d. for 12 weeks acute treatment	Itraconazole 200 mg PO q.d.	Fluconazole may be effective
Coccidioidomycosis	None recommended	Initially, amphotericin B 1 mg/kg IV q.d. until clinical response seen, then fluconazole 400 to 800 mg PO q.d. Mild disease: Fluconazole 400 to 800 mg PO q.d.	Fluconazole 200 to 400 mg PO q.d.	Itraconazole may be effective; optimal treatment regimen not yet established

per cubic millimeter. Two agents, gancyclovir and foscarnet, are currently available for the treatment and maintenance of CMV (Table 4), although they are only effective in limiting the progression of disease and must be given parenterally. Documented CMV disease eventually progresses in most patients despite continued intravenous maintenance treatment. Both agents have significant toxicities: gancyclovir causes neutropenia, especially in patients on concomitant zidovudine, and foscarnet is nephrotoxic. Both are equivalent as anti-CMV agents; however, studies have suggested a survival benefit with the use of foscarnet, possibly associated with its intrinsic antiretroviral activity. CMV viruria or viremia may precede the development of end-organ disease, but without orally available, less toxic agents, treatment in the absence of organ dysfunction is not warranted. Recently completed studies suggest that an oral formulation of gancyclovir may be useful in the prevention of CMV disease in persons with low CD4 counts.

Recurrent herpes simplex (HSV) infections cause appreciable morbidity in patients with HIV infection, most commonly presenting as perianal ulcerations or esophagitis. Suppressive therapy with daily oral acyclovir may benefit patients who have poorly healing or frequent infections, although this use may promote the development of viral resistance. Foscarnet is the treatment of choice where clinical or virologic resistance is documented. Acyclovir resistant strains of HSV are generally resistant to gancyclovir as well.

In adults, varicella zoster virus (VZV) is most commonly seen as classic zoster, which can present in HIV-infected individuals with normal CD4 counts. Dissemination may rarely occur, requiring the use of intravenous acyclovir. Uncomplicated zoster does not require treatment unless the ophthalmic division of the trigeminal nerve is involved. Famciclovir, which has an antiviral spectrum similar to acyclovir, has recently been licensed for treatment of VZV (see Table 4) and may decrease the incidence of postherpetic neuralgia. Other viral illnesses encountered in HIV infection include oral hairy leukoplakia (OHL), associated with Epstein-Barr virus. OHL does not require treatment, although acyclovir may occasionally be useful. Progressive multifocal leukoencephalopathy occurs in persons with a very advanced HIV infection, with CD4 counts of fewer than 50 cells per cubic millimeter, and is caused by a papovavirus, JC. There is no known treatment, and prognosis is very poor for these individuals.

Table 4 Management of Viral Infections in HIV-Infected Persons

Disease	*Treatment*	*Maintenance*	*Comments*
CMV	Gancyclovir 5 mg/kg IV q12h × 14 days, *or* Foscarnet 90 mg/kg IV q12h × 14 days	Gancyclovir 5 mg/kg IV q.d. or foscarnet 90 to 120 mg/kg IV q.d.	No effective licensed prophylaxis Oral gancyclovir may be effective Higher doses of gancyclovir with colony stimulating factors (i.e., G-CSF) or combination gancyclovir/foscarnet may be considered for refractory disease
HSV			
Mild mucocutaneous	Acyclovir 200-400 mg PO 5 × daily for 7 to 10 days	None	Prophylaxis for frequently recurrent VZV/HSV: consider acyclovir 200-400 mg PO b.i.d. to t.i.d.
Severe	Acyclovir 5 mg/kg IV q8h × 7 days	None	
VZV			
Zoster	Acyclovir 800 mg PO 5 × daily × 7 days Famciclovir 300 mg PO t.i.d. × 7 days	None None	For severe or recurrent HSV or VZV disease with documented acyclovir resistance, treatment with foscarnet 60 mg IV q12h induction, then 60 mg daily maintenance
Disseminated	Acyclovir 10 mg/kg IV q8h × 7-10 days	None	

BACTERIAL INFECTIONS

Mycobacterium tuberculosis has been undergoing an epidemic of its own in addition to its association with the AIDS epidemic since the mid-1980s. One-third of the world's population is infected with *M. tuberculosis,* with 8 to 10 million new cases of active tuberculosis yearly, of which a significant portion may have concomitant HIV infection. Of critical importance is that *M. tuberculosis* is one of the few HIV-related pathogens that can be transmitted via a respiratory route to immunocompetent hosts in a community or health care setting.

HIV infected individuals are prone to developing active tuberculosis after exposure, with an estimated 10 percent annual risk of disease in persons with known positive tuberculin skin tests, underscoring the critical need for chemoprophylaxis in this population. Skin reactions of larger than 5 mm to the standard PPD are considered positive in HIV-infected individuals, and as HIV progresses, relative or absolute cutaneous anergy may develop, decreasing the utility of a negative skin test. Twelve months of chemoprophylaxis is indicated for HIV-infected individuals with a positive skin test, as well as for anergic patients with a significant exposure.

Active tuberculosis has varied manifestations in HIV-infected individuals, and since it can occur at any level of immunosuppression, it may be the first clinical presentation of HIV infection. In addition to commonly recognized pulmonary manifestations, tuberculosis may involve any tissue and organ system. Treatment (Table 5) should initially include 3 or 4 agents, based on the geographic prevalence and likelihood of exposure to drug-resistant organisms, for at least 2 months, with total treatment continued for at least 9 months, and at least 6 months after cultures are negative. All persons with tuberculosis should have their *M. tuberculosis* isolates tested for drug sensitivity.

Disseminated *Mycobacterium avium* complex (MAC) infection occurs in at least 25 percent of persons with AIDS and CD4 counts less than 50 cells per cubic millimeter. The presentation is that of a systemic illness most often associated with fevers, night sweats, weight loss, and gastrointestinal symptoms. Recent studies have indicated that prophylaxis of persons with CD4 cell counts of fewer than 75 cells per cubic millimeter with rifabutin, 300 mg daily, may decrease the incidence of disseminated MAC by 50 percent. Recent studies suggest that the macrolide antibiotic clarithromycin may also be effective as prophylaxis. Despite the documented efficacy of rifabutin, many experts are wary of using this agent because of the concern of other mycobacteria developing resistance to the rifamycins, the multiple drug-to-drug toxicities associated with rifabutin, and its cost. Treatment of documented MAC infections (see Table 5) should be administered lifelong, and include either azithromycin or clarithromycin, ethambutol, and one or more of the following: ciprofloxacin, clofazimine, rifampin, or rifabutin. Other atypical mycobacterial infections are also seen in HIV-infected patients, including *M. kansasii, M. hemophilum, M. xenopi,* and others.

Many bacterial infections seen in immunocompetent hosts, such as the encapsulated organisms *(S. pneumoniae* and *H. influenzae),* are seen more commonly in HIV-infected individuals, and should be treated conventionally. The AIDS epidemic has led to increased recognition of new bacterial pathogens, particularly of the *Bartonella* species, which have been found to be the etiologic organisms of cat-scratch disease (in immunocompetent hosts, particularly children), and bacillary angiomatosis and peliosis hepatis in persons with AIDS.

Table 5 Management of Mycobacterial Disease in HIV-Infected Persons

Disease	*Patient Population*	*Initial Regimen*	*Maintenance*	*Duration*	*Comments*
M. tuberculosis	Positive skin test, no active disease	INH 300 mg PO q.d. For suspected INH resistance: add 2 drugs from: rifampin 600 mg PO q.d., ethambutol 15 mg/kg PO q.d., pyrazinamide 15-30 mg/kg PO q.d.		12 mo	Defined as >5 mm induration: consider treatment with 2 to 5 mm induration, and with suspected exposure in setting of anergy
	Active disease, sensitive strain	INH plus rifampin plus pyrazinamide or ethambutol × 2 mo	INH plus rifampin	Total of 9 mo, or 6 mo after culture conversion	
	Active disease, resistant strain suspected, or prevalent geographically	INH plus rifampin plus ethambutol plus pyrazinamide or streptomycin 15 mg/kg IM q.d. If known, total of 4 drugs to which organism susceptible × 2 mo	3 drugs to which organism sensitive	Total of 12 mo after culture conversion	Alternatives include amikacin 7.5 mg/kg IV q12h; ofloxacin 600 to 800 mg PO q.d.
Mycobacterium avum complex	Stool, resp. colonization	No treatment recommended			
	CD4 cell count $<75/mm^3$	Prophylaxis with rifabutin 300 mg PO q.d.			Macrolides may be effective
	Disseminated	Clarithromycin 500 mg PO b.i.d. or azithromycin 500 mg PO q.d., plus 2 or 3 of the following: ethambutol 15 mg/kg PO q.d., plus ciprofloxacin 750 mg PO b.i.d. or clofazimine 100 mg PO q.d., rifampin 600 mg PO q.d., or rifabutin 450 mg PO q.d.	Same as initial regimen	Lifelong	

INH, Isoniazid.

B. henselae is associated with cat exposure, unlike *B. quintana,* and both pathogens cause similar systemic illnesses. The diagnosis of bacillary angiomatosis may often be missed since its skin manifestations may resemble other HIV-associated diseases. Treatment is effective with indefinite courses of doxycycline or erythromycin, although many other agents are likely to be effective, including the newer macrolides and ciprofloxacin. Another bacteria to receive increasing attention is *Rhodococcus equi,* which causes both pulmonary (usually with abscess formation) and systemic illness, and can be treated with a prolonged course of vancomycin. These two newly described entities are examples of the evolving nature of the AIDS epidemic, and one would expect many further changes in the bacterial pathogens described in this patient population.

The management of opportunistic infections in persons with HIV infection is a rapidly changing and complex task. Appropriate prophylaxis, treatment, and maintenance therapy is critical to optimize the quality of life for HIV-infected individuals. The task of the primary caregiver includes monitoring the immune status of an HIV-infected patient and maintaining a high degree of suspicion for the infections that may occur as the disease progresses. As the epidemic continues to evolve, further attention will likely focus on less frequently described pathogens, as well as the identification of new, undescribed pathogens. Finally, the complexity of medical regimens that patients receive as their disease progresses should not be underestimated, and the relative risks and benefits of various prophylactic therapies will require close evaluation in each individual. On a global scale, consideration needs to be given to limiting the development of resistant organisms and to limiting progression of concomitant epidemics such as tuberculosis.

SUGGESTED READING

Gallant JE, Moore RD, Chaisson RE. Prophylaxis for opportunistic infections in patients with HIV infection. Ann Intern Med 1994; 120: 932–944.

Glaser CA, Angulo FJ, Rooney JA. Animal-associated opportunistic infections among persons infected with the human immunodeficiency virus. Clin Infect Dis 1994; 18:14–24.

Hoover DR, Saah AJ, Bacellar H, et al. Clinical manifestations of AIDS in the era of pneumocystis prophylaxis. N Engl J Med 1993; 329: 1922–1926.

Katz MH, Hessol NA, Buchbinder SP, et al. Temporal trends of opportunistic infections and malignancies in homosexual men with AIDS. J Infect Dis 1994; 170:198–202.

Lane HC, moderator. Recent advances in the management of AIDS-related opportunistic infections. Ann Intern Med 1994; 120: 945–955.

Wheat J. Histoplasmosis and coccidioidomycosis in individuals with AIDS. Infect Dis Clin North Am 1994; 8:467–482.

HUMAN IMMUNODEFICIENCY VIRUS INFECTION: POTENTIAL THERAPIES FOR IMMUNOLOGIC RECONSTITUTION

SMRITI K. KUNDU, M.D.
THOMAS C. MERIGAN, M.D.

ENHANCEMENT OF HIV-SPECIFIC IMMUNE RESPONSES

The development of effective therapies for the treatment of HIV infection is an ongoing process. Much work has suggested that antiretroviral chemotherapy has only limited efficacy. This has focused more attention towards the potential for immunologic interventions. HIV infection leads to progressive depletion of the number and function of $CD4^+$ T lymphocytes, which are the main effector cells of the immune system. This results in a variety of immunologic abnormalities, including defective soluble antigen recognition, defective specific and nonspecific cytotoxicity, abnormal monocyte macrophage function, altered lymphokine production, polyclonal B-cell activation, and hypergammaglobulinemia. Therefore, modalities to boost the specific immunologic responses to HIV and general immune responses to HIV-infected individuals may be useful immunotherapeutic strategies (Table 1). It is also possible that only combined antiretroviral therapy and immunotherapy may ultimately be successful in limiting disease progression.

The potential approaches to enhance HIV specific immune responses are (1) the use of HIV vaccines; (2) passive immunotherapy using polyclonal and monoclonal antibodies; and (3) the adoptive transfer of specific cell populations to boost the immune system against HIV.

HIV VACCINES

Therapeutic vaccines have been used in HIV infection to boost the HIV-specific immune responses that may be responsible for controlling virus replication; however, so far there is little evidence that they will decrease the virus load in an enduring manner. This approach was adopted from the speculation that both cellular and humoral immune responses control the virus

Table 1 Potential Immunotherapeutic Agents for HIV Infection

Immunostimulant		*Immunosuppressive*
HIV-Specific	*Nonspecific*	
Vaccines	**Cytokines**	Cyclosporins
Envelope	*Immunostimulants*	Glucocorticoids
r-gp160	IL-2, IL-7	
r-gp120	IFN-alfa, gamma;	
V3peptide	*Inhibitors* of IL-6: IL-4;	
Core	TNF-alfa: corticosteroids,	
r-p24	pentoxyfylline, thalidomide	
P24VLP	*Oxidative stress modulative*	
Virus	Procysteine	
Recombinant virus		
Whole killed virus		
Cells		
Antibodies		

load during the asymptomatic phase and as the disease progresses immune responses disappear and virus load increases. Yet the use of vaccine candidates as immunotherapeutic agents to treat HIV disease is in its infancy.

Clinical evaluations of multiple doses of recombinant gp160, gp120, p24 vaccines separately or in combinations have been carried out in HIV-seropositive individuals. These vaccines have been shown to be safe and immunogenic. Safety was measured by clinical events, $CD4^+$ T cell numbers, and drug toxicity. Immunogenicity was measured by HIV specific immune responses such as cytotoxic T lymphocyte (CTL) activities, lymphocyte proliferative (memory T cell) responses, cytokine responses (IL-2, interferon gamma production by helper T lymphocytes), delayed type hypersensitivity (memory T cell) responses, and antibody (B cell) responses.

HIV-1 IIIB r-gp160 from MicroGeneSys Inc., Meriden, Conn., has been studied extensively for several years in HIV-seropositive, asymptomatic individuals. Despite its relative safety and immunogenicity this vaccine did not decrease the virus load significantly. Virus load was measured by serum P24 antigen, virus culture, plasma virion RNA by RT-polymerase chain reaction (PCR), and cellular proviral DNA by PCR. These observations led us to think that the virus may be mutating to avoid the effect of the immune responses. To study this phenomenon, we undertook a study in which $HLA\text{-}A2^+$, HIV-seropositive, asymptomatic patients with $CD4^+$ T cell counts of more than 500 per cubic millimeter were immunized with r-gp160 (ImmunoAG, Vienna, Austria) monthly for 6 months. HLA-A2 restricted, envelope epitope specific CTL responses were measured at regular intervals pre- and postimmunization. Patient virus was also sequenced at the appropriate CTL epitope regions simultaneously. This study also revealed that patients with preimmunization virus of the vaccine sequence had shown enhanced CTL responses, whereas patients with virus of different sequence than the vaccine in the critical epitope sites did not mount these responses. Thus it appears to be a recall response. It is also analogous to the concept of "original antigenic sin," which was first described in relation to influenza immunity in which exposure to the previous strain of the virus determined the immune responses to the newly introduced strain or vaccine. In influenza, this phenomenon was in relation to B-cell responses such as antibodies, whereas in our study it was observed in the context of T-cell responses. In our study during the relatively short course of immunization we did not observe the development of escape mutants. We have designed a clinical trial of this vaccine in a larger group of patients with a longer study period to determine the effect of these enhanced immune responses on the virus.

r-gp120 vaccines (Biocine, Emeryville, Calif., and Genentech, Inc, South San Francisco, Calif., USA), have been shown to be immunogenic and safe in HIV-seronegative individuals (prophylactic vaccines) and are also being evaluated in HIV-seropositive individuals (therapeutic vaccines). The Biocine r-gp120 vaccine induced specific antibody responses to gp120 after several injections in HIV-seropositive individuals with $CD4^+$ T cell counts of more than 600 per cubic millimeter. No evidence of an effect on $CD4^+$ T cell numbers has been reported. The r-gp120 MN and IIIB from Genentech have also proved to be safe and immunogenic in HIV-seropositive individuals with $CD4^+$ T cell counts of more than 500 per cubic millimeter. In patients with a lower number of $CD4^+$ T cells, its immunogenic effect was not detectable. A placebo-controlled trial of this vaccine did not show any difference in the clinical endpoint development between the vaccine recipients and placebo recipients.

A killed HIV vaccine lacking gp120 (Immune Response Corporation, San Diego, Calif., USA) has been proven to be safe and immunogenic and has been associated with a lower virus load in the vaccine recipients at certain times within one study. Larger studies with this vaccine covering the wide range of

$CD4^+$ T cells categories are planned to see if these effects are reproducible and more enduring.

Synthetic peptides are becoming increasingly attractive alternatives to the full-length recombinant envelope glycoproteins. Animal studies have demonstrated that the development of multideterminant peptides linking helper peptides with neutralizing epitopes of the HIV-1 envelope glycoproteins may augment specific immune responses. Another approach is the use of an anti-idiotype vaccine. Two studies have shown that mouse monoclonal antibody against the HIV gp120 (IOTA 4a, Immunotech, France) was well tolerated and produced specific anti-idiotype antibody responses. Another auto-idiotype antibody, 3C9, recognizes a marker on human B cells that produces broadly neutralizing anti-gp120 antibodies. This vaccine was also reported to be safe and immunogenic.

PASSIVE IMMUNOTHERAPY USING ANTIBODIES

People early in infection are able to neutralize primary field isolates belonging to the same clade to a greater extent than most initially seronegative HIV vaccine recipients. This activity is lost with progression to clinical AIDS. The most well-explored antibody treatment approach so far has been the use of HIV-specific immunoglobulin as passive immunotherapy in HIV-infected persons. This reagent can be prepared from individuals infected with viruses of a similar clade or through the development of monoclonal antibodies directed against specific epitopes of the virus. Potential advantages of antibody therapy over traditional drugs include the fact that antibodies have longer half-lives so that they can be given intermittently. They not only neutralize virus directly, but also they enhance cellular immunity via antibody-dependent or complement-mediated cellular cytotoxicity. The disadvantages include the possibility that the virus may mutate to escape the effect of the antibody, or the patient may develop an immune response to the nonhuman products when nonhuman monoclonal antibody is being used. Finally, the distribution of antibody to all body sites may not be equal; for example, they may penetrate the central nervous system poorly.

Several trials have been designed to study the effect of polyclonal HIV immune plasma on the course of HIV disease. Some studies have shown positive effects on disease progression, whereas others have shown no effect. Intravenous immunoglobulin that lacks anti-HIV antibodies has also been tested with conflicting results in several studies. The most likely value of such therapy is in the reduction of bacterial or other viral infections, particularly in children. Further investigations are underway to determine their applicability. Monoclonal antibodies or cocktails of several monoclonal antibodies are under development, directed at more than one neutralizing epitope, including C3 loop, CD4 binding site or gp41 epitopes. Clinical therapy trials of these antibodies have been designed and are being implemented.

ADOPTIVE CELL TRANSFER

The ability to expand lymphocytes ex vivo has recently been recognized as an important development. It should permit the infusion of specific cell populations into HIV-infected individuals. Several studies have been started in recent months. Hence, data on the fate of the infused cells as well as their immunologic capabilities and antiviral activity should be reported soon.

In a study of HIV-discordant identical twins, the lymphocytes from the uninfected twin was expanded and reinfused into the HIV-positive twin. This approach was safe and increased his $CD4^+$ T cell count. The adoptive transfer of $CD8^+$ T cells following expansion and then reinfusion into the syngeneic recipient has been tried in several centers. Currently one study is underway using ex vivo expanded HIV-specific CTL for therapy. Preliminary results have shown that the procedure is safe, HIV-specific CTL activities have increased, and the study is continuing.

Recent reports suggest that $CD4^+$ T cells can be expanded in vitro in the presence of three antiretroviral drugs. Preliminary data indicate that it is possible to increase the number of $CD4^+$ T cells after 6 to 8 weeks by 4 to 6 $\log_{10}$ and that at least two-thirds of the cells expanded are identifiable as $CD4^+$ T cells. The cultures can be maintained in the presence of triple drug combination antiviral therapy and show no evidence of active virus replication following the procedure. Such techniques could allow the reinfusion of autologous expanded $CD4^+$ T cells into HIV-infected people.

There is growing interest and activity in the field of bone marrow transplant and hematopoietic cell therapy. A protocol is currently being proposed to evaluate the use of granulocyte-colony stimulating factor (G-CSF) in stem-cell mobilization and the function of these cells at different time points after cryopreservation. Another protocol is being developed to cryopreserve autologous cord blood in order to transduce cells with transdominant Rev protein, which acts at the transcriptional level of the HIV life cycle, and later reinfuse hematopoietic stem cells into a pediatric population. The development of a comprehensive study design on the role of the thymus in HIV infection is of utmost importance in defining mechanisms to optimize bone marrow transplant and stem-cell therapy approaches as well as in determining the role of thymus transplant and thymic hormones such as thymopentin-5 or Thymosin alpha-1 in treating HIV. Because cells from nonhuman primates are less susceptible to infection by HIV, xenogeneic cell transfer (e.g., baboon to human) may provide an alternative for immune reconstitution techniques with cell therapy without the need for genetic manipulation. These recent efforts in cellular therapy involving expanding specific cell populations in vitro and reinfusing them into patients in an attempt to reconstitute the immune system could produce new insights bearing on HIV pathogenesis and/or therapy.

GENERAL IMMUNE MODULATION

The ability to nonspecifically manipulate the immune system is also an important HIV therapeutic approach. The availability of substances that inhibit specific cytokines, which may be produced in excess, in HIV infected individuals, as well as the availability of general immune stimulators including certain cytokines, has made development in this area possible.

INHIBITION OF PROINFLAMATORY CYTOKINES

Evidence that certain cytokines are produced in excess has led to therapy with drugs known to decrease their production. The most extensively studied cytokine is tumor necrosis factor (TNF)-alfa which is produced in excess in HIV infection and up-regulates HIV expression in vitro. The major interventions include pentoxifylline, thalidomide, tenadap, and corticosteroids, all of which at least partially inhibit TNF production and other immunologic activities. Pentoxyfylline has been tried on HIV-infected patients with active pulmonary tuberculosis because these individuals can have high levels of TNF-alfa.

Thalidomide is being evaluated in regard to inhibition of TNF expression and subsequent decrease in HIV virus load. This compound has been shown to positively influence the course of patients with manifestations of erythema leprosum. It has been suggested that HIV patients with aphthous ulcers may benefit from thalidomide. A large scale placebo-controlled trial is underway to study this phenomenon in detail, specifically in patients with late-stage HIV disease.

Corticosteroids appear to benefit patients with HIV-associated nephropathy. In a preliminary trial, four patients appeared to show improvement in renal function. Because of concerns regarding the toxicity and immunosuppressive effects of corticosteroids, a carefully designed placebo-controlled trial is being undertaken in patients with biopsy-proven nephropathy.

IL-4 has also appeared to show some benefit in HIV-infected patients with Kaposi's sarcoma by inhibiting the inflammatory cytokine IL-6.

Cytokines That Potentially Enhance Immune Responses

Various cytokines have been used over the past several years to enhance immune responses. The results are mixed, with some showing benefit and some none. Interferon-alfa has been tried along with antiretrovirals in HIV-infected individuals. Results are matched with a general impression that its best action is in early disease. Interferon-gamma given with an anti-retroviral is also to be evaluated in clinical trials.

Beneficial effects of IL-2 have been tested in several clinical trials using different preparations of IL-2 with antiretrovirals. Intermittent use of intravenous IL-2 showed short-term increase in $CD4^+$ T cell numbers, which goes back to baseline value within 2 weeks. However, one recent study showed that patients with $CD4^+$ T cell counts of more than 200 per cubic millimeter showed a much more sustained increase in $CD4^+$ T cells associated with intermittent treatment, whereas patients with $CD4^+$ T cell counts of fewer than 100 cubic millimeter did not show such benefit. IL-2 may also be useful as an adjuvant in active immunization trials to enhance immune responses.

IL-12 and IL-15, novel T-cell growth factors, will also be tested for their clinical usefulness. Stem cell factor (SCF) is also being tried to mobilize stem cells; however, it appears that G-CSF is more potent and less toxic in stem-cell mobilization. IL-7 is another cytokine of interest since it has shown immune enhancement in in vitro assays.

DEFECTS IN OXIDATIVE METABOLISM

There is considerable interest in repairing the decreased oxidative pathways that have been described in HIV infection. Replenishment of glutathione, which has been shown to be decreased in patients with AIDS, might inhibit HIV replication. It has been shown that increases in glutathione can decrease reverse transcriptase activity in vitro. Intravenous and oral procysteine administration have been shown to increase $CD4^+$ T cells. But additional clinical trials are underway to evaluate the effect of procysteine on virus load, as well as the pharmacokinetics and intracellular levels of glutathione in blood.

IMMUNOSUPPRESSIVE THERAPY

There has been speculation that overstimulation of the immune system may enhance HIV disease progression. Cyclosporin A was used to counteract the immune stimulation effect. Anecdotal reports have shown that HIV-infected patients who received organ transplants have done better with cyclosporin as compared to those who did not receive the cyclosporin. A derivative of cyclosporin that has no immunosuppressive effect but has an antiviral effect has been under development and may be tried in HIV patients. In another study, 44 HIV-infected, asymptomatic patients with $CD4^+$ T cell counts of 200 to 799 per cubic millimeter received oral prednisolone for 6 months. It was safe and led to sustained increases in $CD4^+$ T cell counts and to improvement or stabilization of other biologic markers of disease activity. For example, DR^+, $CD25^+$ phenotypes in $CD4^+$ T cells and serum beta$_2$ microglobulin levels decreased; apoptosis of peripheral blood mononuclear cells decreased as well. However, concerns about the potential adverse virologic consequences of attempting to down-regulate the immune response in HIV-infected individuals has caused some hesitation in developing such interventions.

SUGGESTED READING

Fauci AS, Rosenberg ZF. Immunopathogenesis. In: S Broder, TC Merigan, D Bolognesi, eds. Text book of AIDS Medicine. 1994:55–75.

Merigan TC, Kundu SK. HIV envelope glycoproteins. J Acquir Immune Syndr 1994; 7(S):S14–S20.

Schooley RT. Immune-based therapies for HIV-1 infection. In: S Broder, TC Merigan, D Bolognesi, eds. Text book of AIDS medicine. 1994:713–719.

Walker BD. The rationale for immunotherapy in HIV infection. J Acquir Immune Syndr 1994; 7(S):S6–S13.

ACQUIRED IMMUNODEFICIENCY SYNDROME: THERAPY FOR NEOPLASTIC COMPLICATIONS

ALEXANDRA LEVINE, M.D.

Kaposi's sarcoma (KS) was the first malignancy associated with acquired immunodeficiency syndrome (AIDS), and remains the most common of the AIDS-related malignancies. The disease is seen primarily in homosexual or bisexual men and is rare in women. Although the incidence of KS appears to be decreasing in recent years, the clinical characteristics of KS diagnosed during the second decade of the epidemic appear somewhat distinct from those encountered earlier. Thus, it is now more common for patients to present with advanced and disseminated disease in the setting of more profound immunodeficiency.

Malignant lymphoma was first recognized as an AIDS-defining condition in 1985, and represents a later manifestation of HIV-induced immune dysfunction. The disease is seen with equal frequency in all population groups at risk for infection by the human immunodeficiency virus (HIV). While approximately 3 percent of all initial AIDS-defining conditions are lymphoma, the incidence increases as individuals live longer with HIV disease; recent data from Europe indicate that the overall incidence may be as high as 10 to 15 percent. Patients with systemic AIDS-lymphoma are moderately immunocompromised, with median CD4 cells at lymphoma diagnosis of approximately 100 to 200 per cubic millimeter. In distinction, patients with lymphoma primary to the central nervous system (CNS) often present with extreme degrees of immunocompromise, with history of AIDS prior to the CNS lymphoma in approximately 75 percent and median CD4 cell counts of fewer than 50 per cubic millimeter.

Cervical cancer became an AIDS-defining condition in 1993, with recognition that HIV-infected women were more likely than their uninfected controls to be infected by human papilloma virus (HPV) types 16 and 18, which are associated with development of cervical intraepithelial neoplasia (CIN) and invasive cervical carcinoma. Although not currently AIDS-defining, an increasing incidence of HPV-induced anal intraepithelial neoplasia (AIN) has also been reported in HIV-infected homosexual men.

KAPOSI'S SARCOMA

Background

Pathogenesis of Disease, in Terms of Therapeutic Implications

The actual malignant nature of KS has been questioned because of the polymorphous nature of the cellular infiltrate and the lack of specific and reproducible chromosomal or molecular biologic aberrations. Nonetheless, the disease is certainly proliferative in nature and behaves in a malignant fashion, with multifocal onset and eventual wide dissemination to essentially all organs. The abnormal cell appears to be a spindle cell of vascular endothelial origin, which may be driven to proliferation by the HIV-tat protein. Once established, these spindle cells are capable of producing a variety of angiogenic factors such as basic fibroblast growth factor (bFGF). These angiogenesis-promoting factors together with the chronic, HIV-induced production of various inflammatory cytokines such as IL-6, promote the development of the full KS lesion, characterized by numerous slit-like vascular spaces, along with spindle cells, fibroblasts, and inflammatory cells. The environment of the KS lesion, then, is rich in inflammatory cytokines and angiogenesis promoting factors, which are required for the initial establishment and eventual growth of the tumor. The blocking of these factors may provide a means to abrogate KS growth, and this hypothesis is currently being tested.

Presentation of AIDS-Related KS

KS most commonly presents with lesions on the skin. These may be quite variable in appearance, but are most often pink, red, or violaceous nodules or irregularly shaped, papular lesions. The lesions are usually painless and nontender, and may occur in any area, including the gingiva, tongue, or hard and soft palate of the oral cavity. The lesions are often symmetric on the body and may follow normal skin lines.

KS may also present in visceral organs, most commonly the gastrointestinal tract, which is involved in as many as 50 percent of patients at diagnosis. Asymptomatic involvement of the GI tract does not mandate therapeutic intervention. The lung may also be involved, and may be associated with rapid demise, unless systemic chemotherapy is promptly instituted.

The patient with KS may first present with lymphoedema, which may be quite extreme, involving the face or extremities. The edema may be seen in the absence of overlying skin lesions and is thought to be secondary to a local capillary leak syndrome due to the release of inflammatory cytokines and angiogenic factors. The presence of such lymphoedema is usually an indication for use of systemic chemotherapy. KS can also first present with lymphadenopathy, even in the absence of documented skin involvement; the diagnosis in these cases requires lymph node biopsy.

Therapy of AIDS-Related KS

Treatment Options for Localized KS

In patients with relatively few lesions, the initial management may be restricted to use of cosmetics without specific therapy, while the physician ascertains the pace of disease over time. In some individuals, this pace is quite slow, and "watchful waiting" may proceed for a number of years without adversely affecting the overall outcome of disease.

If a given patient is uncomfortable without treatment or if the disease is cosmetically unacceptable or is shown to be progressing, several types of local therapy may be effective. First, one can surgically excise the lesion. Second, liquid nitrogen cryotherapy may be used, employing open spray or cyroprobes, with thaw times ranging from 30 to 60 seconds. Since normal melanocytes are also sensitive to freezing, hypopigmentation may result, limiting the use of this modality to fair-skinned individuals or to lesions in nonvisible sites. Laser therapy employing argon or carbon dioxide has been used with success in AIDS-related KS, although the former may be quite time consuming.

Local injections of various chemotherapeutic agents have also been effective in treating the lesions of KS, although pain at the site of injection is common, and local skin irritation may occur. Additionally, the patient may be left with a hypo- or hyperpigmented scar. Vinblastine has been employed at doses ranging from 0.01 to 0.8 mg per lesion, injected every 2 weeks for a maximum of approximately three injections per lesion, with response rates of over 90 percent. Vincristine has also been used successfully, at doses of approximately 0.1 to 0.2 mg per injection. Interferon-alpha (IFN-α) may also be injected intralesionally, employing doses ranging from 1 to 5 million units of recombinant IFN alfa-2b, administered at intervals ranging from 1 to 3 times per week. Again, response rates in excess of 90 percent have been reported, and placebo-controlled trials have demonstrated the clear efficacy of this approach.

Radiation therapy may also be effective for local lesions of AIDS-related KS, although results are far less dramatic than reported in the classic variant of disease, and complications are more profound. Thus, relatively small doses of radiation have been complicated by severe mucositis in patients with AIDS-related KS who are receiving radiation to the oral cavity or oropharynx; this may be obviated by fractionation or slow administration. A variety of types of radiation have been employed, including orthovoltage, photons, and electrons, and dose schedules have varied from single doses of 800cGy in one fraction, to 2,000 to 3,000 cGys administered over 2 to 3 weeks. Overall, radiation may be successful in approximately 60 to 75 percent of patients, although most responses are incomplete, and eventual retreatment is often necessary. Radiation appears most successful when used to treat periorbital edema, cosmetically unacceptable lesions on the eyelids or face, or painful KS lesions. In general, however, radiation is considered a palliative modality of therapy.

Recombinant Interferon-Alpha (IFN-α) Alone or With Antiretroviral Agents

Various interferon preparations have been tested in patients with AIDS-related KS because of their known antiproliferative, immunomodulating, and antiviral effects. Although interferon-beta and interferon-gamma have been found to have little or no efficacy, recombinant interferon-alfa (2a or 2b) is currently licensed in the United States for the therapy of patients with AIDS-related KS.

When used as a single agent, IFN-α induces responses in approximately 40 percent of patients with good prognostic indicators of disease, including those with a CD4 cell count greater than 200 per cubic millimeter, no history of opportunistic infection, and absence of systemic "B" symptoms. However, a response rate of less than 10 percent is expected in patients who present with any of these poor prognostic signs, and single agent IFN-α is therefore not indicated in this circumstance. Regression of lesions may begin after 1 to 2 months of therapy, with maximal response achieved after approximately 3 to 6 months. Although most responses are not complete, major partial remissions that are clinically significant are expected. When used as a single agent, high doses of IFN-α are required for optimal response, employing subcutaneous injections of approximately 36 million units per day of IFN alpha-2a, or 50 million units per day for IFN alpha-2b. The toxicities of IFN-α at these doses may be quite substantial, with onset of a "flu-like" syndrome, consisting of fever, malaise, fatigue, myalgias, and a decreased sense of well-being. These symptoms decrease or disappear over time, with continued therapy.

Recently, IFN-α has been used in combination with zidovudine in patients with AIDS-related KS, and results have been superior to those achieved with IFN-α alone. Thus, by employing zidovudine at a dose of 500 mg per day together with 10 million units of daily subcutaneous IFN alpha-2a, response rates of approximately 60 percent have been achieved in patients with good prognostic indicators, while 30 percent of patients with poor prognostic signs have also responded. The reduced dosage of IFN-α has served to decrease the subjective toxicities of this agent, while the combination may be safely administered in terms of organ toxicity. Furthermore, the combination has been shown to have significant antiretroviral activity. Recent trials have substituted zidovudine with other antiretroviral agents, including didanosine (ddI) and zalcitibine (ddC); preliminary data appear promising.

Systemic Chemotherapy in AIDS-Related KS

Since systemic chemotherapy may itself lead to immunosuppression with resulting opportunistic infections, the use of such therapy in the setting of AIDS-related KS has been restricted to certain specific indications. In general, systemic chemotherapy is reserved for patients with rapidly progressive disease, presence of symptomatic visceral involvement, pulmonary KS, and/or significant lymphoedema.

Several drugs have known efficacy, when used as single agents in patients with AIDS-related KS. These include vinblastine, vincristine, doxorubicin (Adriamycin), etoposide, and bleomycin. Using an average of 6 mg of vinblastine, given intraveneously each week (range 3 to 8 mg), a response rate of 26 percent was reported in a group of 38 patients; median duration of response was 3+ months. Single-agent vincristine (2 mg) given weekly or biweekly resulted in a partial remission rate of 61 percent in a group of 18 patients, with responses lasting 4+ months. The use of vincristine (2 mg), alternating with vinblastine (0.1 mg per kilogram), given in alternating fashion once each week resulted in an objective response rate of 43 percent, lasting a median of 9+ months as noted in a group of 21 subjects. Etoposide, used intravenously at a dose of 150 mg per square meter on 3 consecutive days each month, has resulted in a response rate of almost 90 percent, lasting a median of 9 months, although neutropenia was common as was gastrointestinal toxicity and alopecia. Single-agent etoposide has also been used orally, with promising early results. Bleomycin, employed at a dose of 20 mg per square meter daily for 3 consecutive days each month, has resulted in a partial response rate of approximately 40 to 60 percent, although fever was a common complication. Doxorubicin, at doses of 10 to 20 mg per square meter every other week has led to partial remissions in approximately 50 percent of patients.

Use of combinations of drugs may be more effective than single agents as shown by a trial comparing doxorubicin alone, resulting in a 53 percent partial remission rate versus an 87 percent response rate with the combination of doxorubicin (20 mg per square meter), vincristine (2 mg), and bleomycin (10 mg per square meter), all administered by vein every other week. Although no case of complete remission was documented in the 31 patients who received single-agent doxorubicin, complete responses were seen in 37 percent of the 30 patients who received the combination (ABV). Median survival in the two groups was similar, perhaps because of the cross-over design, which allowed a switch to ABV in those patients failing doxorubicin (A) alone. A combination of doxorubicin (40 mg per square meter) and vinblastine (6 mg per square meter) on day 1, with bleomycin (15 units) on days 1 and 15 resulted in an overall response rate of 84 percent, including 23 percent complete remissions. However, hematologic toxicity was significant, and opportunistic infections occurred in approximately 75 percent of patients. Another combination, employing the relative marrow-sparing agents vincristine (2 mg) and bleomycin (10 mg per square meter), given by vein every other week, has resulted in an objective response rate of 72 percent, with minimal toxicity. While each of these combination regimens has thus demonstrated some degree of efficacy, no regimen has yet produced long-term, disease-free survival, and the KS will eventually recur when the chemotherapy is discontinued. No particular regimen of maintenance therapy has yet been able to prevent relapse of disease.

Newer Chemotherapeutic Agents

Recently, various liposomal forms of doxorubicin have been generated and tested in preliminary fashion. These preparations have the potential advantage of more specific delivery of chemotherapy directly into the KS cells. Early phase I trials, employing escalating doses of 10, 20, and 40 mg per square meter, have resulted in major responses in approximately 90 percent, although hematologic toxicity was significant at the highest dose level. Additional trials and studies of liposomal doxorubicin in combination with other agents are currently ongoing.

Paclitaxel (Taxol), a new chemotherapeutic agent derived from the Pacific Yew tree, which interferes with microtubule function (similar to vincristine and vinblastine), has recently been administered in escalating doses (maximum of 175 mg per square meter), given as 3- or 96-hour infusions. Although myelosuppression has been the dose-limiting toxicity, definite efficacy has been reported.

Use of Antiangiogenesis Compounds and Growth Factor Inhibitors

With the understanding that multiple angiogenic factors and inflammatory cytokines are necessary for initiation and subsequent growth of the KS lesion, several ongoing trials are attempting to define the clinical activity of such compounds. In this regard, Tecogalen, a sulfated polysaccharide isolated from Arthrobacter species AT-25, has been shown to have novel antiangiogenesis effects, with both in vitro and in vivo antitumor activity. The compound is currently undergoing clinical testing in patients with AIDS-KS, with some preliminary evidence of activity. Another antiangiogenesis compound, the fumagillan analogue TNP 470, is also undergoing clinical testing at this time, and results are awaited with great interest. Studies of IL-4 are also in progress, to determine if the inhibitory effect of this cytokine on IL-6 may have clinical benefit in AIDS-KS.

Overall Approach to the Management of the Patient with AIDS-KS

An approach to the overall management of patients with AIDS-related KS is shown in Table 1. As shown, no specific treatment is currently considered as the therapy of choice, and individualized decisions must be made, based upon the extent of disease, presence of other coexisting illnesses, and the overall degree of HIV-induced immunocompromise.

AIDS-RELATED LYMPHOMA

Primary Central Nervous System Lymphoma

Patients with AIDS-related primary CNS lymphoma are extremely fragile, with far advanced HIV-induced immunodeficiency. These patients may present with focal neurologic deficits, seizures, and/or altered mental status. Any site in the brain may be involved, and 1 to 4 space-occupying lesions are usually seen on MRI or CAT scans. The majority of lymphomas are of large cell or immunoblastic subtype, and uniform presence of Epstein-Barr Virus (EBV), with expression of EBV-related latent proteins, has been demonstrated.

At this time, the optimal therapy for patients with AIDS-related primary CNS lymphoma is unknown. The usual standard of treatment has been whole brain radiation, which results in complete remission rates (CR) between 20 to 50 percent, after delivery of approximately 4,000cGy, with an additional 1,000cGy to the specific site(s) of tumor. Despite achievement of CR, however, the median survival of these patients has only been in the range of approximately 2 to 4 months, with death often being attributable to complicating opportunistic infections. Survival is not substantially changed by withholding therapy altogether, although radiation has been associated with an improvement in the quality of survival in approximately 75 percent of patients. Ongoing trials are evaluating the use of short courses of multiagent chemotherapy, or use of less myelosuppressive single agents, followed by whole brain radiation. Although such approaches appear efficacious in non-HIV infected patients with primary CNS lymphoma, no data are currently available with regard to AIDS-related disease.

Systemic AIDS-Related Lymphoma

Clinical and Prognostic Characteristics of Disease

Patients with AIDS-related systemic lymphoma usually present with widespread disease involving one or more extranodal organs. Such advanced stage disease has been reported in 80 to 90 percent of patients. Involvement of the CNS is extremely common, presenting as leptomeningeal disease, with lymphoma cells in the CSF; leptomeningeal lymphoma occurs in approxi-

Table 1 Approach to the Management of Patients with AIDS-Related Kaposi's Sarcoma

Clinical Setting	*Treatment Options*
Localized disease	Cosmetics with "watchful waiting"; surgical excision; liquid nitrogen cryotherapy; laser therapy; intralesional injections of vincristine, vinblastine, or interferon-alpha
More advanced mucocutaneous involvement	Interferon-alpha plus zidovudine, or other antiretroviral agents
Rapidly progressive disease; symptomatic visceral KS; pulmonary KS; or significant lymphoedema	Single-agent chemotherapy: Vincristine Vinblastine Doxorubicin Bleomycin Etoposide Combination chemotherapy: Doxorubicin, vincristine, bleomycin Vincristine and bleomycin Vincristine alternating with vinblastine
Promising new or experimental therapies	Liposomal doxorubicin; paclitaxel (Taxol) Anti-angiogenesis compounds Tecogalen Fumagillin derivative (TNP-470)

mately 20 percent of asymptomatic individuals at diagnosis and in as many as 66 percent throughout the course of disease. Systemic "B" symptoms, such as fever, drenching night sweats, and/or weight loss, are expected in 60 to 90 percent of patients at diagnosis, and must be differentiated from similar symptoms occurring because of an occult opportunistic infection.

Certain clinical features have been associated with shorter survival and decreased likelihood of chemotherapeutic response. Thus, history of AIDS prior to the lymphoma; CD4 cell counts of fewer than 200 per cubic millimeter; poor performance status; and stage IV disease, especially if it is due to bone marrow involvement, have each been associated with shorter survival. Elevated lactic dehydrogenase (LDH) and an age of 35 years or more have also been associated with decreased survival.

Treatment for Newly Diagnosed Patients

Although occassional patients may be diagnosed with early stage disease, the vast majority will relapse shortly after receipt of local radiation, indicating that the lymphoma was probably more extensive than initially believed. The use of multiagent chemotherapy is therefore indicated in patients with AIDS-related systemic lymphoma, even though such disease may appear to be relatively localized. Although standard regimens of dose-intensive, multiagent chemotherapy were initially employed, results were disappointing, with low rates of complete remission and high rates of complicating opportunistic infections.

In an attempt to ascertain if "less might be better," the AIDS Clinical Trials Group (ACTG) embarked upon a study of a low-dose modification of the m-BACOD regimen, with early use of intrathecal cytosine arabinoside to prevent CNS relapse, and a total treatment period consisting of 4 to 6 cycles, given monthly, as depicted in Table 2. With 35 evaluable patients, a complete remission rate of approximately 50 percent was achieved; these responses were rapid in onset and durable in approximately 80 percent. Median survival of complete responders was 18 months. With use of intrathecal cytosine arabinoside, isolated CNS relapse was not observed. Opportunistic infections were seen in approximately 20 percent of patients during the course of therapy. It became apparent from this trial that patients with AIDS-lymphoma could be treated effectively and could experience long-term lymphoma-free survival.

Table 2 Low-Dose m-BACOD Regimen

Bleomycin	4 mg/m^2, day 1, IV
Doxorubicin	25 mg/m^2, day 1, IV
Cyclophosphamide	300 mg/m^2, day 1, IV
Vincristine sulfate	1.4 mg/m^2, day 1, IV (not to exceed 2 mg)
Dexamethasone	3 mg/m^2, days 1-5, PO
Methotrexate (MTX)	500 mg/m^2, day 15, IV with folinic acid rescue, 25 mg PO q6h × 4, beginning 6 hr after completion of MTX
Cytosine arabinoside	50 mg, intrathecal, days 1, 8, 21, 28, cycle 1
Helmet-field radiotherapy	4,000 cGy with known CNS involvement
Zidovudine	100 mg q4h for 1 yr; starting after chemotherapy
Total treatment	4-6 cycles, at 28-day intervals

Addition of Hematopoietic Growth Factors

Use of the CHOP regimen, either with or without granulocyte-macrophage colony stimulating factor (GM-CSF) was studied by the group in San Francisco, resulting in a clear benefit for the GM-CSF treated patients, in terms of nadir granulocyte counts, development of fever, and number of days hospitilized for fever. A complete remission rate of 70 percent was reported in 11 patients receiving GM-CSF from days 4 through 13 of each chemotherapy cycle. Although serum HIV p24 antigen levels rose to 243 percent of baseline during the third week of therapy in these patients, the clinical significance of this finding could not be determined.

The ACTG also explored the use of GM-CSF with escalating doses of M-BACOD, noting that full dose m-BACOD could be given safely without clinical progression of HIV disease.

In an attempt to ascertain the role of dose intensity in the setting of AIDS-related systemic lymphoma, the ACTG has recently completed accrual to a large, prospective trial in which patients were stratified by prognostic factors and then randomized to receive either low dose or full-dose m-BACOD with GM-CSF support. Preliminary results indicate significantly greater myelotoxicity with full dose m-BACOD, with no differences in complete remission rate, duration of remission, or duration of survival.

Anecdotal reports have employed granulocyte-CSF (G-CSF) with multiagent chemotherapy in patients with AIDS-related lymphoma, noting an amelioration of chemotherapy induced myelosuppression, with no upregulation of HIV. Relatively low doses of G-CSF (1 to 3 μm per kilogram per day) may be effective in this setting.

Addition of Antiretroviral Agents to Chemotherapy

Several studies have now demonstrated that zidovudine cannot be given safely with combination chemotherapy because of serious marrow compromise. However, the low dose m-BACOD regimen has recently been administered with concomitant zalcitibine (ddC) at a dose of 0.75 mg orally, three times per day. Although both ddC and vincristine (Oncovin) may cause peripheral neuropathy, this toxicity was not encountered, and the combination was found to be safe and effective. Of interest, the HIV viral burden, as measured by acid dissociated p24 antigen, was found to decrease significantly, or return to nondetectability in approximately 75 percent of treated patients. Furthermore, use of concomitant ddC was associated with equivalent complete response rates in patients with good or poor prognostic indicators of lymphomatous disease.

Infusional Chemotherapy

A regimen consisting of cyclophosphamide (750 mg per square meter), doxorubicin (50 mg per square meter), and etoposide (240 mg per square meter), administered as a continuous intraveneous infusion over 4 days and repeated every 28 days for up to six cycles, was recently employed in 12 patients with AIDS-related lymphoma, all of whom had at least one poor prognostic feature. Complete remission was achieved in 67 percent, while seven remained alive and disease-free with a median follow-up of 15 months. Granulocytopenia of 500 or fewer cells per cubic millimeter occurred in 47 percent of treatment cycles, and the dose of infusional CDE was reduced in 44 percent of cycles. A total of eight infections occurred in five HIV-infected patients, one of which was lethal. An update of this series was recently provided, after treatment of 21 patients. A complete remission rate of 62 percent was achieved, and the estimated median survival of the study group was 18 months.

Therapy for Patients Who have Failed or Relapse after Initial Chemotherapy

No standard of therapy currently exists for patients who are resistant to first-line therapy or for those who have relapsed after an initial response. Several new modalities may offer help for such patients. Mitoguazone (MGBG) interferes with polyamine biosynthesis, and as such represents a new mechanism of known antitumor activity. Preliminary use of MGBG, given at a dose of 600 mg per square meter by vein on day 1, day 8, and every 2 weeks thereafter has shown promise in patients with relapsed or refractory AIDS-lymphoma. Response rates of approximately 30 percent have been reported in patients with far-advanced disease and significant immunocompromise. The drug crosses the blood brain barrier and has no significant myelotoxicity. The use of an anti-B4 (CD20) monoclonal antibody, conjugated to the potent toxin, ricin, has also shown some efficacy in patients with relapsed or refractory AIDS-related lymphoma. Use of this agent, given as a 28-day continuous infusion, is currently being studied together with combination chemotherapy, consisting of CHOP or the low-dose m-BACOD regimen.

SUGGESTED READING

Krown SE, Gold JWM, Niedzwiecki D, et al. Interferon-alpha with zidovudine: Safety, tolerance, and clinical and virologic effects in patients with Kaposi's sarcoma associated with AIDS. Ann Intern Med 1990; 112:812–821.

Levine AM. AIDS-related malignancies: The emerging epidemic (review). J National Cancer Inst 1993; 85:1382–1397.

Levine AM, Wernz JC, Kaplan L, et al. Low-dose chemotherapy with central nervous system prophylaxis and azidothymidine maintenance in AIDS-related lymphoma: A prospective multi-institutional trial. JAMA 1991; 266:84–88.

Lilenbaum RC, Ratner L. Systemic treatment of Kaposi's sarcoma: Current status and future directions. AIDS 1994; 8:141–151.

Sprarano JA, Wiernik PH, Strack M, et al. Infusional cyclophosphamide, doxorubicin, and etoposide in HIV and HTLV-I related non-Hodgkin's lymphoma: A highly active regimen. Blood 1993; 81:2810–2815.

AUTOIMMUNITY

MULTIPLE SCLEROSIS AND RELATED DEMYELINATING DISEASES

ANTONIO UCCELLI, M.D.
STEPHEN L. HAUSER, M.D.

Multiple sclerosis (MS) is a chronic inflammatory disease of the central nervous system (CNS). MS is a common disorder that affects women more often than men. Pathologically, it is characterized by multifocal inflammation, demyelination, and scarring (gliosis) in CNS white matter pathways. The symptoms of MS, numbness, weakness, visual disturbances, incoordination, or bowel and bladder dysfunction result from disturbances in nerve conduction secondary to tissue damage. Both genetic and environmental factors contribute to susceptibility to MS, and existing data favor an autoimmune pathogenesis. The initial symptoms of MS usually appear between adolescence and midadult life, and a chronic course that may persist for decades ultimately results in significant disability in 90 percent or more of affected individuals.

Several clinical forms of MS have been identified. The first, *relapsing MS,* is characterized by recurrent attacks of neurologic dysfunction. MS attacks generally evolve over days to weeks and may be followed by complete, partial, or no recovery. Recovery from attacks generally occurs within weeks to several months from the peak of symptoms. The second form of the disease, *chronic progressive MS,* results in gradually progressive worsening without intervals of stabilization or improvement. This form most often develops in individuals with a prior history of relapsing MS, and in this setting, is referred to as *secondary progressive MS.* In this group, acute relapses may also occur during the progressive course. In approximately 20 percent of patients with chronic progressive MS no history of relapses at any time can be identified *(primary progressive MS).*

Proper care of the MS patient requires that serial assessments of neurologic function be performed by the use of validated measures. Many therapeutic decisions will be based upon estimates of clinical status derived from these scores. Two useful scales, the Expanded Disability Status Scale (EDSS) of Kurtzke and the Ambulation Index (AI), are reproduced in Table 1. They may appear complicated to those unaccustomed to their use, but with a little practice they can be accurately measured in 5 to 10 minutes.

Therapy for MS has traditionally been divided between treatments that may favorably modify the underlying disease process and symptomatic treatments.

TREATMENT OF ACUTE RELAPSES

Established MS (Fig. 1)

Acute relapses may be treated with a short course of intravenous methylprednisolone (MePDN) followed by oral prednisone (PDN) (Table 2). This treatment has largely replaced adrenocorticotropic hormone (ACTH) (see Table 2) as the mainstay of treatment, but courses of ACTH may still be used in selected patients or in cases of MePDN/PDN treatment failure. Pulse therapy with these agents speeds the tempo of recovery from acute relapses and may modestly improve the degree of recovery noted to occur over a short follow-up period. Both MePDN/PDN and ACTH courses appear to have equivalent therapeutic effects. In a recent trial of MePDN/PDN for acute optic neuritis, this therapy was associated with improvement of visual outcome at 6 months, but this effect was no longer present at 1 year.

Which attacks should be treated? For patients with established MS, MePDN/PDN is generally used to treat moderate or severe attacks that result in significant functional disability that can be measured by changes on the EDSS. Mild attacks such as subjective sensory symptoms unaccompanied by objective changes on examination, Lhermitte's symptom, or worsening of bladder function are generally not treated. When neurologic worsening occurs in patients with relapsing MS, it is useful to consider whether it reflects new inflammatory lesions in the CNS or whether it is a nonspecific consequence of infection (commonly a viral infection or UTI) or other intercurrent illness. MS patients typically worsen transiently following exposure to heat, stress, or infection. "Nonspecific" MS worsenings may consist only of recrudescences of old symptoms

Table 1 Scoring Systems for MS

	A. Expanded Disability Status Score (EDSS)
0.0	Normal neurologic exam (all grade 0 in FS*)
1.0	No disability, minimal signs in one FS* (i.e., grade 1)
1.5	No disability, minimal signs in more than one FS* (>1 grade 1)
2.0	Minimal disability in two FS (two FS grade 2, others 0 or 1)
2.5	Minimal disability in two FS (two FS grade 2, others 0 or 1)
3.0	Moderate disability if one FS (one FS grade 3, others 0 or 1) or mild disability in three or four FS (three or four FS grade 2 others 0 or 1) though fully ambulatory
3.5	Fully ambulatory but with moderate disability in one FS (one grade 3) *and* one or two FS grade 2; *or* two grade 3 (others 0 or 1) *or* 5 grade 2 (others 0 or 1)
4.0	Fully ambulatory without aid, self-sufficient, up and about some 12 hours a day despite relatively severe disability consisting of one FS grade 4 (other 0 or 1), or combination of lesser grades exceeding limits of previous steps and the patient should be able to walk ≥500 m without assistance or rest
4.5	Fully ambulatory without aid, up and about much of the day, may otherwise require minimal assistance; characterized by relatively severe disability usually consisting of one FS grade 4 (others or 1) or combinations of lesser grades exceeding limits of previous steps and walks ≥300 m without assistance or rest
5.0	Ambulatory without aid for at least 50 meters; disability severe enough to impair full daily activities (e.g., to work a full day without special provision). (Usual FS equivalents are one grade 5 alone, others 0 or 1; combinations of lesser grades) Patient walks ≥200 m without aid or rest
5.5	Ambulatory without aid for at least 50 meters; disability severe enough to preclude full daily activities. (Usual FS equivalents are one grade 5 alone, others 0 or 1; or combinations of lesser grades). Enough to preclude full daily activities. (Usual FS equivalents are one grade 5 alone, others 0 or 1; or combinations of lesser grades). Patient walks ≥100 m without aid or rest
6.0	Intermittent or unilateral constant assistance (cane, crutch, brace) required to walk at least 100 m. (Usual FS equivalents are combinations with more than one FS grade 3)
6.5	Constant bilateral assistance (canes, crutches, braces) required to walk at least 20 m. (Usual FS equivalents are combinations with more than one FS grade 3)
7.0	Unable to walk at least 5 m even with aid, essentially restricted to wheelchair; wheels self and transfers alone; up and about in wheelchair some 12 hours a day. (Usual FS equivalents are combinations with more than on FS grade 4+; very rarely pyramidal grade 5 alone)
7.5	Unable to take more than a few steps; restricted to wheelchair; may need aid in transfer; wheels self but cannot carry on in wheelchair a full day. (Usual FS equivalents are combinations with more than one FS grade 4+; very rarely pyramidal grade 5 alone)
8.0	Essentially restricted to chair or per ambulated in wheelchair, but out of bed most of day; retains many self-care functions; generally has effective use of arms. (Usual FS equivalents are combinations, generally grade 4+ in several systems)
8.5	Essentially restricted to bed most of day; has some effective use of arm(s); retains some self-care functions. (Usual FS equivalents are combinations generally 4+ in several systems)
9.0	Helpless bed patient; can communicate and eat. (Usual FS equivalents are combinations, mostly grade 4+)
9.5	Totally helpless bed patient; unable to communicate effectively or eat or swallow. (Usual FS equivalents are combinations almost all grade 4+)
10.0	Death due to MS
	Functional Status (FS) Scores
FS1	*Pyramidal Functions* 0. Normal 1. Abnormal signs (e.g. increased reflexes) without weakness 2. Mild weakness (in one limb 4−, 4+): Weakness evident on stressed functions (e.g., hopping, writing or buttoning), but patient able to complete without any adaptation 3. Moderate paraparesis or hemiparesis (strength 4/5 or 4−/5; stressed functions require some adaptation to be completed e.g., can hop but only if holding the wall); or severe monoparesis—grade ≤3/5 4. Severe paraparesis or hemiparesis; moderate quadriparesis; or monoplegia; there still may be movement somewhere; there may be severe weakness in three limbs—grades 3 or 2 (stressed function cannot be completed even with adaptation) 5. Paraplegia, hemiplegia, or marked quadriparesis; there is no movement in the limbs. For example, both lower extremities or there is movement or severe weakness in four but not three limbs 6. Quadriplegia. No movement in four limbs 7. Untestable. Use this if strength cannot be tested for any reason 9. Unknown. Use this if not tested by oversight
FS2	*Cerebellar Functions* If one or more limbs can't be tested for cerebellar dysfunction (e.g., paraplegia or hemiplegia), but the remaining limbs can be tested, score only the remaining limbs 0. Normal—no evidence of cerebellar dysfunction (e.g., paraplegia or hemiplegia), more limbs are incoordinated due to weakness, apraxia, or sensory loss but not due to cerebellar dysfunction 1. Abnormal signs without disability—slight abnormality on formal testing but does not interfere with ADLs 2. Mild ataxia—limb or gait ataxia in any or all limbs adequate to noticeably interfere with function when the targeted function is stressed, including stressed gait hopping, toes, heels 3. Moderate ataxia. Use this if there is moderate ataxia in any or all limbs, in gait, or stressed gait. This is also used if there is severe ataxia of one limb. A moderate ataxia requires some physical or mechanical adjustment for the targeted activity to be completed (e.g., the patient must hold the wall to hop or be steadied by the examiner, fastening a button cannot be completed without a button holer)

Table 1 Scoring Systems for MS—cont'd

	4. Severe ataxia ≥2 limbs for routing activities and/or routine gait; stressed functions cannot be completed even with adaptation The patient may be marginally functional (e.g., may still be able to walk with aids and feed self). Use also if only remaining testable limb(s) is severely ataxic 5. Unable to perform coordinated limb or routine gait movements for ADLs due to ataxia. Use also if only remaining testable limb(s) is unable to perform coordinated movement due to ataxia 7. Untestable. Use this if weakness will not permit testing of coordination 9. Unknown. Use this if not tested by oversight
FS3	*Brainstem Functions* 0. Normal 1. Signs only (unsustained nystagmus, detectable impairment of saccadic pursuit or ocular dysmetria, facial numbness) 2. Sustained conjugate nystagmus, or incomplete disconjugate nystagmus (INO), or other disability that is noticeable but does not cause a functional impairment in speech, swallowing, or facial expression 3. INO or severe extraocular weakness, or moderate disability of other cranial nerves, which causes a functional impairment but does not result in choking or unintelligible speech 4. Severe dysarthria (marginally intelligible speech or worse) or facial paralysis 5. Inability to swallow or speak 7. Untestable for any reason 9. Unknown. Not tested by oversight
FS4	*Sensory Function* 0. Normal 1. Detectable vibration or figure; writing decrease only in one or two limbs 2. Mild decrease in touch or pain or position sense, and/or moderate decrease in vibration in one or two limbs; or vibratory decrease alone in three or four limbs 3. Moderate decrease in touch or pain or position sense, and/or essentially lost vibration in one or two limbs; or mild decrease in touch or pain and/or moderate decrease in all proprioceptive tests in three of four limbs 4. Marked decrease in touch or pain or loss of proprioception, alone or combined, in one or two limbs, or moderate decrease in touch or pain and/or severe proprioceptive decrease in more than two limbs 5. Loss (essentially) of sensation in one or two limbs, or moderate decrease in touch or pain and/or loss of proprioception for most of the body below the head 6. Sensation essentially lost below the head 7. Untestable 9. Unknown
FS5	*Bowel and Bladder Function:* Ask about both bladder and bowel; score the worst, as follows: *Bladder* 0. Normal bladder function 1. Bladder symptoms but no incontinence 2. Incontinence ≤ once per week 3. Incontinence > once per week but < daily 4. ≥ daily incontinence 5. Indwelling bladder catheter 6. Grade 5 bladder function *plus* grade 5 bowel function 7. Untestable for any reason 9. Unknown. Not tested by oversight X. Intermittent catheterization (use this letter in addition to number that best describes bladder function) *Bowel* 0. Normal bowel function 1. Mild constipation but no incontinence 2. Severe constipation but no incontinence 3. Rare (≤ once per week) bowel incontinence 4. Frequent (> weekly but < daily) bowel incontinence 5. No bowel control 6. Grade 5 bladder function *plus* grade 5 bowel function 7. Untestable for any reason 9. Unknown. Not tested by oversight
FS6	*Visual Functions* (all visual acuity is best corrected) 0. Normal visual acuity better than 20/30 and no sign of optic nerve disease 1. Visual acuity (corrected) better than or equal to 20/30 with signs of optic nerve disease. For example, if there is an afferent pupil defect 2. Worse eye with maximal visual acuity (corrected) of 20/40 or 20/50 3. Worse eye with maximal visual acuity (corrected) of 20/70; check both eyes 4. Worse eye with maximal visual acuity (corrected) of 20/100 or 20/200 5. Worse eye with maximal visual acuity (corrected) worse than 20/200 and maximal acuity of better eye of 20/60 or better 6. Grade 5 plus maximal visual acuity of better eye of 20/60 or worse 7. Untestable for any reason 9. Unknown. Not tested by oversight

Continued.

Table 1 Scoring Systems for MS—cont'd

FS7	*Cerebral (or Mental) Function* 0. Normal 1. Mood alteration only (does not affect DSS score) 2. Mild decrease in mentation 3. Moderate decrease in mentation 4. Marked decrease in mentation (chronic brain syndrome—moderate) 5. Dementia or chronic brain syndrome—severe or incompetent 7. Untestable for any reason 9. Unknown. Not tested by oversight
FS8	*Other Function* (Any other neurologic findings attributable to MS) *Spasticity** 0. None 1. Mild—detectable only 2. Moderate—minor interference with function 3. Severe—major interference with function 7. Untestable for any reason 9. Unknown. Not tested by oversight *Other* 0. None 1. Any other neurologic findings attributed to MS: Specify 9. Unknown
	B. Ambulation Index
	0. Asymptomatic; fully active; no gait abnormality reported or observed 1. Walks normally but reports fatigue or difficulty running, which interferes with athletic or other demanding activities 2. Abnormal gait or episodic imbalance; gait disorder is noticeable to family and friends and is evident to examiner. Able to walk 25 feet in 10 seconds or less 3. Walks independently; requires ≥10 seconds, but able to walk 25 feet in 20 seconds or less 4. Requires unilateral support (cane, single crutch) to walk; uses support more than 80% of the time. Walks 25 feet in 20 seconds or less 5. Requires bilateral support (canes, crutches, walker) and walks 25 feet in 20 seconds or less; or, requires unilateral support but walks 25 feet in more than 20 seconds 6. Requires bilateral support and walks 25 feet in more than 20 seconds. May use wheelchair on occasion 7. Walking limited to several steps with bilateral support; unable to walk 25 feet; may use wheelchair for most activities 8. Restricted to wheelchair; able to transfer independently 9. Restricted to wheelchair; unable to transfer independently

Note: DSS steps below 5 refer to patients who are fully ambulatory, and the precise step is defined by the Functional System score(s). DSS steps from 5 up are defined by ability to ambulate, and *usual* equivalents in Functional System score are provided.
*A Mental Function grade of 1 does *not* enter in FS scores for DSS steps.

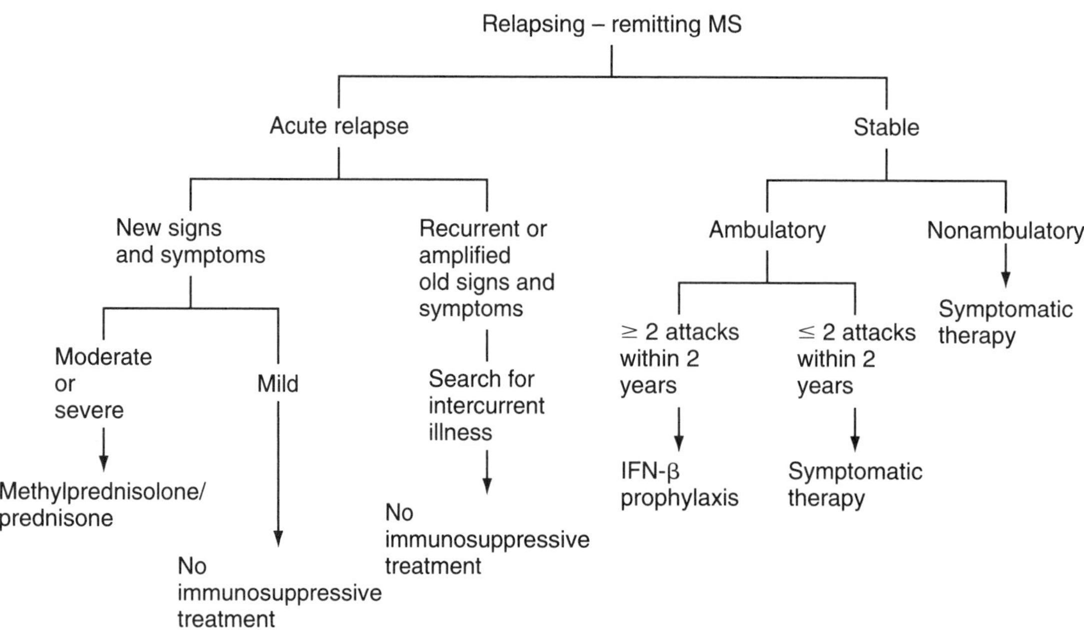

Figure 1 Therapeutic approach to established relapsing multiple sclerosis.

and may be short-lived (i.e., <48 hours in duration). Patients with relapsing MS experience on average fewer than one and one-half true relapses per year. The presence of a high frequency of attack-like events should raise the possibility that symptomatic worsenings unrelated to new disease activity are occurring.

Table 2 Steroid Therapy Regimens

I. *Methylprednisolone-Prednisone*
Methylprednisolone, 1,000 mg IV daily for 3 days, followed by oral prednisone (1 mg/kg per day) for 11 days.

II. *ACTH*
1. Aqueous ACTH (20 U/ml), 80 U is given IV in 500 ml of 5% dextrose and water (D_5W) over 6-8 hr for 3 days
2. ACTH gel (U/ml) is then given IM in a dose of 40 U q12h for 7 days. The dose is then reduced every 3 days as follows:
   35 U b.i.d. for 3 days
   30 U b.i.d. for 3 days
   50 U q.d. for 3 days
   40 U p.d. for 3 days
   30 U q.d. for 3 days
   20 U q.d. for 3 days
   20 U every other day for 3 doses

III. *Methylprednisolone/Prednisone: 8-Week Course*
Methylprednisolone is mixed in 500 ml D_5W and administered slowly, over 4-6 hours, preferably in the morning:
1,000 mg daily for 3 days
500 mg daily for 3 days
250 mg daily for 3 days
Followed by oral prednisone:
60 mg for 7 days; then
60-40 mg alternate days for 7 days; then
60-20 mg alternate days for 7 days; then
60 mg every other day for 7 days; then
40 mg every other day for 7 days; then
20 mg every other day for 7 days; then
10 mg every other day for 7 days

Side effects of short-term corticosteroid therapy include fluid retention, potassium loss, weight gain, gastric disturbances, acne, and emotional lability. With longer term use, clinically important risks of infections and osteoporosis must be considered. Salt and fluid retention are managed with a low-salt, potassium-rich diet and avoidance of potassium-wasting diuretics. In patients with heart disease or who require concurrent diuretic therapy, oral potassium supplementation is advised. We recommend low dosages of lithium carbonate (300 mg orally twice a day) as prophylaxis for emotional lability and insomnia associated with corticosteroid therapy. In patients with a history of peptic ulcer disease, cimetidine or ranitidine (150 mg twice daily) are advised.

The Initial Attack (Fig. 2)

A modified approach is employed for treatment of an initial attack of demyelinating disease. In this setting, MS may represent a diagnostic possibility, but a chronic course, which is required for a diagnosis of clinically definite MS, has not yet occurred. Recommendations for different clinical settings follow.

Acute Optic Neuritis

As previously noted, MePDN/PDN modestly speeds the tempo of recovery from acute optic neuritis (ON) but has little effect on the ultimate degree of recovery that occurs. It may also protect against evolution to clinically definite MS over a 2-year period. In optic neuritis patients, the risk of evolution to MS is high (35 percent over a 2-year period) when the MRI indicates disseminated disease, whereas the risk is low (5 percent over 2 years) in patients with normal MRI scans at the time of presentation.

Based on these results, MePDN/PDN is indicated in

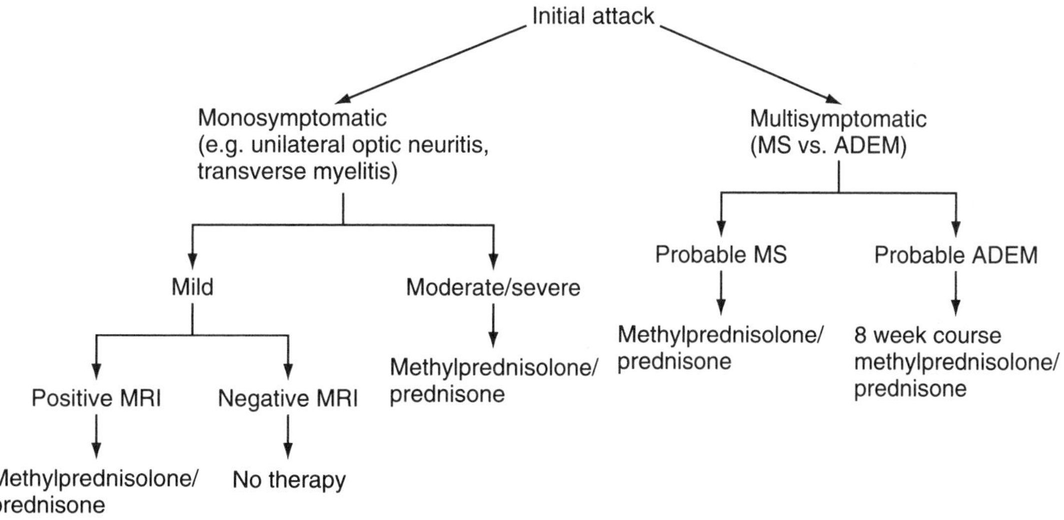

Figure 2 Therapeutic approach to the initial attack.

the treatment of moderate or severe episodes of ON or when MRI findings indicate the presence of disseminated disease. Oral PDN alone should probably not be used for treatment of uncomplicated optic neuritis, because its use in one study was associated with an increase in the frequency of new attacks of optic neuritis.

Transverse Myelitis and Other Monosymptomatic Presentations

Treatment of acute demyelinating disorders, including transverse myelitis or isolated brainstem syndromes, is largely empirical. In these patients, MRI may also predict the future clinical course. In one study, evolution to MS occurred in only 5 percent of patients with scans that were normal or provided evidence of only the solitary lesion detected clinically. By contrast, when disseminated abnormalities were detected by MRI, more than half of these patients evolved to develop clinically definite MS over a 3- to 5- year follow-up period. It is reasonable, based upon these findings, to perform cranial MRI on patients with all monosymptomatic presentations of demyelinating disease, and to treat moderate to severe symptoms, or presumptive disseminated disease detected by MRI, with MePDN/PDN.

Explosive Presentations

Occasional patients present with the acute onset of diverse and rapidly evolving neurologic symptoms and signs indicating the simultaneous involvement of multiple white matter pathways. These syndromes, grouped under the name acute disseminated encephalomyelitis (ADEM), may appear without an obvious antecedent event, or they may follow vaccination or infection, especially viral or mycoplasmal infection. Unlike MS, in ADEM the vast majority of cases are monophasic and do not evolve into a chronic illness. In some cases, it may be difficult to distinguish between an initial attack of MS and ADEM.

ADEM is treated empirically with a modified MePDN/PDN regimen. The author recommends a 9-day course of IV MePDN followed by a slow taper of oral PDN (see Table 2). The taper is scheduled so that alternate-day therapy is ideally begun within approximately 1 month, and therapy is continued for a total of 2 months. The therapeutic regimen may need to be lengthened if symptoms recrudesce during the course of the taper.

Neuromyelitis optica, or Devic's syndrome, is another acute form of demyelinating disease. It is characterized by the development of acute bilateral optic neuritis, followed within days to weeks by transverse myelitis, in a previously healthy individual. In some cases, optic neuritis may be unilateral or myelitis may be the initial symptom. Devic's syndrome may be treated with the same regimen employed for ADEM.

Prophylaxis for Relapses

Interferon-beta (IFN-β) is now known to be partially effective in the prophylaxis of relapses in MS. In one study, subcutaneous injections administered every other day reduced the relapse rate by one-third and reduced severe relapses by one-half. In a recently reported second trial of IFN-β, a reduction in both the relapse rate and (perhaps more significantly) in neurologic disability was present in the treated group. IFN-β is well tolerated in most patients. A transient flulike illness may occur with initiation of therapy, but generally disappears after 4 to 6 weeks. Other side effects may include local skin reactions or abnormalities in blood counts or hepatic enzyme levels.

Chronic Progression (Fig. 3)

At this time, chronic immunosuppression represents the best available option for the specific treatment of progressive MS. These treatments should be administered only with the understanding that they carry a variety of short- and long-term risks and that their therapeutic efficacy in MS is modest. Monotherapy with either methotrexate or azathioprine given orally is a reasonable initial approach.

Methotrexate is a relatively well-tolerated therapy for progressive MS. It has been shown to slow the progression of neurologic disability as measured by tests of upper limb function. Low-dose methotrexate therapy is easily administered as a single oral 7.5 mg dose; some centers prefer higher dosages, up to 20 mg weekly. An important practical advantage of methotrexate is the simplicity of a weekly dosing schedule. Most patients experience few or no side effects from low-dose methotrexate therapy. Nausea, diarrhea, headache, myalgia, or fever may require discontinuation of the drug, or these side effects may be treated symptomatically. Laboratory monitoring should include a complete blood count (CBC) and tests of hepatic and renal function at 8-week intervals. Methotrexate is currently our first choice for therapy of progressive symptoms.

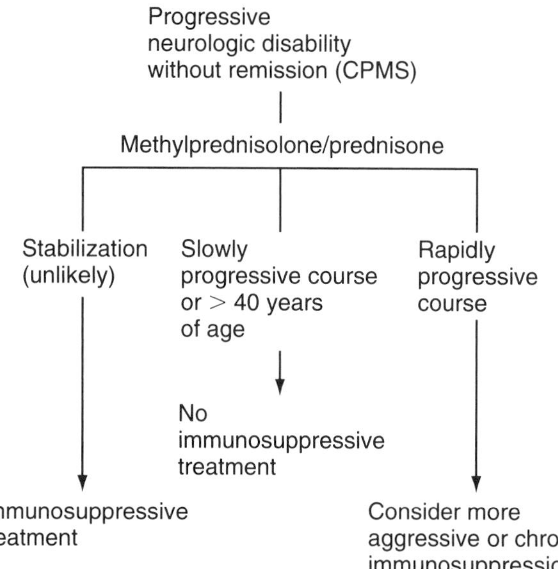

Figure 3 Therapeutic approach to progressive multiple sclerosis.

Azathioprine is a purine analogue that has potent suppressive effects on the immune system. Meta-analysis of individual trials indicates that chronic azathioprine therapy has a small beneficial effect on the slowing of MS disease progression. It is administered as a single daily oral therapy at a dose of 2 to 3 mg per kilogram. A CBC and tests of liver function should be performed initially at monthly intervals and then bimonthly in patients who receive azathioprine. In patients who experience a fall in the white blood count (WBC) – an inconsistent finding in our experience – the dosage is then adjusted in order to maintain the WBC between 3,500 and 4,000 cells per microliter. We empirically begin oral methotrexate therapy following a course of MePDN/PDN. The most frequent side effects of methotrexate therapy are nausea and abdominal pain that may require a lower dosage or cessation of therapy. The most serious long-term consequence of methotrexate therapy is the development of irreversible liver disease. Asymptomatic elevations of hepatic enzymes are frequent in patients receiving methotrexate and need not result in termination of therapy if the level of transaminase elevation is less than one and one-half times the upper limit of normal. Transaminase values above this level generally require a lower daily dose. Should methotrexate therapy be continued for more than 2 years, we recommend that a blind liver biopsy be performed so that drug-induced liver damage can be detected early. Other potential side effects of methotrexate immunosuppression include skin rash, an increased susceptibility to infection, and a possible increase in cancer risk, in particular non-Hodgkin's lymphoma.

Cyclophosphamide is a potent alkylating agent with both cytotoxic and immunosuppressive effects. In contrast to methotrexate and azathioprine, it is highly toxic and its use should be restricted to practitioners experienced with its use. An initial induction regimen consists of IV cyclophosphamide infusions administered daily for 10 to 14 days at a dosage of 500 mg per day. Large volumes of fluid are given with cyclophosphamide to minimize bladder toxicity. IV ACTH is coadministered. Bimonthly cyclophosphamide booster injections (700 mg per square meter) are advocated by some as maintenance therapy. Side effects include alopecia, severe nausea and vomiting, an infectious risk from acute severe immunosuppression, and hemorrhagic cystitis. In addition, serious risks of this therapy include an increased incidence of bladder and possibly other cancers, and sterility that is dose dependent. It is reasonable to consider cyclophosphamide therapy only in a small subset of young MS patients (< 40 years of age) who are ambulatory, have a secondary progressive course, and have exhausted reasonable alternative therapies.

It must be again emphasized that the modest clinical efficacy of immunosuppression for progressive MS does not justify its use in all progressive patients. Patients with relapsing-progressive MS are probably more safely treated with IFN-β than with an antimetabolite or alkylating agent. Older (> 60 years of age) or severely disabled, nonambulatory patients should also, in most cases, not be treated aggressively. For all patients who receive immunosuppression, a yearly re-evaluation of its value – its beneficial and deleterious effects – is appropriate.

SYMPTOMATIC THERAPY

Any comprehensive care plan for patients with MS must strive to maximize therapy for painful or disabling symptoms.

Spasticity

MS patients may complain of muscle stiffness, spasms or clonus that may be painful or functionally disabling. The GABA agonist baclofen (10 to 80 mg per day in divided dosages) is the most useful drug available. Some patients require higher dosages, up to 240 mg per day. For refractory cases, intrathecal baclofen may be administered via an indwelling catheter. Fatigue and sedation are the most important side effects of baclofen. For treatment of nocturnal spasms, low dosages of diazepam (2 mg at bedtime) may be helpful. Dantrolene (25 to 100 mg per day) relaxes muscle via a direct effect on the sarcolemmal membrane; it often results in unacceptable weakness, thus its use is generally limited to nonambulatory patients with painful or disabling spasticity. Dantrolene may be hepatotoxic, thus monitoring of liver function is essential.

Pain

Dysesthetic pain is common in MS; it may take the form of trigeminal or occipital neuralgia or paresthesias. Pain may respond to carbamazepine (up to 1,200 mg per day), amitriptyline (50 to 200 mg per day), or phenytoin (300 mg per day). We recommend that carbamazepine be tried initially; we begin with low dosages, generally 100 mg twice daily, with gradual increase thereafter by 200 mg per day every 3 days until there is 50 percent relief of pain or a total daily dose of 1,200 mg (200 mg, 6 times daily) is reached. Side effects include sedation or transient paresthesias. Baseline and periodic CBC and liver function tests are required in patients on carbamazepine because of the rare agranulocytosis, aplastic anemia, and hepatitis that may occur.

Paroxysmal Symptoms

"Tonic seizures" are recurrent, brief, stereotyped attacks consisting of tonic contractions, dysesthesias, or other symptoms. They respond to acetazolamide (125 to 250 mg three times daily) or carbamazepine (dosages as above). Side effects of acetazolamide may include dry mouth, sedation, or paresthesias; liver function should also be monitored in patients who receive this drug.

Emotional Lability

Pathologic laughter or crying, manifestations of pseudobulbar palsy in MS, respond to amitriptyline in most cases. Depression should be aggressively sought out and treated appropriately.

Fatigue

Severe or disabling fatigue is reported to occur in up to 88 percent of patients with MS. Afternoon fatigue may be managed by a shift to an earlier work schedule or by a regular afternoon nap. Amantadine (100 mg twice daily) may transiently benefit a small proportion of patients with fatigue.

Bladder Dysfunction

Specific symptoms of bladder dysfunction correlate poorly with physiologic findings, thus urodynamic evaluation is required to define and adequately treat this problem. The pathophysiology of bladder dysfunction may also change over time in MS. Bladder hyper-reflexia is treated with anticholinergics (oxybutynin, 5 mg two to three times per day, or proanthyline 7.5 to 15 mg four times daily). Urinary retention due to bladder hyporeflexia may respond to the cholinergic drug bethanechol (10 to 50 mg three to four times per day). Dyssynergia between detrusor and external sphincter muscles is common in MS, difficult to treat, and may require a combination of anticholinergic medication to decrease bladder contractions and intermittent catheterization. Supravesical urinary diversion or placement of a chronic indwelling catheter may be required in cases of severe bladder disturbance. Ascorbic acid may reduce the risk of urinary tract infections.

Bowel Dysfunction

Regimentation of bowel function with laxatives or enemas may be required for constipation. A low-fiber diet to decrease bulk may be advised for incontinence.

Sexual Dysfunction

In males, erections may be achieved pharmacologically using papaverine and phentolamine injections in the corpora cavernosa. In some patients, penile implantation may be useful. Women may experience vaginismus, which may be helped by antispasticity medications, or decreased vaginal lubrication leading to dyspareunia, which may be treated with lubricants.

SUGGESTED READING

Beck RW, Cleary PA, Anderson MM, et al. A randomized, controlled clinical trial of corticosteroids in the treatment of acute optic neuritis. N Engl J Med 1992; 326:581.

Goodkin DE, Rudick RA, VanderBerg Medenorp S, et al. Low-dose (7.5 mg) oral methotrexate reduces the rate of progression in chronic progressive multiple sclerosis. Ann Neurol 1995; 37:30.

Hauser SL. Multiple sclerosis and other demyelinating diseases. In: Isselbacher KJ, Braunwald E, Wilson JD, et al, eds., Harrison's principles of internal medicine. 13th ed. New York: McGraw Hill, 1994.

Paty DW, Li DKB, the UBC MS/MRI Study Group, and the IFNB Multiple Sclerosis Study Group, et al. Interferon beta-1b is effective in relapsing remitting multiple sclerosis. I: Clinical results of a multicenter, randomized, double-blind, placebo-controlled trial. Neurology 1993; 43:655.

Weiner HL, Mackin GA, Orav EJ, et al. Intermittent cyclophosphamide pulse therapy in progressive multiple sclerosis: Final report of the Northeast Cooperative Multiple Sclerosis Treatment Group. Neurology 1993; 43:910.

Yudkin PL, Ellison GW, Ghezzi A, et al. Overview of azathioprine treatment in multiple sclerosis. Lancet 1991; 338:1051.

MYASTHENIA GRAVIS

ANDREA M. CORSE, M.D.
RALPH W. KUNCL, M.D., Ph.D.

Myasthenia gravis (MG) is an autoimmune disorder with an antibody-mediated pathogenesis. Antibodies directed against the nicotinic acetylcholine receptor (AChR) on skeletal muscle are responsible for impaired transmission at the neuromuscular junction, resulting in muscle fatigability and weakness. The prevalence of MG is approximately 5 per 100,000 population. Autoimmune MG affects all ages. Peak incidence occurs in young women and older men. Neonatal MG affects approximately 15 percent of babies born to myasthenic mothers. It is a transient, potentially life-threatening condition resulting from the passive transfer of immunoglobulin from the mother to the baby. By contrast, congenital myasthenic syndromes are nonautoimmune gene defects, usually affecting AChR ion channels or acetylcholinesterase.

PATHOGENESIS

The defect in myasthenia gravis is a reduction in the number of available acetylcholine receptors at the neuromuscular junction. Anti-AChR antibodies reduce the number of available receptors via three mechanisms: increased receptor degradation by accelerated receptor endocytosis, receptor blockade, and complement-mediated receptor damage. Additional morphologic alterations of the neuromuscular junction also occur, including simplification of the postsynaptic membrane folds and increased distance between the pre- and postsynaptic membranes.

In MG the amount of acetylcholine released from the presynaptic terminal both at rest and after sustained activity is normal. However, because of the reduced number of acetylcholine receptors available, the amplitude of motor endplate potentials triggered by the acetylcholine is reduced. Normally, the amplitude of the endplate potentials is more than large enough to trigger an action potential. This excess amplitude, termed the "safety margin," is estimated to be three to four times greater than the threshold needed to generate a muscle action potential. However, because of insufficient AChRs in MG the endplate potential amplitudes at some neuromuscular junctions may be too low to trigger an action potential, and if transmission is sufficiently impaired at enough neuromuscular junctions, the muscle will be weak.

Normally, with sustained muscle activity the amount of acetylcholine released from the presynaptic nerve terminal is reduced with each successive impulse. Because of the large "safety factor," transmission is not affected and strength is sustained. However, in MG the reduced acetylcholine results in further impaired impulse transmission at even more neuromuscular junctions. This is the basis of muscle fatigability and electrophysiologic decrement in MG.

Anti-AChR antibodies are detectable in about 85 percent of patients with myasthenia gravis using the most sensitive radioimmunoassay detection. The antibody titer does not correlate well overall with disease severity, though for an individual patient, a significant reduction in serum antibody titer (≥ 50 percent) is often associated with clinical improvement. Evidence indicates that "antibody-negative" MG is nonetheless autoimmune, because it responds to immunotherapy and pheresis and can be passively transferred. Therefore, anti-AChR antibodies appear to be present that are not detectable by conventional radioimmunoassay methods.

The thymus gland appears to play a role in the origin and perpetuation of MG. The high incidence of pathologic abnormalities of the thymus gland in patients with MG and the favorable response to thymectomy initially suggested a pathogenetic role for the thymus. The anti-AChR antibody response is T cell–dependent. T cells obtained from thymus glands of myasthenic patients are more responsive to acetylcholine receptors than T cells derived from peripheral blood. Furthermore, the thymus contains myoid cells, which are striated, multinucleate "muscle-like" cells bearing AChRs on their surface. Because of their proximity to the immunocompetent cells of the thymus, the myoid cells may be particularly vulnerable to immune attack and might serve as an antigenic stimulus in MG.

DIAGNOSIS

Every attempt should be made to establish the diagnosis of MG *unequivocally* before the initiation of chronic therapies.

Clinical Features

The hallmark clinical features of MG are weakness and muscle fatigability. The latter must be differentiated from tiredness or depression. Symptoms may include diplopia, ptosis, difficulty chewing and swallowing, dysarthria, proximal limb weakness, and shortness of breath. The most common muscles involved, in descending frequency, are the extraocular muscles and levators of the eyelids; proximal limb muscles, especially deltoid, iliopsoas, triceps; muscles of facial expression, mastication, and speech; and neck extensors. Weakness is often worsened by repetitive or prolonged activity and improved with rest. Rarely, MG can *present* with respiratory insufficiency.

Diagnostic Tests

Confirmatory laboratory tests are generally performed in the following order: edrophonium (Tensilon) test, determination of anti-AChR antibody titers, repetitive nerve stimulation, and single-fiber electromyography.

Tensilon is a short-acting inhibitor of acetylcholinesterase. Acetylcholinesterase inhibitors potentiate the effects of acetylcholine at the neuromuscular junction by inhibiting its degradation. An initial 2 mg test dose of Tensilon is followed by 8 mg, using a double-blind control if possible. If a patient has demonstrable weakness due to MG, intravenous injection of Tensilon should result in transient improvement in strength lasting 1 to 3 minutes. Quantitative measures of endpoints should be used. As an alternative, 1 mg of neostigmine can be given by intramuscular injection, which allows for approximately 30 minutes of observation.

Repetitive nerve stimulation can identify abnormalities in neuromuscular transmission in approximately 80 percent of patients when clinically affected muscles are tested. The typical electrodiagnostic features on repetitive nerve stimulation in MG are decremental responses greater than 10 percent, comparing the amplitude or area of the fourth to the initial compound motor unit potential; postactivation facilitation; and later postactivation exhaustion.

Single-fiber electromyography provides the highest sensitivity in the detection of neuromuscular junction defects, detecting abnormalities in 88 to 99 percent of patients with MG. The hallmark feature of a neuromuscular junction defect by this technique is increased jitter, where jitter is the varying time interval between the triggered muscle action potentials in two muscle fibers belonging to the same motor unit. In patients undergoing evaluation for MG who are antibody negative and in whom repetitive nerve stimulation is normal or equivocal, single-fiber electromyography is routinely performed.

Chest CT or MRI to investigate the thymus should be performed in all patients diagnosed with MG. Thymic abnormalities occur in nearly 75 percent of patients with MG and include thymic hyperplasia in 85 percent and thymomas, benign tumors of the thymus gland, in 15 percent.

Screening for other autoimmune diseases often linked with MG such as hyper- or hypothyroidism, systemic lupus erythematosus, rheumatoid arthritis, or polymyositis should be performed; these disorders may add to the diagnostic picture of immune dysregulation and may complicate therapy.

TREATMENT

Cholinesterase Inhibitors

Anticholinesterase agents are the first-line therapy for MG. These drugs prolong the action of acetylcholine by slowing its degradation at the neuromuscular junction, thereby enhancing neuromuscular transmission. Although most patients experience some benefit from anticholinesterase agents, the response is often incomplete, necessitating the addition of immunotherapy.

Pyridostigmine bromide (Mestinon) is the most widely used anticholinesterase. The onset of action occurs within 30 minutes and peaks at 1 to 2 hours. The usual starting dosage is one tablet (60 mg) orally every 3 to 4 hours while awake. Dosages higher than 120 mg 5 to 6 times daily are not often useful. A sustained-release anticholinesterase preparation, Timespan 180 mg, is available; however, because of its irregular absorption, it should be used only for nighttime dosing in patients who have weakness during the night or upon awakening.

Anticholinesterases are safe, well-tolerated drugs, though they should be used with caution in patients with asthma or cardiac conduction defects. The most common side effect is diarrhea, which is dose-related and which can be controlled with diphenoxylate (Lomotil) or loperamide (Imodium) once or twice a day. Other symptoms of cholinergic excess are tearing, sialorrhea, and fasciculations. Excessive amounts of anticholinesterases may cause increased weakness that is reversible after decreasing or discontinuing the drug.

Thymectomy

Thymectomy is recommended for patients with MG in two instances. First, patients between puberty and age 50 who are inadequately controlled with Mestinon monotherapy may benefit (because of involution, no significant thymic tissue remains beyond middle age). Thymectomy results in clinical improvement in probably 85 percent of patients, with drug-free remission in up to 35 percent and reduced medication requirements in up to 50 percent. The benefit from thymectomy is delayed, rarely occurring within 6 months and requiring up to 2 to 5 years for demonstrated efficacy. Second, at any age thymomas should be removed, because these tumors may spread locally and become invasive, though they rarely metastasize.

Thymectomy is an elective procedure and should be performed when the control of myasthenia is optimal. Patients with significant weakness often benefit from a course of plasmapheresis during the weeks to days before thymectomy. Postoperative plasmapheresis may also be necessary if patients have significant weakness. We prefer thymectomy *before* other immunosuppressive therapy. This avoids poor wound healing related to steroids and the potential risk of infections postoperatively because of immunosuppression. If immunosuppressive therapy after thymectomy is indicated, it is generally begun 2 to 6 weeks postoperatively for prednisone or 1 to 2 weeks postoperatively for Imuran.

Median sternotomy and limited transcervical or transcervical endoscopic approaches for thymectomy have been used. Despite a cosmetic disadvantage, we advocate a "maximal" transternal dissection of all thymus, because thymic tissue can extend throughout the mediastinum from the diaphragm to the neck. This is particularly true in cases of thymoma, which can spread throughout the thoracic cavity. If thymomatous tissue cannot be completely excised, nonferromagnetic clips should be placed at the site of remaining tumor and postoperative radiotherapy administered.

The risks of surgery include injury to the phrenic or recurrent laryngeal nerves, atelectasis, pleural effusion, pneumonia, myasthenic crisis, intercurrent pulmonary embolism, impaired wound healing, and later sternal instability. Therefore, thymectomy should always be performed in an institution where this procedure is performed expertly and regularly and where the staff is experienced in the anesthetic care and pre- and postoperative management of MG.

Immunosuppressive Drugs

The prognosis for myasthenic patients has improved strikingly as a result of advances in immunotherapy; most myasthenic patients can be returned to full productive lives with proper therapy. Three agents can now be considered as first-line drugs for chronic immunosuppressive therapy in MG—prednisone, azathioprine, and cyclosporine. The choice among them is made by considering two facts: (1) how the toxicity profile fits the patient, and (2) how fast the patient has to improve. Factors by which to compare their use are outlined in Table 1.

We see patients who are not immunosuppressed potently enough, not treated long enough, or are treated without adequate management of side effects or infections. The predictably poor outcomes may end up souring both the patient and doctor on a particular drug, or convincing both that it is ineffective, when it may not be.

Before immunosuppression is begun, the patient's history of tuberculosis (TB) exposure and tuberculin skin testing must be obtained. If the patient has a significantly positive skin reaction, alternative immunomodulatory therapies, such as maintenance plasmapheresis or human immune globulin therapy, should be reconsidered. Alternatively, empiric TB prophylaxis should be given concurrent with immunosuppressive treatment.

Table 1 Standard Immunotherapy in Myasthenia Gravis

Drug	*Usual Adult Dosage*	*Time to Onset of Improvement*	*Time to Maximal Improvement*	*Toxicity/Efficacy Monitoring*
Prednisone	Gradually ascending to 60 mg q.d. orally followed by q.o.d. regimen	2-3 wk	3-6 mo	Weight; blood pressure; fasting blood glucose; electrolytes; ophthalmic examination; bone density; 24-hr urine calcium; 25-OH vitamin D (especially in postmenopausal women)
Cyclosporine (Sandimmune)	5 mg/kg/day orally, divided b.i.d. (125-200 mg b.i.d.)	2-12 wk	3-6 mo	Blood pressure; serum creatinine; blood urea nitrogen; cyclosporine level, 12-hr trough by RIA; amylase; cholesterol
Azathioprine (Imuran)	2-3 mg/kg/day orally (100-250 mg daily)	3-12 mo	1-2 yr	WBC (maintain >3,500); differential (goal <1,000 lymphocytes); MCV (goal >100 fl); platelets; liver function tests; amylase

Corticosteroids

Indications. Corticosteroids have been the mainstay of MG therapy for over 20 years. Corticosteroids are indicated when MG symptoms are insufficiently controlled by anticholinesterase agents and are sufficiently disabling to the patient that the frequent side effects of these drugs are worth risking. "Sufficient control" is best defined functionally by each individual patient. For example, some patients are willing to live with moderate generalized weakness, whereas for others even mild ptosis or diplopia is intolerable. Corticosteroids can produce improvement in patients with all degrees of weakness, from diplopia to severe respiratory involvement. Diplopia, which is rarely corrected by anticholinesterase agents alone, usually responds well to steroid treatment. Older men with MG seem to respond particularly well to steroid therapy. Steroids may improve overall results following removal of a thymoma because of their lympholytic effects.

More than 80 percent of myasthenic patients can be expected to improve with steroid treatment alone; the clinical effect usually begins within 2 to 3 weeks or occasionally longer, though maximal benefit may not be realized for up to 6 months or more.

Contraindications. There are no absolute contraindications to the use of corticosteroids. Relative contraindications include severe obesity, diabetes mellitus, uncontrolled hypertension, ulcer disease, osteoporosis, or ongoing infections. These problems can usually be circumvented by appropriate medical measures. Long-term treatment with steroids requires medical attention by an experienced physician; patients who are unable or unwilling to be followed closely should *never* be treated with steroids. Nursing mothers should be warned that steroids may pass into breast milk.

Many of the immunosuppressive effects of corticosteroids may last far longer than the maximal suppression of ACTH secretion by the pituitary. This allows effective *alternate-day* therapy in MG. If the drug is administered as a single dose in the morning at a time when the normal endogenous cortisol level would peak, by evening the administered dose is no longer present in the circulation, and the hypothalamus-pituitary-adrenal axis should secrete ACTH. This, in turn, will stimulate secretion of endogenous cortisol the next morning. The longer immunopharmacologic effect maintains disease control, while the single alternate-morning dose schedule mimics the normal diurnal cortisol cycle, reduces side effects, and facilitates eventual tapering of total dose.

Induction. Patients with moderate to severe generalized weakness or significant respiratory insufficiency or bulbar weakness are at risk of a transient steroid-induced exacerbation and should be admitted to the hospital for initiation of steroid therapy and observation. Nearly 50 percent of such patients have an exacerbation, which lasts days and occurs most commonly during the second 5 days of induction. The cause of this initial steroid-induced deterioration is not clear.

We prefer a gradually increasing schedule, since larger doses may exacerbate weakness. Prednisone is begun at a dosage of 15 to 20 mg per day and is increased gradually by about 5 mg every 2 or 3 days until the patient reaches a satisfactory clinical response or a level of 60 mg daily is reached. Only if the patient is already on a ventilator do we begin with a high dose. Prednisolone is chosen only if a problem in the hepatic metabolism of prednisone to prednisolone is known or suspected. The rate of increase must not be preprogrammed but should be guided by the patient's response. Increasing weakness is a signal to backtrack or proceed more slowly in raising the dose of prednisone.

If a patient has mild MG or purely ocular involvement and can be reliably monitored at about weekly intervals, outpatient initiation of prednisone may be done as follows: begin with 5 to 10 mg per day, and increase every week by 5 mg until a response is seen. This usually occurs at a dose of 35 to 60 mg per day.

Maintenance. High-dose prednisone is maintained until clinical improvement levels off or for 3 months, whichever comes first. Then the same total dose is maintained but the dosage schedule is gradually tapered to an alternate-day regimen. The amount on the "on" day is increased by 5 mg, while the amount taken on the "off" day is decreased by the same amount. Eventually an alternate-day regimen is established in most patients; occasionally a small dose of prednisone must be given on the "off" day to prevent fluctuations in strength. Although corticosteroids are effective in lowering the AChR antibody levels, one should avoid treating the antibody level. What is important is the patient's index symptoms and quantitatively measured signs, which served as the original indication for immunotherapy.

Finally, when the patient reaches a plateau of improvement on an alternate-day regimen, the total dosage is tapered gradually to seek the *smallest effective dosage.* The goal is not to eliminate all medication, because steroid treatment must be continued indefinitely in nearly all (>90 percent) patients, though the dose may be substantially reduced. We recommend reducing the dosage at a rate no faster than 10 mg every 2 months, until a dosage of about 50 mg every other day is reached, after which the reduction should be at a rate of about 5 mg every 2 months. It usually takes more than a year to determine the minimum requirement for a given patient. It is extremely important to taper the drug very gradually because the disease may exacerbate with too rapid a taper. The consequences of lowering the dosage too far may not be apparent for several months, and higher dosages may be needed to achieve the same effect as before the exacerbation. As an alternative to the above scheme, when the patient has responded rapidly to steroids, the dose may be decreased on the "off" day and maintained on the "on" day, a gradual process that usually takes 3 to 6 months or longer, depending on the clinical course.

Corticosteroids should not be used in divided daily doses; this need arises mainly in painful, inflammatory, arthritic, or vasculitic diseases, never in MG.

Follow-up visits are usually required every 6 to 12 weeks. Muscle strength should be measured quantitatively by the physician at interval visits. The most useful measurements include forced vital capacity, forward arm abduction time (arms sustained forward, extended, palms down, parallel to the floor), ptosis time (sustained upgaze until lid fatigues down to predetermined level, e.g., top or middle of the pupil), and measurements of individual muscle strength using a dynamometer.

The following patients should be considered candidates for other forms of immunotherapy such as azathioprine, cyclosporine, or thymectomy if not already performed: those who have an exacerbation when prednisone is slowly tapered; those who fail to respond; those requiring more than 40 to 50 mg every other day; and those in whom toxicity exceeds benefit.

Toxicity. Physicians must make their patients familiar with the unfortunately long list of side effects of chronic steroid therapy and of their potential seriousness. Of course, not every patient will develop every symptom, but most patients will have some side effect and almost every patient will gain weight and develop part of the Cushingoid habitus.

In handling toxicity, cooperation and communication between the patient's internist and neurologist is essential. Fortunately, many of the side effects can be minimized with alternate-day dosing and scrupulous attention to follow-up. We routinely monitor weight, blood pressure, the lens, fasting blood glucose, and electrolytes. Much of the toxicity can be prevented. We suggest the following:

Osteoporosis: Preventative treatment, especially in postmenopausal women, includes exercise, calcium supplements (1,500 mg per day, monitoring 24-hr urinary calcium), vitamin D (50,000 units twice weekly, monitoring serum 25-OH vitamin D levels), and replacement of gonadal hormones. Use of calcitonin or etidronate should be considered in patients who develop steroid osteopenia (detected by monitoring baseline and follow-up quantitative bone mineral densitometry) or fractures.

Obesity, hypertension, and diabetes: Monitor caloric intake to prevent weight gain. Restrict sodium intake. Supplement potassium as needed. Monitor fasting serum glucose.

Ulcer and dyspepsia: Give antacids (Tums and Rolaids double as a calcium supplement), H-receptor antagonists, or both in susceptible individuals.

Adrenal insufficiency: Double any low maintenance steroid doses during acute periods of stress.

General: Use the smallest effective dose—no more than once daily therapy—and gradually switch to alternate-day dosing when possible.

Azathioprine

Pharmacology. Since a completely intact immune response requires antigen processing and presentation (dependent in part on RNA synthesis) as well as proliferation and differentiation of immunocompetent cells (dependent on DNA and RNA synthesis), purine analogues like azathioprine can interrupt the immune response potently at multiple sites. A tight relationship exists between azathioprine dose and biologic effects on dividing cells like lymphoid and erythroid cells. Leukopenia and macrocytosis occur predictably and are monitored as guides to azathioprine dosage. The drug is extensively oxidized and methylated in liver and red blood cells. Concurrent administration of allopurinol (for treatment of gout) can increase the toxicity of azathioprine by interfering with its metabolism by xanthine oxidase, an important degradative pathway. Therefore, azathioprine dosage must be reduced by as much as 75 percent in patients who take allopurinol.

Indications. Azathioprine can be used effectively as initial therapy in MG. The manner in which azathioprine is most often used derives from its chief disadvantage—beneficial effects may take 6 months or more to appear. It therefore tends to be used as additional therapy in patients whose myasthenia has not been adequately controlled by thymectomy and corticosteroids. The combination affords the relatively rapid onset of immunosuppression produced by the steroids and allows tapering of corticosteroids once the azathioprine has had time to take effect. Finally, the addition of azathioprine allows a reduction of steroid dosage in otherwise well-controlled patients with excessive toxic effects of prednisone or in those who require a chronic maintenance dose of prednisone of more than about 50 mg on alternate days.

Contraindications. Patients who are unable or unwilling to be followed medically should *never* be treated with azathioprine. Only approximately 10 percent of patients are unable to tolerate azathioprine because of abnormal liver function, bone marrow depression, or an idiosyncratic reaction consisting of flulike symptoms of fever and myalgia. The question of a small increased risk of malignancy in azathioprine-treated patients has not been resolved; experience with azathioprine in organ transplantation suggests an increased risk of malignancy. However, patients with myasthenia or rheumatoid arthritis have been treated for years with the drug, and no increase in the incidence of malignancies has been found.

Induction. The usual *target* dosage of azathioprine is 2 to 3 mg per kilogram per day. It is important to realize that in obese patients, the optimum dose depends on the *total body weight,* not on lean body weight. A test dosage of approximately 50 mg per day should be given for the first week. If this is well tolerated, the dose should be gradually raised by 50 mg each week, while the WBC, differential count, platelets, and liver function tests are monitored closely. To establish the optimum dosage, several end points may be used. A total WBC of 3,000 to 4,000 per cubic millimeter is a safe end point. Azathioprine should be briefly discontinued if the WBC falls below 2,500 per cubic millimeter or the absolute neutrophil count is less than 1,000 per cubic millimeter, then reintroduced at a lower dose. This measure cannot be used in patients receiving prednisone because of the steroid-induced leukocytosis. In that situation, an absolute lymphocyte count of 5 to 10 percent is the appropriate target. A rise in the RBC mean corpuscular volume to greater than 100 fl also provides a useful gauge of biologic activity, and in MG, usually correlates with clinical improvement, but macrocytosis does *not* require discontinuation of therapy.

Maintenance. An adequate therapeutic trial of azathioprine as sole therapy must last at least 1 to 2 years, since the lag to onset of effect may range from 3 to 12 months, and the point of maximum benefit may be delayed until 1 to 3 years. Although azathioprine is decidedly slow to act, it is well tolerated by most patients. Close monitoring for toxicity should continue indefinitely, and patients should be seen at a minimum every 3 months after a stable, nontoxic dosage is reached. Although most myasthenic patients require lifelong immunosuppression, it is worthwhile to attempt to taper azathioprine to establish a minimal effective dose. A doubling of the anti-AChR antibody titer (optimally, in sera from two different dates measured in simultaneous assay) may predict clinical relapse. Based on European experience with the drug as sole therapy, only a minority of myasthenic patients remain in remission after discontinuation of azathioprine, so continued close follow-up is necessary after therapy is stopped.

Toxicity. As with other immunosuppressive agents, azathioprine increases susceptibility to opportunistic infections, which should be treated promptly and vigorously. The hematologic toxicity discussed above—leukopenia, anemia, and thrombocytopenia—are all reversible upon reduction of the dose of azathioprine. Hepatic toxicity, with mild elevation of transaminases, is common and responds to lowering the dose. A rise in transaminase levels up to two-fold is usually well tolerated by patients. Gastrointestinal discomfort, with nausea and anorexia is usually mild and responds to the use of divided doses taken after meals.

Cyclosporine

Mechanisms. Cyclosporine inhibits the activation of helper inducer ($CD4^+$) T cells and their production of IL-2, while relatively sparing suppressor ($CD8^+$) T cells. Its therapeutic effect in MG is thus explained, because the activation of B cells and production of anti-AChR antibodies are T-cell dependent. This relatively selective immunomodulatory action contrasts with the broad spectrum effects of corticosteroids, azathioprine, and cyclophosphamide. Unlike cytotoxic immunosuppressants, cyclosporine does not cause generalized myelosuppression, thereby limiting the risk of opportunistic infections.

Pharmacokinetics and Drug Interactions. Cyclosporine reaches peak plasma concentrations within 3 to 4 hours after ingestion. The drug has a large volume of distribution and is sequestered in tissues. It is cleared from blood with a half-life of about 19 hours. Most of the drug is metabolized in the liver and excreted in the bile. This accounts for its ability to potentiate greatly the risk of necrotizing myopathy or myoglobinuria due to lovastatin, which also depends on biliary excretion. Because cytochrome P-450–mediated oxidation of the drug is extensive, hepatic dysfunction or concomitant administration of agents that affect the cytochrome P-450 system can cause dramatic changes in the elimination of cyclosporine. Cyclosporine's independent mechanism of action produces an effect that is additive to that of corticosteroids. Because of evidence that the combination of cyclosporine with azathioprine and prednisone for suppression of organ rejection causes an increased risk of malignancies and infectious complications, most centers prefer to use only prednisone in combination with cyclosporine. It should be noted that corticosteroids increase plasma cyclosporine levels.

Indications. Cyclosporine is the only drug that has been shown to be effective primary immunotherapy for the treatment of MG in a prospective double-blinded, randomized, placebo-controlled trial. Improvement began at about 2 weeks, with maximal improvement by 4 months, correlating with a reduction in anti-AChR antibody levels. Although that original trial was small and limited, reported experience with the drug in open trials for MG has also been generally positive, and a large multicenter controlled trial has been completed and awaits publication. The efficacy of cyclosporine is similar to that of azathioprine but it has the advantage of a more prompt effect, usually occurring within weeks.

It is becoming more and more justified to use cyclosporine as a first-line drug because of its more targeted immunomodulatory effects. It is also indicated in patients in whom corticosteroids or azathioprine treatment has either failed or been excessively toxic. The general indications for use of the drug in MG are the same as for any immunosuppressant—the severity of the MG must not be functionally trivial, the expected benefit must outweigh the risks of toxicity, and the patient must be reliable.

Induction. The efficacy of cyclosporine relates to the lowest ("trough") plasma levels, whereas toxicity depends on peak concentrations. Therefore, the drug is given in a divided dosage schedule, twice a day. Because it is lipid soluble and variably absorbed, cyclosporine should be taken with a fat-containing meal or snack. The initial dose is 2.5 mg per kilogram twice a day. With this dose and schedule, nephrotoxicity and hypertension occur in fewer than 8 percent of patients.

Maintenance. Although the dose is eventually guided by clinical efficacy, it is initially adjusted by monitoring plasma cyclosporine levels and side effects. Plasma levels should be measured every 2 weeks until stable, and then approximately monthly. Trough levels are measured in the morning, 12 to 14 hours after the last dose. The reported levels depend on the method of assay; using the RIA with a specific monoclonal antibody, the trough level should be maintained between 100 and 200 ng per milliliter. The blood pressure, serum creatinine, and BUN are monitored, and the dose of cyclosporine is decreased if the creatinine level rises above 1.4 times the baseline level.

Toxicity. Compared with corticosteroids, cyclosporine has less frequent serious chronic toxicity. The most worrisome side effects are nephrotoxicity and hypertension. It should therefore only be used with great caution in patients with pre-existing uncontrolled hypertension or significant renal disease. There is an increased risk of nephrotoxicity in elderly patients. Nonsteroidal anti-inflammatory drugs that inhibit prostaglandin generation will potentiate cyclosporine nephrotoxicity. Other side effects include facial hirsutism, gastrointestinal disturbance, headache, tremor, convulsions, and rarely, hepatotoxicity. These are related to drug level and are reversible with dose reduction. Hypertension usually responds either to dose reduction or, if levels are appropriate, to institution of weight reduction, salt restriction, and/or an antihypertensive drug. Calcium channel blockers are preferred. As with other immunosuppressive agents, there is a theoretically possible increase in the long-term risk of malignancy. With close attention to management, cyclosporine can be used safely in nearly 90 percent of patients.

Short-Term Immunotherapies

Plasma Exchange. Plasma exchange, which depletes circulating antibodies, can produce short-term improvement in ongoing MG. Several uncontrolled trials, as well as long experience, have proven its effectiveness. Plasma exchange is now used primarily to stabilize patients in myasthenic crisis or for short-term management of patients undergoing thymectomy to avoid using corticosteroids and immunosuppressants. Less commonly it is used as adjuvant therapy in severely ill patients who are slow to respond to immunosuppressants. Repeated plasma exchange as a *chronic* form of therapy, either because the patient is intolerant or unresponsive to conventional immunosuppressant treatment, is rarely indicated. Plasma exchange works rapidly, with objective improvement measurable within days of treatment. Improvement (in the individual patient) correlates roughly with reduction in anti-AChR antibody titers. The beneficial effects of plasma exchange are temporary, lasting only days to weeks, unless concomitant immunosuppressive agents are used. Even "antibody-negative" patients may improve after plasma exchange.

Many protocols for plasma exchange have been advocated. Five exchange treatments of 3 to 4 liters each over a 2-week period is a typical program at our institution. In centers with adequate experience, plasma exchange is safe. The vital signs and the serum concentrations of potassium, calcium, and magnesium should be monitored. The major risks are due to problems of vascular access. Blood flow from peripheral veins is frequently insufficient for processing by modern high-volume hemapheresis machines. Therefore, indwelling catheters in large veins are used, and can cause infection, thrombosis, perforation, and even pneumothorax. Sepsis, arrhythmia, anaphylactic shock, pulmonary embolism, and systemic hemorrhage from disseminated intravascular coagulation, among other hazards, have also been reported. The benefit of plasma exchange must be weighed against problems of vascular access, the risks of pheresis, and the high cost of the procedure.

Intravenous Human Immune Globulin. The indications for use of intravenous human immune globulin (HIG) are the same as those for plasma exchange, that is to produce rapid improvement so as to get the patient through a difficult period of myasthenic weakness. The largest review of the efficacy of HIG summarized eight independent studies of 60 patients and reported overall improvement in 73 percent, but this figure is likely to be biased by the selective reporting of positive uncontrolled trials. The usual dose is 400 mg per kilogram per day on each of 5 consecutive days. When patients respond, the onset is within 4 to 5 days and the maximal response occurs within 1 to 2 weeks of initiation of HIG. The effect is transient but may be sustained for weeks to months, allowing intermittent chronic therapy. The mechanism of action of HIG in MG is not known, but it has no consistent effect on the measurable amount of AChR antibody in vivo or in vitro. Possible mechanisms that have been suggested to explain the immunomodulatory action of HIG include blockade of Fc receptors on macrophages and other cells and inhibition of the immune response to AChR by specific anti-idiotypic antibodies in the HIG pool.

Adverse reactions occur in fewer than 10 percent of patients and are generally mild, including allergy, headache, fluid overload, and various GI symptoms. The process of preparation of HIG has been shown to inactivate HIV and hepatitis B. HIG is very expensive, and this factor as well as the possible risks should be carefully weighed against the potential of rapid benefit.

COMPARISONS

Each of the available treatment options has its own advantages and disadvantages. Prednisone generally acts rapidly, is tried and true, but is beset by the problems of prevention and treatment of side effects. Azathioprine is safe and moderately effective, but slow. Cyclosporine is about equal to azathioprine in effectiveness; it is rapid in onset, but expensive to use. Cyclophosphamide is potent but highly toxic and is therefore reserved for special cases. Plasmapheresis or intravenous immunoglobulin are often useful for the short-term management of acute problems, or as pre- or postoperative therapy. However, the effects of both are transient, and their costs are extremely high. The therapeutic armamentarium now available provides a broad spectrum of effective treatment modalities. However, more specific and long-lasting treatments are still needed.

MYASTHENIC CRISIS

A patient with MG is said to be in myasthenic crisis when significant respiratory insufficiency or dysphagia results. Any patient with MG who reports dyspnea or dysphagia should be evaluated promptly. The two most helpful measurements of respiratory function in myasthenic patients are forced vital capacity (FVC) and negative inspiratory force. Arterial blood gas measurements are not a good determinant because they may be normal despite imminent respiratory failure. If the forced vital capacity is reduced to approximately 25 percent of normal or about 1 liter, the patient should be admitted to an intensive care unit for continuous monitoring and intubation if necessary. If the FVC is greater than 1 liter, the patient should be hospitalized for close observation of respiratory parameters and pharyngeal function. Anticholinesterase dose and route are optimized. For intravenous or intramuscular administration, neostigmine (Prostigmin) is available. Neostigmine 1 mg is equivalent to 60 mg of pyridostigmine. Neostigmine is given as a continuous IV infusion. Acute immunotherapeutic intervention begins usually with plasmapheresis or, less commonly, HIG in patients known to be HIG-responsive. In patients already on steroids, the dose can be increased abruptly concurrent with the start of pheresis. The beneficial effect of pheresis typically lasts only weeks, by which time the increased steroid dose should be effective. Ventilated patients who have not previously been on steroids can be started on high doses of prednisone (60 mg daily). Steroid dose must be accelerated slowly as previously described in patients not on steroids at the onset of the crisis. Steroids must be used with caution, however, in the setting of infection.

One should have a high suspicion of infection as a potential precipitating cause of myasthenic crisis. These patients are frequently immunosuppressed; furthermore, reduced respiratory function increases their vulnerability to pneumonia. MG patients with respiratory insufficiency (or post-thymectomy) can benefit from periodic inflation of the lungs with intermittent positive pressure therapy (three times daily) to reduce atelectasis and the risk of pneumonia. Incentive spirometry is discouraged because it is probably ineffective and may contribute to respiratory muscle fatigue.

NEONATAL MYASTHENIA GRAVIS

Preparations for the contingency of neonatal myasthenia should be made in the delivery room for all myasthenic mothers, because it is not possible to predict from the severity or laboratory features of the mother's myasthenia (even antibody positivity) whether an infant will be affected. Affected infants have weak suck and cry and may have generalized weakness or impaired swallowing and breathing. The clinical diagnosis is confirmed by repetitive nerve stimulation. The disorder may be recognized anytime in the first 72 hours and abates spontaneously after 2 to 3 weeks. Treatment requires only anticholinesterase agents and support of vital functions. Neostigmine (Prostigmin), 0.005 to 0.020 mg per kilogram per hour, is given by continuous intravenous infusion. Alternatively, 4 to 10 mg pyridostigmine (Mestinon) syrup may be used orally or by nasogastric tube every 4 hours. Cholinergic symptoms should be monitored to prevent overmedication.

The authors wish to acknowledge their support from the Jay Slotkin Fund for Neuromuscular Research. We thank D.B. Drachman for critical review of portions of the manuscript.

SUGGESTED READING

Arsura E. Experience with intravenous immunoglobulins in myasthenia gravis. Clin Immunol Immunopathol 1989; 53:S17–S179.

Drachman DB. Myasthenia gravis. N Engl J Med 1994; 330:1797–1810.

Drachman DB, Kuncl RW. Myasthenia gravis. In: Hohlfeld R, ed. Immunology of neuromuscular disease. Immunology and medicine series. Dordrecht, The Netherlands: Kluwer Academic Publishers, 1994:165.

Lisak R. Handbook of myasthenia gravis and myasthenic syndromes. New York: Marcel Dekker, 1994.

Matell G. Immunosuppressive drugs: Azathioprine in the treatment of myasthenia gravis. Ann NY Acad Sci 1987; 505:588–594.

Penn AS, Richman DP, Ruff RL, Lennon VA, eds. Myasthenia gravis and related disorders: Experimental and clinical aspects. vol 681. New York: Annals New York Academy of Sciences, 1993.

Tindall RSA, Rollins JA, Phillips JT, et al. Preliminary results of a double-blind, randomized, placebo-controlled trial of cyclosporine in myasthenia gravis. N Engl J Med 1987; 316:719–724.

Younger DS, Jaretzki A III, Penn AS, et al. Maximum thymectomy for myasthenia gravis. Ann NY Acad Sci 1987; 505:832–835.

AUTOIMMUNE UVEITIS

C. STEPHEN FOSTER, M.D., F.A.C.S.

Intraocular inflammation (uveitis) literally means inflammation of the uveal tract, the highly vascular coat of the eye (iris, ciliary body, and choroid). Inflammation may be localized to the iris (iritis), iris and ciliary body (iridocyclitis), ciliary body (cyclitis), or choroid (choroiditis). Uveitis can be referred to as anterior, intermediate, or posterior, depending on the portion of the eye predominantly involved with the inflammation, that is front, middle, or back.

Autoimmune uveitis is a general term for many forms of intraocular inflammation unrelated to any infectious agent. For instance, toxoplasmosis and toxocariasis are major causes of uveitis but are not autoimmune.

Uveitis causes approximately 10 percent of blindness in the United States. The visual loss associated with uveitis can be related to many factors. These include decompensation of the cornea from injury to the corneal endothelial cells; cataract formation induced by persistent inflammation, or treatment with glucocorticoids (see following); glaucoma secondary to inflammatory damage to the normal physiologic mechanisms maintaining pressure within the eye; vitreous clouding related to inflammatory cells or inflammatory-induced changes in the vitreous gel; retinal and subretinal neovascularization with hemorrhage; cystoid macular edema related to the release of inflammatory mediators and the resulting vascular changes; or damage to the optic nerve resulting from inflammation or persistent edema leading to optic atrophy. Any one or combination of these pathogenic conditions caused by persistent inflammation can result in permanent structural damage and vision loss.

One general approach to the treatment of autoimmune uveitis is the stepladder use of anti-inflammatory agents, beginning with glucocorticoids but with limited total amount of steroid use, since steroid-induced pathogenesis can be just as blinding as uveitis. It is best not to tolerate any level of chronic inflammation, to suppress inflammation quickly through aggressive use of steroids, and to add steroid-sparing agents if each attempt at steroid discontinuation is associated with recurrence of uveitis. Glucocorticoid preparations can be delivered topically, locally by injection, or systemically. The method of drug delivery is often dictated by the location of the inflammation in the eye or by the severity of the inflammation.

GLUCOCORTICOID THERAPY

Anterior uveitis (the most common type) usually responds to topical glucocorticoid therapy. Table 1 lists the various topical ocular steroid preparations available in the United States. Prednisolone sodium phosphate appears to be the best treatment, although animal studies have shown superior penetration of 1 percent prednisolone acetate preparations into rabbit cornea and anterior chamber. The acetate preparations must be vigorously shaken, however, before application of the medication. If not vigorously shaken, the drop delivered is not a 1 percent drop. Patients administering drops frequently (this is almost always the cases in patients with uveitis) are noncompliant with the requirement for shaking. Rimexolone 1 percent is a "soft" steroid for use in patients who have a tendency toward intraocular pressure elevations associated with the use of topical steroids.

In cases with very mild inflammation and few symptoms, 8 drops per day in the involved eye spaced at equal intervals is recommended, with subsequent taper. More severe cases will require topical application of glucocorticoids every half hour, with subsequent taper. The pain associated with anterior uveitis is related to spasm of the ciliary body, and this can be lessened by paralysis of the ciliary muscle with a cycloplegic agent such as 5 percent homatropine.

Patients treated with topical glucocorticoids should be examined within 4 days of therapy initiation. Then slowly taper the medication with weekly re-evaluations. Topical glucocorticoid administration is associated with both inevitable and potential side effects. Sufficient steroid (topical or systemic) inevitably induces cataract formation. Glaucoma, secondary to steroid-induced elevations of intraocular pressure in the susceptible individual, is a potential risk of topical steroid use that can generally be avoided, *if* regular and frequent

Table 1 Topical Ophthalmic Corticosteroid Preparations

Drug	*Preparation*	*Common Trade Name*	*Formulation*
Prednisolone	Acetate	Pred Forte (Allergan) Econopred Plus (Alcon) AK-Tate (Akorn)	1.0% suspension
	Sodium phosphate	Inflamase Forte (Iolab) AK-Pred (Akorn)	1.0% solution
Dexamethasone	Alcohol	Maxidex (Alcon)	0.1% suspension 0.05% ointment
	Sodium phosphate	Decadron Phosphate (MSD)	0.1% suspension 0.05% ointment

monitoring of the patient and his or her intraocular pressure has detected the earliest evidence of pressure elevation, and the appropriate therapeutic measures have been taken. Increased susceptibility to ocular infection (bacterial, fungal, parasitic, or viral) is an additional potential, though remote, risk of topical ocular corticosteroid use. Individuals with a past history of herpes simplex keratitis, however, are at high risk of recurrence of the herpes keratitis if treated with topical steroids without the concomitant use of the topical antiviral agent. Occlusion of the lacrimal punctum for 2 minutes after the application of each drop of corticosteroid should minimize even the most remote potential risk of sufficient systemic absorption of steroid to produce systemic side effects.

Periocular

The injection of glucocorticoid preparations into tissues surrounding the eye is effective treatment for uveitis. Injection therapy is typically considered in severe uveitis and for cystoid macular edema. Table 2 lists the available injectable preparations of corticosteroids in the United States. The preferred technique for administration of periocular steroids in most instances is to mix 1 cc of triamcinolone acetate (40 mg/ml) with 0.5 cc of 2 percent xylocaine (without epinephrine), and to inject this 1.5 cc mixture through the inferior preorbital septum, just above the inferior orbital rim, while elevating the globe, through the lower lid, with the index finger of one's nondominant hand. A three-eighths inch 30 gauge needle is recommended. The patient should compress the entire inferior portion of the globe for 3 minutes following the injection. In instances of particularly severe uveitis, add 1 cc of dexamethasone sodium phosphate (24 mg per milliliter) to the above mixture, and administer the 2.5 cc preparation as described above. If a patient has macular edema that responds to such injections but recurs, necessitating reinjection of steroid, administer a trans-septal injection of 80-mg depo-preparation of methyl prednisolone acetate, *provided* the patient has shown no propensity toward intraocular rises associated with frequent topical steroid applications or the aforementioned trans-septal injections of triamcinolone acetate.

Potential risks of periocular steroid injections include those mentioned above for topical steroid use (cataract, glaucoma, and enhancement of potential for infection). Other risks are globe perforation, periocular hemorrhage, and orbital fat prolapse through sites of multiple perforations in the preorbital septum when multiple injections have been administered. Build-up of depo-preparations is a risk if multiple injections of depo-steroid have been administered, resulting in fibrosis of extraocular muscles and/or mechanical restriction of globe movement.

Systemic

Patients with severe uveitis may require systemic glucocorticoids for control of the intraocular inflammation. Prednisone 1 mg per kilogram of body weight per day given with breakfast is administered after careful questioning regarding potential contrary indications to oral steroid use (e.g., hypertension, diabetes, history of tuberculosis, and history of peptic ulcer disease). In the case of patients with systemic lupus erythematosus, split-dosage is more appropriate. Informed consent is obtained, and a drug information sheet published by the American Medical Association is dispensed to the patient. The patient is counseled regarding the effect of the drug on appetite and mood, and advised about techniques to minimize the consequences of increased appetite, insomnia, emotional lability, and so on. Subsequent tapering of the medication is predicated on the basis of patient response, with tapering typically beginning 7 days after initiation of therapy. A switch from daily to alternate-day therapy is usually made once the patient has reached the 15 mg per day level; 30 mg every other day is then administered, with subsequent tapering of the alternate-day dose every 2 weeks. Limited tolerance for steroid use is especially acute for systemic steroids, and therefore it is uncommon, on the Immunology Service of the Massachusetts Eye and Ear Infirmary, for any patient to be on chronic systemic steroid therapy. Even patients with ocular manifestations of sarcoidosis are offered steroid-sparing strate-

Table 2 Injectable Corticosteroid Preparations

Drug	*Common Trade Names*	*Formulation*	*Typical Dose*
Triamcinolone			
Diacetate	Aristocort (Fugisawa)	25 mg/ml, 40 mg/ml suspension	40 mg
Acetonide	Kenalog (Westwood-Squibb)	10 mg/ml, 40 mg/ml	40 mg
Methylprednisolone			
Sodium succinate	Solu-Medrol (Upjohn)	40 mg/ml, 125 mg/2 ml, 2 g/ 30 ml solution	40-125 mg
Acetate	Depo-Medrol (Upjohn)	20-80 mg/ml Depot suspension	40-80 mg
Dexamethasone			
Acetate	Decadron-LA (MSD)	8-16 mg/ml suspension	4-8 mg
Sodium phosphate	Decadron Phosphate (MSD)	4, 10, 24 mg/ml solution	4-24 mg
Betamethasone acetate and sodium phosphate	Celestone Soluspan (Schering)	3 mg/ml suspension	1-3 mg

Table 3 Topical Nonsteroidal Anti-Inflammatory Agents

Drug Name				
Generic	*Commercial*	*Mfr.*	*Supplied*	*Typical Doses*
Flurbiprofen	Ocufen	Allergan	0.03% solution	One drop every 30 minutes, 2 hours preoperatively (total dose 4 drops)
Suprofen	Profenal	Alcon	1.0% solution	Two drops at 1, 2, and 3 hours preoperatively or every 4 hours while awake on the day of surgery
Diclofenac	Voltaren	Ciba Vision	0.1% solution	q.i.d.
Ketorolac	Acular	Syntex	0.5% solution	t.i.d.
Indomethacin	Indocin	MSD	0.5-1% suspension	q.i.d.

Table 4 Systemic Nonsteroidal Anti-Inflammatory Agents

	Drug Name			
Drug Class	*Generic*	*Commercial (Mfr.)*	*Supplied (mg)*	*Typical Adult Daily Dosage (mg)*
Salicylates	Aspirin	Multiple	325-925	650 every 4 hours
	Diflunisal	Dolobid (MSD)	250, 500	250-500 b.i.d.
Fenamates	Mefenamate	Pronstel (Parke-Davis)	250	250 q.i.d.
	Meclofenamate	Meclomen (Parke-Davis)	50, 100	50-100 q.i.d.
Indoles	Indomethacin	Indocin (MSD)	25, 50, 75 (SR)	25-50 t.i.d.-q.i.d., 75 b.i.d.
	Sulindac	Clinoril (MSD)	150, 200	150-200 b.i.d.
	Tolmetin	Tolectin (McNeil)	200, 400, 600	400 t.i.d.
Phenylalkanoic Acids	Fenoprofen	Nalfon (Lily)	200, 300, 600	300-600 t.i.d.
	Ketoprofen	Orudis (Wyeth)	25, 50, 75	75 t.i.d.-50 q.i.d.
	Piroxicam	Feldene (Pfizer)	10, 20	10 b.i.d., 20 q.d
	Flurbiprofen	Ansaid (Upjohn)	50, 100	100 t.i.d.
	Ketorolac	Toradol (Syntex)	10	10 q.i.d.
	Naproxen	Naprosyn (Syntex)	250, 375, 500	250-500 b.i.d.
		Anaprox (Syntex)	275, 550	275-550 b.i.d.
	Ibuprofen	Motrin (Upjohn)	300, 400, 600, 800	300-800 t.i.d.
	Nabumetone	Relafen (SmithKline)	500, 750	500-750 b.i.d.
Phenylacetic Acids	Diclofenac	Voltaren (Geigy)	25, 50, 75	50-75 b.i.d.

gies, such as systemic methotrexate or azathioprine or cyclosporin, if every attempt at systemic steroid therapy is associated with recurrence of uveitis.

Nonsteroidal Anti-Inflammatory Drug Therapy

Various cyclooxygenase inhibitors have been evaluated in the care of patients with uveitis. Nonsteroidal anti-inflammatory medications available for topical ophthalmic use are shown in Table 3, and a representative listing of systemic nonsteroidal anti-inflammatory drugs (NSAIDs) and their typical dosages are listed in Table 4. Abundant evidence from well-controlled clinical studies now exists regarding the efficacy of topically applied NSAIDs, given before and immediately following cataract surgery, in the prevention of or management of postoperative inflammation. Indocin 1 percent, flurbiprofen 0.3 percent, ketorolac 0.5 percent, and diclofenac 1 percent have been shown to be effective in randomized, double-blind, placebo-controlled trials. More important, however, is that NSAID therapy has been unequivocally shown to be an important adjunct in the care of patients with uveitis. At the very least, topical and systemic NSAIDs have a steroid-sparing effect, reducing the total amount of corticosteroid required to control uveitis. Five percent tolmetin was compared with 0.5 percent prednisolone and saline in a double-blind, randomized controlled trial of 100 patients with acute nongranulomatous anterior uveitis. Tolmetin and prednisolone were equally effective in eliminating the inflammation. A similar trial, comparing 1 percent topical indomethacin with 0.1 percent dexamethasone also showed equivalence 2 weeks after the institution of therapy. Systemic nonsteroidal anti-inflammatory drugs have been proven to be steroid-sparing in children with chronic iridocyclitis. They have also been shown to be effective in preventing attacks of iridocyclitis in a substantial number of children with juvenile rheumatoid arthritis–associated iridocyclitis.

Every patient must be appropriately apprised of the relative risks and benefits of the systemic use of NSAIDs. If the patient has no past history of gastrointestinal disease (peptic ulcer or otherwise), nor any documented past sensitivity to nonsteroidal drugs, the likelihood of a drug-associated serious complication (provided the medication is taken properly, after a full meal) is quite small. The benefits from this therapeutic approach in patients with chronic or recurrent uveitis are obvious to

Table 5 Immunosuppressive Agents

Class	*Drug*	*Dose and Route*
Alkylating Agents	Cyclophosphamide	1-2 mg/kg/day, PO, IV
	Chlorambucil	0.1 mg/kg/day, PO
Antimetabolites	Azathioprine	2-3 mg/kg/day, PO
	Methotrexate	2.5-15 mg every 1-4 weeks over 36-48 hours, PO, IM, IV
Antibiotics	Cyclosporine	2.5-5.0 mg/kg/day, PO

us. Extensive use of this approach in well over 1,000 patients with steroid-dependent uveitis, and the available controlled, randomized, blinded clinical studies support the usefulness of this drug class in the care of patients with uveitis. Patients with a history of steroid-dependent, recurrent uveitis should be kept on an oral nonsteroidal anti-inflammatory drug for at least 1 year, provided the patient has no recurrent attacks of uveitis while on the medication and tolerates the medication without significant side effect.

IMMUNOSUPPRESSANTS

Immunosuppressive agents (Table 5) are the final rung in a stepladder approach to the medical treatment of patients with uveitis, *except* in selected instances where an immunosuppressant must be used (i.e., not to use one would be negligent) such as in uveitis associated with Wegener's granulomatosis, polyarteritis nodosa, retinal vasculitis associated with Behçet's disease, and systemic lupus erythematosus). Patients with autoimmune uveitis that has been inadequately responsive to aggressive corticosteroid therapy and patients who have developed significant complications from the use of glucocorticoids are also candidates for immunosuppressive chemotherapy for their uveitis. Examples of patients with problems that often fall into these categories include children with juvenile rheumatoid arthritis–associated iridocyclitis, patients with sympathetic ophthalmia, Vogt-Koyanagi-Harada syndrome, inflammatory bowel disease, relapsing polychondritis, and strictly ocular autoimmune inflammation (birdshot retinochoroidopathy and multifocal choroiditis with pan uveitis). The prudent use of the medications begins with the exclusion of infection, mechanical, or other treatable cause of uveitis.

The appropriate monitoring of the patient requires the involvement of an expert chemotherapist who is qualified to manage the chemotherapeutic aspects of the patient. The potential risks and benefits are discussed candidly with patient and family, and the need for strict compliance with medication dosage and follow-up appointments is stressed. The choice of immunosuppressant is individualized for each patient, and depends on the underlying disease, the patient's age, sex, and medical status. The patient is screened for potential exclusions for use of any particular agent (liver disease or excess alcohol intake in the potential methotrexate candidate, renal disease in the potential cyclosporin candidate, and so on). A close collaboration between the ophthalmologist and the chemotherapist is essential in the care of these patients, with the ophthalmologist evaluating the therapeutic response, apprising the chemotherapist of the need for increased vigor of therapy, and the chemotherapist making the judgment about whether or not the patient can safely tolerate increased drug dosage. We avoid depressing the white count below 3,500 cells per cubic millimeter, the neutrophil count below 1,500 cells per cubic millimeter, or the platelets below 75,000 per cubic millimeter. Liver enzymes, urine analysis, blood urea nitrogen, and serum creatinine are obtained before therapy and at intervals of 1 to 4 months thereafter, depending upon the medication. Hemograms are typically monitored every 2 weeks. A listing of immunosuppressive agents is shown in Table 5.

Cytotoxic Agents

The first choice of a steroid-sparing immunosuppressant, in most instances, is once-a-week low-dose methotrexate, provided the patient has no contraindications to its use. Its safety record, including in the care of children with juvenile rheumatoid arthritis, is extraordinary, and because of its safety and efficacy, rheumatologists are turning to it with increasing frequency earlier on in their care of patients with rheumatologic disorders. We typically begin with a 5 to 7.5 mg oral or intramuscular dose once a week, either as a single bedtime dose or divided over a 36- to 48-hour period. Concomitant use of 1 mg per day of folic acid reduces the likelihood of a methotrexate-induced complication. The drug dosage is adjusted upward as needed for control of the inflammatory problem. Doses as high as 25 mg per week can be safely used, though it is extremely uncommon to advance a patient above 15 mg per week. Hematologic and hepatologic parameters are monitored regularly (every 2 to 4 weeks, depending on the clinical circumstances). The uveitic problems for which methotrexate is found to be most predictably effective include the seronegative spondyloarthropathies, JRA-associated iridocyclitis, pars planitis, sarcoidosis, and uveitis associated with systemic lupus erythematosus.

Azathioprine (2 mg per kilogram of body weight per day) has also been shown to be generally well tolerated and effective in the care of patients with uveitis of various autoimmune etiologies. It has been recently shown, in a controlled, randomized, blinded clinical trial, to be effective in the care of patients with ocular manifestations of Beçhet's disease. Used alone or in combination with cyclosporin, it can achieve the goal of total abolition of all intraocular inflammation in patients with Vogt-Koyanagi-Harada syndrome, sympathetic ophthalmia, pars planitis, and sarcoidosis. The usual caveats, bone marrow suppression, interstitial pneumonitis, and hepatitis, apply to this drug, as they do to methotrexate and the alkylating agents.

We generally reserve the alkylating agents (cyclophosphamide and chlorambucil) for the care of patients with blinding uveitis unresponsive to all other modalities, with the exception that they are the agents of choice in the care of patients with ocular inflammation associated with Wegener's granulomatosis and polyarteritis nodosa. Further, chlorambucil is the only well-documented agent to be capable of inducing frank, permanent cures in patients with Behçet's disease. The chemotherapist should inform the prospective patient being considered for treatment with an alkylating agent of the potential benefits and risks, including not only the aforementioned ones but also sterility, alopecia, and hemorrhagic cystitis and bladder malignancy (for cyclophosphamide) and a possible increased likelihood of malignant disease later in life.

Cyclosporine

Cyclosporine is not cytotoxic, and hence does not have the bone marrow depression potential of the cytotoxic agents. It is, however, nephrotoxic and hepatotoxic. The original optimism about the efficacy of this drug for patients with uveitis, at a time when 10 mg per kilogram body weight per day was being employed, has been reduced by the discovery that this dose of cyclosporine invariably produces irreversible kidney damage. The current recommended dose is 5 mg per kilogram body weight per day; at this dose cyclosporine is less effective than some of the cytotoxic drugs for care of patients with certain inflammatory diseases, including Behçet's disease. Still, it has a prominent role to play in the care of patients with uveitis. For some diseases it is the drug of choice. For example, patients with birdshot retinochoroidopathy rarely respond adequately to any agent other than cyclosporine. Used in combination with azathioprine and low-dose prednisone, cyclosporine is also effective in the care of patients with sympathetic ophthalmia, Vogt-Koyanagi-Harada's syndrome, multifocal choroiditis and pan uveitis, sarcoidosis, and the uveitis associated with Behçet's disease. However, this drug is potentially as dangerous as the cytotoxic drugs, and should be administered and regulated by an individual who is expert in the use of the medication, and in recognition and management of its earliest side effects.

SUGGESTED READING

Nussenblatt RB, Palestine AG. Uveitis: Fundamentals in clinical practice. Chicago: Year Book, 1989.

O'Brien JM, Albert DM, Foster CS. Anterior Uveitis. In: Albert DM, Jakobiec FA, eds. Principles and practices of ophthalmology: Clinical practice. Philadelphia: WB Saunders, 1993:407.

O'Brien JM, Albert DM, Foster CS. Juvenile Rheumatoid Arthritis. In: Albert DM, Jakobiec FA, eds. Principles and practices of ophthalmology: Clinical practice. Philadelphia: WB Saunders, 1993:2873.

Opremcak EM. Uveitis: A clinical manual for ocular inflammation. New York: Springer-Verlag, 1995.

Smith RE, Nozik RM. Uveitis: A Clinical approach to diagnosis and management. Baltimore: Williams & Wilkins, 1983.

IMMUNOLOGIC DISEASE OF THE EXTERNAL EYE

PAUL S. IMPERIA, M.D.
BARTLY J. MONDINO, M.D.

The external eye consists of the eyelids, conjunctiva, cornea, episclera, and sclera. These structures may be involved in all types of immunologic disease (Table 1). The eye can be affected primarily or as part of a systemic process. The external eye is critical in maintaining vision and protecting the intraocular contents. Immunologic external eye disease can be a source of major morbidity, including pain and permanent loss of vision. We provide a brief description of each disease and concentrate on the therapeutic modalities we employ with specific agents and dosages outlined.

Three important new therapeutic agents have become available since the last edition of this publication (Table 2). Lodoxamide tromethamine 0.1 percent solution is a mast cell stabilizer approved for vernal keratoconjunctivitis. Disodium cromoglycate 4 percent, the original mast cell stabilizer, is no longer available. Ketorolac tromethamine 0.5 percent solution is a nonsteroidal anti-inflammatory agent approved for seasonal allergic conjunctivitis. Levocabastine hydrochloride 0.05 percent suspension is a selective histamine H_1-receptor antagonist approved for seasonal allergic conjunctivitis. These agents are also mentioned for indications not approved by the FDA but for which clinical experience suggests they are useful. Individual clinician judgment is advised.

Table 1 Immunologic Disease of the External Eye Classified by Presumed Type of Immune Reaction

Type 1: Immediate, IgE-mediated
Vernal keratoconjunctivitis
Giant papillary conjunctivitis
Atopic keratoconjunctivitis
Hay fever conjunctivitis
Type 2: Tissue Fixed Antibodies and Complement
Cicatricial pemphigoid
Mooren's ulcer
Catarrhal infiltrates and ulcers
Type 3: Circulating Immune Complexes
Erythema multiforme
Reiter's syndrome
Marginal corneal ulcers associated with systemic diseases
Sjögren's syndrome
Scleritis and episcleritis
Type 4: Cell-mediated
Contact dermatoconjunctivitis
Disciform keratitis
Corneal transplant rejection
Phlyctenulosis
Atopic keratoconjunctivitis
Graft-versus-host disease

Table 2 Examples of Therapy in Immunologic Disease of the External Eye (see individual disease for details)

Artificial tears (solutions or ointments)
With preservatives, up to every 4 hours
Without preservatives, no frequency limit
Topical vasoconstrictor
Naphazoline hydrochloride, 0.5%-1.0% q.i.d.
Topical antihistamine
Levocabastine hydrochloride, 0.05% q.i.d.
Mast cell stabilizer
Lodoxamide tromethamine, 0.1% q.i.d.
Antibiotic ointments
Bacitracin, erytrhomycin, gentamycin, tobramycin
Antibiotic drops
Trimethoprim plus polymixin B (Polytrim)
Gentamycin, tobramycin, sulfacetamide
Ciprofloxacin, norfloxacin, ofloxacin
Topical steroids
Strong, prednisolone acetate suspension 1.0%
Weak, fluoromethalone suspension 0.1%, 0.25%
Ointment, dexamethasone 0.1%
Topical nonsteroidal anti-inflammatory
Ketorolac tromethamine, 0.5% q.i.d.
Systemic nonsteroidal anti-inflammatory
Indomethacin, 25-50 mg t.i.d.
Systemic steroid
Prednisone, 1 mg/kg/day starting dose with taper
Dapsone, 25-50 mg once daily, up to 300 mg/day oral
Immunosuppressives
Cyclophosphamide, 1-2 mg/kg/day oral
Azathioprine, 1-2 mg/kg/day oral
Cyclosporine, 5-10 mg/kg/day oral, 2% topical q2-6h
Methotrexate, 5-15 mg once weekly, oral or intramuscular

CONTACT DERMATITIS

The conjunctiva and eyelid skin are common sites of contact allergic reaction to topical drugs, cosmetics, jewelry, plastics, or chemicals. Patients present 24 to 48 hours after allergen exposure with tearing and itching. The eyelid skin shows edema, erythema, induration, papules, and vesicles. The conjunctiva demonstrates hyperemia and edema. It is important to rule out periorbital cellulitis.

Therapy is first directed at removing the allergen, which can be determined through a careful history or patch testing. Cool compresses provide symptomatic relief. Eyelid skin can be treated with dexamethasone ophthalmic steroid ointment four times a day for 5 to 10 days. The ophthalmic preparation is preferable to dermatologic agents since inadvertent ocular contact is possible with application to the eyelids. More potent fluorinated steroids should be avoided to prevent skin depigmentation and atrophy. Conjunctivitis responds to a weak topical steroid four times a day for 5 to 10 days, adjusting for severity. When using topical ocular steroids, one must monitor patients carefully for the following: increased intraocular pressure (reversible), cataract formation (irreversible), enhancement of viral replication (particularly herpes simplex), secondary infections, and inflammatory rebound from abrupt withdrawal. Fluoromethalone is less likely to cause these complications, particularly increased intraocular pressure, than stronger topical steroids such as prednisolone acetate. Ketorolac tromethamine and levocabastine hydrochloride can be used as alternatives to steroids or as steroid-sparing agents.

SEASONAL ALLERGIC CONJUNCTIVITIS

Seasonal allergic conjunctivitis is a recurrent, seasonal inflammation of the conjunctiva secondary to airborne allergens such as pollens, molds, and dusts. Symptoms include itching, tearing, and burning, with signs of eyelid edema and conjunctival hyperemia, edema, and papillae. The cornea is typically spared.

Treatment includes eliminating or minimizing allergen exposure and using cold compresses. Initial drug therapy consists of 1 to 2 weeks of ketorolac tromethamine, levocabastine hydrochloride, or naphazoline hydrochloride. If disease severity or duration warrant, a weak topical steroid may be substituted or added, starting four times a day for 4 to 5 days and then tapering off over 5 to 7 days as indicated by signs and symptoms. Systemic desensitization may be helpful in some patients with concurrent rhinitis or asthma.

ATOPIC KERATOCONJUNCTIVITIS

Patients with atopic dermatitis develop dry, indurated skin that may show fissures, excoriations, and scaling. The symmetrical, persistent lesions are located in the antecubital and popliteal areas, sides and back of the neck, face, head, axillae, shoulders, thorax, and retroauricular area. Examination may show typical skin involvement of the eyelids and frequently an ulcerative staphylococcal blepharitis (i.e., inflammation of the eyelids). Keratoconjunctivitis (i.e., inflammation the cornea and conjunctiva) is found in approximately 25 percent of patients during the teens through forties, with symptoms of tearing, itching, and burning. The conjunctiva shows hyperemia, edema, papillae, and occasionally scarring. Corneal involvement includes punctate epithelial breakdown, ingrowth of blood vessels, ulceration, and scarring.

Acute exacerbations may first be treated with cool compresses, systemic antihistamines, and topical naphazoline hydrochloride, ketorolac tromethamine, or levocabastine hydrochloride. A weak topical steroid usually results in dramatic improvement in more severe or resistant exacerbations. However, topical steroids may aggravate cataracts, which develop in 10 percent of atopic patients, and herpes simplex viral keratitis, which occurs in atopic patients as a result of depressed cellular immunity. Chronic treatment for several months with lodoxamide tromethamine can decrease the frequency and severity of exacerbations in very active cases.

A bandage soft contact lens may help protect the cornea from keratinized eyelid margins. Careful monitoring is necessary since contact lenses increase the risk for infectious keratitis, particularly in an already compromised eye. In the event of corneal epithelial breakdown in this or any of the conditions listed in this chapter, prophylactic therapy with a topical antibiotic solution four times daily or an antibiotic ointment every evening should be instituted to help prevent secondary bacterial keratitis.

VERNAL KERATOCONJUNCTIVITIS

Vernal keratoconjunctivitis is a recurrent, bilateral, seasonal condition of childhood occurring in warm climates. There is a male preponderance and a history of atopy. Patients present with tearing, photophobia, and severe itching. Signs include a thick mucoid discharge, large upper palpebral papillae (cobblestones), limbal (i.e., the junction of the cornea and conjunctiva) gelatinous elevations, visible limbal accumulations of eosinophils (Horner-Trantas dots), conjunctival pseudomembranes, punctate corneal epithelial breakdown, sterile corneal ulceration, and calcific corneal plaques.

Moving the patient to a cool environment, if possible, and using cool compresses are helpful. Naphazoline hydrochloride or levocabastine hydrochloride may help in mild cases but are often ineffective. Lodoxamide tromethamine four times a day for up to 3 months is a therapeutic mainstay and should be started initially so as to maintain the control achieved with steroids and to facilitate steroid withdrawal. Oral antihistamines are of no proven benefit. Initial control is often only achieved with a strong topical steroid, at least four times daily up to every hour, tapering by 1 drop every several days as allowed. Prednisolone acetate is favored as a strong topical steroid because of its superior penetration into the tissues of the external eye.

In severe cases, systemic steroids can be used until a response is achieved and then rapidly tapered off over 1 to 2 weeks as indicated by signs and symptoms. Acetylcysteine 10 percent solution four times a day is a mucolytic that dissolves the discharge and provides symptomatic relief. Oral aspirin has been recommended as a useful adjunct therapy because of its inhibition of the prostaglandin pathway, which may be involved in the pathogenesis of the condition. Patching or a bandage soft contact lens can relieve symptoms and help heal cases of sterile corneal ulcers. Topical cyclosporine A 2 percent every 4 to 6 hours has also been reported to be effective.

GIANT PAPILLARY CONJUNCTIVITIS

Giant papillary conjunctivitis is an allergic reaction of the upper eyelid conjunctiva, usually secondary to soft contact lens wear. An allergic reaction to lens deposits and mechanical trauma from the lens itself may be important factors in the etiology of this condition. It results less commonly from hard contact lenses, ocular prosthesis, exposed scleral buckles after retinal detachment surgery, and exposed nylon sutures. Symptoms include excess mucus, mild itching, irritation, and contact lens intolerance. The characteristic sign is papillae greater than 1 mm in diameter on the upper eyelid conjunctiva.

Early in the disease attempts at decreasing lens wearing time, cleaning and treating the lenses with enzyme to remove deposits, and/or switching to a new lens, especially disposable contacts, may be helpful. Lodoxamide tromethamine may be useful in mild cases. Giant papillary conjunctivitis will disappear gradually with discontinuation of lens wear. A short course of a weak topical steroid four times daily can be used to accelerate resolution once lens use is discontinued.

CATARRHAL CORNEAL INFILTRATES AND ULCERS

Catarrhal infiltrates and ulcers may represent a hypersensitivity reaction in the peripheral cornea to staphylococcal antigen(s) in patients with chronic staphylococcal blepharitis. Associated blepharitis should be treated with eyelid scrubs followed by an antibiotic ointment at bedtime. Eyelid scrubs are performed by rubbing of the eyelashes with a cotton tip applicator soaked in warm water. If the meibomian glands of the eyelid margin become involved, a 4- to 6-week course of tetracycline, 250 mg four times a day can be helpful. The corneal lesions themselves are very responsive to a weak topical steroid four times a day with a gradual taper over 1 to 2 weeks.

PHLYCTENULOSIS

Phlyctenules are subepithelial inflammatory nodules of the conjunctiva and cornea that can ulcerate and scar. Like catarrhal infiltrates, most cases of phylctenulosis are a reaction to antigens associated with staphylococcal blepharitis. Treatment of blepharitis and the phlyctenules themselves is similar to that outlined for catarrhal infiltrates and ulcers. In particular, topical steroids and a course of tetracycline are often helpful.

SJÖGREN'S SYNDROME

Primary Sjögren's syndrome is characterized by keratoconjunctivitis sicca (dry eye) and xerostomia (dry mouth). The secondary form is associated with a collagen vascular disease such as rheumatoid arthritis. The dry eye results from autoimmune destruction of the lacrimal gland. Ocular findings are related to the dry eye syndrome and include punctate breakdown of the corneal epithelium, peripheral corneal infiltrates, corneal thinning, and even perforation.

Keratoconjunctivitis sicca is primarily treated with artificial tear preparations. Ointments are more long-lasting than solutions, but blur vision. Preservatives in artificial tear preparations can be toxic to the cornea, limiting application to every 4 hours. Artificial tears without preservatives can be given as often as necessary although the single dose vials are generally more expensive and inconvenient. The tear film may be improved by obstructing lacrimal drainage from the eye with lacrimal punctal occlusion either permanently with cautery or temporarily with plugs. Corneal drying and breakdown can be treated by extended-wear bandage soft contact lenses. Creating a moist chamber for the ocular surface with swim goggles or plastic wrap held on to the skin with petrolatum ointment is helpful but often impractical.

OCULAR CICATRICIAL PEMPHIGOID

Ocular cicatricial pemphigoid (OCP) is a variably progressive autoimmune disease presenting in late adulthood with a female preponderance. The disease produces blisters or bullae of the skin and mucous membranes, notably including the conjunctiva, resulting in chronic scar formation. Chronic ocular sequelae include progressive shrinkage of the conjunctiva, inturning of the eyelid and eyelashes against the eye, dry eye, secondary bacterial eye infections, and corneal opacification. Treatment must address disease activity as well as the chronic ocular complications.

Mechanical epilation, electrolysis, cryotherapy, or hyfrecation can be used to treat inturning eyelashes. Mechanical epilation has the least tendency to exacerbate scarring but recurrence is likely and repeated treatments are necessary. Inturning of the eyelid may be successfully treated early in the disease course by ocular plastic surgical techniques. Mucous membrane grafts can be used to expand and reconstruct fornices obliterated by conjunctival shrinkage. However, any ocular surgical procedure may trigger acute disease activity and should not be attempted unless disease activity is quiescent or controlled by systemic medications. Systemic prednisone, 1 mg per kilogram per day for several weeks, may suppress postoperative inflammatory disease activity.

Dry eye can be treated with artificial tears, lacrimal punctal occlusion (if the puncta are not already obliterated by the disease), sewing the eyelids partially closed, a bandage contact lens, and/or moist chambers as described for Sjögren's syndrome.

Staphylococcal blepharitis is a frequent complication that can be treated by eyelid scrubbing and an antibiotic ointment at bedtime. Chronic treatment with oral tetracycline, 250 mg 4 times daily, may be necessary in cases with meibomian gland dysfunction.

Acute disease activity can be treated with systemic steroids, such as prednisone. Topical steroids are of no proven benefit. Dapsone has also been shown to help control disease activity. Systemic immunosuppressives, such as cyclophosphamide and azathioprine with or without prednisone, may be necessary on a long-term basis to reduce conjunctival inflammation and shrinkage. Early stages of OCP are more likely to respond. Immunosuppressive therapy does not affect existing scarring. Patients on immunosuppressives must be monitored for such serious complications as pancytopenia, hemorrhagic cystitis, dermatitis, anorexia, weight loss, and gastrointestinal bleeding. Elderly patients with limited life spans or complicating medical problems should not be subjected to immunosuppressives if they are at an early stage of the disease.

In the late stages of OCP, vision may be lost from corneal opacification. A keratoprosthesis may restore some vision in these cases, but it is frequently complicated by glaucoma, infection, and retinal detachment.

ERYTHEMA MULTIFORME

Erythema multiforme (EM) is an acute, self-limited bullous inflammatory disease of skin and mucous membranes that develops as a reaction to a wide variety of exogenous precipitating factors such as infections and drugs. The minor form primarily affects the skin, whereas the major form (the Stevens-Johnson syndrome) can involve mucosa and skin with associated toxemia, fever, prostration, and death.

Ocular effects include swollen, ulcerated, and crusted eyelids and conjunctivitis. In severe cases, pseudomembranous or membranous conjunctivitis may result in scarring, with associated complication of inturned eyelids and eyelashes, inability to fully close the eyelids, fibrosis of lacrimal puncta, dry eye, and keratinization. As a result, corneal erosions, ulcers, opacification, and even perforation can occur. Ocular EM is self-limiting in 2 to 3 weeks and, unlike OCP, conjunctival scarring is not chronically progressive.

Treatment of acute disease consists of removing any possible offending etiologic agent such as drugs and treating concurrent infections. Management of acute cutaneous and systemic manifestations is dealt with elsewhere. Wet dressings are used to debride crusted lesions, intravenous hydration compensates for fluid losses, and systemic broad-spectrum antibiotics are often necessary for sepsis. Systemic steroids with a gradual taper over 3 to 4 weeks have been advocated but have not been proven to be beneficial. They may also prolong recovery and predispose patients to complications such as sepsis. Lysis of symblephara (conjunctival adhesion) should be attempted as they develop, but it is often ineffective. Other methods used to prevent adhesion of raw conjunctival surfaces include suturing a lining of household plastic wrap to the inside of the eyelid or inserting a symblepharon ring with a bandage contact lens.

Late ocular complications depend on disease severity and are not prevented by local treatment. The chronic ocular sequelae of conjunctival scarring, dry eye, secondary bacterial conjunctivitis and keratitis, inturning of the eyelids, and corneal opacification are treated as outlined for OCP. Topical tretinoin may reverse conjunctival keratinization.

REITER'S SYNDROME

Reiter's syndrome consists of conjunctivitis and/or iritis, urethritis, arthritis, and mucocutaneous lesions. It most commonly occurs in young men who are HLA-B27 positive and have had exposure to dysentery or venereal disease, especially *Chlamydia.* Conjunctivitis is noninfectious and requires no specific therapy. Iritis is treated with a weak topical steroid and a topical cycloplegic agent, such as homatropine 5 percent twice daily. Other less common external eye manifestations include episcleritis, scleritis, and keratitis. Keratitis, if severe, is treated with a weak topical steroid four times a day.

INTERSTITIAL KERATITIS

Interstitial keratitis is an inflammation of the corneal stroma (i.e., the layer between the outer epithelium and inner endothelium), resulting in intracorneal infiltration of leukocytes and blood vessels. The keratitis is thought to represent a hypersensitivity reaction to a previous infection, most commonly congenital syphilis. Other causes include tuberculosis, mumps, herpes simplex and herpes zoster, influenza, lymphogranuloma venereum, trypanosomiasis, and Cogan's syndrome (interstitial keratitis, deafness, vertigo, and tinnitus). A strong topical steroid every 3 to 4 hours with a gradual taper over several weeks is the mainstay of therapy.

DISCIFORM KERATITIS

Disciform keratitis is a disc-shaped area of corneal edema thought to represent a cell-mediated immune response most commonly to previous herpes simplex virus infection. Pain, tearing, photophobia, and eventual corneal opacification can develop.

The disease responds well within 7 to 10 days to a strong topical steroid every 1 to 6 hours depending on severity and proximity to the central visual axis with a gradual taper over several weeks. There is less urgency to treat peripheral, mildly symptomatic lesions. Symptoms of concurrent anterior uveitis are treated by a topical cycloplegic such as homatropine 5 percent twice a day. Recurrent herpetic keratitis is possible at any time. If it occurs during topical steroid therapy, a particularly severe keratitis can result. To cover for this possibility, the topical antiviral trifluridine is given 5 times daily along with steroids or on a drop-for-drop basis.

MOOREN'S ULCER

Mooren's ulcer is a rare autoimmune disease resulting in chronic, painful ulceration of the peripheral cornea. It can advance centripetally and circumferentially, leaving a thinned, vascularized cornea. Treatment proceeds in a stepwise fashion. Initial therapy includes a strong topical steroid hourly. If unsuccessful, a resection of 3 to 4 mm of adjacent conjunctiva may facilitate healing by removing conjunctival enzymes and plasma cells that produce autoantibodies. Repeated resection may be necessary.

If the ulcer is unresponsive to the previous measures, immunosuppressives such as azathioprine, cyclophosphamide, or cyclosporine should be used. Penetrating or lamellar keratoplasty and conjunctival flaps have been attempted to arrest disease or avoid perforation, but these usually fail in the face of active disease and may themselves ulcerate from the same process. Bandage soft contact lenses and cycloplegia with homatropine 5 percent twice a day are useful in relieving pain but do not affect disease progression.

SCLERITIS AND EPISCLERITIS

Episcleritis denotes inflammation of the connective tissue under the conjunctiva adjacent to the sclera. Scleritis involves the deeper, thicker scleral tissue. Either can exist alone or in association with a known systemic immune disorder such as rheumatoid arthritis, Wegener's granulomatosis, periarteritis nodosa, influenza, scleroderma, lupus erythematosus, relapsing polychondritis, Cogan's syndrome, and cranial arteritis.

Episcleritis is frequently recurrent, mildly painful, and self-limited. As such, no specific treatment may be required. Severe or chronic cases may respond to a systemic nonsteroidal anti-inflammatory agent such as indomethacin or to a strong topical steroid four times a day with a taper over 1 to 2 weeks.

Scleritis is much more painful and can be associated with intraocular inflammation and threaten vision. Systemic therapy of scleritis is necessary to control pain and prevent ocular complications. In the case of necrotizing scleritis, systemic therapy is also necessary to decrease morbidity and mortality from the associated disease. Topical therapy is usually ineffective. Oral indomethacin is the usual initial therapy. Prednisone can be used with a slow taper over several weeks to months if there is no response to indomethacin and is particularly useful in necrotizing scleritis. Use of a combination of indomethacin and prednisone can produce a response in disease that is resistant to either agent alone. This combination also allows for a lower total dose of steroid. Cyclophosphamide or other immunosuppressives are indicated for scleritis resistant to indomethacin or prednisone or for necrotizing scleritis. Scleral patch grafting with donor sclera can be used for severe scleral thinning or perforation.

MARGINAL CORNEAL ULCERS ASSOCIATED WITH SYSTEMIC DISEASES

Marginal corneal ulcers may be associated with the immune disorders listed under scleritis as well as bacillary dysentery, influenza, and acute leukemia. The initial sign is usually a peripheral corneal infiltrate that ulcerates and can progress to involve the entire corneal circumference.

Resolution of the corneal infiltrates and ulcers is dependent on treating the associated systemic disease with nonsteroidal anti-inflammatory agents, systemic steroids, or immunosuppressives. Bandage soft contact lenses, cyanoacrylate adhesives, conjunctival resection, and other surgical procedures can be used and have similar results as described for Mooren's ulcer.

CORNEAL TRANSPLANT REJECTION

A lack of vascularity and lymphatic drainage makes the cornea an immunologically privileged site. However, rejection of a transplanted cornea can occur, especially when contact between the cornea and blood vessels of the conjunctiva or iris exists.

Fortunately, in most cases, allograft rejection can be easily recognized clinically and successfully treated. The mainstay of therapy is topical steroids, which have a lympholytic effect on the killer lymphocytes that mediate the rejection by destroying the corneal endothelial cells. Initially, a strong topical steroid is used hourly until inflammation subsides and the rejection halts. A slow taper over several weeks to months is then carried out. In severe or resistant cases, a subconjunctival injection of triamcinolone diacetate, 40 mg, can be effective. Oral prednisone is used in the most severe cases, with a gradual taper over several weeks and continuation of topical steroids for months. Topical cyclosporine A has been shown to be ineffective, although systemic cyclosporine A is currently being investigated to treat and prevent rejection in high-risk cases. Tissue matching does not decrease the risk of rejection.

GRAFT-VERSUS-HOST DISEASE

Graft-versus-host disease is a major cause of morbidity and mortality in patients undergoing bone marrow transplantation for malignancies such as acute leukemia. It affects the skin, mucous membranes, gastrointestinal tract, and liver in an acute or chronic form. Ocular involvement in the form of an acute pseudomembranous conjunctivitis and a chronic Sjögren's-like syndrome is common. Patients with active disease are treated with systemic immunosuppressives and steroids. Local ocular treatment with lubricants is similar to that for Sjögren's syndrome. Infectious ocular complications are common.

SUGGESTED READING

Brown SI, Mondino BJ. Therapy of Mooren's ulcer. Am J Ophthalmol 1984; 98:1–6.

Foster CS, Forstot SL, Wilson LA. Mortality rate in rheumatoid arthritis patients developing necrotizing scleritis or peripheral ulcerative keratitis: effects of systemic immunosuppression. Ophthalmology 1984; 91:1253–1263.

Mondino BJ. Immunologic disease of the external eye. In: Spoor TC, ed. Modern management of ocular disease. Thorofare, NJ: Slack, 1985:153–164.

Mondino BJ. Cicatricial pemphigoid and erythema multiforme. Ophthalmology 1990; 97:939–952.

Mondino BJ, Phinney RB. Treatment of scleritis with combined oral prednisone and indomethacin therapy. Am J Ophthalmol 1988; 106:473–479.

CHRONIC LYMPHOCYTIC THYROIDITIS

ROBERT VOLPÉ, M.D., F.R.C.P.(C), F.A.C.P., F.R.C.P.(EDIN. & LOND.)

Chronic lymphocytic thyroiditis has many synonyms (such as autoimmune thyroiditis, struma lymphomatosa, and Hashimoto's thyroiditis), and several variants, including postpartum thyroiditis (PPT), lymphocytic thyroiditis of childhood and adolescence, at least some cases of silent thyroiditis, and atrophic thyroiditis. Autoimmune thyroiditis is also closely related to Graves' disease, which is another of the autoimmune diseases.

In past generations, lymphocytic thyroiditis was considered uncommon and the diagnosis was often made at thyroidectomy. Increased awareness, coupled with improved diagnostic procedures, has resulted in improved recognition. The disease appears also to have increased in frequency, perhaps owing to the sharp increase in iodine intake that has occurred in the Western world in the past two generations. It is now considered that approximately 3 to 4 percent of the population has significant autoimmune thyroiditis, often with functional deficiency of the thyroid gland. The disorder is much more common in females (female-male ratio, 4:1), and increases with age; in elderly women, about 16 percent are found to have thyroid autoantibodies that correlate with at least some degree of lymphocytic infiltration of the thyroid gland. There is also a definite increase in both compensated and overt hypothyroidism in elderly women. The malady tends to aggregate in specific families and is clearly genetically induced.

The disease is consequent to an immunoregulatory defect, which in turn may prove to be secondary to reduced specific antigenic activation of regulatory thymic-dependent (T) lymphocytes (presumably from genetic abnormalities in antigen-presenting genes) and from additive environmental insults to the immune system; these events result in an immunologically mediated lymphocytic infiltration of the thyroid gland with destruction of thyroid follicular cells. This cytolysis is due to activation of thyrocyte-directed cytotoxic T lymphocytes, antibody dependent cell-mediated cytotoxicity, and killer cell activation, with the participation of various other immunologically active molecules and cytokines. Bursa-equivalent (B) lymphocytes and plasma cells are stimulated by helper T lymphocytes (primarily locally within the thyroid), and consequently may produce antibodies to certain thyroid antigens, such as thyroglobulin (Tg), thyroperoxidase (TPO), the thyrotrophin receptor (TSHR), and others.

The histology is characterized by an inflammatory infiltrate with areas of follicular hyperplasia and tall columnar follicular cells, although often the follicles are small and contain scant colloid. Follicular cells may be vacuolized with very eosinophilic cytoplasm (Hurthle or Askanazy cells). Widespread lymphocytic infiltration, usually replete with germinal centers is a hallmark, and plasma cells are common. A variable degree of fibrosis is noted, from minimal to predominant.

CLINICAL ASPECTS

A wide variation in clinical expression and presentation is observed in this condition. Some patients may have no clinical signs or symptoms whatever, and the diagnosis may be made by screening in geriatric institutions, or by inadvertent testing for thyroid function and/or thyroid autoantibodies, or by finding lymphocytic infiltration within the thyroid gland unexpectedly at operation or autopsy. Others may be found to have enlarged thyroid glands (usually diffuse goitres) as their only clinical manifestation. At the opposite extreme, patients may present with overt evidence of thyroid dysfunction, usually hypothyroidism. Either iodide or lithium ingestion can unmask occult thyroiditis, rendering it overt, with goiter, thyroid antibodies, or both, with or without thyroid dysfunction. Amiodorone, which contains large amounts of iodine, is another drug worthy of special mention because of its widespread use; it may certainly aggravate pre-existent autoimmune thyroiditis.

Pressure symptoms within the neck are occasionally encountered, with mild discomfort, hoarseness, dysphagia or cough; however, usually there are no local symptoms in the neck. Severe pain in the thyroid region, radiating to the ear(s), reminiscent of subacute thyroiditis, is seen in about 5 percent of patients, and in this circumstance, the gland may be correspondingly tender. More moderate pain may also occasionally occur.

Hyperthyroidism may occur in autoimmune thyroiditis and may be of two types. The first of these is due to Graves' disease, which may coexist concomitantly with Hashimoto's thyroiditis. This condition is clearly a combined disorder and is indistinguishable from other cases of Graves' disease, with the exception of the firmness of the goiter and the high titers of thyroid antibodies. Some patients with euthyroid or hypothyroid Hashimoto's thyroiditis will have exophthalmos, with or without thyroid stimulating antibodies (TSAb). When TSAb are present in a patient with Hashimoto's thyroiditis, the thyroid functional status will depend on the state of parenchymal cell integrity. That is, the number of remaining intact thyroid follicular cells will dictate whether the patient is hyperthyroid, euthyroid, or hypothyroid.

The second form of hyperthyroidism may occur transiently in the initial phase of Hashimoto's thyroiditis, once again simulating subacute thyroiditis. This form may or may not be associated with a painful thyroid gland. The hyperthyroid phase is due to destructive thyroiditis, with a discharge of preformed thyroid hormone resulting from the inflammatory process. In "silent" or "painless" thyroiditis, which is often a forme fruste of Hashimoto's thyroiditis, and in postpartum thyroiditis, which is similarly due to autoimmune thyroiditis, the hyperthyroid phase often precedes a hypothyroid phase, or conversely, the patient may manifest only a transient hypothyroid phase.

An atrophied thyroid gland as an expression of autoimmune thyroiditis is commonly associated with hypothyroidism and may be due to an antibody to the TSH receptor that blocks the action of TSH. Less commonly, goitrous Hashimoto's thyroiditis is also associated with hypothyroidism (usually less severe than in the atrophic form). The most common cause of spontaneous compensated hypothyroidism (characterized by normal plasma concentrations of thyroid hormones, but elevated TSH values) or spontaneous overt hypothyroidism, is autoimmune thyroiditis. In compensated hypothyroidism, patients are clinically euthyroid, and the diagnosis is made by virtue of the elevated TSH levels.

The thyroid functional state may vary considerably with time in this condition. Patients may remain clinically euthyroid for years, or there may be considerable variation in thyroid function or serology over time; remissions may occur not infrequently. Moreover, patients who have Hashimoto's thyroiditis and even severe hypothyroidism may recover and even later develop hyperthyroidism due to Graves' disease. Conversely, hyperthyroidism due to Graves' disease may ultimately culminate spontaneously as hypothyroidism secondary to autoimmune thyroiditis.

In most patients with goitrous Hashimoto's thyroiditis, the goiter is diffusely but not necessarily symmetrically enlarged, and varies considerably in size and firmness. It is characteristically associated with firmness and bosselation without discrete thyroid nodules. The gland is only occasionally tender, and bruits are not heard. The disorder may be associated with other organ-specific autoimmune disease such as insulin-dependent diabetes mellitus, pernicious anemia, Addison's disease, vitiligo, and others in the patient or in relatives. Indeed there is often a family history of autoimmune thyroid disease, and relatives should be tested for this disorder.

As mentioned, there is an increased incidence of autoimmune thyroiditis in the older population, particularly females. Because of the frequent subtleness of expression of this disorder, there has been a suggestion that screening procedures in geriatric institutions might be useful to detect mild or occult forms of autoimmune thyroiditis.

In children or adolescents, lymphocytic thyroiditis is the cause of diffuse goitre in about two-thirds of instances. In such patients, thyroid antibodies are not detected as often or in the same titers as in adults, and often the diagnosis can only be verified by biopsy. It may also be mentioned that transient neonatal hypothyroidism may result from the passive transplacental transfer of thyroid blocking antibodies.

Although there is no evidence that thyroid carcinoma is increased with Hashimoto's thyroiditis, discrete thyroid nodules coexisting with Hashimoto's thyroiditis must be treated on their own merits. Lymphoma of the thyroid, a rare condition, is nevertheless definitely increased in incidence in conjunction with Hashimoto's thyroiditis.

Practically, the observation of a patient with a diffuse goiter, associated with moderate or high titers of thyroid antibodies, with or without any degree of hypothyroidism, would permit a presumptive diagnosis of autoimmune thyroiditis. Biopsy procedures are generally unnecessary, but would be a final and definitive means of establishing such a diagnosis.

MANAGEMENT

It is clear from the previous discussion that chronic lymphocytic thyroiditis is indeed an autoimmune disease. Theoretically, therefore, one would like to interfere with the immunologic process by utilizing drugs or treatments designed for this purpose. Indeed, large doses of prednisone have been shown to improve thyroid function and reduce thyroid swelling in this condition. Moreover, under experimental conditions, drugs such as FK-506 have been shown to improve the histology and serology of this disorder. However, neither prednisone or other immunosuppressive drugs are of practical importance in the management of chronic lymphocytic thyroiditis because a simpler, more effective, and nontoxic agent is available in the form of thyroid hormone, primarily levothyroxine (T4), therapy. Thyroid hormone therapy is effective for three reasons: (1) it acts as replacement when insufficient thyroid hormone is being produced by the thyroid gland itself; (2) it suppresses TSH, thus allowing the goitre to regress in size; and (3) by suppressing TSH, thyroid antigen expression is reduced, which in turn inhibits thyroid autoantibody production, and presumably also, T helper cell responses in this condition; this tends to reduce the immune response within the thyroid gland.

T4 is one of the 13 most commonly prescribed medications in North America, with more than 15 million prescriptions filled annually. Sensitive means of measuring serum TSH now permit equally precise means of determining the dosage of T4, either for replacement therapy (where the serum TSH concentration should be maintained within the normal range), or for suppression of TSH with somewhat larger dosages provided so as to cause regression in the goiter. This is discussed further in the following discussion. Suppression of TSH has been reported to induce decreased bone mineral density, thus resulting in considerable concern about prescribing such dosages. However, more recently, studies have failed to confirm such bone loss; thus anxiety over this point has been generally allayed. However, there may be subtle effects on cardiac function (shortening of systolic time intervals, increased nocturnal heart rate) and hepatic enzymes that might possibly have long-term implications.

As mentioned, the form of thyroid hormone now generally prescribed is levothyroxine (T4). In previous generations, desiccated thyroid was employed, but the means of assaying its potency left something to be desired; moreover, its content of T4 and triiodothyronine (T3) was variable from lot to lot, thus making for some variability in its effects. On the other hand, T3 is also available; however, it has a very short half-life, such that the serum values of T3 will actually vary considerably during each day, making it much less effective for long-term management when compared to T4. T4 as now available is synthetically produced, but is identical to T4 secreted by the thyroid gland. The T4 content of tablets must be between 90 and 110 percent of the stated amount as measured by high pressure liquid chromatography.

T4 is absorbed along the course of the human small intestine, with a decrease in absorption distally. About 80 percent of T4 is absorbed whether the patient is euthyroid or hypothyroid. Since about 75 percent of circulating T3 comes from monodeiodination of T4 to T3, serum concentrations are generally stable in long-term T4 therapy (in contrast to the situation with T3 treatment). In North America, T4 is available in many strengths (25, 50, 75, 88, 100, 112, 125, 150, 175, 200, and 300 μg) thus permitting precision in dosage with a single daily oral tablet. There are a few situations in which there may be changes in the requirement for T4, necessitating more frequent TSH determinations. These include pregnancy, in which the T4 requirement may rise as much as 45 percent, particularly during the last trimester. Other circumstances in which T4 requirements may be altered are listed in Table 1.

As mentioned, chronic lymphocytic thyroiditis may result in hypothyroidism whether compensated or overt. The relatively narrow normal range for serum TSH makes its normalization a reasonable goal in managing hypothyroid patients. With appropriate therapy, the TSH values should be between 0.35 and 5.0 mU per liter. In younger patients, one may commence with a full replacement dosage in the order of 1.6 μg per kilogram of ideal body weight. The average dose for adult females is about 100 μg per day, and about 150 μg daily in most adult males. However, the dosage must be individualized, with the attainment of a normal TSH as an objective of treatment. It may take a few months for the TSH to drop into the normal range. If the TSH is not normal after 4 months of treatment, the daily dose of T4 should be increased by 25 μg. There is no need to retest more often than about every 8 weeks. Once the TSH has been stabilized, the dosage of T4 may be left as it stands, and it only occasionally requires further adjustment. After an appropriate dosage is established, usually only an annual TSH determination is needed to monitor treatment. A serum free T4 measurement is generally not required once stabilization has been brought about. At times problems of bioavailability, compliance, or absorption may confound precise control.

In older patients, or in those who have cardiovascular disease, hypothyroidism must be treated more cautiously. T4 may augment cardiac rate and contractability and increase myocardial oxygen consumption.

Table 1 Circumstances in Which Levothyroxine Requirements May Be Altered

Increased levothyroxine requirements
Malabsorption
Gastrointestinal disorders
Mucosal diseases of the small bowel (e.g., sprue)
After jejunoileal bypass and small-bowel resection
Diabetic diarrhea
Cirrhosis
Pregnancy
Therapy with certain pharmacologic agents
Drugs that block absorption
Cholestyramine
Sucralfate
Aluminum hydroxide
Ferrous sulfate
Possibly lovastatin
Drugs that increase nondeiodinative T4 clearance
Rifampin
Carbamazepine
Possibly phenytoin
Drugs that block T4 to T3 conversion
Aminodarone
Selenium deficiency
Decreased levothyroxine requirements
Aging (65 years and older)

Reproduced from Mandel SJ, Brent GA, Larsen PR. Levothyroxine therapy in patients with thyroid disease. Ann Int Med 1993; 119:492-502; with permission.

Some patients will develop angina initially after beginning T4 therapy. However, with pre-existing angina, the symptom may be alleviated in over one-third of patients, possibly because of improved cardiac contractability. In any event, T4 therapy for hypothyroid patients with cardiac disease or even for older patients without overt cardiac disease (e.g., >75 years of age), should be initiated cautiously with small doses of 25 μg per day with increments of 25 μg at 8-week intervals. The objective in such individuals should be suboptimal, not full replacement; it is quite appropriate under such circumstances to leave the TSH levels somewhat elevated, so as to ease the burden of work on the heart; this is particularly apt if angina develops or is worsened. The addition of a beta-adrenergic blocker may help to alleviate the angina.

Therapy for primary hypothyroidism is generally permanent and lifelong. It may be recalled, however, that a minority of patients with Hashimoto's thyroiditis may have spontaneous remissions (but also later relapses). Because of the variability of such courses, it is preferable not to interrupt the treatment, which usually succeeds only in making the patient feel insecure.

Rarely, patients with autoimmune thyroiditis may present with myxoedema coma, a very dangerous condition with a mortality rate of about 80 percent in untreated patients. Clinical features include hypothermia, lethargy, respiratory acidosis, hyponatremia, hypoglycemia, shock, and coma. Intravenous l-thyroxixne in bolus doses of 300 to 500 μg have been successfully administered. Patients have been successfully treated with T3 alone, but some fatal outcomes have also been reported. Correction of the hypothermia should be very cautious and slow. Cardiorespiratory support is also necessary, and glucocorticoids are usually given.

In contrast, subclinical hypothyroidism is one of the more common forms of presentation of lymphocytic thyroiditis, often with virtually no clinical evidence to suspect it. Often it is detected inadvertently by TSH screening or by the palpation of a goiter. Patients who have both an elevated TSH value and detectable thyroid autoantibodies have a 5 percent annual incidence of developing overt hypothyroidism. In elderly patients, the incidence of progression to overt hypothyroidism is higher. Moreover, as mentioned, there may be subtle metabolic changes resulting from even compensated hypothyroidism that may prove to be deleterious over years. It is thus my practice to treat such patients with T4 with the objective of normalizing TSH. The means for doing this have been described previously.

T4 is also prescribed for the purpose of causing regression in a goiter. Thyroid enlargement associated with autoimmune thyroiditis may occur in the context of euthyroidism or hypothyroidism. In either instance, suppression of TSH is likely to cause the goiter to regress. Sometimes this regression is striking and relatively quick (e.g., over 6 months time), particularly when TSH is initially elevated. Complete regression in the size of the goiter is unusual due to the persistence of the inflammatory component; however, even this is ameliorated by suppression of TSH, resulting in reduced expression of thyroid autoantigen and the immune response thereto. With T4 dosages adjusted to suppress the serum TSH concentrations somewhat below the normal range, dosages will often be in the order of 0.125 mg daily for the average female, and 0.175 mg daily in the average male.

There may be some circumstances in which the continued administration of T4 for life may not be entirely necessary. As mentioned above, some patients with autoimmune thyroiditis will spontaneously remit, although as also mentioned, it is not good practice to frequently interrupt treatment in the often false hope of "encountering" a remission. In postpartum thyroiditis, a forme fruste of autoimmune thyroiditis, recovery is the rule, and one could discontinue T4 after 1 year's therapy. However, patients with this condition will usually suffer a recurrence following future pregnancies, and may ultimately culminate in chronic thyroiditis years later. Thus it might be useful to initiate T4 therapy while the patient is in her hypothyroid phase and continue on this through life. This would inhibit new formation of colloid, thus preventing a hyperthyroid phase during a subsequent bout of postpartum thyroiditis; it would, of course, also prevent the hypothyroid phase of subsequent episodes of postpartum thyroiditis.

Some patients with hypothyroidism due to Hashimoto's thyroiditis will rarely go on to spontaneously develop hyperthyroidism. Thus, if a patient becomes overtly hyperthyroid while taking long-term T4 therapy, the T4 can be weaned away from the patient, and thyroid function then retested. Patients being treated with long-term therapy should be considered to have unstable thyroid metabolism, thus requiring at least some degree of lifelong monitoring.

SUGGESTED READING

Franklyn JA, Betteridge J, Daykin J, et al. Longterm thyroxine treatment and bone mineral density. Lancet 1992; 340:9–13.

Helfand M, Crapo LM. Monitoring therapy in patients taking levothyroxine. Ann Int Med 1990; 113:450–454.

Mandel SJ, Brent GA, Larsen PR. Levothyroxine therapy in patients with thyroid disease. Ann Int Med 1993; 119:492–502.

Toft AD. Drug therapy: Thyroxine therapy. New Engl J Med 1994; 331:174–180.

Volpé R. Autoimmune thyroiditis. In: Braverman LE, Utiger RD, eds., Werner's and Ingbar's the thyroid, a fundamental and clinical Text. 6th ed. Philadelphia:JB Lippincott, 1991:921–933.

Volpé R. Immunoregulation in autoimmune thyroid disease. Thyroid 1994; 4:373–377.

Yoshikawa N, Arreaza G, Mukuta T, et al. Effect of FK-506 on xenografted human Graves' thyroid tissue in severe combined immunodeficient mice. Clin Endocrinol (Oxf) 1994; 41:31–39.

POTENTIAL TREATMENTS OF IMMUNOLOGIC DISEASES

IMMUNOTHERAPY FOR TYPE 1 DIABETES

H. PETER CHASE, M.D.

Insulin-dependent (Type 1) diabetes is now believed to result from an autoimmune destruction of the insulin-producing beta cells in the pancreatic islets of Langerhans in individuals who have a genetic predisposition to develop the disease. Environmental factors are also known to be important, as only 30 to 50 percent of identical twins are concordant for the disease. The genetics have been further delineated in recent years, with about 40 percent of the genetic risk associated with HLA DR3, DR4 on chromosome 6 and another 10 percent associated with the insulin gene on chromosome 11p15 (particularly in children negative for DR3, DR4). Using DNA typing, the high risk DQA1/DQB1 alleles associated with DR3 are 0501/0201 and with DR4 are 0301/0302. Protective alleles are also known to be important and include DQB1*0602 and DQA1*0102.

It is now realized that, at least for some people, the destruction of beta cells is a gradual process taking place over many years. Unfortunately, by the time a person is diagnosed to have Type 1 diabetes, approximately 90 percent of the beta cells have already been destroyed. Thus, although two forms of treatment have been shown to increase remissions in newly diagnosed subjects, it is unlikely that the 10 percent of remaining tissue will ever afford a lasting remission or cure at this late stage in the disease process. The two treatments that have been shown to have an effect are oral cyclosporine A (see 1991 edition of this book) and high-dose intravenous insulin therapy with tight control of blood glucose levels for 2 weeks after diagnosis. Both treatments are discussed in more detail in the following discussion, although neither treatment allowed noninsulin requiring remissions after 3 years.

The importance of preventing Type 1 diabetes is apparent in that along with Type 2 diabetes (with both types contributing equally) it is the leading cause of renal failure, loss of vision, and extremity amputations in the United States and Europe. Fortunately, it is now possible to predict Type 1 diabetes with accuracy, at least in people who have a relative with the disease, before the onset of insulin dependence. This state will be referred to as "prediabetes," although technically the term prediabetes can only be used in a person followed to insulin dependence. Conversely, one might now ask when diabetes should be considered present, at the onset of insulin dependence, or when islet destruction is ongoing and insulin dependence can be predicted? The accurate prediction of prediabetes has now led to the initiation of three large intervention trials involving somewhat different theoretical immunologic approaches. The condition of prediabetes is discussed first, followed by a discussion of the different immunologic approaches for prevention, and finally, a discussion of the three specific interventions trials that have now started.

PREDIABETES

Prediabetes can now be predicted with a 95 percent positive predictive value in a subset of relatives of people with Type 1 diabetes (and possibly in the general population, although studies are just starting). Diagnosis involves a combination of immunologic, genetic, and metabolic tests.

The immunologic tests, and realization that the disease was at least in part autoimmune, followed the description by Botazzo and associates in 1974 of the presence of islet cell antibodies (ICA) in the serum of newly diagnosed patients. Subsequently, approximately 12 other antibodies (Table 1), including insulin autoantibodies (IAA), glutamic acid decarboxylase (GAD) antibody, CD45 related islet tyrosine phosphatase ICA-512, and the ICA-69 antibody have been described both in newly diagnosed and in prediabetic subjects. Combinations of these later antibody tests have now been shown to be more accurate than the original ICA test while being more quantitative and reproducible among laboratories.

The genetic tests essential for prediction involve determination of the protective alleles HLA DQB1*0602 and DQA1*0102. It is now known that some people develop positive serum antibodies but do not develop diabetes, and that this is most likely related to the presence of protective genes. Testing for HLA DR3,

Table 1 Serum Antibodies Used in the Detection of (Type 1) Prediabetes*

Islet cell antibody (ICA)
Insulin autoantibody (IAA)
Glutamic acid decarboxylase antibody (GAD-A)
GAD-65 antibody
GAD-67 antibody
37 kD islet antigen antibody (37k-A)
ICA 69 kD antibody (ICA-69)
ICA 512 kD antibody (ICA-512)
Bovine albumin (and ABBOS peptide) antibodies
Heat shock protein 65kD (hsp-65-A)
Carboxypeptidase H antibody
GM 2-1 islet ganglioside antibody
(and others)

*These antibodies are believed to reflect cell damage rather than to be the cause of damage.

Table 2 One-Plus Three-Minute Insulin Levels (FPIR) Required for Entry into DPT-1*

A. Siblings and offspring 4 to 45 years old (or second-degree relatives 4 to 20 years old)	*Tenth percentile**
Age 4 to 8 years	<60μU/ml
>8 years	<100μU/ml
B. Parents (≤45 years old)	<60μU/ml

*These values must be present in two consecutive, or in 2 of 3, IVGTTs for the person to be eligible for the trial. They are approximately the lower tenth percentile of normal for each group.

DR4 will also be important in identifying high-risk subjects in the general population. A study has now started in Denver to identify newborns (using cord blood) at high risk genetically for Type 1 diabetes, and to follow them at regular intervals to detect the development of antibodies in their serum. Because 70 to 90 percent of people developing Type 1 diabetes do not have a first-degree relative with the disease, the general population screening will be very important if the disease is to be prevented.

The metabolic test that is important in increasing the prediction rate from approximately 33 (using antibodies alone) to 95 percent, assuming genetic susceptibility, is the intravenous glucose tolerance test (IVGTT). If the sum of the 1- and 3-minute insulin levels (the first phase insulin release or FPIR) after giving IV glucose is below the tenth percentile for age (given in Table 2) the risk for developing diabetes in the next 5 years is greater than 50 percent. With a FPIR below the fifth percentile of normal, this risk can increase to 95 percent or higher. By defining patients with similar levels of risk, it is possible to design meaningful intervention trials.

IMMUNOLOGIC APPROACHES TO PREVENTION

Immunologic approaches currently being tried, or under consideration to prevent or cure Type 1 diabetes, include (1) generalized immunosuppression, (2) immunomodulation, and (3) antigen-based therapies.

Generalized Immunosuppression

As discussed in the 1991 edition of this book, cyclosporine A therapy during the first year after onset of Type 1 diabetes leads to insulin-free remissions at 1 year in 23 percent of treated subjects compared to 10 percent of controls. However, by 3 years, all subjects are again insulin dependent. Cyclosporine A also prevents diabetes in prediabetic mice and rats.

In an abstract titled "Preliminary Results of a Trial of Low-Dose Cyclosporine in Preclinical Type 1 Diabetes," physicians from Paris, France, concluded that "Cyclosporine can restore insulin secretion and glucose tolerance in three out of four cases of preclinical diabetes." Although this approach may work, it is associated with the following: (1) the dangers of possible secondary malignancy or infection, (2) possible renal damage, with further renal risk if diabetes develops, (3) how long to treat someone, and (4) whether the T-lymphocytes causing the islet cell damage (diabetes is considered to be cell mediated) will be reactivated once treatment is discontinued.

Most physicians in the United States do not believe treatment of prediabetic people (those who do not yet have a clinical disease) with cyclosporine A is warranted at this time. Perhaps opinions will change in the future if treatment with less toxic agents (or combinations of agents) is shown to be effective.

Immunomodulation

Immunomodulation for some investigators refers to therapies that enhance or diminish an immune response without cytotoxicity. Others have used the term to refer to agents that stimulate and expand a specific population of T lymphocytes. The BCG vaccine (or Freund's adjuvant) has been effective in preventing diabetes in prediabetic mice. In a preliminary trial of 17 newly diagnosed children with Type 1 diabetes, a remission was reported to occur in 65 percent (11 of 17) by 12 weeks compared to only 7 percent (2 of 29) in historical controls (see references). A proper double-blind trial of BCG vaccine in 100 newly diagnosed children is currently in progress in Denver. There are no reports of trying BCG vaccine in prediabetic humans as of yet. In animal models, Freund's adjuvant and the BCG vaccine are reported to change islet infiltrating T lymphocytes from predominating Th1 (interleukin-2 and interferon-γ), to Th2 lymphocytes (interleukin-4 and interleukin-10).

It should be noted that it has been the general rule in diabetes prevention research that agents would not be tried in humans unless first shown to have an effect in prediabetic mice or rats. It has also been the rule that agents would not be tested in prediabetic humans unless they had first been tested in newly diagnosed subjects (presumably to make sure the agent does not accelerate the diabetegenic process). There is no absolute sound scientific rationale for these current therapeutic principles.

Nicotinamide may also work through immunomodulation, although its mechanism of action in vivo is uncertain. In vitro, it prevents beta cell damage from the cytokines IL-1 and TNF-α and IFN-γ, and limits damage from free radicals such as nitric oxide. Nicotinamide was shown in 1984 to reduce the incidence of diabetes in nonobese diabetic (NOD) mice. Studies of nicotinamide in newly diagnosed humans with Type 1 diabetes have only shown an effect in adults in whom a larger percentage of beta cells still function. A pilot trial of 14 prediabetic children (see references) suggested nicotinamide might delay or prevent Type 1 diabetes. A large multinational double-blind trial of nicotinamide is now in progress (see Trials, following).

Insulin therapy is discussed in the following section, Antigen Therapy. However, the exact mechanism of immunologic effect is unknown. In prediabetic rats treated with insulin, "smaller quiescent beta cells" are described on histology, and it was suggested that they might be "less immunogenic" and have reduced susceptibility to killing by T lymphocytes or cytokines. In human studies, it has been suggested that "resting the beta cell" is a likely mechanism of the insulin activity. Thus, insulin may also have an immunomodulatory effect.

Antigen Therapy

Two of the three trials under way in people with prediabetes (see following sections) are based on either antigen avoidance (cow's milk) or on antigen administration (insulin). The latter may possibly "tolerize" or immunize the person to the insulin molecule, or more likely, to peptides from the insulin molecule.

Cow's Milk

NOD mice given casein develop diabetes more rapidly than do NOD mice fed an amino acid diet. Children who are newly diagnosed with Type 1 diabetes are reported to have increased levels of serum antibodies to bovine serum albumin (and to one of its peptides, referred to as ABBOS). Epidemiologic studies have suggested that children with diabetes were more often exposed to cow's milk before 4 months of age and were more apt to have breast feeding terminated before 2 months of age, than for age-matched controls (see references). Unfortunately, most data rely on long-term recall and are retrospective and possibly inaccurate or biased.

Some investigators have suggested that the effect of cow's milk might be due to "molecular mimicry" in stimulating production of an antibody that resembles a beta-cell surface antigen, which thus leads to beta-cell destruction.

Although results of studies excluding cow's milk from the diet at the time of diagnosis of Type 1 diabetes or from the diet of a pilot group of subjects with prediabetes are not available, these studies would be irrelevant and not needed. The large neonatal trial in Finland (described in the final section) will be an important prevention trial.

Insulin

The second potential antigen therapy utilizes insulin. Insulin reduces the incidence of diabetes when given to either prediabetic mice or rats. Insulin antibodies are present at the time of diagnosis and before giving insulin therapy in many people with Type 1 diabetes. Two weeks of large intravenous dosages of insulin (via the Biostator artificial pancreas) increased the remission rate of newly onset diabetic patients to a level similar to giving cyclosporine A in newly diagnosed patients. It is not known if this effect is related to beta cell rest, reduction of glucose toxicity, an immune mechanism, or a combination of all of these. It has been suggested that the exogenous insulin may "tolerize" or alter the cytokine profile of T cells from the vicinity of the islet and reduce secondary cytokine or free radical damage to the beta cell as a result.

Intravenous insulin plus twice daily subcutaneous insulin were given to five prediabetic subjects while seven others declined treatment. Only one of the treated subjects and all seven of the controls developed insulin dependence within 3 years (see references). This pilot trial is the basis for the U.S. prevention trial described later.

Other investigators have suggested other antigens (particularly GAD) to be primary autoantigens. The GAD and insulin molecules have both been shown effective in prediabetic NOD mice in preventing diabetes when given orally (see trials below). Most investigators at this time believe there is more than one primary antigen. Any or all may exert their influence via a "bystander" effect when administered orally. The antigens need not be beta cell specific, but they do need to show HLA restricted T-cell activity.

PREVENTION TRIALS

There are three large prevention trials currently under way. These involve (1) the use of the B-vitamin derivative, nicotinamide, (2) intravenous and subcutaneous insulin treatment, and (3) restriction of cow's milk.

Nicotinamide Trials

Nicotinamide is being evaluated in the European Nicotinamide Diabetes Intervention Trial (ENDIT), a multinational trial of primarily European countries, and in the smaller Deutsche Nicotinamide Intervention Study (DENIS). Both are double-blind randomized and placebo-controlled studies. Both involve first-degree relatives of patients with Type 1 diabetes. DENIS is restricted to children 3 to 12 years of age, with the total number of patients to be calculated based on the severity of risk of the children entered. ENDIT will screen 30,000 first-degree relatives to identify 550 high-risk relatives, 5 to 40 years of age, who have two positive ICA tests (with one positive at ≥ 20 JDF units and one positive at ≥ 4 JDF units). An initial IVGTT will be done (no preset admission criteria) and the oral glucose tolerance test (GTT) must be shown to be nondiabetic before entry. The dose of nicotinamide is the same (1.2 g/per square meter) for both studies, although the source of the nicotinamide is different. Enrollment is well under way for both studies and the results should be available in the next 5 years.

In addition to the studies of nicotinamide in first-degree relatives, Dr. Robert Elliott in Auckland, NZ screened 20,195 school-age children, 5.0 to 7.9 years of age. Those with ICA $\geq$ 20 JDF units or FPIR $\leq$ 100 μU/ml and ICA of 10 JDF units were treated with nicotinamide. After 1.7 to 4.7 years of treatment, treated children were compared to 13,463 children who refused testing and to 48,335 children followed as controls. The diabetes rates in the two latter groups respectively were 15.1 and 20.1 per 10^5 treatment years compared to 8.1 per 10^5 treatment years for the treated children. It was concluded that a protective effect of nicotinamide was present, although not as great as described in the NOD mouse. The lesser effect was attributed to the variability in age when given to the human as well as the smaller dose per kilogram body weight used in the humans.

Insulin Trials

Insulin is being evaluated in the NIH-sponsored U.S. Diabetes Prevention Trial (DPT-1). The trial will screen 60,000 first- or second-degree relatives of people with Type 1 diabetes over a 4-year time period to detect 340 study patients who have a greater than 50 percent chance of developing diabetes within 5 years. The entrants must have two positive ICA tests (10 JDF units or greater), two IVGTTs below the tenth percentile (see Table 2), a nondiabetic oral GTT, and be negative for the protective molecules, DQA1*0102 and DQB1*0602. An insulin autoantibody test is also being done, but entry is not dependent on positivity. Age limits are shown in Table 2 and are 4 to 45 years of age for first-degree relatives and 4 to 20 years for second-degree relatives. Half of the participants (170 subjects) will receive IV insulin for 4 days once yearly and twice daily subcutaneous insulin (0.25 units per kilogram per day) of Humulin ultralente insulin. The design considers a 10 percent drop-out rate and gives an 80 percent likelihood of showing an effect if there is a 35 percent reduction in the need to start insulin. The major problem likely to occur with the DPT will be with the 170 subjects randomized to no treatment. Some of these families may select treatment on their own. The study will be terminated early if treatment is found effective, but results will otherwise be available in the year 2001.

At the time of starting the DPT, a four-arm trial was in progress between the Joslin Clinic in Boston and the Barbara Davis Center For Childhood Diabetes in Denver to evaluate the combination of subcutaneous and IV insulin (as originally described) or of just IV insulin, or of just subcutaneous insulin or of IV placebo (saline). In contrast to the DPT, this study was double blinded. The design would have helped determine if both the IV and subcutaneous insulin were necessary. Although entry into the study was terminated at the start of the DPT, 21 patients were entered and may give some pilot information as to whether both IV and subcutaneous insulin are necessary.

The DPT also has plans to start an oral antigen trial in 1996. This will study people judged to have a 30 to 50 percent risk for developing diabetes in the next 5 years. Oral insulin will be utilized because it has been shown to reduce the incidence of diabetes in NOD mice. No data are available for giving agent to humans as of yet.

Infant Feeding Trial

A study to evaluate the effects of feeding cow's milk versus a casein hydrolysate formula for the first 6 to 8 months of life will soon start in Finland. Mothers in both groups may breast feed their infants, but all supplements (and all milk when nursing is discontinued) will depend on the group to which the infant has been randomized. Approximately 6,000 infants who have a parent or sibling with Type 1 diabetes will be screened for high-risk HLA DQ genes. It is estimated that 2,000 infants will be entered into the trial and will be followed for 10 years. The dietary restrictions will cease 6 to 8 months after birth. Additional venous blood samples will be collected every 2 years for ICA, GAD 65 antibodies, cow's milk antibodies, beta-lactoglobulin antibodies, bovine serum albumin antibodies, glycated hemoglobin levels, and blood glucose values. The end point will be the development of diabetes before 10 years. Drawbacks to the study are (1) breast milk may be protective; (2) cow's milk proteins are not being restricted in the mothers and could be passed through nursing; and (3) it may be very hard to be certain that someone does not inadvertently give cow's milk formula or products to a test infant. The study will be very important in finally delineating the role of cow's milk in causing Type 1 diabetes.

SUGGESTED READING

Elliott RB, Chase HP. Prevention or delay of Type 1 (insulin-dependent) diabetes mellitus in children using nicotinamide. Diabetologia 1991; 34:362–365.

Gerstein HC. Cow's milk exposure and Type 1 diabetes mellitus. Diabetes Care 1994; 17:13–19.

Keller RJ, Eisenbarth GS, Jackson RA. Insulin prophylaxis in individuals at high risk of Type 1 diabetes. Lancet 1993; 341:927–928.

Shehadeh NN, Calcinaro F, Bradley BJ, et al. Effect of adjuvant therapy on development of diabetes in mouse and man. Lancet 1994; 343:706–707.

Zhang ZJ, Davidson L, Eisenbarth G, et al. Suppression of diabetes in nonobese diabetic mice by oral administration of porcine insulin. Proc Natl Acad Sci USA 1991; 88:10252–10256.

IMMUNOSUPPRESSIVE TREATMENT OF CHRONIC ASTHMA

SARA H. LOCK, M.B., B.S., M.R.C.P.
A. BARRY KAY, Ph.D., F.R.C.P.

Asthma affects between 5 and 10 percent of the population and is characterized by cough, shortness of breath, and wheeze associated with variable airflow obstruction. Bronchial biopsy studies have revealed infiltration of the bronchial mucosa by inflammatory cells, most notably lymphocytes and eosinophils. The mechanisms maintaining this chronic eosinophilic desquamative bronchitis are complex, but the consequence is believed to be epithelial damage resulting from the release of eosinophil basic proteins. The intense local eosinophilia is probably under the control of activated CD4 T lymphocytes, which release cytokines such as interleukin-3 (IL-3), interleukin (IL-5), and granulocyte-macrophage–colony stimulating factor (GM-CSF), which provoke eosinophil differentiation, chemotaxis, and enhanced survival. This supposed central role for the T lymphocyte in chronic asthma suggests that this cell type might be an attractive target for treatment by immunosuppressive agents.

When treating patients with asthma specific precipitating factors should be identified and removed or reduced where possible. The role of allergens should be investigated with skin prick tests and avoidance instigated as appropriate. Occupational exposure to sensitizing agents such as isocyanates should be considered. Drugs such as beta-blockers and nonsteroidal antiinflammatory agents can induce or exacerbate asthma.

Mild asthma confirmed by variable airflow obstruction can be relieved with bronchodilators; however, regular daily requirement of these agents indicates that an anti-inflammatory agent needs to be added for "prevention." Thus the mainstay of modern treatment for chronic asthma is inhaled corticosteroid therapy, although, especially in children, sodium cromoglycate (cromyln) may be considered as first-line treatment. As disease becomes more severe a stepwise increase in medication is advocated with the introduction of high-dose inhaled corticosteroids, long-acting bronchodilators, theophyllines, inhaled ipratropium or oxitropium, and oral or high-dose inhaled beta-agonists. Compliance with medication and inhaler technique should always be assessed. In a small proportion of patients, these measures will not be sufficient to control the disease, and regular oral corticosteroids are required. Despite regular oral corticosteroids some patients remain symptomatic with reduced lung function (in some instances because of corticosteroid resistance) and these patients are at risk of developing corticosteroid-related side effects, including (importantly) osteoporosis. It is in these individuals that alternatives to regular oral corticosteroids such as immunosuppressive therapy should be considered.

AZATHIOPRINE

Double-blind, placebo-controlled studies of azathioprine, a purine antagonist, in chronic severe asthma did not demonstrate any significant benefit, and azathioprine therapy was associated with unwanted effects. Purine antagonists have relatively little effect on T-lymphocyte proliferative responses in vitro. Their primary mechanism of action appears to be at the level of killer cell activity and antibody production. There is little support for its use in the treatment of asthma.

Methotrexate

The antimetabolite, methotrexate (MTX), is a folic acid antagonist that inhibits synthesis of purine and thymidine and also impairs neutrophil chemotaxis at low dosage. The half-life of MTX varies from 6 to 69 hours, and the drug is excreted mostly unchanged in the urine. There have been several studies evaluating MTX in chronic severe asthma. An initial double-blind, crossover study of 14 patients using low dosage therapy (15 mg per week as 3 divided doses 12 hours apart) over 12 weeks suggested a 36.5 percent reduction in prednisolone usage for MTX as compared with placebo. All patients had been taking oral prednisolone for 1 year at an average dosage of 10 mg per day or more, which maintained forced expiratory volume in one second (FEV_1) within 70 percent of the predicted value. They were taking inhaled corticosteroids and bronchodilators at least 3 times daily and maximum tolerated theophylline. Patients with other serious illness, kidney or liver disease, insulin-dependent diabetes, morbid obesity, abnormal full blood count, or alcoholism were excluded. There were no changes in lung function, although subjective assessment of symptoms improved. Side effects included nausea, rashes, and abnormal liver function tests.

A more recent double-blind placebo-controlled parallel group study of 60 asthmatics found that MTX therapy (15 mg once a week after food) resulted in an average reduction in corticosteroid dosage of 50 percent as compared with 14 percent in the placebo group. Corticosteroid dependence was defined as a requirement for oral prednisolone 7.5 mg per day in addition to 800 or more micrograms inhaled corticosteroid, regular bronchodilators, and maximum tolerated theophylline. Patients with renal, hepatic, or hematologic diseases were excluded. There was a 16 percent reduction in prednisolone dosage in both the MTX and placebo groups after 12 weeks. The further significant reduction in the MTX group occurred in the last 12 weeks of the study. This improvement was not maintained in the 10-week run-out period. There were no significant changes in lung function or symptom scores. Side effects included hepatic toxicity (necessitating three withdrawals) and nausea (necessitating two withdrawals).

Open studies of more long-term treatment have been performed. Twenty-five patients received oral or intramuscular MTX 7.5 to 50 mg per week for 18 months. Twenty-four of these patients reduced their prednisolone dosage by more than 50 percent, and 15 stopped regular prednisolone usage. Twelve patients developed abnormal liver function tests, five had nausea, two suffered a rash, and one patient had recurrent stomatitis.

Low-dose methotrexate can be a useful corticosteroid-sparing agent in some patients with corticosteroid-dependent asthma, although it has not been shown to improve lung function. It should be used in carefully selected patients, and they should be closely monitored throughout therapy. Liver biopsy has been recommended after 1,500 mg cumulative dose, although recently doubts, have been expressed regarding the necessity for this. Cases of pneumocystis pneumonia following MTX therapy have been reported. Thus the risk-benefit ratio has to be considered very carefully when recommending this form of treatment in chronic asthma, especially because certain side effects such as liver fibrosis are nonreversible.

GOLD SALTS

The precise mode of the anti-inflammatory action of gold salts is uncertain, although in vitro studies have demonstrated inhibition of mitogen-induced proliferation of T lymphocytes. Both parenteral and oral preparations have been evaluated in asthma. Parenteral gold is associated with significant adverse effects (e.g., proteinuria) and a blinded, cross-over study, while suggesting some benefit, concluded that side effects may preclude its continued use.

A more recent double-blind, placebo-controlled parallel group study of oral gold salts, auranofin 3 mg once daily for 2 weeks then twice daily given for an additional 24 weeks, in 32 asthmatics taking 2.5 or more milligrams per day prednisolone for 1 year or more has shown a significant corticosteroid-sparing effect. Over the last 14 weeks of the study, daily prednisolone dosage was reduced by 4 mg in the auranofin-treated group as compared with 0.3 mg in the placebo group. Lung function (FEV_1) improved by 6.4 percent in the auranofin group and symptoms were reduced, but two patients were withdrawn because of serious exacerbations of constitutional eczema, and an additional two patients with eczema required treatment with topical corticosteroids. Gastrointestinal symptoms occurred in four other patients, but they improved with a dose reduction. A longer term study is needed to determine the safety and efficacy of this medication if used regularly for chronic disease. Thus at the present time this form of treatment is not recommended for routine use.

CYCLOSPORIN A

Cyclosporin A (CsA) is a lipophilic, cyclic undecapeptide which, like corticosteroids, is thought to exert its immunosuppressive effects predominantly via inhibition of T lymphocytes, although it does have effects on other cells (e.g., mast cells and basophils). CsA binds to a ubiquitous cytoplasmic protein named cyclophilin and the CsA-cyclophilin complex then binds to calcineurin, which is a calcium and calmodulin-dependent serine threonine phosphatase. Inhibition of this activity by CsA-cyclophilin complexes prevents the formation of a transcription factor NF-AT (nuclear factor of activated T-lymphocytes) in the nucleus. Reduced binding of NF-AT to cytokine gene promoter regions reduces the transcription of mRNA for various cytokines (e.g., IL-2, IL-3, GM-CSF, IFN-γ), which is believed to be the major mechanism of action of CsA. The increasing evidence for the central role of the T lymphocyte in the pathogenesis of asthma and the predominantly T-lymphocyte effects of CsA led to the initiation of a double-blind placebo-controlled cross-over study of CsA in chronic severe asthma.

Thirty-three chronic severe asthmatics taking oral corticosteroids for at least 3 months in a dosage of at least 5 mg were given 12 weeks of CsA (5 mg per kilogram per day divided into twice daily dosage) and identical placebo in a cross-over, double-blind design. Subjects were nonsmokers, with no contraindications to CsA therapy such as renal or hepatic impairment, uncontrolled hypertension, epilepsy, a history of malignancy, chronic infection, or essential therapy that interacts with CsA (e.g., aspirin/aminoglycosides, which increase the risk of renal impairment). Isotope glomerular filtration rate measurements were performed before starting trial medication and were repeated after each limb of the study. Subjects were chosen whose FEV_1 was less than 75 percent of predicted and their FEV_1 and/or PEFR had shown 20 percent or more reversibility in lung function in response to bronchodilator (5 mg nebulised salbutamol) or spontaneously. Maintenance corticosteroid therapy was kept constant throughout the entire study period unless it was increased to treat disease exacerbations. One female patient withdrew from the study because of hypertrichosis (a known reversible side effect of CsA) and two patients failed to complete the protocol. CsA therapy resulted in a mean increase above placebo of 12 percent in morning peak expiratory flow rate ($p < 0.004$) and 17.6 percent in FEV_1 ($p < 0.001$). There was a mean reduction in diurnal variation in PEFR of 27.6 percent ($p = 0.04$). The frequency of disease exacerbations requiring an increased prednisolone dosage was reduced by 48 percent in patients taking CsA as compared with placebo ($p < 0.02$).

In view of these encouraging results and the fact that CsA was well tolerated during the 12-week treatment phase a longer term study of CsA as a corticosteroid-sparing agent was initiated. This double-blind, placebo-controlled, parallel group study has recently been completed. Thirty-nine corticosteroid-dependent asthmatics participated; nineteen received CsA (5 mg per kilogram per day) and 20 received identical placebo. There was a four-week run-in period during which prednisolone dosage was kept stable at minimum maintenance levels and then a 36-week treatment phase. An attempt was made to reduce prednisolone dosage at 14-day intervals if patients' asthma had been stable or improved as judged from the diary cards and spirometry. Three patients withdrew during the first 12 weeks of the study (one because of exacerbation requiring high-dose prednisolone, another because of hypertrichosis, and a third, because of non–asthma-related death); they were all receiving CsA. In the remaining patients there was a median reduction in prednisolone dosage of 62 percent in the CsA-treated group as compared with 25 percent in the placebo-treated group ($p = 0.043$). Morning PEFR prebronchodilator increased in the CsA-treated group by a mean of 9.4 percent despite the reduction in their prednisolone dosage ($p < 0.01$) as compared with no significant change in the group taking placebo ($p = 0.026$ between groups).

The major side effects of CsA are nephrotoxicity and hypertension while less serious adverse effects include hypertrichosis and gum hypertrophy. There is evidence that renal toxicity remains largely reversible provided trough blood concentrations are maintained in the range of 100 to 200 ng per milliliter (average concentrations in the two studies described were 152 ng per milliliter and 144 ng per milliliter). An elevation in serum creatinine of greater than 25 percent above baseline values should lead to a dose reduction. Hypertension should be treated with calcium antagonists as far as possible and renal and hepatic function monitored closely. During the corticosteroid reduction study there was an expected decrease in glomerular filtration rate (median 18.4 percent; $p = 0.06$); eight patients taking CsA and one taking placebo required treatment for hypertension, and there was a small rise in diastolic blood pressure (mean 5.48 mm Hg $p < 0.01$).

These studies suggest that cyclosporin A is an effective corticosteroid-sparing agent and improves lung function in corticosteroid-dependent asthmatics. It was also well tolerated over a 36-week period, and although expected rises in blood pressure, urea, and creatinine occurred, they resolved on cessation of CsA therapy. Groups treating patients with transplanted lungs have been investigating the feasibility of using nebulized cyclosporin A. There are technical difficulties due to the lipophilic nature of the drug, but as with inhaled corticosteroids inhaled CsA therapy should have less systemic side effects and should increase the range of asthmatics who could be treated with this medication. Nevertheless a trial of oral CsA can be recommended in patients with corticosteroid-dependent asthma ($\geq$ 15 mg per day prednisolone or equivalent) who have normal renal and liver function, are normotensive, and have no other contraindications for receiving the drug. Blood levels must be carefully monitored and the treatment given for at least 12 weeks before deciding whether or not the patient has responded.

OTHER IMMUNOSUPPRESSIVE AGENTS

FK-506 is a macrolide derived from a soil organism *Streptomyces Tsukudaiensis* that, despite having a different structure to CsA, has similar immunosuppressant properties, although it is more potent. FK-506 is being evaluated in transplantation medicine with promising results and may have advantages over CsA in treating severe asthma such as greater potency and a better safety profile. However, there is no evidence at present for believing that FK-506 is of value in this disease.

Rapamycin is also a macrolide that is derived from *Streptomyces hygroscopius;* it binds to the same cytosolic receptor as FK-506 in competition with the latter. Despite these similarities rapamycin has a different mode of action than FK-506. Thus in vitro it is effective even when added 12 hours after the initiation of T-cell activation. Hence, unlike CsA and FK-506, it can inhibit T lymphoblasts, which have already been activated, and this might theoretically result in a more rapid onset of therapeutic benefit in inflammatory disease. It inhibits the cell signal transduction pathway following cytokine (e.g., IL-2) binding to cytokine receptor (IL-2R). T lymphocytes are sensitive to rapamycin because they rely on IL-2/IL-2R interactions for proliferation. There is evidence to suggest that CsA and rapamycin may have synergistic effects leading to increased therapeutic potential for this combined drug regimen.

Other new immunosuppressive agents such as brequinar sodium and mycophenolic acid, which are inhibitors of de novo synthesis of pyrimidine and purine synthesis, respectively, are being studied as potential advances in transplantation therapy and may be evaluated for use in other autoimmune diseases in the future.

SUGGESTED READING

Alexander AG, Barnes NC, Kay AB. Trial of cyclosporin in corticosteroid-dependent chronic severe asthma. Lancet 1992; 339:324–328.

Hodges NG, Brewis RAL, Howell JBL. An evaluation of azathioprine in severe chronic asthma. Thorax 1971; 26:734–739.

Iacono AT, Keenan RJ, Duncan SR, et al. Aerosolized cyclosporine as additional therapy for the treatment of refractory chronic rejection in lung transplant recipients. Am Rev Resp Dis 1994; 149(4):A730.

Nierop G, Gijzel WP, Bel EH, et al. Auranofin in the treatment of steroid-dependent asthma: A double-blind study. Thorax 1992; 47:349–354.

Shiner RJ, Nunn AJ, Chung FK, Geddes DM. Randomised, double-blind, placebo-controlled trial of methotrexate in steroid-dependent asthma. Lancet 1990; 336:137–140.

Thomson AW, Starzl TE. New immunosuppressive drugs: Mechanistic insights and potential therapeutic advances. Immunol Rev 1993; 136:71–98.

NEW VACCINES FOR IMMUNOLOGIC DISEASES

HOWARD B. DICKLER, M.D.

Vaccines are the most effective medical intervention, in terms of both cost and efficacy, for preventing disease and resulting mortality. While we are used to thinking of vaccines solely as a means of preventing infectious diseases, the definition of the term vaccine is evolving to include agents for preventing and treating immune system–mediated diseases such as autoimmune and allergic diseases. This evolution is based on advances in the fields of immunology and molecular and cell biology and by an increased understanding of the pathogenic role of the immune system in many diseases.

Originally, the definition of vaccine was restricted to cowpox virus (vaccinia) preparations used for immunization. Over time the term evolved to include all preparations of microorganism origin, including killed or attenuated whole organisms or molecules derived from them, which were administered to generate or increase immunity to that microorganism and thereby prevent infection and disease. Currently, the definition of vaccine is being further expanded to include any material that is administered to generate *or abrogate* a specific immune response(s) for the purpose of preventing or treating disease. Agents that generate an immune response are called immunogenic vaccines. These would include all the currently used microorganism-based vaccines, as well as naked DNA, which allows production of the immunizing antigen after administration, and anti-idiotypes, which are antibody molecules used as surrogates for an infectious agent based on resemblance to an antigen of that agent. Conversely, molecules used to abrogate a response(s) are called tolerogenic vaccines and would include such agents as the target self-antigens in autoimmune disease or the allergen (or portions thereof) in allergic diseases. Tolerogenic vaccines abrogate the pathogenic immune response thereby interrupting or preventing the disease process.

Recently, remarkable progress has been made in the use of self-antigens as tolerogenic vaccines to prevent and/or treat autoimmune diseases, and this approach appears to offer unusual promise for successful intervention in these diseases. In this chapter, I review the immunologic basis for this approach, the results of studies in animal models of human autoimmune diseases, and the results of the published clinical trials that utilized self-antigens as an intervention.

IMMUNOLOGIC BASIS FOR USING SELF-ANTIGENS AS VACCINES IN AUTOIMMUNE DISEASES

Autoimmune diseases affect approximately 5 percent of the adults in North America and Europe and can affect any organ system. Any universal approach to prevention and treatment in this polymorphic group of diseases must therefore focus on a required event common to the pathogenesis of each of these diseases. Such an event is the activation of T lymphocytes, which recognize self-antigens expressed in the affected organ. In broad terms, there are three main mechanisms of tissue damage in autoimmune disease: antibody mediated, cytotoxic T–lymphocyte mediated, and phagocyte mediated. Some autoimmune diseases are mediated solely by antibody such as autoimmune hemolytic anemia and myasthenia gravis. Others are more complex and involve all three mechanisms, one example being multiple sclerosis. In this disease, antibodies bind to oligodendroglial cells and cause cell death via the complement attack complex. Cytotoxic T lymphocytes cause demyelination via release of tumor necrosis factor, lymphotoxin, and interferon-gamma. Macrophages directly attack the myelin sheath and also release tumor-necrosis factor. All three pathogenetic mechanisms involve T lymphocytes. Most pathogenetic autoimmune antibodies are of the IgG class and require helper T lymphocytes for their production. Similarly, phagocytes are recruited and directed by T lymphocytes. Thus, the destructive process can be interrupted by preventing the activation of T lymphocytes, which recognize self-antigens in the affected tissues.

The interaction of the T lymphocyte with either the antigen presenting cell or the target cell and its subsequent activation is a complex process involving several sets of molecules (Table 1). Interventions that interrupt any of these interactions might have a beneficial effect in autoimmune disease. Interferon-beta has recently been approved for use in multiple sclerosis because it has been shown to reduce the number of attacks by 30 percent. It is thought to act by decreasing expression of major histocompatibility complex (MHC) molecules in central nervous system white matter thereby protecting the tissue from recognition and attack by autoimmune lymphocytes. Currently, monoclonal antibodies against other molecules such as ICAM-1 and CD4 are being developed and tested for efficacy in various autoimmune diseases. However, because these interventions are not antigen specific, it is possible that non–disease-related immune responses will also be affected. In order to select only those T lymphocytes involved in the disease process, one must interrupt the interaction between the antigen-specific T-cell receptor (TCR) and the target self-antigen. One approach to this goal is to generate an immune response against the T-cell receptor(s), which recognizes the target self-

Table 1 Molecules that Mediate Interaction between T Lymphocytes and Antigen Presenting Cells (APC) or Target Cells

T Lymphocyte Molecule	*Ligand on APC or Target Cell*
Antigen-specific T-cell receptor (TCR)	Major histocompatibility complex (MHC) molecule plus antigen peptide
CD4 or CD8	MHC molecule
CD28	B7.1, B7.2, B7.3
LFA-1	ICAM 1 or 2
CD2	LFA-3
CD5	CD72

antigen, thereby preventing the function of the pathogenic T lymphocytes. Clinical trials are in progress to determine if this approach will alter the course of multiple sclerosis. However, this approach is only feasible when there are only a few TCRs used by the pathogenic T lymphocytes, a situation which may not exist in a number of autoimmune diseases. A second approach, which appears to be more widely applicable, is to tolerize (render nonresponsive) the pathogenic T lymphocytes by appropriate administration of the target self-antigen.

The first requirement for successful intervention in autoimmune diseases using target self-antigens is the identification of the individuals at risk. This is clearly evident in individuals whose autoimmune disease is clinically active or has been well documented during previous clinical attacks. However, in some cases the first episode of an autoimmune disease can be life threatening, and in certain diseases clinical symptoms only become manifest after the autoimmune process has completely or nearly completely destroyed the target tissue such as pancreatic beta-islet cells in insulin-dependent diabetes mellitus (IDDM). Ideally then, one would be able to screen the population for individuals at high risk for developing various autoimmune diseases. Progress towards this goal has been substantial as a result of improved identification of MHC molecules using molecular genetic techniques and improved techniques for the rapid identification of pathogenetic T lymphocytes or antibodies in many diseases. In IDDM, it has been found that the combination of the presence of significant levels of islet cell antibodies (ICA+) plus a decreased first-phase insulin response to an IV glucose tolerance test indicates a greater than 80 percent risk of developing IDDM within 3 years. The presence of several antibodies (ICA, insulin autoantibodies, and antibodies against glutamic acid decarboxylase) can also accurately predict a high risk of developing IDDM.

A second requirement for the use of target self-antigens as an intervention is the conclusive identification of those antigens. The evidence required includes the molecular identification of the antigen recognized by autoreactive antibodies and T lymphocytes; correlation of the presence of the target self-antigen specific antibodies or T cells with disease or disease activity; and production of disease by transfer of the autoantibody or autoreactive T cells (generally in animals). In some diseases the target self-antigen is definitively known (e.g., the acetylcholine receptor is the target in myasthenia gravis). In other diseases the situation is less clear. In IDDM there are a number of candidate self-antigens including insulin and the enzyme glutamic acid decarboxylase (GAD), but the evidence is not definitive.

Multiple sclerosis (MS) can provide a useful example of the difficulties involved. It has been known for a number of years that injection of a component of myelin called myelin basis protein (MBP) into animals could produce a disease (experimental autoimmune encephalomyelitis [EAE]) that resembled MS pathologically. However, if one looked at the peripheral blood of MS patients, the frequency of cells responding to MBP was not greater than in normal subjects. It was only when one looked at the activated T lymphocytes (those that expressed receptors for and responded to the cytokine IL-2) that one saw a higher frequency of MBP-specific T cells in MS patients versus normal controls. Moreover, the percentage of IL-2 responsive cells that were specific for MBP was much higher in cerebral spinal fluid (CSF) than in the peripheral blood of MS patients and this was not true in individuals with other neurologic diseases. Another correlation was obtained by painstaking analysis using polymerase chain reaction of the TCR of cells found at sites of inflammation in the brains of MS patients. These studies revealed that the receptors were specific for an antigen complex that contained a peptide of MBP. Finally, disease resembling MS has been produced in immunodeficient mice (which do not reject human cells) by T cells from the CSF of MS patients but not from controls.

The third requirement for successful intervention in autoimmune diseases using target self-antigens is the ability to render the T lymphocytes specific for those antigens tolerant or nonresponsive. Evidence exists to support two main mechanisms for achieving this end. The first is the induction of anergy or inactivation of the T lymphocyte. This occurs when the T cell encounters the antigen on an antigen presenting cell in the form of a complex with an MHC molecule but does not receive a required second signal. The inactivated T cell will then not respond when subsequently presented with both antigen and the required second signal. In mice, it appears that the second signal is delivered mainly through CD28 upon binding one of the forms of the B7 molecule on the antigen presenting cell. In man, it seems that the second signal can be delivered by several sets of molecules. How anergy is induced in vivo is not yet clear. One theory is that when antigen is presented by non-activated B lymphocytes, the second signal is absent.

The second mechanism for generating nonresponsiveness in T lymphocytes specific for self-antigens is by the induction of suppressor cells. Such cells can be induced by oral administration of the self-antigen in appropriate amounts, and these suppressor cells can transfer nonresponsiveness in adoptive transfer experiments. They are antigen specific in terms of their

Table 2 Examples of Successful Intervention Using Self-Antigens in Animal Models of Human Autoimmune Disease

Human Diseases	*Animal Models*	*Antigen Used*
Rheumatoid arthritis	Collagen-induced arthritis Adjuvant-induced arthritis	Type II collagen
Insulin-dependent diabetes mellitus	Nonobese diabetic mouse	Insulin Glutamic acid decarboxylase
Multiple sclerosis	Experimental autoimmune encephalomyelitis	Myelin basic protein
Uveitis	Experimental autoimmune uveoretinitis	S-antigen

activation, but their effect is antigen nonspecific and appears to involve the cytokine transforming growth factor beta (TGF-β) (see next section).

USE OF TARGET SELF-ANTIGENS AS INTERVENTIONS IN ANIMAL MODELS OF HUMAN AUTOIMMUNE DISEASE

Although the methods for inducing antigen specific unresponsiveness have been known for decades, it is only a bit more than 10 years ago that induction of unresponsiveness to a target self-antigen was first used as an intervention in an animal model of human autoimmune disease. Since that time, considerable data has been accumulated in a number of models (Table 2). I will summarize the results as a whole rather than detail individual studies. The majority of studies have induced unresponsiveness by administration of the self-antigen via the oral route. However, the intravenous, subcutaneous, and intrathymic routes have also been utilized successfully. Intervention with self-antigens has been successful both for prevention and for treatment, that is when given prior to induction of disease or (in the case of spontaneous disease) before clinical symptoms; or alternatively, when given after onset of the disease. Responses have most often been partial rather than total. In prevention studies this means delayed onset, decreased incidence, decreased severity, or some combination thereof. In treatment studies, there has generally been decreased severity rather than remission. In agreement with these findings, histologic examination of target organs revealed decreased but persistent inflammatory responses. No side effects from the treatment itself were noted.

In a number of animal studies, the mechanism underlying successful intervention with self-antigens appeared to be suppression because cells from treated animals could adoptively protect naive animals. In one model (oral administration of MBP as an intervention in EAE) suppressor cells were generated that were specific in their stimulation (MBP was required) but operated through the antigen nonspecific cytokine TGF-β. This is important because it theoretically means that one can successfully intervene in an autoimmune disease by induction of this type of suppression in the target organ using a single self-antigen even if many self-antigens are involved in the disease process. One might even be able to use one that is not related to the pathogenic process. Consistent with this line of reasoning are the observations that both adjuvant-induced and collagen induced-arthritis can be suppressed by type II collagen, proteolipid protein induced EAE can be suppressed by another self-antigen (i.e., MBP), and both GAD and insulin can successfully delay or prevent onset of diabetes in NOD mice. These considerations played an important role in shaping the subsequent clinical trials in human autoimmune diseases.

CLINICAL TRIALS USING SELF-ANTIGENS TO TREAT OR PREVENT AUTOIMMUNE DISEASES

Based on the success of this approach in animal models of human autoimmune diseases, clinical trials were begun. To date, the results of three trials have been published. One was a phase II trial in rheumatoid arthritis (RA), whereas the other two were pilot trials, one in MS and one in individuals at high risk of developing IDDM.

A phase II randomized, double-blind trial to determine the effect of oral administration of type II collagen on rheumatoid arthritis was conducted by David Trentham and his colleagues in Boston. Type II collagen is the most abundant structural protein of cartilage, and immunization of animals with this protein produces a disease resembling RA. Sixty patients were enrolled who met the following criteria: American Rheumatism Association (ARA) criteria for classic or definite arthritis; onset at age 16 or older and at least 18 years old at entry; ARA functional class II or III; synovitis unresponsive to at least one immunosuppressive drug; and evidence of severe active disease. Immunosuppressive drugs were withdrawn at the beginning of the trial but patients were permitted to stay on nonsteroidal anti-inflammatory drugs and/or prednisone if dosage was less than or equal to 10 mg per day. The treatment group received 0.1 mg of type II collagen daily for 1 month, then 0.5 mg daily for 2 months. The control group received an indistinguishable placebo.

At study end, 59 patients were evaluable, of whom 28 had received collagen and 31 placebo. The two groups were similar in terms of demographic, clinical, and laboratory parameters. Collagen-treated patients showed a significant ($p < 0.05$) decline (compared to entry) in the number of swollen joints, tender joints, and joint-swelling and joint-tenderness indices, while no such improvement was seen in the placebo-treated group. The two groups also differed significantly in the percentage of patients who worsened and who required analgesic use (in both cases placebo > collagen). Remarkably, (because complete responses had not been seen in animal models), four of the collagen treated group (but none of the control group) had complete resolution of disease. No side effects or significant changes in laboratory values were observed.

While this study might be criticized for lack of a washout period to eliminate immunosuppressives (64 percent of the collagen group and 58 percent of the placebo group were on such agents at entry), the investigators were concerned about the possibility that the patients would receive ineffective therapy or placebo. In fact, it seems impressive that so many collagen-treated patients improved while off immunosuppression, whereas the placebo-treated patients tended to deteriorate. No evidence was obtained that would bear on the hypothesis (based on animal studies described previously) that tolerance was induced.

Although efficacy and safety were demonstrated in this trial, questions concerning long-term effects on the disease and optimization of this form of intervention remain. A phase III pivotal trial using oral type II collagen in RA in now underway.

A pilot double-blind 1-year trial of oral administration of myelin in multiple sclerosis was conducted by Howard Weiner and his colleagues. Thirty individuals with early relapsing-remitting MS and at least two attacks in the previous 2 years were randomized in pairs matched for age, disease duration, disability, and number of attacks in the previous 2 years. The treatment group received 300 mg of bovine myelin (which contains both myelin basic protein and proteolipid protein) daily, while the placebo group received bovine dry milk.

The two groups were similar for the characteristics noted above, but the placebo group contained more females (80 percent versus 47 percent) and more HLA-DR2–positive individuals (73 percent versus 60 percent). The primary outcome measures were the number of major exacerbations and changes in disability status. Fewer patients in the myelin-treated group had major attacks (6/15) versus the placebo-treated group (12/15) ($p = 0.06$). There was no significant difference in disability status between the two groups. However, subgroup analysis revealed some striking gender and MHC phenotype differences in the myelin-treated group. While the myelin-treated males had no major attacks (0/8) and a marked improvement in disability status, 6 of 7 myelin-treated females had attacks and their disability status worsened. Similarly, DR2-negative myelin-treated individuals had no attacks (0/6) and improved disability status, while DR2-positive myelin-treated participants had the opposite response (6/9 attack, worsened disability status). The relative roles of gender and MHC phenotype in response to therapy could not be distinguished because patients were not prospectively randomized by these criteria and there was great overlap (6/8 myelin-treated males were DR2-negative and 7/7 myelin-treated females were DR2-positive). No side effects were seen clinically or in laboratory tests. No correlation was seen between clinical responsiveness and changes in frequency of T cells responding to MBP.

Although this trial did not demonstrate efficacy, it did demonstrate safety and positive trends. A larger, double-blind randomized trial of oral myelin in patients with MS is currently underway.

As noted earlier, it is now possible to identify individuals at high risk for developing IDDM. Richard Jackson and his colleagues have conducted a pilot trial using low-dose parenteral insulin to prevent onset of IDDM in such individuals. High-risk individuals were identified by a combination of islet cell antibodies, insulin autoantibodies, and their insulin response to IV glucose. They were between 7 and 40 years of age, were first-degree relatives of patients with IDDM, and had a normal oral glucose tolerance test. Twelve individuals were offered the prevention protocol, which consisted of twice daily subcutaneous low-dose insulin combined with 5-day courses of low-dose intravenous insulin every 9 months. Five eligible subjects chose treatment while seven declined and became contemporary controls. The two groups were similar with respect to the tests mentioned above.

All seven control patients developed clinical diabetes (based on oral glucose tolerance test or high fasting plasma glucose) within 2.5 years from time of eligibility. At the time the trial was reported, one of the five treated individuals had developed IDDM (at 2.5 years) while the other four were free of disease with follow-ups ranging from 2.8 to 3.7 years. Subsequently, a second insulin-treated individual developed IDDM at 4 years, while the other three were nondiabetic with follow-up beyond 4 years. No side effects were seen, including no episodes of hypoglycemia with altered consciousness. This promising pilot result is being followed up with a large multicenter randomized trial to evaluate efficacy.

SUGGESTED READING

Friedman A, al-Sabbagh A, Santos LM, et al. Oral tolerance: A biologically relevant pathway to generate peripheral tolerance against external and self antigens. Chem Immunol 1994; 58:259–290.

Keller RJ, Eisenbarth GS, Jackson RA. Insulin prophylaxis in individuals at high risk of type I diabetes. Lancet 1993; 341:927–928.

Trentham DE, Dynesius-Trentham RA, Orav EJ, et al. Effects of oral administration of type II collagen on rheumatoid arthritis. Science 1993; 261:1727–1730.

Weiner HL, Mackin GA, Matsui M, et al. Double-blind pilot trial of oral tolerization with myelin antigens in multiple sclerosis. Science 1993; 259:1321–1324.

A NEW GENERATION OF ANTIGENS FOR IMMUNOTHERAPY

MALCOLM L. GEFTER, Ph.D.

Discoveries made within the past several years on the nature of antigen presentation have provided new opportunities for intervention in the immune system. Specifically, the work of Unanue, Grey, and ourselves as well as that of Wiley and colleagues has established that the transplantation antigens (major histocompatibility complex, human leukocyte antigen) molecules present on cell surfaces act as peptide receptors. The bound peptide is in turn displayed to T cells for recognition and reactivity within the immune system. It has become apparent from recent experiments that manipulation of immunity through alteration of the peptide complex is possible and that such manipulation can lead to effective therapies for a variety of immune-related disorders. In this chapter I restrict the discussion to class II transplantation antigens that exist constitutively on the monocyte-macrophage line of cells as well as B lymphocytes.

The specialized class II bearing "professional" antigen-presenting cells select a peptide from the invading antigen that has selective affinity for the surface transplantation antigen and then the bimolecular complex is presented on the cell surface. In conjunction with other antigen nonspecific signals, this complex is displayed to T cells, usually of the helper CD4 variety. It is this complex that is essential for the reactivity that the immune system will display to the parent antigen.

Proteins (antigens) that do not contain peptides displaying affinity for the host transplantation antigen fail to elicit immune responses. This is because T–helper cell activation is required in order to stimulate other T cells or B cells, which in turn make antibody against the parent antigen. Similarly, a high affinity peptide contained within an antigen can lead to vigorous immune responses. Other factors as discussed are also involved in the quantitative nature of the response. It has further been shown that display of peptide in the thymus during immune system development results in the death of responding T cells. Thus, the mechanism of self-tolerance is also governed by the peptide-transplantation antigen complex. It follows that the totality of self-peptides displayed in the thymus governs the surviving T-cell repertoire (i.e., that population of T cells with which we are able to recognize the biologic universe). It is presumed, therefore, that peptide specificity with respect to any given transplantation antigen be rather precise to ensure survival of sufficiently large numbers of T cells. The consequences of this specificity is that avoidance of immunity to a given protein would occur if mutation in the binding sequence occurred. It is for the latter reason that we presume that extreme polymorphism exists within the transplantation antigens of the species. Experiments have indeed demonstrated that in the mouse species inbred strains are very precise in the peptides they respond to, and that the entire species as a whole can react to a large array of peptides, but any single individual has a very limited peptide recognition capacity. Humans, as studied by their peptide reactions to several antigens, appear to have a diverse response but to a more limited extent than inbred mice. The benefits of being able to identify the precise peptides that lead to immune responses to specific antigens, or allergens, provides us with a precise set of molecules with which to alter immunity. The knowledge of this relationship and those described in the following discussion also readily account for, on a chemical basis, the HLA association with disease.

The peptides that are able to bind to transplantation antigens are able to stimulate cellular as well as humoral immune responses against themselves or the parent antigens from which they were derived. Thus many experiments have been done to study the behavior of these "pure" antigens. As stated previously, infusion of these peptides intraperitoneally leads to killing of responding T cells in the thymus. Administration of these peptides in the presence of Freund adjuvant leads to vigorous immune responses. A most critical observation relevant to this discussion is that if peptides are administered intravenously in the absence of adjuvants, then responding T helper cells are apparently rendered inactive or anergic. It has become clear through the use of peptides as T cell antigens that anergy rather than immunity (activation of the T cell in a manner consistent with it providing "help") can be readily achieved in vitro and in vivo. The biologic basis for this response is presumably to provide a post-thymic (postdevelopmental) mechanism to generate and maintain self-tolerance to antigens not available for creating tolerance by the mechanism of cell death in the thymus.

It is the latter observation that primarily opens up new avenues to intervene in immune disorders, specifically to use precise immunotherapy for allergic desensitization.

THE MOLECULAR BASIS OF ALLERGIC DISEASE

The peptide-dependent T-cell response readily explains the on/off switch of the immune response. What is not contained within this switch is the control of the qualitative immune response, that is, for humoral responses, what governs the isotype of antibody induced by the antigen? Considering that the nature of the infecting organism should dictate the nature of the immune response, we can suppose that molecular structures displayed by distinct organisms (bacteria, viruses, parasites) or their mode of access to the body is "read" by the system in a manner that ultimately translates to the induction of particular isotype expression. Studies conducted primarily in the murine system strongly suggest that control of isotype expression is mediated by the particular set of lymphokines produced by responding T helper cells. The helper T cells probably receive hormonal signals from the antigen-presenting cells that "instruct" the T cell as to which lymphokine program to express. There clearly are special receptors on these cells, but the details of the biochemical translation are as yet obscure.

Experimentally, we do know that parasitic infection leads to the selective synthesis of IgE, an apparently critical element in allergic disease. Furthermore, in murine models, it seems clear that parasitic infection produces a systemic signal such that concomitant immune responses also lead to IgE production, which on their own would not. In addition, antibodies that block the action of the lymphokine interleukin-4 prevent the systemic signal from functioning, thus, no IgE is made. These types of results demonstrate the link between infection and isotype expression. How does this relate to allergic disease?

Considering that the antigen itself (its amino acid sequence) does not impart the isotype signal and that in complex mixtures of allergens (i.e., pollen, insect venom) several proteins induce IgE synthesis, it is plausible to assume that in a manner similar to parasitic infection, a "systemic" signal is generated by the nature, chemical or mechanical, of the complex allergen (i.e., pollen grain, dust mite particle, venom mixture, and so on). Delivery of the "second signal," "systemic signal," "inflammatory signal" is perhaps avoided if a soluble extract is made of the complex allergen and the former is delivered to the immune system. We consider some aspects of this description relate to the efficacy (and sometimes lack thereof) of current immunotherapy.

HOW DOES IMMUNOTHERAPY WORK?

A clear explanation for the efficacy of immunotherapy has so far been elusive. Clearly, in the short term at least, reduction in the IgE/IgG ratio is unlikely to explain the desensitization process. Following the argument that lymphokine production controls isotype expression and that lymphokines have multiple effects on many cell types, an alteration of lymphokine production could readily explain the short- and long-term benefits of immunotherapy. We would propose that "natural" exposure involves both the antigen (peptide) signal and the inflammatory signal in order to induce and maintain the allergic state. Subcutaneous administration of "extract" alters or removes the constituent responsible for the second signal. We would propose, therefore, that responding T cells do not, in the latter case, release lymphokines (and/or express other gene products) necessary for maintenance of the allergic state. In fact, T cells may release factors that actively inhibit the action of allergy-related molecules (lymphokines, adhesion molecules, mast cell growth and activation factors, chemotactic factors, and so on). Such effects are seen in in vitro systems in that one lymphokine not only is an agonist for a given gene expression system, but is simultaneously an antagonist for another gene expression system. Thus, the near term effects of immunotherapy could readily be observed and after prolonged therapy, the effects on IgE synthesis would follow. It is worth mentioning that in addition to soluble molecules, T cells also express a variety of surface molecules that are crucial to their geographic distribution. Thus, T cells may also be recruited away from the site of natural antigen exposure by administration of the antigen at an "ectopic" site. In fact, any or all of these factors may play a role in successful therapy.

This sort of analysis can also be used to explain the failure of the therapy in many cases. Current extracts used for therapy in the United States are mixtures of native and partially degraded antigens. The fractions that are native and/or at least can react with IgE have the capacity to bind to and release mast cell mediators. It is likely that among the mediators released are those that create a positive feedback loop, further enhancing the production of allergy-related molecules (not just IgE). This situation is likely to recreate the "systemic signal" as described previously. Thus, there are two competing events occurring during therapy. In addition, the dose of antigen given "ectopically" may be so low, considering the patient's sensitivity, that effective therapy is unlikely.

Various attempts have been made to modify complex allergen mixtures to improve the efficacy relative to the side effects associated with conventional therapy. Some of these modifications, such as denaturation, or partial degradation, support the notion that the native structure is not important in therapy. Since T cell–reactive peptides are devoid of the structural integrity of the native molecule in that they are typically approximately 20 amino acids in length, it is plausible that therapeutic benefits are derived from T-cell reactivity.

THE STRATEGY FOR A NOVEL THERAPY

A relatively straightforward strategy for allergy therapy based on the arguments presented previously would be to treat allergic individuals with the peptides that activate their specific T cells to specific allergens. Such peptides can be prepared in pure form and administered in the absence of second signals. In addition, their size and valency would presumably not allow them to cause mast cell degranulation. The most important aspect of this strategy is that it can be tested directly and the absence of side effects can be determined ex vivo.

IMPLEMENTATION OF THE THERAPEUTIC STRATEGY

Until recently, the precise molecular identity of most allergens was unknown. The advent of convenient cloning strategies allowed various groups to begin to identify the genes and then the molecules produced by them to which the bulk of human IgE is directed. Once the sequences of these allergens are known, it becomes possible to determine the T cell–reactive sequences within them for individuals and the human population at large. To date, the genes encoding the major allergens responsible for ragweed, wasp venom, house dust mites, certain grass and tree pollens, and cat allergies have been cloned and sequenced. No doubt, others will follow shortly.

The technology is at hand to determine which amino acid sequences are responsible for T-cell reactivity in human patients. This is done by examining fragments of the allergens for their ability to stimulate a patient's T cells taken from a small peripheral blood sample. By narrowing down these sequences, the precise epitopes can readily be identified. Examination of large numbers of individuals with diverse HLA types provides the information needed to produce a simple mixture of peptides suitable for the human population at large. We have done this work, and it is clear that the number of amino acids expressed in convenient peptides is small enough to provide the T-cell reactivity of virtually all patients. In addition, it has been readily demonstrated that these peptides do not interact with pooled human IgE taken from patients with positive skin tests. These peptides can be shown to not result in histamine release from peripheral basophils of the same patients. Thus, it seems possible to treat human allergic disease with such peptide preparations. Considering the number of amino acids comprising the major allergenic proteins (derived from cloning) and the distribution of T cell–reactive sequences, this strategy will be possible in all cases examined to date.

CLINICAL TRIALS

The first and most obvious result to be expected is that patients can be treated safely with these peptide preparations. Judging from the doses required to anergize antigen-specific T cells in the mouse, it would seem that one or a very small number of treatments would be required, and that the total amount of material needed would be several milligrams per patient. The clinical endpoint desired of course is loss of clinical symptoms of allergy. In looking at this type of therapy for the first time, however, it would be crucial to collect the data necessary to establish the mechanism of effective desensitization. Accordingly, surrogate endpoints can be looked at during therapy in order to determine if the presumed mechanisms stated previously are operative.

Specifically, we would like to know if T cells reactive to the allergens have been anergized (loss of interleukin-2 production and loss of autocrine growth ability) or modified with respect to their lymphokine profile (e.g., acquisition of interleukin-II, interleukin-X production, and/or loss of interleukin-4 production). These parameters can readily be examined. It is also straightforward to examine adhesion molecule expression on the cell surface. Preliminary experiments done with patients desensitized with conventional therapy suggests that the former mechanism is operative.

To date, limited clinical trials have been conducted using chemically-synthesized peptides derived from the cat allergen *Fel d* 1. Although still incomplete, several conclusions can be drawn at this time. Peptides with the properties described above can be safely administered to humans in doses up to milligram amounts. In molar terms, these levels of "antigen" are 100 to 1,000 times greater than can be administered safely with conventional extracts. Preliminary indications support the thesis that T-cell products appear to be relevant to the expression of allergic symptoms, and in turn these may be controlled by this mode of therapy.

It is also quite feasible to treat a select group of patients who, by analysis, respond to only a single peptide present within an allergen. Such patients could be expected to be desensitized (assuming of course that the model is correct) with a single peptide. The analysis of their T-cell reactivity would be easier. In addition, controls can show that in fact only peptides to which they are reactive result in desensitization.

GENERAL CONSIDERATIONS

It is clear that if such therapy would work as expected, then we could conclude that already activated T cells can be turned off or at least diverted from participation in a deleterious immune reaction. This would open the window to treat a variety of other conditions. Specifically, we could expect to turn off any untoward response to an antigen that could be identified. Autoimmune diseases such as myasthenia gravis immediately come to mind as candidates. Current research is active in the areas of trying to identify target antigens in most autoimmune diseases. Thus, it is possible that the treatment of allergy may be the proving ground for therapies for autoimmune diseases.

SUGGESTED READING

Scherer MT, Chan BMC, Ria F, et al. Control of cellular and humoral immune responses by peptides containing T-cell epitopes. Cold Spring Harbor Symp Quant Biol 1989; 54:497–504.

Finkleman FD, Katona IM, Urban JF Jr., et al. Suppression of in vivo polyclonal IgE responses by monoclonal antibody to the lymphokine B-cell stimulatory factor-1. Proc Natl Acad Sci USA 1986; 83:9675.

Bond JF, Garman RD, Keating KM, et al. Multiple Amb a I allergens demonstrate specific reactivity with IgE and T cells from ragweed-allergic patients. J Immunol 1991; 146:3380–3385.

BENEFIT OF INTRAVENOUS IMMUNOGLOBULIN IN THE TREATMENT OF STEROID-DEPENDENT ASTHMA

ERWIN W. GELFAND, M.D.

The changes associated with airway obstruction in asthma are initiated by inflammatory events in the airways, which are infiltrated by cells, have epithelial disruption, and show evidence of mucosal edema. Once present, altered airway responsiveness may be increased and perpetuated by agents that cause airway inflammation. These stimuli include common viral respiratory infections, occupational agents, air pollutants, including cigarette smoke, and allergens. Various types of inflammatory cells, including eosinophils and mast cells, have been observed in the airways. Initially, the products of these cells were the focus of attention for producing the abnormalities linked with asthma. Presently, lymphocytes and IgE production are attracting attention.

The association between asthma and allergy is well recognized. Roughly 40 to 85 percent of patients with asthma have positive immediate skin-test reactions to common inhalant allergens. Allergic reactions in asthmatic airways are important for several reasons. Inhalant allergens can cause an immediate reaction with bronchial obstruction. Furthermore, they are capable of precipitating a late bronchial obstructive reaction, the late-phase response, several hours after the initial exposure. Central to this late bronchial response and altered airway responsiveness are inflammation and secondary epithelial damage in these airways. T lymphocytes play a central role in the allergic, asthmatic inflammatory response. First, they provide essential growth factors for the induction of IgE production (IL-4 and IL-13). Second, activated T cells express a surface protein, gp39 or CD40 ligand, which is also essential for IgE production through its interaction with B cell CD40. T cells also contribute more than simply promoting IgE synthesis. A number of T cell–derived cytokines play major roles in directing the nature of the airway inflammatory response in asthma. Among these are IL-5, IL-3 and granulocyte-macrophage–colony stimulatory factor (GM-CSF), which enhance eosinophil differentiation, maturation, adherence to endothelial surfaces, activation, and degranulation. The T-cell cytokine TNF-α has significant proinflammatory properties on neutrophils and eosinophils. T cells have been identified in the airways and lung parenchyma of asthmatics. Analysis of bronchoalveolar lavage (BAL) fluid has revealed the presence of $CD4^+$ and $CD8^+$ lymphocytes with these cells expressing increased levels of T-cell activation markers. Additional studies have observed increased numbers of activated T cells in the central airways of asthmatics.

THERAPEUTIC ALTERNATIVES

Control of airway inflammation represents the primary goal of treatment of airway hyper-responsiveness (AHR) in asthma. As an approach to controlling airway inflammation, treatment has concentrated on anti-inflammatory agents or methods to modify AHR. Corticosteroids are the most effective anti-inflammatory drugs for the treatment of AHR. Inhaled corticosteroids are safe and effective in the majority of patients. Nevertheless, a number of patients persist with severe symptoms, necessitating administration of systemic corticosteroid therapy. This has the potential to evoke a host of significant adverse effects, including growth suppression, weight gain, Cushingism, hypertension, cataracts, osteoporosis, and spontaneous bone fractures. A major goal remains the identification of drugs that relieve the need for prolonged systemic corticosteroid use. Some of these approaches have attempted to increase the effectiveness of corticosteroids using troleandomycin or reducing inflammation with the administration of gold, methotrexate, or dapsone. Unfortunately, none of these approaches has provided consistent benefit or the ability to reduce systemic corticosteroid use.

RATIONALE FOR USING IVIG IN ASTHMA

The rationale for initiating intravenous gammaglobulin (IVIG) in the treatment of severe steroid-dependent asthma was the recognition that (1) asthma is an inflammatory disease; (2) IVIG may have potent anti-inflammatory activity; and (3) passive therapy with IVIG may mimic some of the benefits achieved following active immunotherapy with defined allergens.

Anti-inflammatory Potential of IVIG

Despite little direct information on the mechanism of action, there is increasing support for IVIG exhibiting anti-inflammatory activity. Reduction of signs and symptoms of inflammation have been observed in patients with poly/dermatomyositis and systemic juvenile rheumatoid arthritis. Following infusions of IVIG, improvement in erythrocyte sedimentation rate, fever, rash, and lymphadenopathy have been observed. Perhaps the best support for anti-inflammatory activity has been observed following IVIG therapy in Kawasaki disease. Within a

This work was supported in part by Grant HL-36577 from the National Institutes of Health and Bayer Pharmaceutical Corporation. I am grateful to my many colleagues, Drs. Bruce Mazer, Lawrence Landwehr, and John Jeppson, as well as Beth Esterl, R.N., for their help in carrying out these studies.

short time after infusion, there is a remarkably rapid effect on several acute inflammatory parameters, including fever, granulocyte count, acute phase reactants (e.g., C-reactive protein), and levels of serum soluble IL-2 receptors.

Passive Immunotherapy with IVIG

Administration of IVIG may mimic some of the effects of active immunotherapy with known allergens. There are a number of possible mechanisms by which IVIG may modulate IgE-mediated responses. IVIG may inhibit the differentiation of B cells to antibody-secreting cells. Allergen-specific IgG present in the IVIG may neutralize the allergen, preventing (blocking) their interaction with cell-bound IgE. IVIG may also down-regulate allergen-specific IgE production through anti-idiotypic antibodies, which have been shown to be present in IVIG preparations.

The concept of passive transfer of gammaglobulin in the management of asthma is not a new one. Even in the 1950s, this form of therapy was proposed when monthly injections in patients with hypogammaglobulinemia were shown to reduce the incidence of infection. This was followed by conflicting reports surrounding the capacity of pooled gammaglobulin (given intramuscularly) to prevent respiratory infections, thereby benefiting the management of asthma. In a more recent evaluation of IVIG, five patients with alleged subclass deficiency and asthma were treated with IVIG. Four of them appeared to benefit to some degree from IVIG given every 4 weeks using 100 to 300 mg per kilogram. Indeed, all five patients had low total IgG levels, and although IgG1 levels were said to be deficient in four out of 5 cases, IgG1 still accounted for more than 65 percent of the total IgG, questioning the diagnosis of subclass deficiency. Using these low doses of gammaglobulin, the results were somewhat inconsistent from patient to patient.

RESPONSE TO IVIG IN STEROID-DEPENDENT ASTHMATICS

Patient Selection

We initially studied eight patients with severe steroid-dependent asthma who received high dose IVIG (2 g per kilogram body weight) every 4 weeks. The patients ranged from 6 to 17 years of age. All patients had severe asthma and had been receiving oral prednisone therapy for 1 to 8 years. The patients experienced a minimum of one exacerbation of their asthma each month, requiring bursts of oral corticosteroids. Prior to the trial, optimization of therapy was coupled with attempts to decrease steroid usage. Excluded from the study were patients with a second complicating respiratory illness, those receiving immunotherapy, and individuals with abnormal antibody responses following immunization with specific antigens.

Protocol

Each patient received 1 g per kilogram per day IVIG for 2 days every 4 weeks for 6 months. During the initial 2 months before IVIG treatment (pre-IVIG) each patient underwent full pulmonary function testing, including body plethysmography. A panel of skin-prick tests to common Colorado antigens was performed. Up to five antigens eliciting the most positive reactions were chosen for repeated testing by end-point titration. Reactions were outlined by felt pen and tape transferred to score sheets. Wheal surface areas were calculated with a program to outline and measure the tape-transferred wheal tracings. Peak expiratory flow rates (PEFR) were measured twice daily, before and after inhaled medication, and then logged. Symptom scores, monitored from 0 (no symptoms) to 4 (severe, incapacitating symptoms), were also logged for cough, shortness of breath, chest discomfort, wheezing episodes, medication changes, and numbers of inhaled treatments with beta-agonists. Before each infusion and following the final infusion, symptom scores, PEFR, and skin-test responses were evaluated. Medication adjustments were performed by the patient's primary physician and were based on the patient's clinical status. Statistical analysis was carried out by the student's t-test for comparison of before and after measures, and ANOVA was used for any multiple comparisons with a repeated measures analysis.

THERAPEUTIC RESPONSE

Reduction in Steroid Usage

The average alternate-day steroid dosage during the 2-month observation period for the eight patients before IVIG therapy was 32 ± 6.0 mg (Table 1). By the conclusion of 6 months of IVIG, the average alternate-day steroid dose was 12.4 ± 2.5 mg, a significant reduction. In addition to the need for a regular intake of corticosteroids, these patients often required brief pulses of corticosteroids for acute exacerbations of their asthma. As illustrated in Table 1, during the evaluation period before IVIG therapy, this group of patients required 154 ± 21 mg of oral steroids monthly for exacerbations, but only 49 ± 11 mg on average for each month while on IVIG. In an ongoing study of adolescents and adults with steroid-dependent asthma, we observed an 82 percent reduction in steroid usage.

Peak Expiratory Flow Rates

Monitoring of peak expiratory flow rates revealed two groups of patients. In one group normal PEFR were maintained but high doses of oral corticosteroids were required (Table 2, Group I). In this group, IVIG permitted a marked reduction in steroid usage, with maintenance of normal PEFR. In the second group (Table 2, Group II), in the face of low doses of oral corticosteroids, PEFR were abnormally low. However,

Table 1 Reduction in Steroid Requirements

	*Pre-IVIG**	*IVIG*
Average alternate-day steroid dose (mg)	32 ± 6.0	12.4 ± 2.5
Average monthly steroid dose (mg) for asthma exacerbations	154 ± 21	49 ± 11

*Effect of intravenous immunoglobulin (IVIG) on steroid requirements. Values are means ± SE.

Table 2 Normalization of Peak Expiratory Flow Rates Despite Steroid Reduction

		Average Alternate-Day Steroid Dose (mg)	*Peak Expiratory Flow Rate (l/min)*
Group I	Pre-IVIG	38	340
	Post-IVIG	11	346
Group II	Pre-IVIG	15	225
	Post-IVIG	12	255

Effect of intravenous immunoglobulin (IVIG) on peak expiratory flow rates (PEFR). PEFR were continuously monitored on a daily basis and average monthly PEFR are shown along with average alternate-day steroid dose. Two groups were distinguished: Group I required high doses of corticosteroids to maintain normal peak flow rates; Group II had low PEFR while being maintained on lower doses of the drug

on IVIG, PEFR results normalized without increasing the need for oral steroids.

Symptom Scores

All subjects completed daily symptom diaries rating symptoms from 0 (no symptoms) to 4 (incapacitating symptoms). Table 3 illustrates that analysis of individual diary symptoms scores, maintained for each 4-week period, revealed a marked improvement while on IVIG. This improvement was also accompanied by a 50 percent decrease in the need for extra treatments with inhaled beta-agonists while on IVIG.

Skin-test Responses

Of the eight patients initially enrolled in the trial, seven responded to one or more antigens by prick testing. During the course of IVIG therapy, there was a progressive reduction in skin-test reactivity in these individuals. Of the 30 initially positive reactions measured, a single response in one patient worsened over the course of the study, two remained unchanged and 27 improved. At the completion of 6 months of therapy, this decrease in skin-test reactivity was highly significant, averaging a 100-fold decrease in reactivity to each antigen. At the same time, in the skin-test responses to histamine or compound, 48 out of 80 were unaffected.

Table 3 Improvement in Monthly Symptom Scores on IVIG

Month	*Symptom Score Rating*
Pre-IVIG	32 ± 2.5
1	17 ± 2.0
2	17 ± 2.0
3	18 ± 2.5
4	17.5 ± 2.5
5	17 ± 2.5
6	16 ± 2.0

Effect of intravenous immunoglobulin (IVIG) on monthly symptom scores. Patients maintained a daily diary monitoring symptom scores for six parameters: cough, shortness of breath, chest discomfort, morning wheezing, nocturnal wheezing, and wheezing during daytime activities. The average monthly symptom score rating decreased significantly after the first infusion and was maintained throughout the trial ($p < 0.005$). Values indicated are mean ± SE

Follow-Up of Patients

Seven of the patients who completed one cycle of IVIG were followed during the 6 months off IVIG, and a second cycle of IVIG was reintroduced for 6 months. Following cessation of IVIG, symptom scores deteriorated, especially noted were an increase in cough and wheezing. In parallel, increased use of inhaled beta-agonist treatments was recorded. We accumulated data on five patients who restarted therapy; these individuals had a rapid stabilization of their asthma symptoms and steroid requirements once IVIG was reintroduced. They then exhibited further improvement, surpassing that achieved during the first 6 months of IVIG treatment. Reintroduction of IVIG rapidly resulted in an improvement in symptom scores and reduction in steroid usage.

MECHANISM OF ACTION

The mechanism whereby IVIG reduces the need for corticosteroid therapy or improves symptom scores is clearly not defined. It is tempting to speculate that the benefits of IVIG are related to controlling airway or cutaneous inflammation, a key component in the pathogenesis of asthma. Whether the mechanism is similar to what has been observed in reducing the inflammatory parameters observed in Kawasaki's disease or systemic juvenile rheumatoid arthritis is not known. Data from our laboratory and others indicate that IVIG can affect cytokine production. Recently, IVIG has been shown to reduce production of the proinflammatory cytokine tumor necrosis factor-alpha. In vitro, IVIG also triggers the production of IL-1 receptor antagonist, a potent anti-inflammatory protein. IVIG may have improved host defense against infection, consequently reducing asthma exacerbations. Although we could not demonstrate any impairment of antibody production in our patients, subtle effects of IVIG in this regard cannot be discounted. Intriguingly, IVIG is reported to neutralize the affects of bacterial and viral exotoxins, superantigens, which have the capacity to trigger large numbers of T cells to release cytokines, that may contribute to the inflammatory response. Persistent low-grade infection with such infectious agents releasing such toxins could be responsible for chronic inflammation. The toxin-neutralizing effects of IVIG may contribute to their anti-inflammatory potential.

Support for an immunomodulatory effect of IVIG in asthma was gained by the reduction in skin-test reactivity to defined allergens, which we observed in all patients. Whether this reflects a direct reduction in specific IgE synthesis is now being investigated. We could not demonstrate any evidence for IgG-blocking antibodies or anti-idiotypic antibodies to the specific allergens used in skin testing in the preparations of IVIG we used.

PROS AND CONS OF TREATMENT

In these studies, IVIG appeared to provide an alternative therapy in our attempt to reduce the need for systemic corticosteroids and associated adverse effects while maintaining normal airway function. Monthly infusions of 2 g per kilogram IVIG had a marked effect on symptom scores and pulmonary function in the treated patients. In the asthmatics, the need for regular corticosteroids or bursts for exacerbations was reduced approximately threefold, importantly without deterioration of lung function. Institution of IVIG also had a marked impact in reducing utilization of hospital resources. Although the studies were carried out in an open fashion, the data on cessation and reinstitution of IVIG therapy provide further support for its use in the small subgroup of clearly identified, steroid-dependent asthmatics. This potential for IVIG must be confirmed in larger, randomized, placebo-controlled trials. As in other diseases with prominent immune and inflammatory components, IVIG may provide the severe, steroid-dependent asthmatic with a novel approach to reduce steroid morbidity and importantly, reduce corticosteroid dependency.

Two important issues emerge from these and other studies. What is the minimal effective dose of IVIG, especially when determining cost-benefit analyses; and what is the mechanism of action? These questions are linked in that delineation of the mechanism of action would foster more rational decisions concerning dosing and frequency requirements to maximize clinical benefit. Because of the high cost of this form of therapy, careful selection of patients is important as is ensuring that conventional therapy has been optimized. The use of IVIG at a dose of 2 g per kilogram per month appears to be the dose chosen for many autoimmune or vasculitic disorders, including idiopathic thrombocytopenia purpura, Kawasaki disease, or for polydermatomyositis. In Kawasaki disease, reducing the dose by half was less beneficial. In another study in steroid-dependent asthmatic patients, administration of IVIG at 0.4 to 0.8 g per kilogram body weight on a monthly basis appeared to result in some clinical benefit, but perhaps not as complete as observed when higher doses are given. Cessation of IVIG also appears to result in a reappearance of asthma symptoms as we and others have demonstrated. Further study may show that to induce remission of the disease, in a rapid fashion, the higher doses are required, whereas for maintenance the amounts needed may be considerably less. A concerted effort to study these issues is necessary. Overall these large amounts of IVIG appear to be well tolerated, even using 2 g per kilogram in a single infusion. The most troubling side effect we have observed is headache, often occurring 24 to 72 hours after completion of the infusion.

Patients with allergic disorders requiring large doses of oral corticosteroids are in the minority. Most are well controlled without resorting to systemic corticosteroids, avoiding the associated side effects. Advances in inhaled corticosteroids have significantly benefited children and adults with asthma. Nevertheless, a subset of asthmatics persists in their need for systemic steroid therapy for control of their disease. What distinguishes this group from the larger cohort is not known at this time. Since inflammation appears to be the underlying cause of both diseases, new approaches to interrupting the immune-mediated inflammatory cascade are required. In steroid-dependent asthma, IVIG appears to provide a new therapeutic option.

SUGGESTED READING

Amran D, Renz H, Lack G, et al. Suppression of cytokine-dependent human T-cell proliferation by intravenous immunoglobulin. Clin Immunol Immunopathol 1994; 73:180–186.

Busse WW. The role of inflammation in asthma: A new focus. J Resp Dis 1989; 10:72–780.

Dalakas MC, Illa I, Dambrosia JM, et al. A controlled trial of high-dose intravenous immune globulin infusions as treatment for dermatomyositis. N Engl J Med 1983; 329:1993–2000.

Kazatchkine MD, Dietrich G, Hurez V, et al. V region-mediated selection of autoreactive repertoires by intravenous immunoglobulin (I.v.Ig). Immunol Rev 1994; 139:79–107.

Leung DYM. The immunologic effects of IVIG in Kawasaki disease. Int Rev Immunol 1989; 5:197–202.

Mazer BD, Gelfand EW. An open-label study of high-dose intravenous immunoglobulin in severe childhood asthma. J Allergy Clin Immunol 1991; 87:976–983.

Robinson DS, Bentley AM, Hartnell A, et al. Activated memory T helper cells in bronchoalveolar lavage fluid from patients with atopic asthma: Relation to asthma symptoms, lung function, and bronchial responsiveness. Thorax 1993; 48:26–32.

TREATMENT OF ASTHMA AND RHINITIS WITH AGENTS ACTIVE ON THE 5-LIPOXYGENASE PATHWAY

JEFFREY M. DRAZEN, M.D.

The leukotrienes are a family of chemical mediators, derived from arachidonic acid, with the capacity to mediate airway obstruction, glandular secretion, and microvascular leakage. In order to understand the pharmacologic agents that can modify the synthesis or the action of the leukotrienes, we first briefly review leukotriene biochemistry and the current data that indicate a role for leukotrienes in asthma and allergic rhinitis. We then examine the potential for therapeutic use of leukotriene receptor antagonists or synthesis inhibitors.

LEUKOTRIENE BIOCHEMISTRY

Leukotrienes are derived from arachidonic acid, which is commonly found esterified in the *sn-2* position of cell membrane phospholipids; the perinuclear membrane is the most likely source for the arachidonic acid that is subsequently bioconverted into the leukotrienes. Upon cellular activation, cytosolic phospholipase A_2 ($cPLA_2$) is translocated to the perinuclear membrane and activated such that it can cleave arachidonic acid from membrane phospholipids. The arachidonic acid so liberated becomes a substrate for the cytosolic enzyme 5-lipoxygenase (5-LO), which is then translocated upon cellular activation (see following discussion) to the perinuclear membrane where it tightly associates with the protein known as the 5-LO activating protein (FLAP). FLAP is an integral membrane protein, which, when activated by increased intracellular calcium concentrations, develops a high affinity for 5-LO; this high affinity state results in the translocation of 5-LO from the cytosol to the perinuclear membrane. 5-LO operates on arachidonic acid twice in succession, first to form the product known as 5-hydroperoxyeicosatetraenoic acid (5-HPETE) and then to convert 5-HPETE to the unstable epoxide known as leukotriene A_4 (LTA_4). LTA_4 is a branch point in the leukotriene biosynthetic pathway. In polymorphonuclear leukocytes, the predominant enzyme operating on LTA_4 is LTA_4 epoxide hydrolase. This enzyme converts LTA_4 into LTB_4, a dihydroxy derivative of LTA_4. In other cells—most notably for asthma in eosinophils and mast cells—LTA_4 becomes a substrate for another integral membrane enzyme, LTC_4 synthase, which adducts the tripeptide glutathione at the C6 position of the eicosanoid backbone to form the molecule known as leukotriene C_4 (LTC_4).

The precise mechanism whereby LTB_4 exits the intracellular microenvironment is not known, but LTC_4 does so through the action of a specific LTC_4 transmembrane transporter. Once in the extracellular microenvironment, LTB_4 acts at specific receptors, known as BLT receptors, to initiate chemotactic and other cellular responses. In the extracellular microenvironment, LTC_4 is further metabolized by the enzymatic removal of glutamic acid, from the glutathione adducted at the C6 position, by the action of γ-glutamyl transpeptidase to form LTD_4. LTD_4 transduces signals through the $CysLT_1$ receptor, the leukotriene receptor that transduces airway smooth muscle constriction, glandular secretion, and microvascular leak. LTD_4 is subsequently modified, by the action of a variety of dipeptidases, to form LTE_4 by the removal of the glycine moiety from LTD_4. LTE_4 is 100-fold less biologically active then LTD_4 but appears to act at the same receptor.

LTE_4 released into the extracellular microenvironment is inactivated by a variety of pathways. It can be N-acetylated, which results in a loss of bioactivity. LTE_4 is also subject to ω-hydroxylation and subsequent beta-elimination to form a series of bioinactivated molecules, some of which are excreted in the urine. Approximately 10 to 15 percent of bioavailable LTC_4 appears in the urine as authentic LTE_4.

PHARMACOLOGIC AGENTS WITH ACTION ON THE LEUKOTRIENE PATHWAY

Potential biochemical sites of action for agents active on the 5-LO pathway are listed in Table 1. Although this pathway can potentially be inhibited at a variety of sites, agents have actually been developed with only two distinct targets, namely inhibition of the various leukotrienes at their receptors and inhibition of the synthesis of leukotrienes by the inhibition of 5-LO per se or by the inhibition of binding of arachidonic acid to FLAP.

Leukotriene Receptor Antagonists

The antagonists of the action of LTD_4 at its receptor ($CysLT_1$) inhibit signal transduction by leukotrienes D_4 and E_4 by competitive antagonism. Among the agents that have been developed and tested clinically, potency varies approximately fiftyfold. The weakest of the agents, LY171883, causes a fivefold shift of the leukotriene dose response in normal humans, while the most potent agent reported to date, zafirlukast (ICI204219), shifts the leukotriene dose-response curve approximately 200-fold. The antagonists also vary in duration of effect from approximately 6 to 12 hours.

Leukotriene Synthesis Inhibitors

Two classes of agents have been developed to inhibit the synthesis of leukotrienes. The first inhibits the action of the enzyme 5-LO by inhibiting enzyme-directed catalysis of arachidonic acid to leukotriene A_4; zileuton

Table 1 Sites of Potential Drug Action in the 5-Lipoxygenase Pathway

Enzyme/Protein	*Specific Inhibitors Available**	*Inhibitors Tested in Clinical Trials*	*Drug Products Likely to be Available**
$cPLA_2$	No	No	None
FLAP	Yes	Allergen- and exercise-induced asthma	Bay × 1005 MK 886
5-LO	Yes	Allergen, exercise- and aspirin-induced asthma, chronic asthma	Zileuton (Leutrol)
LTC_4 synthase	No	No	None
Receptor Antagonists			
LTC_4 ($CysLT_1$)	Yes	Allergen, exercise- and aspirin-induced asthma, chronic asthma	Zafirlukast (ICI204219, Accolate) MK-478
LTB_4 (BLT)	Yes	Allergen-induced asthma	None

*Availability for clinical testing (Phase 1 or beyond) as of October, 1994.

is in this category. The other class of agents, including MK886 and Bay × 1005, inhibits the interaction of 5-LO with FLAP, thereby inhibiting the translocation and activation of 5-LO. These agents can inhibit from 60 to 90 percent of leukotriene synthesis depending on the dose and test system used. The duration of action varies from approximately 3 to 10 hours.

CLINICAL USE OF AGENTS ACTIVE ON THE LEUKOTRIENE PATHWAY

The major indication for the use of leukotriene receptor antagonists and synthesis inhibitors at this time is asthma. Trials of these agents have shown them to be effective in exercise-induced, antigen-induced, and aspirin-induced asthma.

Exercise-Induced Asthma

Inhaled leukotriene receptor antagonists, oral leukotriene receptor antagonists, or synthesis inhibitors administered before exercise challenge provide approximately 50 percent protection from subsequent bronchoconstriction in exercise-induced asthma, and improved lung function occurs without beta-adrenergic side effects. Current data do not allow distinction among the various agents or insight as to whether treatment with a synthesis inhibitor or a $CysLT_1$ receptor antagonist is superior. There is theoretical reason to believe that treatment with a combination of a 5-LO inhibitor and a $CysLT_1$ receptor antagonist may be superior to treatment with individual agents, although this idea has not been tested directly.

Antigen-Induced Asthma

Antigen-induced asthma, such as may occur when patients are exposed to antigens during the course of their daily life, is another indication for treatment with this class of agents. Antigen-induced asthma can be inhibited by pretreatment with leukotriene receptor antagonists or synthesis inhibitors. Although no "head-to-head" comparisons have been made, current data suggest that the more potent leukotriene receptor antagonists, such as zafirlukast, are more likely to be beneficial than 5-LO inhibitors. The duration of action of the receptor antagonist is important, and it may be necessary to retreat the patient after antigen exposure.

Table 2 Conditions for which Treatment of Asthma with Agents Active on the 5-Lipoxygenase Pathway is Indicated

Treatment of Choice
Aspirin-induced asthma

Effective Primary Treatment
1. Chronic stable asthma trials under marginal control with beta-agonists only
2. Prophylactic treatment of allergen-induced asthma

Aspirin-Induced Asthma

All of the physiological manifestations of aspirin-induced asthma, including bronchospasm and naso-ocular, gastrointestinal, and dermal symptoms, are derived from the activation of the 5-LO pathway following aspirin ingestion (Table 2). Treatment of such individuals with systemic 5-LO inhibitors has been shown to *totally* block the physiological manifestations of aspirin challenge (Fig. 1). It is currently not known whether the asthma that occurs in individuals with aspirin sensitivity in the absence of aspirin exposure will be ameliorated by chronic treatment with 5-LO inhibitors, although in one trial there was a baseline improvement in lung function in such subjects. Anecdotal data from the trials of aspirin challenge indicate that anosmia, which is common in such individuals, is abrogated during treatment with agents active on the 5-LO pathway. This observation suggests that rhinosinusitis, which is also common in these individuals, may be prevented by such treatment, and therefore chronic treatment with agents active on the 5-LO pathway will have a salutary effect.

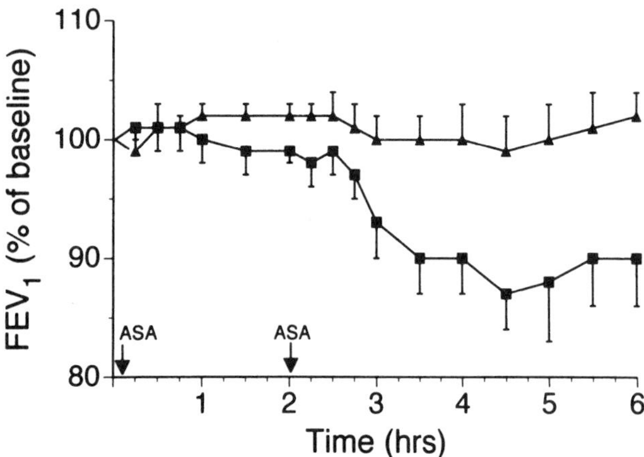

Figure 1 Effect of zileuton on change in FEV_1 after aspirin challenge (*closed triangles* indicate zileuton pretreatment; *closed squares* indicate placebo pretreatment). The FEV_1 expressed as mean percentage of baseline (± SEM) for all eight patients is plotted versus time after dosing. Zileuton pretreatment significantly prevented ($p < 0.02$) the fall in FEV_1 resulting from aspirin challenge. (Reprinted from Israel E, Fischer AR, Rosenberg MA, et al, *Am Rev Respir Dis* 1993; 148:1447-1451; with permission.)

Treatment of Chronic Stable Asthma

A number of trials have been conducted with agents active on the 5-LO pathway, both 5-LO inhibitors and $CysLT_1$ receptor antagonist, in patients with chronic asthma. In general, individuals with moderate asthma (pretreatment FEV_1 values 60 to 70 percent of predicted), who have been treated only with beta-agonists, have been enrolled in such trials. The results of these trials have been remarkably uniform. They demonstrate that chronic treatment with agents active on the 5-LO pathway results in an approximate 15 percent improvement in the FEV_1. Furthermore, such treatment is associated with about a 30 percent decrease both in symptoms and in the use of beta-agonist inhalers. Longer term trials of 5-LO–active agents versus placebo have demonstrated a decrease in the need for oral prednisone therapy. Therefore, for the individual with mild-to-moderate asthma, leukotriene antagonists and synthesis inhibitors may be a useful “second order” treatment when beta-agonist treatment alone is inadequate.

SUGGESTED READING

Chan-Yeung M., Chan H, Tse KS, et al. Histamine and leukotrienes release in bronchoalveolar fluid during plicatic acid-induced bronchoconstriction. *J Allergy Clin Immunol* 1989; 84:762–768.

Christie L, Lee TH. The effects of SKF104353 on aspirin induced asthma. *Am Rev Respir Dis* 1991; 144:957–958.

Cloud ML, Enas GC, Kemp J, et al. A specific LTD4LTE4-receptor antagonist improves pulmonary function in patients with mild, chronic asthma. *Am Rev Respir Dis* 1989; 140:1336–1339.

Dahlen B, Kumlin M, Margolskee DJ, et al. The leukotriene-receptor antagonist MK-0679 blocks airway obstruction induced by inhaled lysine-aspirin in aspirin-sensitive asthmatics. *Eur Respir J* 1993; 6:1018–1026.

Israel E, Fischer AR, Rosenberg MA, et al. The pivotal role of 5-lipoxygenase products in the reaction of aspirin-sensitive asthmatics to aspirin. *Am Rev Respir Dis* 1993a; 148:1447–1451.

Israel E, Rubin P, Kemp JP, et al. The effect of inhibition of 5-lipoxygenase by zileuton in mild to moderate asthma. Ann Int Med 1993b; 119:1059–1066.

INDEX

Note: Page numbers in italics indicate figures; page numbers followed by *t* indicate tables.

N

O

P